Behavioral and Psychological Approaches to Breathing Disorders

Behavioral and Psychological Approaches to Breathing Disorders

Edited by

Beverly H. Timmons
St. Bartholomew's Hospital
London, England

and

Ronald Ley
The University at Albany
State University of New York
Albany, New York

Plenum Press • New York and London

Library of Congress Cataloging-in-Publication Data

Behavioral and psychological approaches to breathing disorders /
    edited by Beverly H. Timmons and Ronald Ley.
        p.   cm.
    Includes bibliographical references and indexes.
    ISBN 0-306-44446-1
    1. Hyperventilation--Psychosomatic aspects. 2. Respiratory
system--Psychophysiology. 3. Respiratory system--Diseases-
-Psychosomatic aspects.   I. Timmons, Beverly H. II. Ley, Ronald.
    [DNLM: 1. Respiration Disorders--physiopathology. 2. Respiration
Disorders--therapy. 3. Respiration Disorders--psychology.
4. Respiration--physiology.   WF 102 B419 1994]
RC776.H9B44   1994
616.2'0046--dc20
DNLM/DLC
for Library of Congress   93-44087
                                                               CIP

ISBN 0-306-44446-1

© 1994 Plenum Press, New York
A Division of Plenum Publishing Corporation
233 Spring Street, New York, N.Y. 10013

Printed in the United States of America

To my many teachers, especially the late Mrs. Magda Proskauer

—BHT

To the memory of my father, August Andreas Ley

—RL

Contributors

PAT A. BARELLI, M.D. • Department of Surgery (Ear, Nose and Throat), University of Missouri–Kansas City School of Medicine, Kansas City, Missouri 64108

CHRISTOPHER BASS, M.D., M.R.C.Psych. • Department of Psychological Medicine, John Radcliffe Hospital, Headington, Oxford OX3 9DU, England

DONALD L. BLIWISE, Ph.D. • Department of Neurology, Emory University Medical School, Atlanta, Georgia 30322

DAVID BOADELLA, M.Ed., M.A.H.P. • Psychotherapy Training, Biosynthesis Center, CH 8049 Zurich, Switzerland

FRANK A. CHANDRA (1925–1993), M.B.B.S., D-P.H. • Formerly, Department of Health, London, England

ASHLEY V. CONWAY, Ph.D. • Department of Psychiatry, Charing Cross and Westminster Medical School, London W6 8RP, England

HERBERT FENSTERHEIM, Ph.D. • Department of Psychiatry, Cornell University Medical College, New York, New York 10021

WILLIAM N. GARDNER, D.Phil., F.R.C.P. • Department of Thoracic Medicine, Kings College School of Medicine and Dentistry, London SE5 9PJ, England

CHRISTIAN GUILLEMINAULT, M.D. • Sleep Disorders Clinic, Stanford University Medical School, Stanford, California 94305

ELIZABETH A. HOLLOWAY, M.C.S.P., S.R.P. • Knebworth Physiotherapy Clinic, Knebworth, Hertfordshire SG3 6HG, England

GRAHAM JACKSON, F.R.C.P. • Cardiac Department, Guy's Hospital, London SE1 9RT, England

SHEILA JENNETT, M.D., Ph.D., F.R.C.P. (Glasg.) • Institute of Physiology, The University, Glasgow G12 8QQ, Scotland

PAUL M. LEHRER, Ph.D. • Department of Psychiatry, Robert W. Johnson Medical School, University of Medicine and Dentistry of New Jersey, Piscataway, New Jersey 08854-5635

RONALD LEY, Ph.D. • Department of Psychology and Statistics, The University at Albany, State University of New York, Albany, New York 12222

L. C. LUM, M.B.B.S., F.R.C.P., F.R.A.C.P. • Department of Chest Medicine (Emeritus), Papworth and Addenbrooke's Hospitals, Cambridge, CB3 8BX, England; and "Summerleas," Dry Drayton, Cambridge CB3 8BX, England

KAREN H. NAIFEH, Ph.D., A.C.P. • Department of Psychiatry, Langley Porter Psychiatric Institute, University of California Medical Center, San Francisco, California 94143

DAPHNE J. PEARCE, Dip.C.S.T. • Speech Therapy Department, St. Bartholomew's Hospital, London EC1A 7BE, England

MAGDA PROSKAUER (1910–1990) • Formerly in Private Practice, San Francisco, California

BEVERLY H. TIMMONS, M.A. • Department of Respiratory Medicine and Allergy, St. Bartholomew's Hospital, London EC1A 7BE, England

JONATHAN H. WEISS, Ph.D. • Department of Psychiatry, New York Hospital, Cornell University Medical Center, New York, New York 10021

ROBERT L. WOOLFOLK, Ph.D. • Department of Psychology, Rutgers State University Piscataway, New Jersey 08854

Foreword

We start life with a breath, and the process continues automatically for the rest of our lives. Because breathing continues on its own, without our awareness, it does not necessarily mean that it is always functioning for optimum mental and physical health. The opposite is true often. The problem with breathing is that it seems so easy and natural that we rarely give it a second thought. We breathe: we inhale, we exhale. What could be simpler? But behind that simple act lies a process that affects us profoundly. It affects the way we think and feel, the quality of what we create, and how we function in our daily life. Breathing affects our psychological and physiological states, while our psychological states affect the pattern of our breathing. For example, when anxious, we tend to hold our breath and speak at the end of inspiration in a high-pitched voice. Depressed people tend to sigh and speak at the end of expiration in a low-toned voice. A child having a temper tantrum holds his or her breath until blue in the face. Hyperventilation causes not only anxiety but also such a variety of symptoms that patients can go from one specialty department to another until a wise clinician spots the abnormal breathing pattern and the patient is successfully trained to shift from maladaptive to normal breathing behavior.

It has long been known that slow, rhythmic, diaphragmatic breathing can soothe our inner storms and make us feel calm and composed. This property of reciprocity has been used by many health care providers to reduce stress and alleviate many stress-related symptoms and disorders. In a number of controlled studies, my colleagues and I have shown that training in diaphragmatic breathing exercise, deep muscle relaxation, visualization, meditation, and other stress management techniques and their integration into daily life reduce hypertension and may also reduce the incidence of coronary heart disease. It is difficult to apportion the benefit contributed by breathing exercise, but I now believe it is likely to be larger than I had originally imagined.

When we investigated the success of our initial training program, using a self-administered questionnaire 4 years after completion of the training, we were disappointed with the degree of compliance. Only a small percentage of subjects were regularly practicing relaxation and meditation techniques 20 minutes once or twice a day as prescribed. However, subjects had retained a significant part of the initial benefit obtained when they were practicing regularly under supervision, apparently through practicing brief one-breath relaxation several times a day and using cognitive strategies. Follow-up group sessions in an ongoing study have revealed that the two components subjects feel they have benefited from most, and that they are willing to continue using, are awareness about stress and breathing exercise. Human nature makes it unlikely that most people, except those strongly motivated, will comply with time-consuming practice in the long term. Breathing exercise is a remarkable therapeutic tool in that it does not make superhuman demands on people's time. It can be practiced anywhere and at any time and while doing almost anything.

Beverly Timmons and Ronald Ley have done an excellent job of putting together an unprecedented and comprehensive book in which experts have contributed chapters on various aspects of normal and abnormal breathing, how disturbed breathing may impair health, and what therapies are appropriate. When technological medicine badly needs to be balanced by a humanistic approach, a book on such a vital subject as breathing is very timely.

Chandra Patel, M.D.

University College, London

Preface

We all know from our experience of emotions—anger, fear, sexual excitement—that our breathing changes with these states. Practitioners of the caring professions have understandably wanted to know more about this prime example of mind–body interaction and how they might best harness it for use in relaxation training, anxiety and stress management, behavior therapy, and other applications.

Therapists and other clinicians encounter problems, however, in extracting the information they need when looking into the vast literature on human breathing and its disorders. One has to survey many different disciplines in order to fully characterize even "normal" human breathing, but only a portion of the knowledge in each of these fields is relevant to behaviorally oriented practice or .research. Then again, textbooks in respiratory medicine are almost exclusively concerned with lung diseases. Finally, other sources—ranging from explications of respiratory physiology to psychoanalytic models to esoteric teachings of breathing practices—can be dauntingly difficult for all but specialists. No wonder we have often been asked over the considerable number of years that we have been involved in this field whether there is a book that "explained breathing."

Our aim has been to fill this gap in the literature by putting together an authoritative, comprehensive sourcebook that introduces the reader to the newly developing field of "respiratory psychophysiology." We have chosen to focus on the clinical aspects: the ways in which breathing may be disturbed and the therapeutic methods currently available. The hyperventilation syndrome and panic attacks are central subjects. In describing a range of therapies, we move from the physical to the behavioral, cognitive, and psychodynamic.

We have adopted a multiauthor approach to ensure that we present current and reliable accounts of each discipline relevant to our topic—although we are, of course, aware that there are omissions, such as dyspnea, the role of breathing in the psychophysiology of exercise, and in pulmonary rehabilitation programs. We invited original contributions from clinicians, therapists, academics, and researchers from both sides of the Atlantic. All but one of the chapters (Proskauer's) are newly published here. We have asked our contributors to focus on those aspects of their specialties that are of interest to our clinician-readers and to present this material in comprehensible form.

The normally functioning human respiratory system and its relationship to other major body systems are outlined. Our terms of reference in discussing dysfunctions of this system have been primarily those conditions for which there are no known organic causes. We have, however, rejected terms such as "functional" or "psychosomatic" because they imply mind–body dualism, rather than the interactive approach we and our contributors endorse. We have instead chosen the nonspecific term "breathing disorders" because we wanted to include some pathological conditions, notably asthma. Even patients with this disease can, as Jonathan Weiss describes in Chapter 14, benefit from a behavioral and educational program used in collaboration with medical care. Other structural and systemic abnormalities, which include those of the nasal passages, those affecting sleep, and those involved in neurological and cardiovascular dysfunctions, are briefly described. We and the contributors to this volume acknowledge, of course, the importance of investigating such abnormalities before initiating behavioral treatment.

It is now more than 10 years since the first editor convened an interdisciplinary meeting of clinicians and researchers interested in breathing patterns. This was the first in a series that is now known as the International Symposia on Respiratory Psychophysiology, coordinated by the first editor and Hans Folgering of the Department of Pulmonary Diseases, University of Nijmegen, The Netherlands. These meetings have resulted in a stimulating mix of clinical and research papers, the abstracts of which are now published regularly in *Biological Psychology* (see Appendix). Research into the diagnosis and treatment of hyperventilation in the United Kingdom and The Netherlands has stimulated interest in the United States, notably among members of the Association for Advancement of Behavior Therapy and the Association for Applied Psychophysiology and Biofeedback. As many readers will know, interest in hyperventilation has also penetrated public consciousness, particularly in the United Kingdom.

We believe that this collection, the first of its kind, will prove a valuable reader on the psychophysiology of breathing for all the helping professions: psychological, medical, paramedical, complementary, and educational. We also recommend the book as an introductory, comprehensive text appropriate for courses in many of these professions. Clinical researchers will find that challenging issues concerning theory as well as treatment are raised by the contributors, who have highlighted areas in which further investigation is needed. The interdisciplinary nature of the book constructively emphasizes both differences in approaches to breathing disorders and current controversies. Hence this first comprehensive, multidisciplinary text will prove useful for researchers as well as for those in or training for the health care professions—to whom we primarily address our book.

An international society for the study of respiratory psychophysiology is being established now and a journal in this field is also planned. The editors welcome proposals for the contents of the journal and also comments and suggestions for a second edition of this book.

Beverly H. Timmons
Ronald Ley

St. Bartholomew's Hospital, London
University at Albany, New York

Acknowledgments

Professor Ley and I have worked with the contributing authors to produce what we hope is a readable book instead of a collection of papers incomprehensible to the nonspecialist. In this prolonged endeavor, I very much appreciate the patience and ever-helpful guidance of Ken Derham, our editor in Plenum's London office. My warmest thanks go also to Maryan Jeffery for her invaluable and insightful editorial assistance over the years. The original and adapted illustrations in Chapters 1, 2, and 15 are by Cathy Clench and colleagues in the Department of Medical Illustration, St. Bartholomew's Hospital, London. I am also grateful to our contributors and many other colleagues for their helpful discussions and comments, especially to Claude Lum. I appreciate the support and encouragement of my managers and colleagues at Barts—Robert J. Davies, Kenneth A.M. Grant, Heather Brown, and Bernard W. Watson. Margaret Christie and Celia Bird provided early encouragement and Elizabeth Carson, generous help. Special acknowledgment is due Richard L. Blanton, Professor Emeritus and former Director of Clinical Training, Department of Psychology, Vanderbilt University, who was one of the first psychologists to recognize the underdevelopment of the field of respiratory psychophysiology.

Finally, I thank Ronald Ley for his astute and genial participation in our transatlantic collaboration since 1989, and for never thinking that facts speak for themselves!

Beverly Timmons

My interest in the psychophysiology of breathing began in 1971 at the Behavior Therapy Unit of the Temple University School of Medicine, on the occasion of a demonstration of the anxiolytic effects of single inhalations of large concentrations of CO_2. I thank Joseph Wolpe for this demonstration, which, together with his many intellectual contributions to behavior therapy, had a significant impact on the direction and development of my scientific and clinical interests.

In subsequent years my research interests led me to L.C. Lum. I wish to thank Dr. Lum for his seminal contributions to the study of hyperventilation-related disorders and for our lengthy discussions that provided me with invaluable lessons in clinical research—research that, I came to learn, requires skills and sensitivity beyond the commonplace approach of nonclinical scientific methodology.

My research interests also led me to Beverly Timmons, the pioneering spirit and coalescing force who, for more than a decade now, has brought scientists and clinicians from all parts of the world together to share their data and critical views at an annual international symposium on respiratory psychophysiology. I wish to thank Beverly for all her good work through the years and especially for offering me the opportunity to share in the writing and editing of this book.

Of the many people who helped in the production of this book, I wish to give my special thanks to Carol Travison and Maribel Gray, State University of New York at Albany, for their clerical assistance with the many documents that an overseas collaboration generates; to Jessica Ley, Bryn Mawr College, for her assistance in indexing a sizable number of chapters; and to my wife, Cindy, for always being on hand to help sort things out.

Ronald Ley

Contents

II. Hyperventilation: Diagnosis and Therapy

7. Hyperventilation Syndromes: Physiological Considerations
in Clinical Management   113

L. C. Lum

8. Psychiatric and Respiratory Aspects of Functional Cardiovascular Syndromes   125

Christopher Bass, William N. Gardner, and Graham Jackson

III. Other Therapeutic Approaches to Breathing Disorders

12. Breathing and Vocal Dysfunction   179

Daphne J. Pearce

13. Respiratory System Involvement in Western Relaxation
and Self-Regulation   191

Paul M. Lehrer and Robert L. Woolfolk

14. Behavioral Management of Asthma   205

Jonathan H. Weiss

Introduction

BEVERLY H. TIMMONS

This book aims to give an overarching view of human breathing, drawing upon a wide range of disciplines relevant to both normal and abnormal breathing. Because the specially written articles cover such a wide range and make new connections between disciplines, the Introduction concentrates on locating the chapters within an explanatory framework. Basic concepts and approaches contained in the chapters are introduced, key issues are highlighted, and certain themes are connected with current thinking in the psychophysiology of breathing. The book as a whole is structured so that the chapters progress from the basic anatomy and physiology of breathing and the discussion of some organic disorders (Part I), to behavioral, psychological and therapeutic aspects (Parts II and III). The reader will find that some of the chapters overlap and cross these broad headings, since analysis and diagnosis are not always separable from discussion of treatment.

In Chapter 1, Karen Naifeh guides the reader who has little or no knowledge of physiology through the structure and function of the respiratory system, giving emphasis to those aspects of most relevance to behavioral practitioners. Trained in both respiratory physiology and clinical psychology, Naifeh is aptly qualified to contribute this first chapter. She describes the interaction of voluntary and involuntary controls of breathing, a central concept in this book. The critical role of *carbon dioxide* (CO_2) in the control of ventilation, a subject that will recur in later chapters, is introduced. Naifeh explains the powerful effects of CO_2 on the nervous system and on blood flow to the brain, which necessitate careful regulation of CO_2 levels. Naifeh next describes the influence of breathing on the

BEVERLY H. TIMMONS • Department of Respiratory Medicine and Allergy, St. Bartholomew's Hospital, London, EC1A 7BE, England.

Behavioral and Psychological Approaches to Breathing Disorders, edited by Beverly H. Timmons and Ronald Ley. Plenum Press, New York, 1994.

1

cardiovascular system. Later in the book, Bass (Chapter 8), following on from the material in this chapter, describes some of the clinical implications of the close interrelationship between the respiratory and cardiovascular systems.

Chapter 1 also includes basic information on the autonomic nervous system since this is needed to understand the regulation of breathing and its interaction with other systems, especially the cardiovascular system. The role of the autonomic nervous system and its neurotransmitters in the fight-or-flight response and the effects of stress on breathing are also described.

Chapter 2 deals with the nose, which is a subject so often, ironically, left out of accounts of breathing. This was the message of Dr. Maurice Cottle, founder of the American Rhinologic Society, who stressed the importance of nasal physiology in many publications dating from the 1950s. There has been all too little progress since then: a 1988 announcement of a session of the Physiological Society on the nose and upper airways stated that these topics "have been relatively neglected by respiratory physiologists." Here, in Chapter 2, Pat Barelli brings the late Dr. Cottle's teachings up to date and describes the ways in which ignorance of nasopulmonary physiology can adversely affect care of patients. He describes the active and powerful role of nasal processes in relation to the lungs, heart, and other organ systems. Quality of sleep, for example, may depend on nasal function: a blocked nose can prevent the cyclic alternation of airflow from one nostril to the other, and thus prevent the cyclic turning of the body necessary for proper rest.

Barelli emphasizes the point that behavioral practitioners should be aware that symptoms similar to those of anxiety states or hyperventilation may originate in the nose. Freud, through the influence of his colleague Wilhelm Fliess, knew of the fascinating links between the psyche and the nose. However, the psychological implications of nasal physiology, like the medical ones, remain generally unrecognized even today, and richly deserve further research.

Therapists should also be aware that symptoms such as daytime somnolence, fatigue, and impairment of intellectual functions may in some clients be associated with *sleep apneas,* which are transient cessations of breathing that can occur repeatedly during sleep. Partners of such patients may report heavy snoring and restless sleep as well as personality changes. This complex of symptoms, the *sleep apnea syndrome,* is described by Christian Guilleminault and Donald Bliwise in Chapter 3. Guilleminault, a pioneer of research in this field, and neuropsychologist Bliwise focus upon the behavioral factors involved in the various treatments for the syndrome; they also provide guidelines for therapists considering possible referral of clients to sleep disorders clinics.

Breathing is the only vital physiological function which is directly subject to both voluntary and involuntary control. The two systems that regulate breathing during wakefulness are introduced in Chapter 1, and in Chapter 3 we learn that these dual controls also prevail during sleep. In rapid eye movement (REM) sleep, breathing is primarily under *behavioral* (or voluntary) control; in non-REM sleep, it is under *metabolic* (or automatic) control. In Chapter 4, Sheila Jennett extends the description of the control of breathing in both normal and disordered states. While the behavioral aspects are, of course, of most interest to therapists, Jennett explains the importance of understanding the automatic controls as well. She describes the latter system as remarkably sensitive and efficient but subject to being overridden by the behavioral system under conditions of excitement or emotional or physical stress.

Chapter 4 also demonstrates, as do the previous two chapters, the importance of investigating for the presence of pathology before behavioral approaches are considered. The reader will find Jennett's review, with its attention to both the voluntary and the automatic nature of breathing, a lucid introduction to a complex subject.

Ronald Ley, in Chapter 5, provides a bridge from the physiological, automatic, and organic aspects of respiration to the psychological and clinical concerns. In the past, psychologists have looked at breathing as a dependent variable that reflects changes in emotion, cognition, and behavior. Ley views these interactions as *bidirectional:* breathing should also be examined as an independent variable affecting psychological processes. The consequences of *hyperventilation,* for example, may have highly significant implications for treatment. Physiologists define hyperventilation as *breathing in excess of metabolic requirements.* Among the effects of such overbreathing are reduced oxygen supply to the brain. The resulting cognitive deficit can diminish a client's ability to understand or remember the details of what transpires during therapeutic sessions.

Of all breathing-related phenomena, the most powerful and frightening is that of suffocation, as anyone who has nearly drowned will attest. Ley calls *dyspnea* (difficulty in breathing) a "harbinger of suffocation," and argues that *dyspneic fear* is a core factor in the etiology of panic attacks. He supports his hyperventilation theory of panic attacks with extensive evidence in this chapter, which is, to our knowledge, the first review of the psychology of breathing.

Before moving on to the chapters concerned specifically with the subject of hyperventilation, some background comments may be helpful. Increased ventilation is a common component of fight-or-flight responses (as explained in Chapter 1), but when our breathing increases and our actions and movements are restricted, we are breathing in excess of metabolic need. Blood levels of CO_2 fall and symptoms may occur. The effects of voluntary overbreathing, even on normal individuals, can be dramatic, as was seen in the original demonstration given by Haldane and Poulton (1908) to the Physiological Society. On this occasion, some of the observers were so distressed by the effects on the subject that they had to leave the room hurriedly.

Table 1 displays the "welter of unpleasant symptoms" that hyperventilators can experience. When these complaints occur in the presence of anxiety states,

Table 1
Symptoms and Signs of Hyperventilation

Cardiovascular: palpitations, missed beats, tachycardia, sharp or dull atypical chest pain, "angina," vasomotor instability, cold extremities, Raynaud's phenomenon, blotchy flushing of blush area, capillary vasoconstriction (face, arms, hands)

Neurological: dizziness, unsteadiness or instability, faint feelings (rarely actual fainting), visual disturbance (occasional blackouts or tunnel vision), headache (often migrainous), paraesthesiae (i.e., numbness, deadness, uselessness, heaviness, pins and needles, burning, limbs feeling out of proportion or "don't belong"), commonly of hands, feet, or face, sometimes of scalp or whole body, intolerance of light or noise, large pupils (wearing dark glasses on a dull day)

Respiratory: shortness of breath (typically *after* exertion), irritable cough, tightness or oppression of chest, "asthma," air hunger, inability to take a satisfying breath, excessive sighing, yawning, sniffing

Gastrointestinal: difficulty in swallowing, globus, dry mouth and throat, acid regurgitation, heart burn, "hiatus hernia," flatulence, belching, air swallowing, abdominal discomfort, bloating

Muscular: cramps, muscle pains (particularly occipital, neck, shoulders, between scapulae; less commonly, the lower back and limbs), tremors, twitching, weakness, stiffness or tetany (seizing up)

Psychic: tension, anxiety, "unreal feelings," depersonalization, feeling "out of the body," hallucinations, fear of insanity, panic, phobias, agoraphobia

General: weakness; exhaustion; impaired concentration, memory and performance; disturbed sleep, including nightmares; emotional sweating (axillae, palms, sometimes whole body); woolly head

Allergies

L.C. Lum, personal communications, 1991

most clinicians use the term *hyperventilation syndrome*. Hyperventilation symptom lists have been published many times in the past, but this compilation by Dr L.C. Lum, a British chest physician, is probably the most comprehensive to date and has been confirmed by his own clinical observations (Chapter 7). The categorization of symptoms by body systems is significant in itself. Because these patients often report symptoms in more than one system, an unusual occurrence in medicine, they are often labeled as hypochondriacs.

Hyperventilators have historically been victims of cruel ironies at the hands of clinicians. They are so often told that nothing is wrong, which induces further puzzlement and exacerbates their anxiety, or they are told to relax and *take a few deep breaths,* which—as we now know—exacerbates their symptoms. Alternatively, they are overinvestigated and overdiagnosed (Kaplan, 1992).

How many people suffer from this disorder? One review indicates that 3.5–28 percent of patients within various medical populations may be hyperventilators (Huey and West, 1983). It could be asked why such a common disorder has not been taken more seriously. Lum's very British explanation is that hyperventilation "fell between the two stools of medicine and psychiatry" (personal communication). Physicians usually failed to diagnose hyperventilation or dismissed the patients' complaints as neurotic. Most psychiatrists have viewed over-breathing as just another manifestation of anxiety, a mere epiphenomenon.

Although full clinical accounts of hyperventilation appeared sporadically in the medical literature from the 1920s onward, it was not until the 1960s that Lum and his physical therapists developed the first structured treatment regimen specifically for this disorder, and not until the 1970s that they began to publish details of their methods (Cluff, 1984; Innocenti, 1987; Lum, 1977). Only very recently has a book specifically on hyperventilation (Bradley, 1991) been written for clients—another sad testimony to the dismissive attitude towards this disorder. If hyperventilators are fortunate enough to see a symptom list such as Bradley's (or Table 1), or are questioned regarding such symptoms, there is often a shock of recognition. They can at last put a name to their symptoms and there is an *explanation* for their years of hitherto inexplicable suffering and invalidism.

Even those patients who are now correctly diagnosed, however, may still find themselves in the victim role, this time in the therapeutic domain. A virtual lottery situation prevails; the type of treatment received may depend arbitrarily on the predominant symptoms and the type of clinician one happens to be referred to (Chapter 19). Some therapists impose their own theoretical models on all patients, and promote unimodal, reductionist approaches ranging from the exclusively physical (e.g., injections of magnesium and vitamins) to the exclusively cognitive (change in belief systems). Thus the tendency to "split" mind and body is being perpetuated. Tavel (1990) talks of another tendency, whereby the hyperventilation syndrome is hidden behind pseudonyms ("aliasing"), which has been going on for more than a century. Currently, many patients diagnosed in the UK as having "ME" (myalgic encephalomyelitis), postviral fatigue syndrome, somatization disorder (Bass, 1990), or various allergies (see Chapter 7) may be hyperventilators. If hyperventilation is subsumed under these other diagnoses, the benefits of direct treatment, including breathing retraining, may be overlooked by both therapists and patients. Studies such as that of Rosen *et al.* (1990), in which patients who have received diagnoses such as those listed above are screened for hyperventilation, are much needed. Similarly, there is a need for research into the prevalence of hyperventilation in, for example, patients diagnosed as having "generalized anxiety disorder," migraine (Dextre, 1982), or "pseudoepilepsy" (Brodtkorb *et al.*, 1990).

At the 1989 International Symposium on Respiratory Psychophysiology (see Appendix), Dr. Herbert Fensterheim claimed that the major reason the hyperventilation syndrome had not been fully recognized was that most clients were still not being taught how to change their breathing. Effective breathing retraining was needed to demonstrate conclusively that hyperventilation was indeed the cause of these clients' symptoms. At this time, there are still only a few specialist trainers available and few technical publications to guide other therapists. Improvement in this situation may be brought about by researchers—

see, for example, a study demonstrating the effectiveness of breathing retraining (DeGuire *et al.,* 1992). In addition, some clinicians are now taking the initiative—British physical therapists have recently organized themselves into a group that aims to raise awareness of, and disseminate information about, the hyperventilation syndrome.* Finally, changes may be patient-led—a patient recently lodged a complaint with a London hospital after he had been referred to a therapist in the hospital who was unfamiliar with the hyperventilation syndrome (Anne Pitman, personal communication, 1993).

These and many other issues are discussed in Part II, which focuses on the etiology, diagnosis, and treatment of hyperventilation; six state-of-the-art accounts are presented by leading practitioners and researchers in the field, providing a number of viewpoints on the subject and a range of useful approaches.

In a series of studies conducted during the past decade, an interdisciplinary team at Kings College Hospital, London, has put forward diagnostic criteria for hyperventilation. In Chapter 6, William Gardner, chest physician and physiologist on that team, describes the problems that confront the diagnostician. Almost all of the symptoms of hyperventilation are nonspecific to this disorder, and some chronic hyperventilators may have *no* symptoms or signs (e.g., no increase in chest wall movement). Overbreathing may originate from psychogenic, organic, or physiological factors, or from some interaction between them. Gardner describes the possible organic causes of hyperventilation and outlines his diagnostic protocols. He advocates that an investigative sequence to detect organic causes should be followed even in the presence of obvious psychopathology. He emphasizes, however, that it is also important to not overinvestigate these patients. Sensitivity, clinical skills, and experience are obviously required.

Gardner recommends that the term "hyperventilation syndrome" be abandoned because its meaning is unclear. In Chapter 7, "Hyperventilation Syndromes," Lum advocates retaining the term that Gardner rejects, but in the plural, in order to indicate the diversity of the sets of symptoms with which these patients may present. There are other differences in viewpoint between these two chest physicians–physiologists. Lum does not, for example, agree that current physiological measurements add significantly to clinical observation by an experienced physician.

Lum's chapter identifies several environmental, nutritional, and physiological factors in hyperventilation that are not commonly recognized. These factors are not only relevant to diagnosis and treatment strategies but are, as is the material in Chapter 6, particularly important for nonmedical practitioners to be aware of. For example, Lum stresses (as does Ley) the importance of *hypoxia.*

---

*For information on this group, "Physiotherapy for Hyperventilation," please contact Anne Pitman, Physiotherapy Department, The Princess Grace Hospital, 42-52 Nottingham Place, London W1M 3FD, England.

Cerebral vascular constriction, a primary response to hyperventilation, can reduce the oxygen available to the brain by about *one-half*. Among the resulting symptoms are dizziness, blurring of consciousness, and, possibly because of a decrease in cortical inhibition, tearfulness and emotional instability. Other effects of hyperventilation that therapists should watch for are generalized body tension and chronic inability to relax. In addition, hyperventilators are particularly prone to spasm (tetany) in muscles involved in the "attack posture"—they hunch their shoulders, thrust head and neck forward, scowl and clench their teeth.

Lum also describes factors that affect symptom thresholds. For example, caffeine stimulates breathing, as does progesterone. Carbon dioxide levels may drop by as much as 25 percent in the week before menstruation. Overbreathing may thus contribute to the common symptoms of premenstrual tension: headache, fatigue, and irritability.

More than one in ten patients attending cardiology clinics are found to have no objective evidence of heart disease despite their complaints of chest pain, breathlessness and other symptoms. Many of these patients with what is now known as *functional cardiovascular syndromes* (FCSs) also have phobic tendencies and suffer from panic attacks. In Chapter 8, Christopher Bass, William Gardner, and Graham Jackson trace the interesting background of these syndromes, first described by an American physician during the Civil War (Da Costa, 1871). Recently, psychiatrists in the United States have suggested that FCSs be subsumed under *Panic Disorder of the DSM-III*. Bass *et al.* point out the inadequacy of this "medical model" categorization, given the complexity of these syndromes in which either cardiovascular, psychiatric, or respiratory symptoms may dominate. They advocate an interdisciplinary approach to both diagnosis and treatment. While many patients with normal coronary arteries have lower than normal PCO_2, Bass *et al.* warn against equating functional heart disease with the hyperventilation syndrome. The authors do, on the other hand, describe the effects of hyperventilation on the cardiovascular system (see also Tavel, 1990; Weiner, 1991; DeGuire *et al.,* 1992).

Herbert Fensterheim is internationally known for his books on behavioral topics, but is also one of the founding members of the Society for Exploration of Psychotherapy Integration, an organization for therapists with both behavioral and analytic training. In Chapter 9 he draws upon this wide experience to formulate the role of breathing disorders in the context of psychopathology. He begins with what, in the editors' opinion, is one of the most important statements in this book.

> Attention to the symptoms of hyperventilation should be a routine part of every psychological examination regardless of the specific presenting complaints.

Fensterheim describes the complex role of hyperventilation in the presence of psychopathology. Hyperventilation may be the primary problem or it may be secondary to psychological or other problems. Diagnosis of hyperventilation is crucial, but the diagnostic requirements of the clinician differ from those of the clinical researcher: the former must minimize false negatives; the latter, false positives. The client who is wrongly diagnosed as a hyperventilator is unlikely to experience side effects as a result of such techniques as relaxation and breathing retraining. On the other hand, denying treatment to patients because they do not meet strict research criteria, can needlessly prolong their suffering. Fensterheim emphasizes, however, that diagnosing hyperventilation is not enough; the clinician must hypothesize the relationship between hyperventilation and the patient's other complaints in order to devise an effective treatment strategy. He also describes how hyperventilation can interfere with treatments such as systematic desensitization, flooding or satiation in imagery, and *in vivo* exposure.

In Chapter 10, Christopher Bass offers another perspective on hyperventilation-related disorders—that of a liaison psychiatrist. Focusing on panic anxiety, Bass reviews the three major types of treatment now available: drug therapy, breathing retraining, and cognitive–behavioral therapy. He stresses the importance and the established effectiveness of the cognitive components of therapy, but describes the need for more research to determine the specific contribution of breathing retraining in the treatment of these patients.

When tranquilizers and electronic instruments became available during the 1950s, skills such as relaxation training, breathing retraining, and massage were neglected, and even dropped from physical therapy curricula in both the United Kingdom and the United States. Thus the treatment described by Elizabeth Holloway in Chapter 11 represents a much-needed return to an earlier tradition. In other respects, however, the regimen recommended does not differ from the ordinary, but not widely recognized, practice of physical therapy. It involves careful assessment, attentive listening, a "hands-on" empathic relationship, and consultation and cooperation with the referring physician, especially regarding organic conditions.

Trained also in the Lum/Papworth tradition, Holloway provides one of the most detailed descriptions of physical therapy for hyperventilating patients available in the literature. Both normal breathing patterns and the initial disturbed patterns presented by these patients are described, as are her methods of retraining. In accord with Lum's observation on the inability of these patients to relax, Holloway emphasizes the need to integrate relaxation and breathing training when treating hyperventilators. The strategies for combining these two components of the program are described. In conclusion, the author sets forth her criteria for the requisite characteristics of therapists who treat hyperventilators.

In this book, the term "breathing pattern," although used somewhat differently by physiologists, will refer primarily to the *mode* or *style* of breathing. In other words, we refer to those external movements that can be *observed* as well as measured by instruments. Breathing patterns will be discussed in Chapter 19 but a clarification of terminology is needed at this point. Readers may have noted that the terms "abdominal breathing" and "diaphragmatic breathing" are used interchangeably in the literature to describe normal breathing, the spontaneous pattern that can be observed in children and relaxed adults. "Diaphragmatic" is the older term. Current usage, however, favors "abdominal" (Chapter 11; Hough, 1991) since muscles other than the diaphragm are involved in quiet, relaxed inspiration, namely, the abdominal, scalene and intercostal muscles (Webber, 1991). The term "abdominal" also has the advantage of describing a movement that is evident to all, whereas many people are not certain of the location or function of the diaphragm. One proviso must be made, however: abdominal movement can occur in early stages of retraining without coordination to breathing (Chapter 11). Another term, "breathing control," is used by some physical therapists (Webber, 1991) as a synonym for "abdominal breathing," thus further confusing the issue. "Breathing control" is also unacceptable to many therapists who retrain breathing because it suggests prolonged voluntary control of breathing. The aim of breathing retraining is to enable clients to regain their natural, spontaneous patterns after initial practice under voluntary control. In this Introduction and in Chapter 19, the term "abdominal breathing" is used, but authors of some chapters retain the traditional term "diaphragmatic."

In Part III, we explore therapeutic approaches to breathing disorders other than hyperventilation, including those involved in vocal dysfunctions, asthma, and the other dysrhythmias of breathing described by somatic psychotherapists. We also look at other, more generalizable, techniques that either include regulation of breathing or affect breathing indirectly: relaxation and biofeedback training, yoga, and methods that integrate psychotherapy and breathing therapy. In the past, hyperventilators' symptoms may have been alleviated by interventions that were not specifically or knowingly intended to reduce ventilation. An example is found in speech therapy. One veteran practitioner of this discipline has surmised that what speech therapists once called "clavicular breathing," which they associated with anxiety states and treated with relaxation and breathing training, was most often hyperventilation. An analogous situation existed with regard to physical therapy. Use of the training skills mentioned above diminished with technological advances and availability of anxiolytic drugs but fortunately is now being revived by some speech therapists.

Few of us are aware of the role of breathing in voice production, and patients with vocal dysfunction are often surprised to learn that the fundamental problem is with breathing rather than the throat. In Chapter 12, Daphne Pearce points out that "a disturbance of the breathing mechanism will inevitably induce a disturbance of laryngeal function." A corollary is that patients with breathing disorders, regardless of etiology, will also have disorders of phonation, usually undetected. Pearce describes retraining of breathing for vocal purposes, once again emphasizing the integration with relaxation training. Since the voice is used in conveying emotion, psychological factors are, of course, important. Counseling, in which speech therapists are trained, is thus another component of their work with many patients. In Chapter 7, Lum points out that hyperventilators must learn to modify their fast and breathless speech. Clinicians treating patients with hyperventilation or other breathing-related disorders should find Pearce's chapter helpful in deciding whether to consult a speech therapist.

Paul Lehrer has published extensively on the behavioral aspects of asthma and on his studies of relaxation. In Chapter 13, he and Robert Woolfolk observe that specific manipulation of breathing is involved in many relaxation techniques and that changes in breathing are brought about by almost all such techniques. In what, to our knowledge, is another unprecedented review, Lehrer and Woolfolk analyze the respiratory components in the major schools of relaxation training: progressive relaxation, autogenic training, hypnosis, and the Alexander method. They also examine the nonsectarian meditation techniques of recent Western origin, including Woolfolk's own breathing method.

As we have seen, specialist clinicians consider relaxation and breathing retraining to be inseparable, but *pacing* of breathing has often been used as an independent variable in psychophysiological laboratories. Lehrer and Woolfolk review these studies as well as clinical applications of abdominal breathing per se. Pioneering applications of various forms of respiratory biofeedback to asthma and chronic obstructive disease are described. The authors also discuss a frequently observed phenomenon: *relaxation-induced anxiety.* (Note that Holloway describes relaxation-induced anxiety as a problem in treatment of hyperventilators in Chapter 11. It is considered again in Chapter 19 and several other chapters; see also Palmer, 1992.)

With few exceptions, such as the work of the late British chest physician hypnotherapist, Gilbert Maher-Loughnan (Mayer-Loughnan and Kinsley, 1968; Mayer-Loughnan *et al.,* 1962), North American researchers have led the way in developing behavioral and educational approaches to asthma. One of the foremost is Jonathan Weiss, who, with the cooperation of the American Lung Association and the American Thoracic Society, has developed *Superstuff,* a self-management instruction kit for asthmatic children. Long-term follow-ups of controlled trials showed decreases in asthma-related problems and school absenteeism in children given this instruction kit (Weiss and Hermalin, 1986). In Chapter 14, Weiss describes the role of cognitive, affective, and behavioral factors in influencing the course of this disease. He emphasizes that the primary treatment must be medical, but argues that the effects of such care can be maximized with behavioral interventions. He describes the ways in which behavioral clinicians can assess patients' needs, teach patients health management skills, and collaborate with physicians in a program of comprehensive care. Detailed descriptions of his protocols for assessment and formulation of treatments are given. Weiss emphasizes the importance of observing every asthmatic patient carefully for a tendency to hyperventilate, a factor that can in itself induce bronchospasm. He uses special exercises to help asthmatics learn abdominal breathing. Once again, we find the importance of learning relaxation skills being emphasized.

Those unfamiliar with yoga may not realize that many contemporary regimens for physical fitness, such as "stretching exercises," in athletics and physical therapy, are very similar to the classical postures of yoga. Originally a spiritual discipline, yoga is now commonly taught and practiced in secular settings as well, as many readers will know. Yogic breathing practices (in Sanskrit, *pranayama*) in their advanced forms are suitable only for expert practitioners. But the basic breathing exercises also have much in common with those used in Western relaxation training and physical therapy. It is these practices, which are appropriate for many patients, that the late Frank Chandra describes in Chapter 15. Qualified in both medicine and physiology, Chandra was well known in the United Kingdom for his lectures on the physiology of yoga. Here, he reviews evidence for the claimed benefits of yoga, drawing mostly upon publications in Western scientific and medical journals. He explores the physiological mechanisms by which such benefits might occur, and reviews studies in which yogic breathing has been taught to asthmatic and hyperventilating patients. The latter may benefit from certain breathing maneuvers that are now known to result in mild *hypercapnia,* that is, carbon dioxide levels slightly above normal. The pervasive effects of this state are described and are, of course, the opposite of those of the fight-or-flight response. Carbon dioxide was, in fact, used as an early form of tranquilizer, administered from gas cylinders to agitated patients in mental hospitals in the nineteenth century.

Self-regulation, or at least awareness of breathing, is at the core of many meditation techniques. While discussion of the many schools of meditation is beyond the scope of this book, Chandra points out that there are two basic types, one leading to physiological hyperarousal and one to hypoarousal. As he goes on to explain, the use of and effects on breathing are different for each.

Those who are interested in the clinical significance of individual differences in or modification of breathing patterns would be well advised to look into the Reichian literature, putting aside, if necessary, any prejudice regarding Reich himself. The influence of this psychoanalyst, one of Freud's colleagues, on many contemporary psychotherapies, group work, and communications has been profound, though often not acknowledged.

David Boadella, preeminent among contemporary Reichian therapists, is the author and editor of many publications in this field, including a biography of Reich (Boadella, 1973). In Chapter 16, Boadella provides a brief introduction to Reich's views on breathing, muscle tone, the autonomic nervous system, and the relationship of these factors to neurotic repression and organic disturbances. For details of methods, the extensive clinical writings of the Reichians and neo-

Reichians should be consulted. Therapists are warned, however, of the danger of altering clients' breathing patterns without themselves first being aware of the underlying meaning of dysfunctional patterns.

Chapter 17, like Fensterheim's, is one of the rare publications in which a psychotherapist addresses the problems of hyperventilation. Ashley Conway, who is also a psychophysiological researcher, describes the influence of emotion on breathing and, specific to hyperventilation, the importance of antecedent events, or triggers. He uses bereavement as an example and looks at the burgeoning research in this field. The author raises the question of why emotion has been left out of some current models of treatment for hyperventilation. Given evidence from bereavement studies of the deleterious effects of failure to express feelings, Conway warns of the inadequacy of treating hyperventilation-related disorders *solely* as problems of behavior or of cognitive function.

Although its title is "Breathing Therapy," Chapter 18 by the late Magda Proskauer takes the reader beyond illness and psychopathology, to describe the role of breathing in the enhancement of insight and creativity. Proskauer was trained as a physical therapist in Munich and in European schools of movement, including Laban and Mensendieck. She became interested in breathing, which, she emphasized, is a movement more than it is anything else. She came to New York in the 1940s and in practice there, found that breathing therapy could help not only patients with respiratory disorders but also those in pain or with postural or emotional problems. Her Jungian analysis allowed her to integrate the various components of her background into an approach that combined breathing training with subtle movements. Proskauer practiced for many years in San Francisco where she became known as "the Jungian analysts' analyst" among her clients, many of whom were artists and dancers.

Proskauer believed that breathing forms a bridge between the conscious and involuntary nervous systems. Breathing to her was meditation, and she said that "by watching it, one can observe an unconscious function at work, learn to exclude interferences, and help self-regulatory processes set in." Her chapter, originally published years ago (Proskauer, 1968), describes her methods and philosophy and is an eloquent statement of the relationship between breathing and psychological processes.

In the final chapter, "Breathing-Related Issues in Therapy," this author presents an overview. Key topics that are of interest to therapists, namely, stress, emotion, and panic attacks, are discussed and related to breathing. The complex and controversial issue of breathing retraining is reviewed in detail. The author then enlarges upon the subject of respiratory measurements and argues the case for use of measurement in therapeutic practice. Finally, breathing is considered in the larger contexts of treatment strategies, clinical outcome studies, and ethical concerns.

References

Bass, C. *Somatization: Physical symptoms and psychological illness*. Oxford: Blackwell, 1990.

Boadella, D. *Wilhelm Reich: The evolution of his work*. New York: Dell, 1973.

Bradley, D. *Hyperventilation syndrome*. Auckland, New Zealand: Tandem, 1991; Berkeley, California: Ten Speed Press, 1992.

Brodtkorb, E., Gimse, R., Antonaci, F., Ellertsen, B., Sand, T., Sulg, I., and Sjaastad, O. Hyperventilation syndrome: Clinical, ventilatory, and personality characteristics as observed in neurological practice. *Acta Neurologica Scandinavica*, 1990, *81*, 307–313.

Cluff, R.A. Chronic hyperventilation and its treatment by physiotherapy: Discussion paper. *Journal of the Royal Society of Medicine*, 1984, *77*, 855–862.

Da Costa, J.M. On irritable heart: A clinical study of a form of functional cardiac disorder and its consequences. *American Journal of Medical Sciences*, 1871, *61*, 17–52.

DeGuire, S., Gevirtz, R., Kawahara, Y., and Maguire, W. Hyperventilation syndrome and the assessment of treatment for functional cardiac symptoms. *American Journal of Cardiology*, 1992, *70*, 673–677.

Dextre, S.L. Rebreathing aborts migraine attacks. *British Medical Journal*, 1982, *284*, 312 (one page).

Haldane, J.S., and Poulton, E.P. The effects of want of oxygen on respiration. *Journal of Physiology*, 1908, *37*, 390–407.

Hough, A. *Physiotherapy in respiratory care: A problem-solving approach*. London: Chapman & Hall, 1991.

Huey, S.R., and West, S.G. Hyperventilation: its relation to symptom experience and anxiety. *Journal of Abnormal Psychology*, 1983, *92*, 422–432.

Innocenti, D.M. Chronic hyperventilation syndrome. In P.A. Downey (Ed.), *Cash's textbook of chest, heart and vascular disorders for physiotherapists*. 4th ed. London: Faber & Faber, 1987.

Kaplan, N.M. Anxiety disorders and hyperventilation. *Archives of Internal Medicine*, 1992, *152*, 413 (one page).

Lum, L.C. Breathing exercises in the treatment of hyperventilation and chronic anxiety states. *Chest, Heart and Stroke Journal*, 1977, *2*, 6–11.

Maher-Loughnan, G.P. and Kinsey, B.J. Hypnosis for asthma—A controlled trial. *British Medical Journal*, 1968, *4*, 71–76.

Maher-Loughnan, G.P., MacDonald, N., Mason, A.A., and Fry, L. Controlled trial of hypnosis in the symptomatic treatment of asthma. *British Medical Journal*, 1962, *2*, 371–378.

Palmer, S. Guidelines and contra-indications for teaching relaxation as a stress management technique. *Journal of the Institute of Health Education*, 1992, *30*, 25–30.

Proskauer, M. Breathing therapy. In Otto, H., and Mann, J. (Eds.), *Ways of growth*. New York: Grossman, 1968.

Rosen, S.D., King, J.C., Wilkinson, J.B., and Nixon, P.G.F. Is chronic fatigue syndrome synonymous with effort syndrome? *Journal of the Royal Society of Medicine*, 1990, *83*, 761–764.

Tavel, M.E. Hyperventilation syndrome—Hiding behind pseudonyms? *Chest*, 1990, *97*, 1285–1288.

Webber, B.A. Evaluation and inflation in respiratory care. *Physiotherapy*, 1991, *77*, 801–804.

Weiner, H. Stressful experience and cardiorespiratory disorders. *Circulation* (Suppl. II), 1991, *83*, 2–8.

Weiss, J.H., and Hermalin, J.A. The effectiveness of a self-teaching asthma self-management training program for school age children and their families. *Prevention in Human Services*, 1986, *5*, 57–78.

I

Anatomy, Physiology, Physiopathology, and Psychology of the Respiratory System

Basic Anatomy and Physiology of the Respiratory System and the Autonomic Nervous System

KAREN H. NAIFEH

1. The Respiratory System

This chapter is designed to provide those readers who have little or no background in physiology, or those who desire a review, with basic knowledge concerning the structure and function of the respiratory system. It is hoped that this chapter will provide a fundamental understanding of respiratory physiology that will form a foundation upon which to integrate the information on various aspects of respiration and behavior presented in later chapters.

From an anatomical and a physiological point of view, the respiratory system is unique. It is the only system in the body subserving a vegetative, or basic life support, function that is under voluntary, as well as automatic, control. The vegetative functions of the respiratory system are to procure the oxygen (O_2) necessary to create energy to "power" the body, and to eliminate carbon dioxide (CO_2) that is produced by metabolism. Metabolism refers to all of the chemical reactions that provide energy to the cells of the body for performing its various tasks. In humans the respiratory system is carefully designed at all levels to provide oxygen and remove CO_2, quickly, efficiently, in the right amounts, and without harm to the overall economy of the body. All of this happens without our being aware of it.

KAREN H. NAIFEH • Department of Psychiatry, Langley Porter Psychiatric Institute, University of California Medical Center, San Francisco, California 94143.
Behavioral and Psychological Approaches to Breathing Disorders, edited by Beverly H. Timmons and Ronald Ley. Plenum Press, New York, 1994.

We also have considerable voluntary control over respiratory movements. We use this control most often in connection with speech. Finally, respiration is intimately connected to the expression of emotion—as in a gasp of surprise, a sigh of sadness, or the irregular, broken breathing of laughing or crying. Thus respiration plays a crucial role in the intellectual, emotional, and basic organic functions of the human organism. Under normal conditions, these varied functions are delicately and precisely integrated. This chapter focuses mainly on the vegetative functions of respiration, with some discussion of speech and emotion as they affect respiratory regulation.

1.1. Basic Anatomy

1.1.1. Respiratory Passages

When we take a breath, air enters the nose or mouth, travels through the *trachea,* the main air passage, to the two main *bronchi,* subdivisions of the trachea, each leading to one lung. Each main bronchus divides into four lobar bronchi, which in turn divide into smaller bronchi. At the 11th subdivision, the airway is called a *bronchiole.* There are also subdivisions of the bronchioles, ending with terminal bronchioles. The final divisions are *respiratory bronchioles* and *alveolar ducts,* with the *alveoli,* or air sacs where gas exchange takes place, arising primarily from the alveolar ducts (Figs. 1 and 2). Airways can be compared to an inverted tree, with the leaves representing the alveoli.

The trachea and bronchi have rings of cartilage as a supporting structure. The rings are not complete, but rather have a band of smooth muscle in one section. As the branches get progressively smaller, they contain less and less cartilage and therefore become more elastic. Bronchioles have no cartilage, only elastic membranes.

The nose functions to warm the air and filter out particles so that they do not reach the lungs. Also provided for this purpose are small hairlike structures called *cilia,* found on the internal surface of the trachea and bronchi.

1.1.2. The Lungs

The two lungs reside within the ribcage in the thoracic, or chest, cavity (Fig. 1). The right lung has three sections, or lobes; the left lung, only two. The structure of the lungs makes them uniquely suitable for efficient passage of gases from the atmosphere into the blood and vice versa. The tiniest of the branching airways end in tiny elastic air sacs, called alveoli (Fig. 2). The walls of the alveoli are extremely thin and are surrounded by tiny *capillaries* (minute blood vessels, also extremely thin-walled). The enormous number of alveoli (millions) provide a large surface area for the exchange of gases to take place—70 square

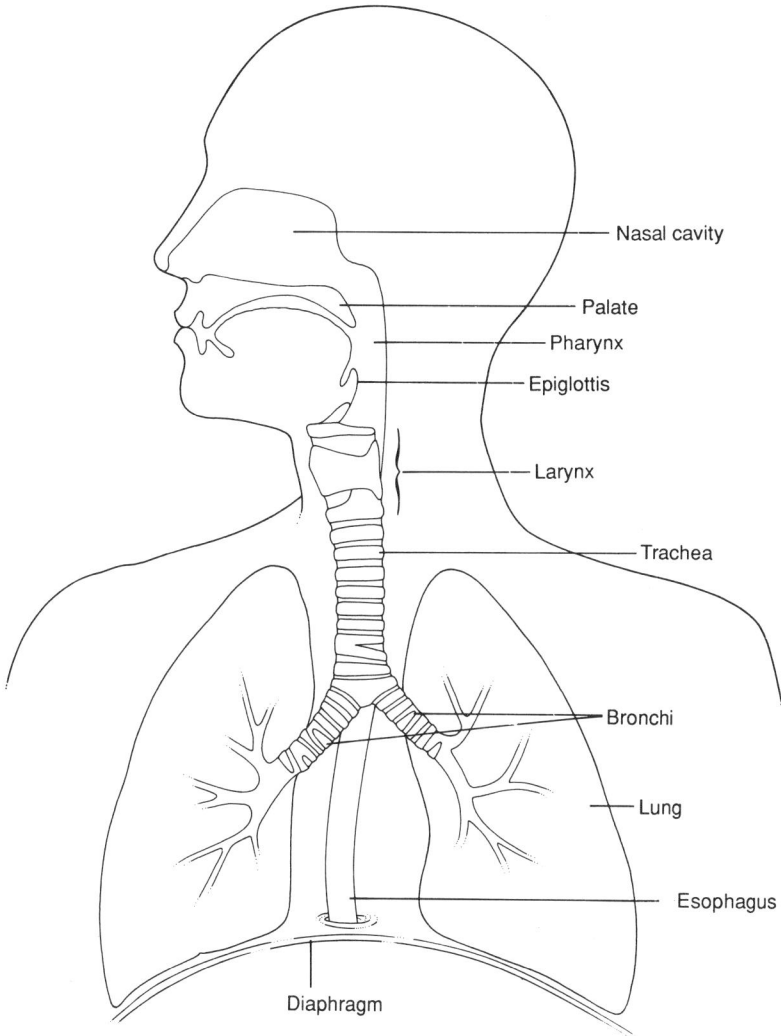

Figure 1. The respiratory system: upper and lower airways and lungs.

meters, to be exact. The process of gas exchange will be examined in more detail later. Each lung is physically attached to the inside of the chest only at the top, or *hilum,* where the bronchus enters. Surrounding each lung, and also lining the inside of the chest wall, is a membrane called the *pleura*. The *intrapleural space* is a very small space that lies between the pleura surrounding the lung and the pleura lining the chest wall.

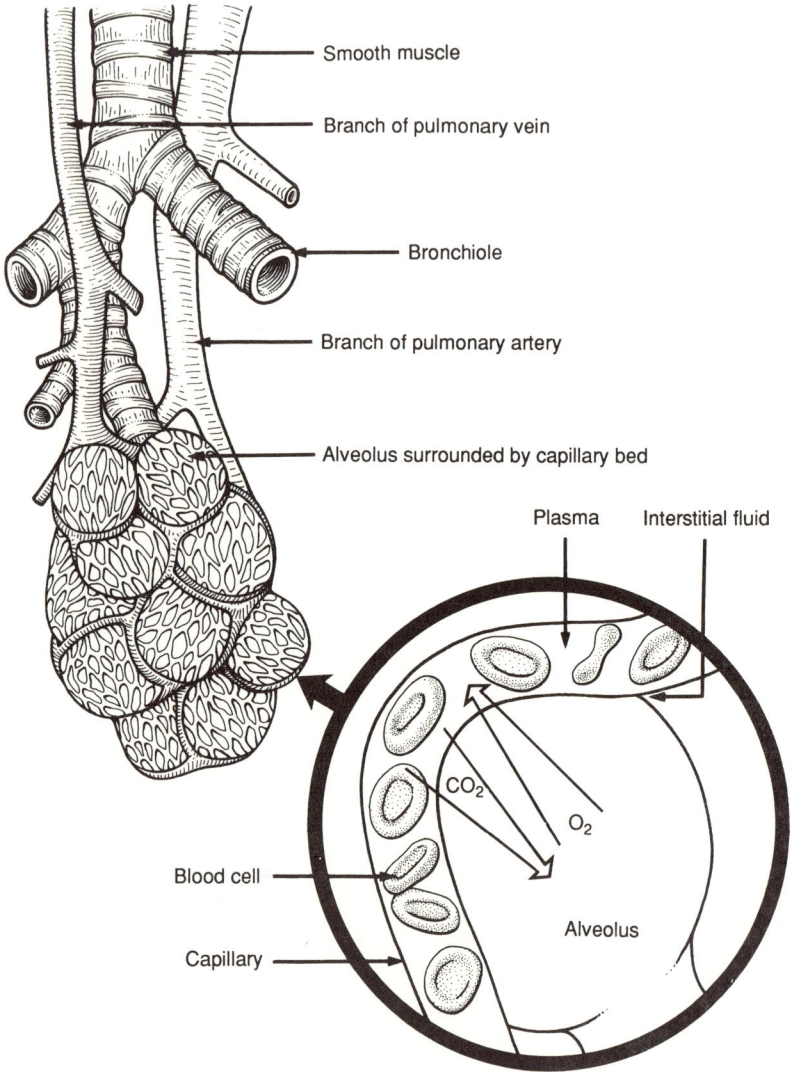

Figure 2. Anatomical relationship between alveoli and pulmonary capillaries in the lung. From Vander *et al.* (1980), with permission.

1.1.3. Respiratory Muscles

When we breathe, our chest rises and falls, and/or our abdominal area moves outward and back inward. The muscles of respiration accomplish these movements. Man uses two different sets of muscles as primary inspiratory muscles. "Primary" refers to the fact that the muscles are the only ones used under normal circumstances. These are the *external intercostal muscles,* located between the ribs, and the *diaphragm,* which forms the floor of the chest cavity and divides it from the abdominal cavity. The intercostals are responsible for chest, or *thoracic,* breathing. They operate by lifting the ribs up and out (Fig. 3). diaphragm is responsible for abdominal, or "belly" breathing and operates by pushing abdominal contents down, allowing the lungs to expand downward.

Accessory muscles are normally used only when one is making a maximal effort at inspiration. These muscles are the *sternocleidomastoids, scapular elevators,* and *scaleni.* They lift the collarbones (*clavicles*) and shoulder blades (*scapulae*). Abnormal use of these accessory muscles is characteristic of certain diseases or malfunctions of the respiratory system, e.g., emphysema or hyperventilation.

At rest expiration is usually passive; we simply relax the inspiratory mus-

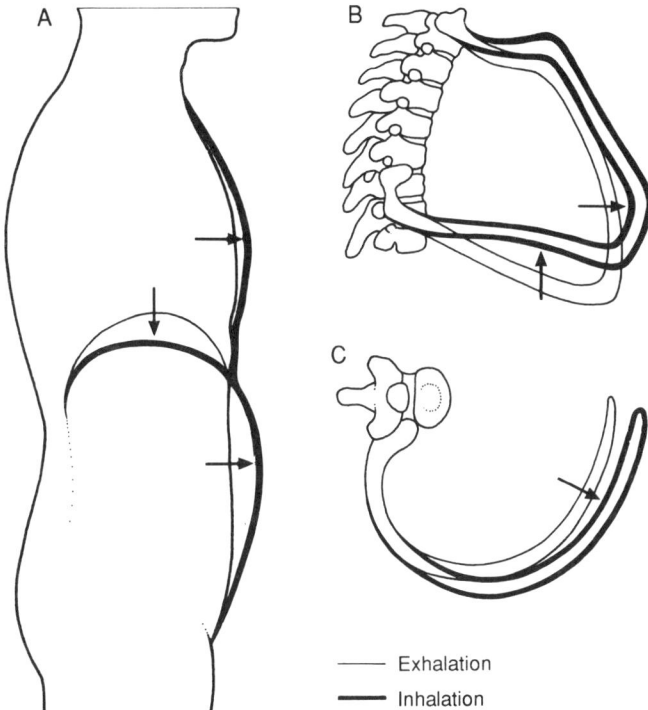

——— Exhalation
■■■ Inhalation

Figure 3. Movement of rib cage and diaphragm during quiet breathing: (A) Descent of the diaphragm and outward movement of rib cage and abdomen during inspiration; (B) a more detailed side view; and (C) a view, from the top looking down, of movement of a rib during inspiration. The ribs move much like bucket handles, up and out. From Selkurt (1976), with permission.

cles and expiration occurs without any muscular effort. During exercise, and other conditions in which an active expiratory effort is required, the *internal intercostals* and the *abdominal* muscles come into play. The former pull the ribs inward and downward; the latter push the abdominal contents inward and upward.

1.2. Mechanics of Breathing

As you can see from this description of the respiratory muscles, they do not pull on the lungs directly in order to enlarge them. How, then, does the activity of the inspiratory muscles result in inflation of the lungs?

Respiratory muscles produce lung inflation indirectly by means of pressure changes within the lung and inside the intrapleural cavity. This phenomenon sounds complicated but the general principle involved is fairly simple. For those not familiar with the physics of gases, let us first cover two basic principles:

1. The amount of gas a container can hold depends on the volume of the container and the pressure of the gas in the container. Therefore, if pressure remains constant, a large container will hold more gas than a small one. If volume is constant (i.e., the containers are the same size) the container with gas at a high pressure will hold more gas than the one with gas at a low pressure will.

2. If two containers with gases at different pressures are connected to each other, gas will flow from the container with higher pressure to the container with lower pressure, until the pressure in both containers is the same. In the situation of breathing, the two containers under consideration are the lungs and the earth's atmosphere. The latter is not a container as we are used to thinking of one, but it acts like a very large container nonetheless. Because it is so large compared to the size of the lungs, its pressure does not change measurably when lung-sized volumes of air are added to or subtracted from it. Therefore, we need only focus on pressure changes in the lung.

Now to simplify this discussion of lung inflation somewhat, let us first consider the analogy of blowing up a balloon. There are two ways to inflate a balloon; one is to blow air into it by some means. To do this we have to raise the pressure of the air with which we are going to inflate the balloon so that it will flow into the balloon, because initially the air inside the balloon is at the same pressure as the earth's atmosphere. Once we have a higher pressure source (e.g., a gas cylinder) and connect the neck of the balloon to it, air will flow in until the pressure inside the balloon equals that of the pressure source. Because the balloon is elastic, it will expand, and this increase in volume allows it to accommodate even more air. There is, however, another way to inflate the balloon. If we place the balloon inside a chamber so that only its neck sticks out, and the chamber is sealed around the neck, then the inside of the balloon will be connected to the atmosphere, but the inside of the chamber (which surrounds the outside of the balloon) will not. If we then create a vacuum inside the chamber, the pressure around the outside of the balloon will be less than that on the inside of the balloon, which is still equal to the atmospheric pressure. The greater pressure inside the balloon will cause it to expand, and its expansion will increase its volume. This, in turn, will cause the pressure inside the balloon to drop, because the same amount of air is now contained in a larger space. The drop in pressure will cause more air from the atmosphere to flow into the balloon (see principle #2, page 22). The stronger the vacuum, the more the balloon will expand and the more air will flow into it. If we then decrease the vacuum by half, the balloon will deflate by half. In a similar way, our respiratory muscles increase and decrease a vacuum in the chest cavity around our lungs in order to produce inspiration and expiration. The chest and lungs are designed so that there is a negative pressure, or vacuum, in the space between the lungs and the chest wall (the intrapleural space). This vacuum creates a suction force, which holds the lungs tightly against the chest wall. Therefore, when the chest cavity expands because the inspiratory muscles pull the ribs up and out, the lungs enlarge also, still being held tightly against the chest wall by the suction force. Now, because the lungs expand, the pressure of the air inside them decreases, becoming lower than the atmospheric pressure; more air then flows in from the atmosphere in order to equalize the pressure between the lungs and the outer environment. And thus inspiration occurs. Expiration is essentially all of this going backwards. When the chest wall goes back to its expiratory position, the chest cavity becomes a smaller container again; this allows the lungs to partially deflate because there is less of a vacuum. The extra air they acquired during inspiration is now filling a smaller space, so the pressure inside the lungs goes up. This forces air to flow out of the lungs until the pressure inside the lungs is again equal to the pressure in the atmosphere.

The above description of the mechanics of breathing has featured two factors: *pressure changes,* and *elasticity* of the lung. We have discussed the former; now let us focus on the latter. The lung's ability to stretch in all its parts and to shrink back down again is crucial to the process of breathing, because without the lung's ability to expand and recoil, there would be no air movement. This elasticity is called *compliance*. Certain structures in the chest, such as the pleural membranes and the lining of the chest wall itself—must also be compliant, of course, because they must also expand and contract. The mechanical system by which the respiratory muscles move air into and out of the lungs depends on the interplay of pressure and compliance.

In summary, the elasticity, or compliance, of the chest wall allows it to increase in size when the inspiratory muscles pull the ribs up and out. The negative pressure, or suction force, between the chest wall and the lungs causes the lungs to expand; because of their compliance, they are able to do so quite easily. Their expansion lowers the pressure inside the lungs; the decrease in pressure causes air from the external atmosphere to flow in. Conversely, when the inspiratory muscles relax, the elasticity of the chest wall and lungs causes them to recoil, or collapse back down to a smaller volume. This produces a rise in pressure inside the lungs, causing the extra air to flow back out. Contraction of the diaphragm produces inspiration through identical mechanisms.

1.2.1. Work of Breathing

Of course it requires some effort and expenditure of energy by the respiratory muscles to inflate the lungs. Because the lungs and chest wall are so elastic, the work involved is really fairly minimal. At rest, only two or three percent of the body's total energy expenditure goes to breathing. Even during heavy exercise it is only three or four percent. The two components that influence the amount of work it takes to inflate (and deflate) the lungs are compliance and *airway resistance*. The first we have discussed already and has to do with how easily the lungs, etc., expand and recoil. The second has to do with air moving through the tubular airways. Most people know that it is necessary to blow harder in order to blow air (or suck liquid) through a narrow straw than through a wide straw. In the same way, more work is required to move air through narrow airways than through wide ones. Any factor that causes the airways to constrict, or narrow, (bronchoconstriction) will increase the work of breathing. The larger airways, such as the bronchi and bronchioles, have muscle tissue that can cause them to constrict (narrow) or dilate (widen) (Fig. 2). One of the problems in asthma is extreme constriction of the airways. Bronchodilator drugs are usually given in order to counteract the constriction.

In addition, any factor which causes the lungs to become less elastic will increase the work of breathing. Certain disease states such as the obstructive lung diseases (bronchitis, emphysema, asthma) affect these two components (compliance and airway resistance) and vastly increase the work of breathing, sometimes to the point that over one third of the body's energy sources are utilized for breathing. Hyperventilation can cause the work of breathing to increase because when CO_2 levels decrease from overbreathing, the airways automatically constrict.

1.2.2. Volumes and Capacities

These terms refer to various degrees of inflation or deflation of the lungs and are used clinically and by research physiologists. Figure 4 depicts the major volumes and capacities and their relationship to each other schematically. In talking about respiratory function, it is often helpful to use these terms to refer to the relative amounts of lung emptying and filling under consideration.

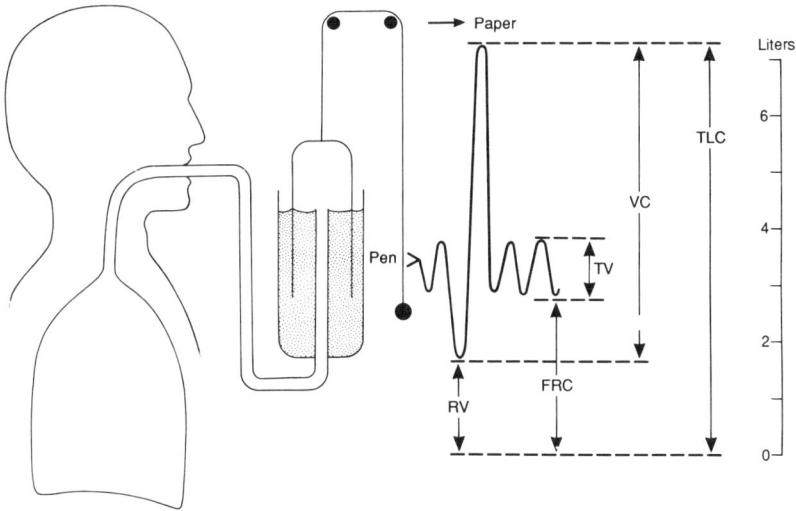

Figure 4. The major lung volumes and capacities at rest. Air from the lungs goes into a volume-measuring device called a spirometer; a pen attached to the top goes up and down as the person breathes, emptying and filling the lungs by different amounts. The pen writes on a rotating drum to give the record seen at the right. The record shows tidal volumes (TV) plus one inspiration and one expiration of maximum volume, or vital capacity (VC). You can see that the other three measures cannot be made with a spirometer because they involve residual volume (RV); this must be measured by a special technique. From West (1979), with permission.

In the resting state the lungs have partially deflated from normal inspiration. This resting level is known as the *resting end-expiratory level*. With a normal inspiration the lungs take in a volume of air called the *tidal volume* (TV). It varies from about 350 milliliters (ml) to about 600 ml. The *functional residual capacity* (FRC) is the total volume of air remaining in the lungs at resting end-expiratory level. *Vital capacity* (VC) is the maximum volume of air that can be moved in and out of the lung. As you can see from Figure 4, even with full exhalation there is still a volume of air left in the lungs and airways; it is called the *residual volume* (RV). Finally, the residual volume together with the vital capacity is called the *total lung capacity* (TLC), the volume of air in the totally expanded lung.

In addition to the volume of air in the lungs themselves, there is a volume of air in the airways leading from the external atmosphere to the lungs, including the air in the nasal passages, trachea, bronchi, bronchioles, etc. Because the air that is in these passages at the end of inspiration never gets into the alveoli where gas exchange takes place, it is called *dead space* air. Of course, dead space air must still be moved in and out. If respiration becomes more shallow (smaller tidal volume) but faster, the work of breathing will be increased because more work will have to go to moving the dead space air.

One other term commonly used clinically and by researchers is *ventilation*. In general it means the movement of air in or out of the lung. *Alveolar ventilation* refers to movement of air in and out of the alveoli, disregarding the respiratory passages. *Minute ventilation* refers to the total volume of air inspired (or expired) in a minute and is expressed in liters per minute. The normal value at rest is 6 liters per minute.

1.2.3. Effect of Posture

The various capacities and volumes just discussed change with the position of the body. Most of them decrease when a person lies down and increase when he or she is standing. This is because (1) in the lying position the abdominal contents push upward against the diaphragm, thus decreasing the expansion of the lungs at the end-expiratory position, and (2) more blood pools around the lungs, which then have less room for expansion.

1.3. Gas Exchange

The O_2 in the air that enters the lungs eventually arrives in all the cells of the body. Conversely, CO_2 produced as a result of the body's metabolism eventually is expelled from the lungs into the atmosphere. In order for O_2 to reach the tissues and CO_2 to reach the lungs they must be transported by the blood. Gas exchange refers to the process by which these gases cross into and out of the blood. A gas moves from a region where it has a high concentration to a region where it has a low concentration by a process called *diffusion,* which is similar to the flow of liquids.

1.3.1. Partial Pressure of Gases

Before we discuss gas exchange in detail, it is useful to introduce the concept of *partial pressure*. Both the lungs and the blood contain mixtures of gases: nitrogen (N_2), O_2 and CO_2 are the most plentiful ones. The composition of gases in a mixture is commonly expressed as "percentages by volume." For example, the composition of atmospheric air is 78% N_2, 21% O_2 and 0.04% CO_2, with traces of other gases. In talking about gases in the body, however, it is more usual to talk in terms of pressures. The pressure of a gas depends on the number of molecules of gas present; that is, the more molecules of gas present in a container, the greater the pressure. This is true whether one gas or a mixture of gases is present. Therefore, the pressure of a mixture of gases is the sum of the separate pressures, each exerted by one of the individual gases in the mixture and equal to the pressure that gas would exert if it were alone in the volume occupied by the mixture. A partial pressure, then, is the pressure contributed by one gas to

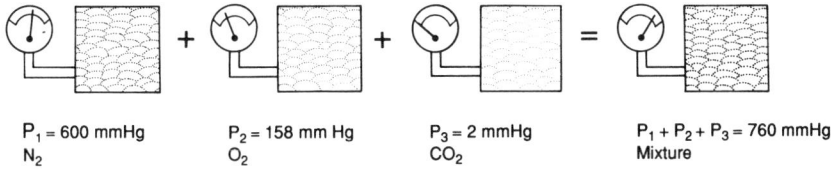

$P_1 = 600$ mmHg $\quad$ $P_2 = 158$ mm Hg $\quad$ $P_3 = 2$ mmHg $\quad$ $P_1 + P_2 + P_3 = 760$ mmHg

N_2 $\qquad\qquad\quad$ O_2 $\qquad\qquad\quad$ CO_2 $\qquad\qquad$ Mixture

Figure 5. The partial pressures (P_1, P_2, P_3) for three gases (for example, N_2, CO_2, and O_2) in a mixture. The partial pressure of each gas is the pressure that gas would exert tif it were alone in the container. Each of the first three containers has a different gas in it, and each gas is at a different pressure, expressed as millimeters mercury (mm Hg). In the fourth container, the contents of the three containers have been combined. Note that the sum of the pressures of the three containers is the same as the pressure in the fourth container, which has all three gases. From Keynes (1973), with permission.

the total pressure exerted by the mixture. The total pressure of the mixture is the sum of the partial pressures of the individual gases in the mixture. These principles are illustrated in Figure 5. The pressures are expressed in millimeters of mercury (mm Hg). Partial pressure is abbreviated "P," often with a letter added to denote the location. For example, the partial pressure of carbon dioxide in alveolar (lung) air would be P_{ACO_2}; a lowercase "a" would symbolize arterial blood. Atmospheric pressure at sea level of 760 mm Hg, and the partial pressures of all gas mixtures in the body must add up this same pressure, since pressures in our body are in equilibrium with atmospheric pressure. For the mixture of gases dissolved in arterial blood being pumped to the cells of the body, the P_{aO_2} is about 105 mm Hg, P_{aCO_2} is 40 mm Hg, P_{aN_2} is 578 mm Hg, and P_{aH_2O} (water vapor) is 47 mm Hg.

1.3.2. The Lung

Let us first examine gas exchange in the lung. Here, all gas exchange takes place between the alveoli and the pulmonary capillaries. As mentioned in Section 1.1.2, alveoli have extremely thin walls and are surrounded on their outer surfaces by tiny capillaries, also with very thin walls (Fig. 2). Capillaries are the smallest of the blood vessels, so narrow that red blood cells literally have to squeeze to traverse them. During inspiration, the alveoli receive atmospheric air, high in O_2 content. In order for O_2 to pass from the alveoli into the red blood cells that carry O_2, it must diffuse across the alveolar wall, the capillary wall, and the walls of the red blood cells inside the capillary. CO_2 produced by metabolism and carried to the lungs by the blood diffuses in the opposite direction. This all happens very quickly because the thin walls and membranes offer almost no impediment, and the full amount of each gas that can diffuse across does so in the second or less during which a bolus of blood passes through the pulmonary capillaries. With each pump of the heart, a new bolus of blood is passed through the capillaries in order for gas exchange to take place.

When the venous blood arrives in the pulmonary capillaries, its Po_2 is only 40 mm Hg, whereas the Pao_2 is 105 mm Hg. O_2 therefore diffuses from the alveolar air into the capillary blood until the blood's Po_2 rises to 105 mm Hg also. Conversely, when venous blood arrives in the pulmonary capillaries, its partial pressure of Pco_2 is 46 mm Hg, whereas the Pco_2 of alveolar air is only 40 mm Hg. CO_2 therefore diffuses from the capillary blood where its concentration is higher, to the alveolar air where its concentration is lower, until the Pco_2 of the capillary blood decreases to 40 mm Hg.

1.3.3. Role of Hemoglobin

As O_2 diffuses from the alveoli of the lung into the red blood cells in the pulmonary capillaries, it attaches itself to molecules of *hemoglobin,* a special protein in red blood cells, which can carry large amounts of O_2. The presence of hemoglobin allows *70 times* more O_2 to be carried by a unit of blood than could be carried without the protein. A small amount of O_2 is dissolved in the blood, but a far greater portion is undissolved and carried bound to hemoglobin. The hemoglobin molecule itself has an iron ion in its centre; this is why iron is important in the diet. The amount of O_2 carried by hemoglobin is normally expressed as percent saturation or the percentage of hemoglobin's total O_2-carrying capacity. The amount of O_2 hemoglobin can carry depends on a number of factors, including the amount of oxygen present (Po_2) and the temperature and pH (acidity) of the blood.

Figure 6 presents the O_2-hemoglobin saturation curve, which shows how saturated the hemoglobin is at different partial pressures of O_2 in the blood. Notice that the curve is shaped sort of like the letter "S," rather flat at the top, and steep at the lower portions. In the steep portion hemoglobin saturation changes a lot, when Po_2 changes a little; in the flat portion hemoglobin saturation only changes a little, when Po_2 changes a lot. The flat portion is where saturation is very high—over 90 percent (Fig 6). In practical terms, this means that hemoglobin keeps on carrying O_2—that is, the O_2 stays bound to hemoglobin—even when Po_2 drops fairly low. Remember that Pao_2 is around 100 mm Hg; Pao_2 can drop to 60 mm Hg and saturation will only drop to 90 percent. Therefore, even when the amount of O_2 present is somewhat less than is normally available, hemoglobin can still carry what there is very efficiently. But it is also important that O_2 can be released from hemoglobin when it gets to where it is needed; this is what the steep part of the curve demonstrates. As Po_2 drops below 50 mm Hg, hemoglobin saturation begins to drop rapidly; e.g., in tissues in which Po_2 is 40 mm Hg, saturation drops to about 73 percent (Fig. 6, point A). Thus, when the hemoglobin arrives in such tissues, it *unbinds* some of the O_2 it had been carrying, freeing the O_2 to diffuse into the tissue cells.

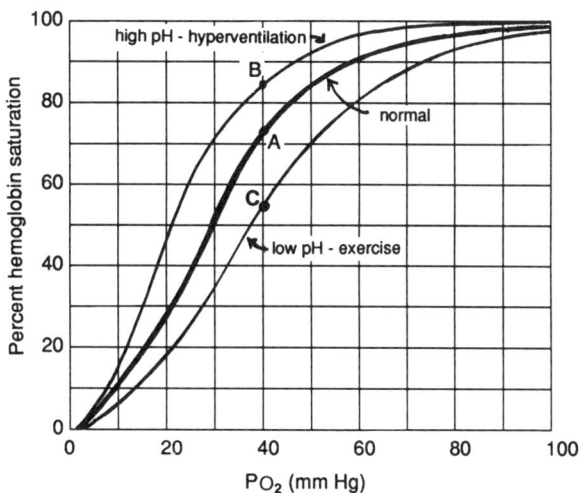

Figure 6. Hemoglobin–oxygen dissociation curve: percent oxygen saturation of hemoglobin at different partial pressures of oxygen in the blood. The bold curve represents normal pH, the one to its left, high pH (alkalosis), and the one to its right, low pH (acidosis). Point A is oxygen saturation with tissues at normal pH; point B is oxygen saturation with tissues at high pH, such as after hyperventilation. Point C is O_2 saturation with tissues at low pH, such as after exercise. From Fox (1987), with permission.

As mentioned above, other factors, such as temperature and pH, can also influence hemoglobin saturation. The shift in the hemoglobin dissociation curve with changes in pH is called *the Bohr effect*. In Figure 6 there are three dissociation curves; one is at normal pH (7.4), one is at low pH (7.2—more acidic), and one is at high pH (7.6—more alkalotic). Normally active tissues are more acidic than normal, and this causes even more O_2 to become unbound from hemoglobin, thus supplying additional O_2 where it is needed (Fig. 6, point C). However, hyperventilation can cause the pH to rise, and this increase in pH can make it more difficult for O_2 to unbind from hemoglobin when blood gets to the tissues (Fig. 6, point B). The figure shows that at a pH of 7.6, hemoglobin saturation only falls to 84 percent at the tissue Po_2 of 40 mm Hg, in contrast with 73 percent at the normal pH. Thus, much more O_2 stays bound and cannot be used by the tissues. So with severe hyperventilation the blood can be fully oxygenated, yet much less of the oxygen will be available to the tissues that need it.

1.3.4. Circulation of Oxygenated Blood

In order to understand how oxygenated blood gets from the lungs to all the cells of the body, some knowledge of circulation is necessary. A short description is included here for those readers not familiar with circulation. Actually, humans

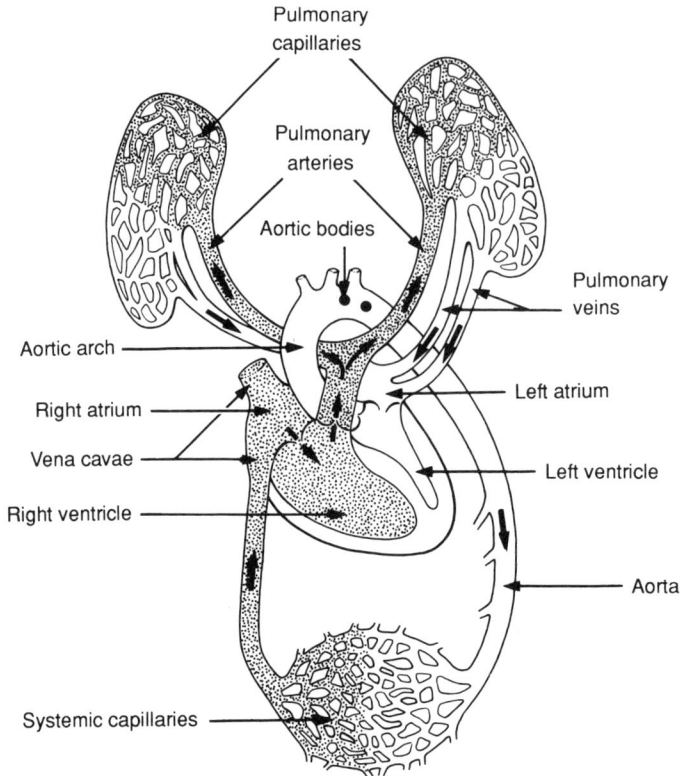

Figure 7. A schematic diagram of the circulatory system. Stippled areas represent blood low in oxygen content. Note the location of the aortic bodies, part of the chemoreceptor system. From Comroe (1965), with permission.

have *(as do all mammals) two circulatory systems (Fig. 7). The pulmonary circulation* travels from the *right ventricle* of the heart, through the pulmonary artery to smaller arteries, then to the arterioles, and then to the pulmonary capillaries, which surround the alveoli of the lung. Here, as mentioned earlier (Section 1.3.2.), the blood receives O_2 from the alveoli and gives up to the alveoli CO_2 it carried from the cells. From the pulmonary capillaries this newly oxygenated blood then travels through pulmonary venules and small veins, then through the pulmonary vein, which empties into the *left atrium* of the heart. The left atrium empties this newly oxygenated blood from the pulmonary circulation into the *left ventricle* of the heart, from where it is pumped into the *systemic circulation,* which will carry it to all the cells of the body. It passes first into the aorta and from there into progressively smaller arterial vessels until it reaches the capillaries supplying blood to the cells of the body (also called *systemic,* or *tissue, capillaries*). Here again the vessels are so tiny and the walls so thin that gas exchange can easily take place. Let us now examine in more detail gas exchange at the tissues.

1.3.5. Gas Exchange at the Tissues

As the oxygenated blood flows into systemic capillaries, O_2 begins to be released by the hemoglobin in the red blood cells and the O_2 diffuses out of those cells, across the capillary wall, and through the cell membranes of the tissues of the body. This diffusion of O_2 out of the blood and into the body cells occurs because the body cells have much less O_2 ($Po_2 = 40$ mm Hg) than does the blood entering the capillaries ($Po_2 = 100$ mm Hg). The body cells have much more CO_2 ($Pco_2 = 46$ mm Hg), which they have produced during their various metabolic processes, than does blood entering the systemic capillaries ($Pco_2 = 40$ mm Hg). Therefore, as O_2 is being released from hemoglobin molecules CO_2 is being taken up into the blood. Part of the CO_2 carried by the hemoglobin molecules and part of it in other forms, including carbonic acid. Thus, as the blood leaves the systemic capillaries it is low in O_2 and high in CO_2.

From the systemic capillaries the blood flows into small venules and then into progressively larger veins until it reaches the *right atrium* of the heart. Here, the systemic circulation ends and the pulmonary circulation begins again, as the blood is emptied into the right ventricle en route to the lungs.

To conclude the section on gas exchange, let us discuss briefly the implications of certain diseases. Any disease that causes the alveolar membrane (across which gas exchange takes place) to thicken will greatly reduce gas exchange; therefore, the amount of breathing that must be done, in order to obtain enough O_2 and eliminate CO_2, would be increased. Diseases such as pulmonary fibrosis do this by producing fibrous tissues, like thick scars, on large portions of the alveolar membranes. Pulmonary edema, or fluid in the lungs, will also decrease gas exchange because the gases must diffuse through the excess fluid. Finally, diseases that reduce the surface area for diffusion by destroying alveoli will reduce gas exchange. Emphysema is such a disease. To asses clinically the ability of a membrane to permit rapid diffusion of gas across it, a measure called the *diffusing capacity* is obtained.

1.4. Regulation of Respiration

So far we have looked at all the parts: the structure of the lungs, the respiratory muscles, the mechanics of inspiration and expiration, and the way in which the circulation interrelates with the respiratory system to get O_2 into, and CO_2 out of, the cells of the body. Now we will turn to the control centers that regulate the firing of *neurons* (nerve cells) that cause the respiratory muscles to

contract. These control centers determine when and how much breathing occurs
in order to best serve the needs of the body.

1.4.1. The Respiratory Centers

The brain stem is the most primitive part of the brain; it begins at the base of
the skull and extends upward 6–8 cm. The lower portion is called the *medulla,*
above which bulges the *pons* (Fig. 8). In the pons and medulla are *respiratory
centers,* aggregates of neurons that drive respiration (Fig. 8). The medulla contains separate *inspiratory* and *expiratory centers.* These two areas are thought to
generate the basic respiratory rhythm. When the neurons of the inspiratory center
fire, or send electrical signals, the impulses, or signals, travel down the spinal
cord, then travel through the *phrenic nerve,* which innervates the diaphragm, and
the intercostal nerves, which innervate the external intercostal muscles. The

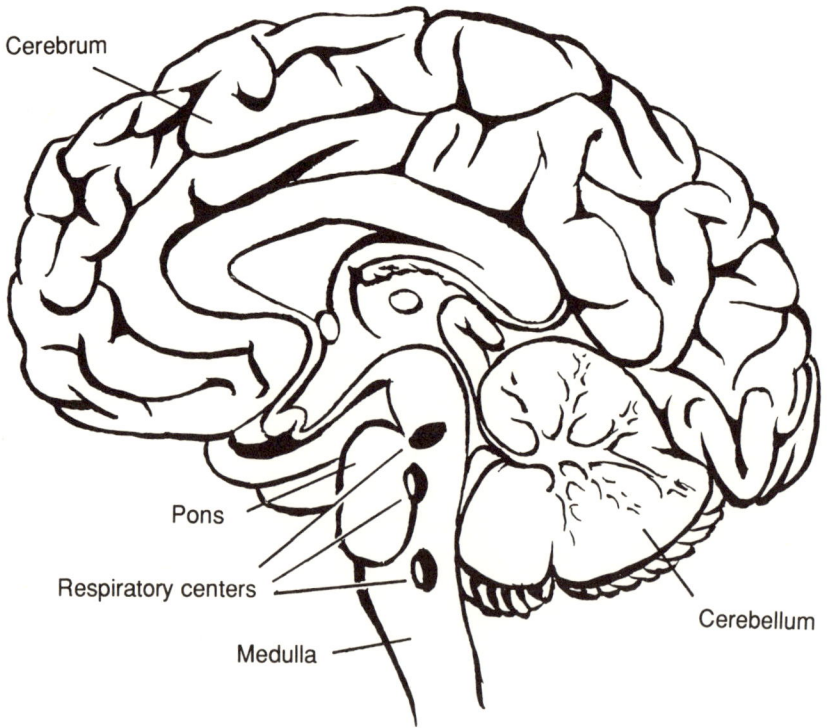

Figure 8. A section of the brain showing the location of the medullary and pontine respiratory
centers. From Hole (1981), with permission.

impulses cause these muscles to contract, producing inspiration. During the time the inspiratory center neurons are firing to produce this sequence of events, they are also sending impulses to inhibit the expiratory center, or make it harder for it to fire simultaneously. At some point, however, the inspiratory center decreases its firing, and the expiratory center begins to fire, sending impulses to inhibit the inspiratory center. This reciprocal inhibition of the two centers ensures that both areas do not fire at the same time, since respiration could not occur if both inspiratory and expiratory muscles fired simultaneously. In this way the two centers set up a basic respiratory rhythm. A variety of other factors then act to modify or modulate this basic rhythm. These factors will be taken up in sequence.

In the pons of the brain stem are located the *apneustic* and *pneumotaxic centers,* two more of the brain stem's respiratory centers. One function of these areas is to smooth out inspiratory and expiratory movements so that there is an even transition from one to the other. If these centers are removed, respiration occurs in jerky gasps. The pneumotaxic center also regulates the respiratory rate.

Two reflexes, known as the *Hering Breuer,* or inflation and deflation reflexes, also modulate basic respiratory rhythm. In the bronchioles of the lungs, there are stretch receptors. When they are stretched during inspiration, they generate signals that travel in the *vagus* nerve to the medullary inspiratory center, where they inhibit its firing; this is the inflation reflex, by which excessive inflation of the lung is prevented. The deflation reflex, although not normally as important, inhibits excessive deflation of the lungs during expiration. If the vagus nerves are cut, respiration becomes deeper (larger tidal volume) and slower.

1.4.2. Chemical or Humoral Control

So far we have examined the way in which a basic respiratory rhythm is established; now we will turn to mechanisms that govern overall ventilation, or how much air is actually breathed. If we breathe too little, we do not meet the body's need for O_2 and for elimination of CO_2. If we breathe too much, some of the energy required by the respiratory muscles is wasted, and the body's chemical balance is disturbed.

Because the main vegetative function of respiration is to provide the body with O_2 and to remove CO_2, these two substances provide the most important moment-to-moment regulation of the volumes of air breathed. Let us first consider the mechanisms underlying control of respiration by CO_2 concentration.

Since CO_2 is an end product of metabolism, its concentration, or partial pressure, strongly influences the chemical reactions in the cells. In addition, because it so easily converts to carbonic acid, it affects cellular pH (acidity). It also has direct effects on the nervous system and on blood flow to the brain. It is therefore necessary for the body to regulate Pco_2 very carefully. Since the primary means of elimination of CO_2 is through respiration, it is through changes in ventilation that a constant CO_2 level is maintained. The normal Pco_2 in the blood is maintained at around 40 mm Hg during wakefulness. An increase in Pco_2 over this level stimulates the medullary inspiratory center neurons to increase their rate of firing (i.e., more impulses are transmitted to respiratory muscles). The increased firing then produces an increase in ventilation, which in turn increases the amount of CO_2 removed from the blood by the lungs; the Pco_2 of the blood therefore decreases. When this happens the respiratory center neurons are no longer stimulated so strongly and they decrease their firing back to normal levels. On the other hand, a decrease in the Pco_2 below 40 mm Hg causes the respiratory center neurons to reduce their rate of firing, to below normal, producing a decrease in rate and depth of breathing (less CO_2 is eliminated) until the Pco_2 rises back to approximately 40 mm Hg. It is important to note that Pco_2 is kept within a very narrow range, and that ventilation is adjusted in order to keep Pco_2 constant. If the metabolic rate increases, and more CO_2 is produced by the body, that will not cause the blood Pco_2 to increase appreciably, because as the blood Pco_2 starts to rise, it will stimulate an increase in ventilation; the increased ventilation will expel the extra CO_2 produced and bring the blood levels back down. Similarly, if the breathing rate slows down, tidal volume will be increased so that the same amount of CO_2 is eliminated per minute, and blood Pco_2 will remain constant at around 40 mm Hg.

Now let us turn to O_2. Under normal circumstances O_2 plays only a small role in the regulation of respiration. This is primarily due to the nature of the hemoglobin molecule, which, as discussed in Section 1.3.3, is able to bind virtually its full load of O_2 (stay virtually fully O_2-saturated) until the Po_2 of the air breathed falls below 70 mm Hg (normal value is 140 mm Hg). Thus even when Po_2 in inspired air drops significantly or ventilation decreases significantly, the amount of O_2 actually delivered to the tissues is still quite high. Ventilation can decrease to half the normal level and O_2 saturation will decrease only 10 percent. This is not, of course, true for Pco_2, which is extremely sensitive to changes in ventilation. Another reason O_2 normally plays a small role in control of breathing is a "braking" effect of CO_2. If breathing increases due to a decrease in Po_2, the increased ventilation will cause increased amounts of CO_2 to be eliminated, thus lowering the Pco_2 of the blood. This will in turn inhibit the respiratory centers (see preceding paragraph) and thereby oppose the stimulatory effect of low Po_2.

The mechanism whereby O_2 controls respiration is the following: *peripheral chemoreceptors,* special neurons located in certain arterial blood vessels called the carotid sinus and aortic arch (the latter shown in Fig. 7), are sensitive to changes in O_2 concentration of the blood. From these receptors, impulses travel in the vagus and glossopharyngeal nerves to neurons of the respiratory centers in the medulla, which then act to increase ventilation.

1.4.3. Behavioral Control

We are all aware of the changes in respiration that occur in response to sudden surprise, fear, or a strong sensory stimulus. These, as well as the control of respiration necessitated by speech, come from the *cerebrum,* or *cerebral cortex,* the most highly developed part of the brain, and responsible for more complex functions (Fig. 8). It is also the source of our voluntary control over respiration; that is, our ability to breathe fast or slowly, or to hold our breath, by a conscious decision to do so. Taken together, these functions may be called the behavioral aspects of breathing. Present evidence indicates that, in addition to these influences on breathing, the cerebral cortex also supplies part of the drive for normal respiratory rhythm during wakefulness. This means that the cortex, as well as the medullary respiratory centers, supply impulses to drive the respiratory muscles for normal rhythmic breathing. These two inputs travel separate paths down the spinal cord, and are integrated in the cord itself to provide the final stimulation to respiratory muscles. Many neurological diseases of breathing affect behavioral and vegetative control differently or even selectively (see Chapter 4). The overbreathing that occurs as part of panic disorders and hyperventilation disorders probably comes from some of these higher centers.

1.5. Influence of Respiration on Cardiac Function

The respiratory and cardiovascular systems are closely interrelated, as demonstrated earlier in this chapter (see Section 1.3.4). Besides the overall coordination of the two systems for proper delivery of O_2 and removal of CO_2, however, there is a constant modulation of cardiac function by respiratory movements. One of the two sources of this modulation is purely mechanical: the increased negative pressure in the thoracic cavity during inspiration actually sucks blood into the thoracic veins, which empty into the right and left atria. This causes increased filling of the heart, which causes it to pump more blood, which raises blood pressure by a few mm Hg during inspiration. So blood pressure cycles up and down a small amount with the respiratory cycle.

The other source of respiratory modulation of cardiac activity is the respiratory centers in the medulla of the brainstem. The *vagus nerve,* a component of the autonomic nervous system (see Section 2 of this chapter), is responsible for slowing the heartbeat. During inspiration the vagus nerve is inhibited, and the heartbeat therefore speeds up. The inhibition of the vagus nerve stops during expiration, and the heartbeat slows back down. Thus, heart rate is faster during inspiration and slower during expiration. This is called *respiratory sinus arrhythmia*, or *RSA*. There are always some signals from the vagus nerve going to the heart, even at rest. They only decrease in frequency during inspiration, due to this inhibition from the respiratory centers, and then increase in frequency during expiration. The degree of change in heart rate depends on the basal number of signals going from the vagus to the heart; this is called *vagal tone*. The greater the vagal tone is, the more the heart rate will be increased by inhibition of the vagus during inspiration, and the more it will slow down during expiration. Therefore, the greater the vagal tone is, the greater the RSA is, and vice versa.

When breathing is very irregular, as in anxiety states and hyperventilation, little RSA is apparent. This is partly because clear phases of speeding and slowing of the heart cannot be seen easily with irregular breathing, but probably also because vagal tone is inhibited as part of the stress response. Recent research has shown that vagal tone, as indexed by measuring RSA, is decreased in response to a number of stressors. This may have implications for biofeedback treatment of stress-related disorders.

2. The Autonomic Nervous System

The autonomic nervous system (ANS) is the part of the nervous system that serves what has traditionally been viewed as the automatic functions of the body: the digestive, urinary, cardiovascular, and glandular systems. The knowledge we have gained in the past twenty years, however, has significantly changed our perceptions of the ANS. We now recognize the crucial role it plays in stress-related disorders; we also know that the functions it serves can be brought under voluntary control—they are not as "automatic" as once believed. The purpose of this section is to outline basic knowledge regarding the structure and function of the ANS, so the reader may more fully understand respiratory regulation, and the interaction of the respiratory system with other systems, especially the cardiovascular one.

2.1. Anatomy

The ANS is part of the *peripheral* nervous system, which means that it does not lie within the brain or spinal cord. The *somatic* nervous system is the other part of the peripheral nervous system, and it includes nerves that go to all the skeletal muscles of the body.

The ANS, unlike the somatic nervous system, which has only one neuron

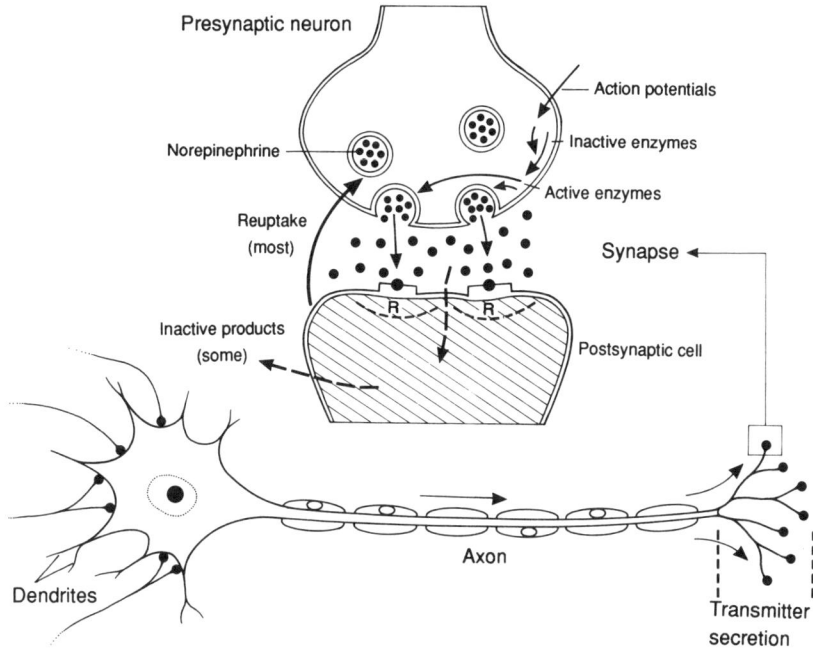

Figure 9. Anatomy of a typical neuron and synapse. R is a receptor on the postsynaptic membrane. From Fox (1987), with permission.

between the central nervous system (CNS) and the muscle, has two neurons between the CNS and what it innervates. The first neuron leaves the CNS and goes to a *ganglion,* where is synapses with a second neuron. A ganglion is ssimply a collection of cell bodies of neurons, located outside the CNS.

Let's take a moment to discuss the basic anatomy and physiology of neurons for those readers with little or no background in neurophysiology (Fig. 9). A neuron has a *cell body,* where the nucleus and most of the other cell "machinery" is; *dendrites,* which are small branches receiving inputs from other neurons; and an *axon,* which is a longer, single branch responsible for conducting signals (*action potentials*). A *synapse* is a place across which these signals are transmitted, by passage of a chemical from the axon of one neuron to another neuron or to a muscle fiber or whatever may be innervated. Such chemicals are called *neurotransmitters,* and are released by the incoming (presynaptic) neuron, at the very end of the axon, to either activate or inhibit the postsynaptic cell. If the postsynaptic cell is a neuron, whether it gets activated or inhibited depends on what neurotransmitter is released by the presynaptic neuron and what kind of *receptor* the neurotransmitter binds to on the postsynaptic neuron. The receptor is a specialized protein that sits on the postsynaptic membrane, receives the neuro-transmitter, and binds to it, thereby setting off a chain of events in the postsynap-tic neuron to produce the *response*. If the response is activation, the postsynaptic neuron then sends a signal along to whatever it innervates; if the response is inhibition, then the postsynaptic neuron becomes harder to activate by other neurons which may also be synapsing (forming a synapse) on it.

The postsynaptic neuron in ANS ganglia is the second neuron mentioned above, and it goes on to innervate a gland or organ. The presynaptic neuron is typically referred to as the *preganglionic* neuron, and the postsynaptic neuron is called the *postganglionic* neuron.

2.1.1. Major Divisions of the ANS

So far we have considered only the basic general anatomy of the ANS. The ANS actually has two divisions: the *sympathetic* nervous system and the *para-sympathetic* nervous system. Let us next talk about the anatomy of each one separately.

2.1.1a. Sympathetic Nervous System Anatomy. It is often called the *tho-racolumbar* division because the preganglionic neurons exit from the spinal cord at the *thoracic* and *lumbar* levels (T1 to L2) of the cord. They form synapses in *paravertebral* ganglia. These are located on both sides of the spinal cord, one at each level. The ganglia on each side are interconnected; often the preganglionic neuron will travel up or down several levels of the chain of ganglia before it forms a synapse. It may also branch and synapse on several postganglionic neurons in different ganglia; this is called *divergence*. Also, one postganglionic neuron can receive inputs from several preganglionic neurons because there are synapses between it and all of them; this is called *convergence*. The upshot of convergence and divergence is that one input can turn on a lot of sympathetic activity, and many different sources of input can turn on similar sympathetic activity.

One exception to the rule of the location of sympathetic ganglia is that many upper thoracic preganglionic neurons travel up to synapse in *cervical* (neck level) sympathetic ganglia. The cervical ganglia do not connect to the cervical spinal cord, only to the thoracic sympathetic ganglia. Another exception is that be-low the diaphragm many of the preganglionic neurons just pass through the para-vertebral ganglia without synapsing, and go on to synapse in *collateral* sym-pathetic ganglia away from the spinal cord—the *celiac* and the *superior* and *inferior mesenteric* ganglia (Fig. 10). A third and very large exception is the *adrenal medulla*. The adrenal gland is really two separate glands; preganglionic sympathetic fibers synapse on the cells of the adrenal medulla, which is com-posed of modified postganglionic cells that do not innervate anything; instead,

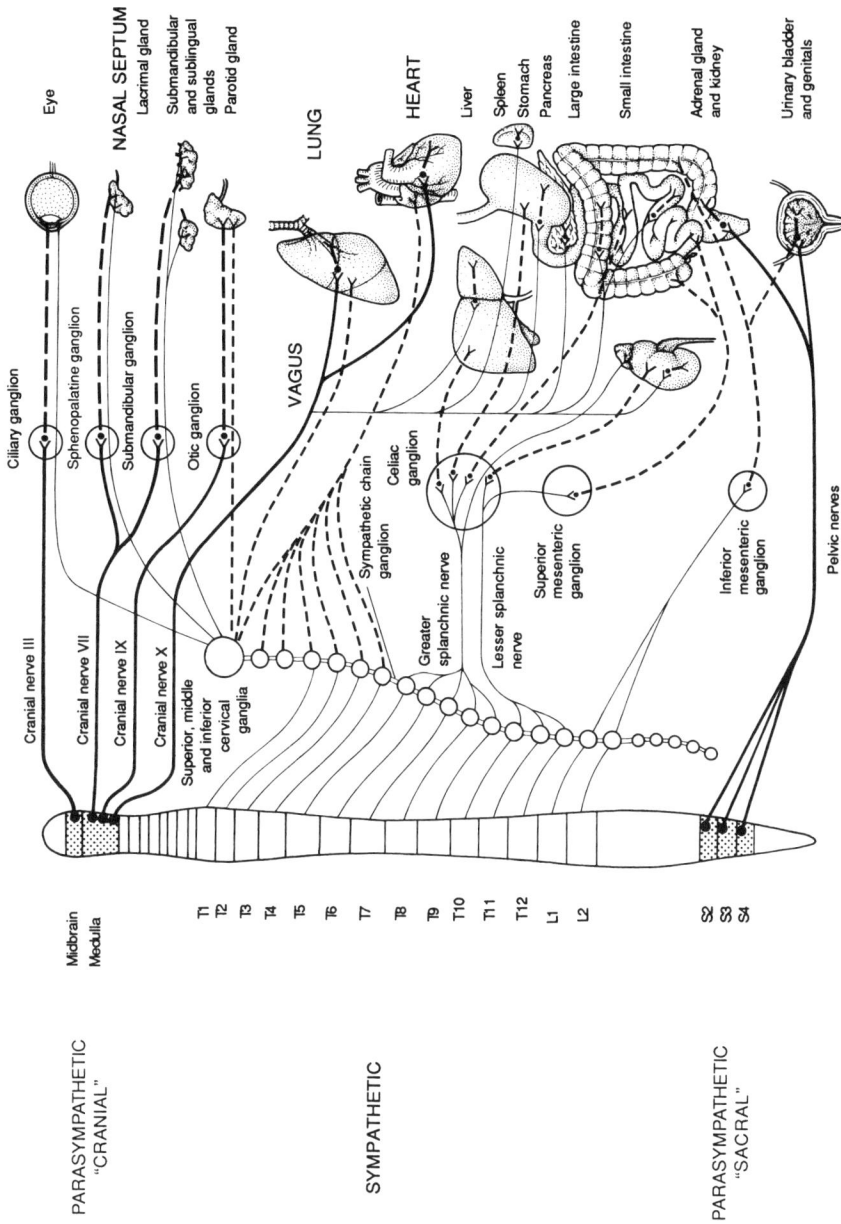

Figure 10. Schematic diagram of the autonomic nervous system. Bold lines indicate the parasympathetic division; light lines, the sympathetic division. Preganglionic fibers are depicted by solid lines; postganglionic fibers, by dashed lines.

they release neurotransmitters into the blood and are therefore considered a gland.

So in summary, the sympathetic nervous system exits from the CNS at the thoracic and lumbar levels of the spinal cord and has its ganglia right next to the cord on both sides. Thus the preganglionic neurons tend to be short and the postganglionic neurons tend to be long. There are some extra ganglia on top of the paravertebral chains in the cervical region, and a few out in the abdomen. The adrenal medulla is really a modified sympathetic ganglion.

2.1.1b. Parasympathetic Nervous System. It is also called the *craniosacral* division because it exits from the brain through *cranial nerves* III, VII, IX, and X (there are twelve in all), and also from the spinal cord at *sacral* levels S2 to S4 (the lowest levels of the cord). Cranial nerve X is the vagus nerve, which has been mentioned several times in this chapter.

In the parasympathetic nervous system, the presynaptic neurons forms synapses in ganglia that are next to or within the organs that the postsynaptic neurons innervate. Therefore, in the parasympathetic nervous system the presynaptic neurons are generally quite long, and the postsynaptic neurons are short.

For an overview of ANS anatomy and the organs innervated, see Figure 10.

2.2. Neurotransmitters

Now that we have covered the general anatomy of the ANS, we need to discuss in some detail the neurotransmitters used by each branch, before we can really cover their functions.

Acetycholine (ACh) is the transmitter at all ganglionic synapses. It is therefore released by all preganglionic neurons, sympathetic and parasympathetic. It is also the neurotransmitter for parasympathetic postganglionic neurons. Synaptic transmission at these sites is called *cholinergic.*

Norepinephrine is the transmitter for most postganglionic sympathetic neurons. The exceptions are (1) the sympathetic neurons innervating the blood vessels in skeletal muscles, and (2) the sympathetic neurons innervating the thermoregulatory sweat glands. Both of these release acetylcholine even though they are sympathetic postganglionic neurons.

Epinephrine is released by the postganglionic sympathetic cells that form the adrenal medulla; as mentioned earlier, the epinephrine is released into the blood. By that method, it is carried to many organs, thus producing a more generalized response—i.e., not just at the site of innervation. Epinephrine and norepinephrine have very closely related chemical structures and both of them are termed *catecholamines.* Sympathetic nervous system stimulation which releases them is termed *adrenergic* stimulation.

2.2.1. Adrenergic Stimulation

Now let's consider adrenergic and cholinergic stimulation in more detail. Adrenergic stimulation can be either excitatory or inhibitory. Its effect depends on the receptors in the organ which is innervated. As we discussed above (section 2.1), when a neurotransmitter is released, it crosses the synapse and binds to a receptor on the postsynaptic neuron. Similarly, at the organ being innervated by the sympathetic neurons, there are receptors for the catecholamine that is released by the particular postganglionic neuron innervating a particular organ. Depending on the type of receptor, the adrenergic stimulation will either activate or inhibit the effector organ.

There are two major classes of adrenergic receptors: alpha and beta. Then within each class there are subtypes: alpha-1 and alpha-2, beta-1 and beta-2. There are some generalities about what happens when there is adrenergic stimulation of the different types of receptors, but there are also a lot of exceptions. In general, alpha-adrenergic receptors are found in *smooth muscle* (the muscle of the gut, blood vessel walls, etc.), and stimulation of those receptors produces constriction of the smooth muscle (activation). In the blood vessels this means they get narrower, and bloodflow is restrained.

Beta-adrenergic receptors, rather than alpha adrenergic receptors, exist in some blood vessel smooth muscle; in those cases, adrenergic stimulation will inhibit muscle constriction, allowing dilation of the blood vessels and less restrained blood flow. Beta-adrenergic receptors are also found in heart muscle and, when they are stimulated, the heart muscle contracts more forcefully. Stimulation of the beta-adrenergic receptors in the specialized tissue of the heart called the *sino-atrial node,* which is the pacemaker of the heart, causes it to beat faster. Finally, stimulation of beta-2 receptors in the smooth muscle of the airways produces bronchodilation (inhibition of contraction), which lets more air get through.

Pharmacologists have developed compounds that selectively bind to one or another of these subtypes of receptors and either promote or block the normal action produced when epinephrine or norepinephrine binds. For example, propranolol is a *beta-blocker.* It binds to beta-adrenergic receptors but doesn't cause the usual chain of events leading to the normal response. And because it is sitting on the receptor, the normal transmitter, epinephrine or norepinephrine, can't bind. As a result, propranolol prevents all the beta-adrenergic effects from occurring; in the case of the heart, it prevents the increase in heart rate that sympathetic stimulation usually produces. Isoproterenol, on the other hand, is a *beta-agonist,* which means that it produces the same effects when it binds to the receptor that epinephrine or norepinephrine would—it activates the receptor. Another example: epinephrine may be given to people with asthma to produce bronchodilation, but it will also cause speeding of the heart (a beta-1 receptor effect). A more selective drug will produce only the beta-2 effect (the bronchodilation).

2.2.2. Cholinergic Stimulation

Cholinergic effects of the preganglionic ANS neurons are always excitatory—ACh always activates the receptors on the postganglionic neuron and causes it to fire. The cholinergic effects of the postganglionic neurons, however, can be inhibitory. For example, in the sinoatrial node of the heart where the heart beat originates, ACh release by the postganglionic parasympathetic neurons causes heart rate to go down.

2.3. Functions of the Autonomic Nervous System

Now that we have talked in detail about the anatomy and neurochemistry of the ANS, let us turn to function. The ANS serves to regulate the visceral, automatic processes of the body. In some ways it is similar to the part of the peripheral nervous system we are all more familiar with—the one that carries information from the senses to the brain and sends messages back from the brain about what muscles to contract. In the ANS too there are nerves from sensors, such as the sensors for blood pressure or amount of inflation of the lungs. But the primary focus in this section has been on the part of the ANS that is akin to the nerves that cause muscles to contract—the *motor* side of it. The ANS causes glands to secrete, smooth muscle to contract or relax, or the heart to speed up or slow down, but, like skeletal muscle contraction, all of these are actions. These actions are the result of integration of sensory and other kinds of information by certain areas of the CNS, just as is the case with skeletal muscle contraction, but the actions are in a different sphere of activity of the organism, normally outside our awareness.

In general, it can be said that sympathetic activation is involved more in "fight-or-flight" activities, while parasympathetic activation is more involved in vegetative functions. It is certainly true that in "fight-or-flight" situations the activation of the sympathetic nervous system readies the organism for a lot of extra movement associated with fleeing or fighting, which is evolutionarily the organism's means of survival from predators. Such activation produces increased heart rate and contractility to increase the perfusion of blood, carrying O_2 and nutrients, to the hard-working muscles. It dilates the airways so air can reach the lungs more easily to supply more O_2 to the blood. It turns off the digestive system so blood can be rerouted to muscles. There are many other effects but these serve to demonstrate a programming of visceral activity to support the needs of the organism as it fights or runs and thereby expends a lot of extra energy. The view of parasympathetic activation as being more vegetative revolves around its central role in activating digestive glands, regulating all other phases of digestion, and slowing the heart, which can safely occur when skeletal muscle activities have diminished. Let's look now at other ways of talking about autonomic function, and then come back to this view as it relates to stress.

Another way to talk about ANS function is to look at the way the two divisions interact with each other. In a number of cases there is dual innervation of an organ by the two branches; the heart, the eye, the digestive system, the airways, the bladder, and the penis are the main examples. In most cases the two branches subserve antagonistic effects (Table 1): sympathetic activation speeds the heart, parasympathetic activation slows the heart; sympathetic activation dilates the pupil, parasympathetic activation constricts it. This type of antagonistic activity gives precise and fine-grained control, just like having an accelerator and a brake on a car. In the case of moment to moment regulation of blood

Table 1

Adrenergic and Cholinergic Effects of Autonomic Nerve
Stimulation on Various Organs (R = receptor)

Organ	Sympathetic		Parasympathetic	
	Effect	R	Effect	R
Eye (pupil)	Dilates	α	Constricts	M
Heart				
Rate	Speeds	β_1	Slows	M
Contractility	Increases	β_1	. . .	.
Blood vessels (affects smooth muscle in vessel walls)				
In skin, viscera	Constricts	α	. . .	.
In skeletal muscles	Dilates	β_2,M	. . .	.
Lungs (bronchioles)	Dilates	β_2	Constricts	M
Gastrointestinal tract				
Motility	Inhibits	β_2	Stimulates	M
Sphincters	Closes	α	Opens	M
Genital and urinary smooth muscle				
Bladder wall	Sets tone	β_2	Contracts	M
Sphincter	Closes	α	Opens	M
Penis	Ejaculation	α	Erection	M
Sweat glands	Stimulates	M	. . .	.

α = Alpha-adrenergic.
β_1 = Beta-adrenergic.
β_2 = Beta-adrenergic type 2.
M = Muscarinic (α-type cholinergic receptor).

pressure, sympathetic and parasympathetic inputs to the heart continuously vary, and the regulation comes from centers in the brainstem, which "turn up" or "turn down" each type of input in order to keep blood pressure constant as the organism changes position or activities. None of this regulation need involve "fight or flight" situations, yet both sympathetic and parasympathetic inputs to the heart are being modulated.

Another way the two branches can interact with each other is cooperatively: one branch subserves one part of the function, and one subserves another. For example, penile erection is the result of parasympathetic activation, while ejaculation is the result of sympathetic activation. Of course, some functions are mediated by only one branch of the ANS, as in the case of sweat gland activity. In this instance, too, there may or may not be a "fight or flight" situation; sweating can be activated by increased environmental temperature, or it can be activated by certain types of stressful situations. Table 1 provides an overview of the effects of sympathetic and parasympathetic innervation, in the major organ systems.

3. Stress

Now that we have covered the basic anatomy and physiology of the respiratory system and the ANS, let's finish by touching on the effects of stress on the ANS and respiration. The stereotype of the stress response is "fight-or-flight," with its massive sympathetic nervous system activation. I was once backpacking and had a firsthand experience of this response. A bear had found our poorly hung food pack about 2 AM and was proceeding to shred it, systematically batting at the pack as it hung (too low) from a tree branch. I lay in my sleeping bag about 30 feet away, unable to either fight or flee (there was nowhere to run), but experiencing my ANS and respiratory system prepare me to do so nevertheless. My heart was pounding (increased rate and contractility), my breath was coming faster and deeper, I had a shutdown feeling in my gut, and my senses were exquisitely tuned. It was remarkable to feel my body respond like that. That extreme a response, however, is not what we normally experience in going through our daily lives. In addition, recent research has made it clear that there are different patterns of responses to different stressors, and that different people show different characteristic patterns of response to stress. All the patterns do include one or more ANS responses (sweating, vasoconstriction, palpitations, etc), and often there is a respiratory response. The respiratory response can be a simple shift from primarily diaphragmatic to primarily thoracic breathing, or it can also involve a large increase in minute ventilation. Hyperventilation, for example, can be part of a pattern of response to stress that is characteristic of certain people. As mentioned in the section on higher nervous system control of respiration (Section 1.4.3), this respiratory component of the stress response probably originates in areas of the cerebral cortex.

4. References

Comroe, J. *Physiology of respiration* (p. 129). St. Louis: Mosby Yearbook, Inc. 1965.

Fox, S. *Human Physiology* (pp. 165, 167, 333, 460). Dubuque, Iowa: Wm. C. Brown, 1987.

Hole, J.W., Jr. *Human anatomy and physiology* (p. 294). Dubuque, Iowa: Wm. C. Brown, 1987.

The Open University. *Systems Behaviour, Module 7, The Human Respiratory System* (p. 226). Milton Keynes, U.K.: The Open University. 1973.

Selkurt, E. *Physiology.* 4th ed. (p. 13). Boston: Little Brown. 1976.

Vander, A.J., Sherman, J.H., and Luciano, D.S. *Human physiology.* 3rd ed. (p. 331). New York: McGraw-Hill. 1980.

West, J. *Respiratory Physiology.* 2nd ed. (p. 13). Baltimore: Williams & Wilkins. 1979.

5. Further Reading

Fox, Stuart, I. *Human physiology.* 2nd ed. Dubuque, Iowa: Wm. C. Brown, 1987.

Guyton, Arthur C. *Human physiology and mechanisms of disease.* 3rd ed. Philadelphia: Saunders, 1982.

Vander, Arthur J., Sherman, James H., and Luciano, Dorothy S. *Human physiology: The mechanisms of body function.* 4th ed. New York: McGraw-Hill, 1985.

Nasopulmonary Physiology

PAT A. BARELLI

The role of the nose in health and in respiration has been greatly neglected by physicians. Ignorance of nasopulmonary activity persists despite more than a century of basic physiological research, clinical experience, and, more recently, availability of specialized equipment for nasorespiratory and nasopulmonary testing. This chapter will attempt to demonstrate that such neglect adversely affects patient welfare, including that of many patients seen outside ear, nose, and throat clinics.

In his many publications and lectures from the 1950s through the 1980s, the late Dr. Maurice H. Cottle attempted to renew interest in nineteenth century history of nasal therapy and surgery. He also pioneered development of an instrument for measuring nasal breathing pressures. He became so closely identified with diagnosis of and surgery for certain nasal problems that they became known as the "Cottle syndromes." He stated repeatedly that many remote rhinologic causes of symptoms that he diagnosed were sometimes not believed by doctors or patients (Cottle, 1987). These causal relationships of nasal origin will be described in this chapter.*

1. The Role of the Nose in Breathing and Respiration

The act of breathing and the function of respiration are not synonymous. *Breathing* is the transport of air in through the upper and lower airways to the

---

*This chapter is based on the teachings of Dr. Maurice H. Cottle (1898–1981), founder of the American Rhinologic Society (Cottle, 1980, 1981), reviewed and updated by Dr. Barelli (Barelli *et al.*, 1987).

PAT A. BARELLI • Department of Surgery (Ear, Nose and Throat), University of Missouri–Kansas City School of Medicine, Kansas City, Missouri 64108.
Behavioral and Psychological Approaches to Breathing Disorders, edited by Beverly H. Timmons and Ronald Ley. Plenum Press, New York, 1994.

alveolar cells with sufficient pressure, moisture, warmth, and cleanliness to ensure optimal conditions for oxygen (O_2) uptake and for elimination of carbon dioxide (CO_2) brought to the alveoli by the blood stream. *Respiration* includes all the processes involved in bringing O_2 to every cell in the body and removing CO_2 from tissues and organs after aerobic cellular metabolism has been completed. Nasal reflex responses play an important role in respiration.

The human nasal aperture consists not only of nostrils but of two noses, right and left, each independent yet coordinated into a single functional unit separated by a nasal septum. These structures, together with the *turbinates* (Fig. 1) and the nasal wall mucosa, combine to provide a regulating mechanism for efficient nasal breathing. In breathing and respiration, the nose has many functions which are important supplements to the roles played by the lungs, heart, and other organ systems. Cottle (1958) stated that there are at least thirty such functions known. To understand nasal function fully, one would need to know the anthropological, embryological, anatomical, and developmental aspects, as well as the effects of injury to the nose. In this chapter, only the major and a few of the less well known, but equally important, roles that the nose subserves will be discussed.

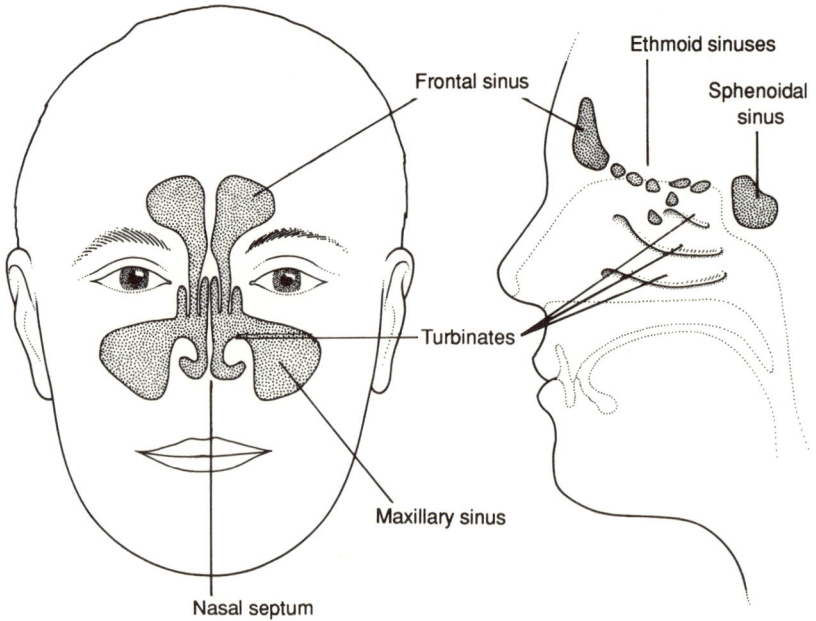

Figure 1. Nasal structures.

1.1. Preparation of Air for the Lungs

The nose warms, humidifies, and cleanses air to prepare it for delivery to the lower airways. The nasal mucosa, with its blanket of cilia and network of arteries, veins, and lymphatics, provides a protective barrier. The autonomic nervous system and anatomic control of the nasal mucosa provide, when contacted by bacteria or by chemical or gaseous stimuli, reflex cholinergic responses which influence the beat and secretions of the mucosa through ciliary activity.

1.2. Control of Air Stream

During both inspiration and expiration, the external nose and the internal nose, with its baffles, culs-de-sac, valves, and turbinates, influence the air stream in many complicated ways. The nose regulates direction and velocity of the air stream to maximize exposure to a network of fine arteries, veins, lymphatics, and sensory and autonomic nerves, and to the mucous blanket (van Dishoeck, 1936). Whirls and eddies cause dust particles to impinge on optimal areas for deposit.

The nose creates pressure differences between the lungs and the external apertures (Chapter 1) which assure flow of the air stream, and consequently O_2, to the heart and lungs (Mink, 1920; Widdicombe, 1986).

The nose alternates the main air stream from one nasal chamber to the other about every 2–4 hours. These changes are brought about by rhythmic, cyclic alterations in the size of the turbinates, whether the head is upright or reclining (Kern, 1986; Stoksted, 1952; Werntz et al., 1983).

1.3. Olfaction

The nose directs, and prolongs the stay of, air over the olfactory receptors. The human nose lost much of its fine ability for olfaction and assumed the more important role of a respiratory receptor area. However, our sense of smell is still integrated through the rhinencephalon, a primitive portion of the brain that remains deeply involved with all bodily structures and functions and is still of great importance.

1.4. Nasal Resistances

Nose breathing imposes approximately 50 percent more resistance to the air stream in normal individuals than does mouth breathing, resulting in 10–20 percent more O_2 uptake (Cottle, 1972; Rohrer, 1915). Resistance during inhalation is regulated by the turbinates in wide noses and by other structures in narrow noses. There must be adequate nasal resistance to breathing to maintain elasticity of the lungs (Cottle, 1980). Breathing through the mouth when the nose is obstructed usually imposes too little resistance and can lead to micro-areas of poor ventilation in the lungs (atelectasis). Alternatively, many years of breathing against excessive resistance, as with nasal obstruction, may also cause micro-areas of poor ventilation (emphysema).

Ogura confirmed that a nasopulmonary nervous system exists by which breathing through a constantly blocked nose can alter pulmonary function in a reflex manner (Cottle, 1981; Ogura et al., 1964). He also found that in nasal obstruction the hemilateral lung complied to this increased resistance (Ogura and Harvey, 1971; Ogura et al., 1964).

1.5. Body Temperature

Through a reflex nasal response, body temperature is influenced by the temperature and moisture of expired air (Scott, 1954; Weiner, 1954).

1.6. Nasal Reflexes

The nose provides constant stimulation by air currents of the trigeminal and other olfactory cranial nerve connections in the nasal mucosa (Nishihira and McCaffrey, 1987). This stimulation engenders many reflex responses. One common nasal reflex is the sneeze, which is a protective mechanism. The trigeminal nerve, with its extensive distribution throughout the nasal mucosa, receiving tactile sensations and often painful impulses with each breath, also has profound and intimate connections with many parts of the brain and spinal cord. The nose is thereby connected with practically all the important structures supplied by the cranial and cervical nerves (Mitchell, 1964). Reflex responses and referred phenomena are well established between the nose and ears, throat, and larynx; the nose and heart, lungs, and diaphragm; and even the nose and abdominal contents (Mink, 1920; Samzelius-Lejdstrom, 1939). Sercer (1930) identified a reflex relationship between each nasal fossa and the corresponding hemithorax. Where there is aberration of this reflex, many clinical symptoms can occur. Voydeville (1951) cited, as important evidence of the effects of nasal phenomena on the act of breathing, the fact that unilateral nasal narrowing (stenosis) can decrease the play of the diaphragm on the same side by 2–5 cm (Cottle, 1980).

1.7. Nasal Reflexes and the Cardiovascular System

Physiologists have noted the striking reflexes that stimulation of the nasal mucosa can evoke, affecting not only respiration but the heart and peripheral blood vessels as well (Allison, 1974). These reflexes are described as among the most powerful of those observed in the experimental laboratory. Responses may depend on the strength of the stimuli. For example, mild olfactory stimulants may cause an increase in breathing, whereas strong irritants can depress respiration or even cause apnea; other irritants can cause bradycardia or hypertension (Angell James and de Burgh Daly, 1969). Exaggerated responses of breathing can occur in patients with certain pathological conditions of the nose and in those with increased irritability of the trigeminal nerve (Angell James and de Burgh Daly, 1969).

In many seagoing mammals, the diving reflex plays an important role. The nose, when closed off, sends certain messages and causes the circulatory system to allow heart and respiration rates to slow or cease, thus allowing more O_2 to the heart and brain for survival. In humans, some reflexes, apparently derived from the diving reflex, have little useful purpose (except for the protective apnea that exposure to noxious fumes evokes), and may even be dangerous. Many doctors and nonmedically trained persons are still woefully ignorant of the fact that these reflexes can cause syncope or sudden death through vagally mediated cardiac inhibition (Allison, 1977; Cottle, 1980).

Nasal reflexes, coupled with the resistance of the nose, increase the efficiency of the lungs and improve the ultimate effectiveness of heart action (Albert and Winters, 1966; Butler, 1960; Edison and Kerth, 1973). This results in a better alkali reserve in the blood, necessary to maintain body chemistry by lowering the percentage of lactic acid in the blood (Luescher, 1930). Lactic acid is an important chemical maintaining a regular rhythm of the heart, rising and falling with breathing. All other body muscles are kept in tone by this mechanism and all the above factors increase the capacity for work (Kreewinsch, 1932).

1.8. Sleep and Postural Adjustment

The nose effects a different type of cycling during sleep than the cycling it effects during the waking state. When one lies with the head to one side, the turbinates of the lower nostril become congested. The chamber narrows and the lumen is closed: thus, breathing during sleep is *unilateral*. The nose initiates movement of the head from one side to the other, which in turn inaugurates a major movement and turning of the body. This head-and-body-moving cycle initiated by the nose ensures maximum rest during sleep (Cole and Haight, 1984). A poorly functioning nose may allow the body and head to remain in one position and can cause symptoms such as backaches, numbness, cramps, and circulatory deficits (Davies *et al.,* 1989; Javorka *et al.,* 1985). Thus, when the normal function of the nose is disturbed or impaired, disturbed sleep may occur.

1.9. Nose versus Mouth Breathing

In addition to those differences described above, another striking physiological difference between nasal breathing and mouth breathing is that the work of lung movement is approximately doubled when breathing is done through the nose, due to increased resistance. Nasal breathing is *involuntary* (Butler, 1960; Cottle, 1981). Mouth, or *voluntary,* breathing occurs when there is difficulty breathing through the nose, such as in exertion, under stress, and—in particular —when cardiac, pulmonary, or other illness hampers the supply of oxygen to the tissues. Thus, nasal versus mouth breathing is a "trade-off." The former increases the work of breathing but provides many benefits in comparison to the latter.

2. The Role of the Rhinologist

As understanding of nasal physiology increases, so does awareness of the special relationship of the function of the nose and upper airways to general health. Our view is that, in addition to the present practice of diagnosing anatomical or physiological aberrations, rhinologists should assess the *functioning* of the nose with nasal pressure (*rhinomanometry*) and nasopulmonary tests. A good nasal history is very important. Cottle (1980, 1981) taught that a thorough history of the patient's complaints will give important information regarding the relationship of the nose to the patient's habits and health. One should know the ethnic background, method of birth delivery, and history of childhood or recent nasal injuries, which might give clues to development of nasal problems. The patient should be asked whether he/she breathes through the nose or mouth at rest and work, how quickly during work or stress, in what conditions must he/she resort to mouth breathing, and when he/she experiences "shortness of breath" or momentary syncope.

Because quality of sleep is in good measure dependent on nasal function, special attention should be paid to sleep habits: Does the patient habitually sleep more on one side? Does the patient awake fatigued? How many pillows are needed? Is the bed torn up? Does the patient snore? The quality of sleep, the quality of breathing, and the quality of life can all depend on adequate nasal function (Issa and Sullivan, 1984; McNicholas *et al.,* 1987).

2.1. Nasal Examination

The outside of the nose is examined: the alignment of the external nose, its width, and its size can affect the resistance and work of breathing. With instruments such as headlamp, speculum, applicator wires, and special endoscopic equipment, the internal nose is examined and the sinuses are transluminated. Observation is made of the vestibule, valves, turbinates, lateral walls, septum, and floor of the nose for pathology or for too little or too much space; the turgescence of the turbinates and their response to shrinkage can give much information about nasal function. X rays, CAT scans of the head, and ultrasound can each add to the final diagnosis of the rhinologic problem.

2.2. Nasal Pressure Tests (Rhinomanometry)

In the process of breathing, the outside air pressure is transmitted through the entire respiratory system, including sinus cavities, eustachian tubes, trachea, bronchi, and alveoli. The pressure measured at the nose in inspiration and expiration is called *nasal pressure*. Abnormal, or absence of, pressure can aggravate nasal and pulmonary problems and exacerbate disabilities due to chronic lung, heart, and vascular problems. Pressure can influence diffusion of O_2 through alveolar and epithelial walls and of hemoglobin through plasma into red blood cells.

Cottle (1980) suggested an objective, accurate method of determining nasal function, easily available and applicable in routine clinical use: with a nozzle in one nostril, the pressure of the air stream as it flows in and out of the other nostril can be observed on a manometer. Recordings obtained with the Cottle nasal pressure-flow-transducer system allow study of a typical nasal breath in detail. Cottle (1958; 1968) identified many aberrations in rhinomanometric graphs, which are useful in diagnosis. Irregularities in breathing pattern amplitude and frequency, and reversal in ratios of pressure and time during inspiration and expiration, can often denote local derangements in the nose. Increases in breathing pressures are associated with nasal obstruction or adenoid hypertrophy. Other conditions such as breath holding, hyperventilation, and exercise, because of their effects on flow, pressure, and rate of breathing, can affect nasal resistance (Hasagawa and Kern, 1978).

When breathing through the nose or even through the mouth becomes difficult, a person automatically assumes a pattern of breathing that most easily fulfils requirements, or else lowers or otherwise modifies his/her requirements and life-style to meet a diminished oxygen supply and other respiratory disturbances. There are more than 100 combinations of ways, positions, and patterns of breathing that disturbed respiration may evoke. Even a superficial survey will reveal that the average person uses 20 to 30 different breathing modes in normal life (Cottle, 1980).

The rate of breathing is an important factor in health and significant aberrations may also be observed on the pressure curve. Negus (1957) claimed that a person must breathe ten times per minute in order to adequately ventilate the lungs (but see Chapters 11 and 15). A rate of more than 20 was considered rapid.

Slow breathing (less than ten per min) may occur with low pressure in Caucasians with long-standing nasal injuries, and with high pressure in young people with chronic nasal blockage. Rapid but typically *regular* breathing is observed in adults with pulmonary disease and in children with adenoid hypertrophy. When breathing is rapid but *irregular,* an emotional disturbance is probable.

Rhinomanometry is increasingly recognized as a valuable adjunct to the examination and diagnosis, and should be used before and after medical or surgical management of rhinologic and upper airway obstructions.

2.3. Sinus (Nasoantral) Pressure Tests

With changes in permeability of the *ostia* (openings to the maxillary sinuses), a variety of symptoms and irritability occur, including headache, sore throat, ear disturbances, cough, and ocular discomfort. Reestablishment of a functioning ostium is so frequently and quickly followed by relief of complaints that it is deemed of prime importance to bring this clinical entity to the attention of clinicians. The permeability of the ostia may be determined with pressure studies. If partial blockage of the aperture occurs, whether in the sinus, the nasal chamber, or the ostium itself, a decrease in antrum pressure is seen. With total obstruction, no pressure recording from within the sinus is obtainable.

2.4. Nasocardiovascular Relationships

Cottle (1981) pointed out that nineteenth century treatises not only recognized the nasal reflexes of sneezing and lacrimation but, astonishingly, the neurological relationship of the nose to the heart and lungs. He awakened much interest in these influences of the nose and upper airways. He demonstrated that pauses in the respiratory cycle ("mid-cycle rests") are sometimes seen in patients with histories of heart disease, with or without discernible nasal pathology (Kern, 1986). Finally, Cottle (1980) suggested that one of the most significant findings from pressure recordings is that the presence of mid-cycle rests in young and older adults can predict development of recognizable cardiac pathology months or even years later. This phenomenon has been recognized by some cardiologists but its predictive value has yet to be formally established by prospective trials. Such observations warrant further nasopulmonary and cardiac studies.

2.5. Nasopulmonary Tests

For further screening of nasal function, nasopulmonary tests using a pressure flow recorder with a spirometer will give tidal volume through each nostril. Additional tests through the nose can be performed with a digital spirometer, to measure forced vital capacity, flow rates, maximum voluntary ventilation, and inspiratory capacity. Parameters measured through the nose may then be correlated with those measured through the mouth. Combined with physical examination and history, these tests provide more accurate diagnoses of upper airway and pulmonary diseases. They also allow periodic comparative evaluations, to assess results of treatment or surgical procedures and to provide medicolegal documentation.

2.6. Middle Turbinate Syndrome

The middle turbinates, neighboring septum, and lateral wall constitute the area where nerves are very abundant. If the middle turbinates are constricted, compressed, or deformed, and thus even more vulnerable to disturbing impulses, the following symptoms can occur: headache, facial pain, colds, sinus disturbances, chest pain, shortness of breath, irritability, poor concentration, cold hands and feet, and other vascular insufficiencies, such as cardiac arrhythmia. Symptom relief is often achieved by anesthetizing the mucosa over the middle turbinate area with a cocaine solution. If relief is immediate, nearly complete, and lasts for at least ten hours, it can be assumed that a morphological, or other pathological, change in or near the middle turbinate is present. Simple medical or appropriate surgical treatment would therefore be expected to alleviate the patient's symptoms.

2.7. Nasal Surgery

When disturbances of the nose are found, subtotal nasal-septal resection and reconstruction, especially in the area of the middle turbinate, is often part of the therapeutic regimen. For example, hyperventilation symptoms can often occur in joggers with partially blocked noses. Following good corrective nasal surgery, the symptoms usually disappear, and following poor surgical techniques, they continue or worsen.

3. Psychological Aspects

The intimate association between the nose and the psyche has often and justifiably been emphasized (Holmes *et al.*, 1950). Anxiety-related disturbances involving nervousness, tension, impaired concentration, and other symptoms may have an origin in the nose and are often similar to symptoms caused by hyperventilation. In our view, rhinologic screening is imperative for patients with such complaints who have typically undergone extensive but unproductive medical surveys and psychiatric workups.

4. Conclusion

Total evaluation of a patient's health should include estimation of nasal function disturbances. Rhinomanometry and nasopulmonary tests have made significant contributions to research and diagnosis of human illness, and should be considered by other clinicians concerned with breathing and the process of respiration.

5. References

Albert, M.S., and Winters, R.W. Acid-base equilibrium of blood in normal infants. *Pediatrics,* 1966, *37,* 7–28.

Allison, D.J. Respiratory and cardiovascular reflexes arising from receptors in the nasal mucosa. *M.D. thesis,* University of London, 1974.

Allison, D.J. Dangerous reflexes from the nose (letter). *Lancet,* 1977, *1* (8017), 909.

Angell James, J.E., and de Burgh Daly, M. Nasal reflexes. *Proceedings of the Royal Society of Medicine,* 1969, *61,* 1287–1293.

Barelli, P.A., Loch, W.E.E., Kern, E.R., and Steiner, A. (Eds.), *Rhinology. The collected writings of Maurice H. Cottle, M.D.* Kansas City, Missouri: American Rhinologic Society, 1987.

Butler, J. The work of breathing through the nose. *Clinical Science,* 1960, *19,* 55–62.

Cole, P., and Haight, J.S. Posture and nasal patency. *American Review of Respiratory Diseases,* 1984, *129,* 351–354.

Cottle, M.H. Rhinology, 1900–1910. *Archives of Otolaryngology,* 1958, *67,* 327–333.

Cottle, M.H. Rhinosphygmomanometry. An aid in physical diagnosis. *Rhinologie Internationale,* 1968 *6,* 7–26.

Cottle, M.H. The work, ways, positions and patterns of nasal breathing (relevance in heart and lung illness). *Proceedings of the American Rhinologic Society,* 1972.

Cottle, M.H. *Rhinomanometry.* Kansas City, Missouri: American Rhinologic Society, 1980.

Cottle, M.H. *Supplement to Rhinomanometry.* Kansas City, Missouri: American Rhinologic Society, 1981.

Cottle, M.H. Clinical benefits and disorders following nasal surgery. In P.A. Barelli, W.E.E. Loch, E.R. Kern, and A. Steiner (Eds.), *Rhinology. The collected writings of Maurice H. Cottle, M.D.* (pp. 425–431). Kansas City, Missouri: American Rhinologic Society, 1987.

Davies, A.M., Koenig, J.S., and Thach, B.T. Characteristics of upper airway chemoreflex prolonged apnea in human infants. *American Review of Respiratory Diseases,* 1989, *139,* 668–673.

Edison, B.D., and Kerth, J.D. Tonsilloadenoid hypertrophy resulting in Cor Pulmonale. *Archives of Otolaryngology,* 1973, *98,* 205–208.

Hasagawa, M., and Kern, E.B. Variation in nasal resistance and man: A rhinonanometric study of the nasal cycle in 50 human subjects. *Rhinology, 16,* 1978, 19–29.

Holmes, T.H., Goodell, H., Wolf, S., and Wolff, H.G. *The nose. An experimental study of reactions within the nose in human subjects during varying life experiences.* Springfield, Illinois: C.C. Thomas, 1950.

Issa, F.G., and Sullivan, C.E. Upper airway closing pressures in obstructive sleep apnea. *Journal of Applied Physiology,* 1984, *57,* 520–527.

Javorka, K., Tomori, Z., and Zavarska, L. Upper airway reflexes in newborns with respiratory distress syndrome. *Bulletin Europeen Physiopathologie Respiratoire,* 1985, *21,* 345–349.

Kern, E.B. The nasal valve: A rhinomanometric evaluation of maximum nasal inspiratory flow and pressure curves. *Annals of Otology, Rhinology and Laryngology*, 1986, *95*, 229–232.

Kreewinsch, P. Die milchsaeure in blute bei experimenteller und pathologischer mundatmung. *Acta Otolaryngologica*, 1932, *17*, 48–72.

Luescher, E. Die alkalireserve des blutes bei behinderter nasenatmug und bei tonsillenhyperplasie. *Acta Otolaryngologica*, 1930, *14*, 90–101.

McNicholas, W.T., Coffey, M., McDonnell, T., O'Regan, R., and Fitzgerald, M.X. Upper airway obstruction during sleep in normal subjects after selective topical oropharyngeal anesthesia. *American Review of Respiratory Diseases*, 1987, *135*, 1316–1319.

Mink, P.J. *Physiologie der oberen luftwege*. Leipzig: Verlag von F.C.W. Vogel, 1920.

Mitchell, G.A.G. Autonomic nerve supply of throat, nose and ear. *Journal of Laryngology and Otology*, 1964, *68*, 495–516.

Negus, V. Observations on the exchange of fluid in the nose and respiratory tract. *Annals of Otology, Rhinology, and Laryngology*, 1957, *66*, 344–363.

Nishihira, S., and McCaffrey, T.V. Reflex control of nasal blood vessels. *Otolaryngology and Head and Neck Surgery*, 1987, *96*, 273–277.

Ogura, J.H., and Harvey, J.E. Nasopulmonary mechanics. Experimental evidence of the influence of the upper airway upon the lower. *Acta Otolaryngologia*, 1971, *71*, 123–132.

Ogura, J.H., Nelson, J.R., Dammkoehler, R., Kawasaki, M., and Togawa, K. Experimental observations of the relationships between upper airway obstruction and pulmonary function. *Annals of Otolaryngology*, 1964, *73*, 381–403.

Rohrer, F. Der stroemungswiderstand inden menschlichen atemwgen und der einfluss der unregelmaessigen verzweigung des bronchialsystems auf den atmungsverlauf in verschiedenen lungenbezirken. *Pfluger's Archiv*, 1915, *162*, 225–299.

Samzelius-Lejdstrom, I. Researches with the bilateral troncopneumograph on the movements of the respiratory mechanism during breathing. *Acta Otolaryngologia (Stockholm)* (Suppl.) 1939, *35*, 1–100.

Scott, J.H. Heat regulating function of the nasal mucous membranes. *Journal of Laryngology and Otology*, 1954, *68*, 308–317.

Sercer, A. Investigations sur l'influence reflectoire de la cavite nasale sur le poumon du meme cote. *Acta Otolaryngologia*, 1930 *14*, 82–90.

Stoksted, P. The physiologic cycle of the nose under normal and pathologic conditions. *Acta Otolaryngologia*, 1952, *42*, 175–179.

van Dishoeck, H.A.E. Die bedeutung der l'usseren nase fuer die respiratorische lufstiomung. *Acta Otolaryngologia*, 1936, *24*, 494–505.

Voydeville, F. *Retentissement des insuffisances mechaniques nasales sur la ventilation pulmonaire*. Nancy: George Thomas, 1951.

Weiner, J.S. Nose, shape and climate. *American Journal of Physical Anthropology*, 1954, *12*, 615–618.

Werntz, D.A., Bickford, R.G., Bloom, F.E. and Shannahoff-Khalsa, D.S. Alternating cerebral hemispheric activity and the lateralization of autonomic nervous function. *Human Neurobiology*, 1983, *2*, 39–43.

Widdicombe, J.G. The physiology of the nose. *Clinical Chest Medicine*, 1986, *7*, 159–170.

Behavioral Perspectives on Abnormalities of Breathing during Sleep

CHRISTIAN GUILLEMINAULT AND DONALD L. BLIWISE

Research on respiration during sleep accelerated in 1965 when Gastaut, Tassinari, and Duron discovered that certain obese patients with daytime somnolence experience abrupt, repetitive obstruction of the airway hundreds of times during a night of sleep. Since then studies of adults and infants have demonstrated that respiratory physiology during sleep differs dramatically from that of wakefulness (Orem and Barnes, 1980; Phillipson, 1978).

1. Sleep and Respiratory Physiology

Sleep can be described in terms of two gross categories: sleep with rapid eye movements (REM) and sleep without such eye movements (NREM). During sleep, modifications in respiration range from increases in airway resistance to changes in the Hering-Breuer reflexes (Chapter 1). Peripheral input, which varies depending upon the state of alertness—wakefulness, NREM, and REM—also modulates the control of ventilation. Breathing is controlled by two functionally integrated systems. One of these, the *metabolic* (or automatic) control system, is driven by chemoreceptors in the brain stem that respond to oxygen (O_2) and

CHRISTIAN GUILLEMINAULT • Sleep Disorders Clinic, Stanford University Medical School, Stanford, California 94305.   *DONALD L. BLIWISE* • Department of Neurology, Emory University Medical School, Atlanta, Georgia 30322.
Behavioral and Psychological Approaches to Breathing Disorders, edited by Beverly H. Timmons and Ronald Ley. Plenum Press, New York, 1994.

carbon dioxide (CO_2). The other system, the so-called *behavioral* (or voluntary) control system, reflects cortical input and is typically involved in activities that use the respiratory system for other purposes (e.g., speech). During NREM sleep, respiration is primarily under metabolic control. During REM, behavioral control predominates.

From the end of the first year of life until old age, nocturnal sleep is organized in a regular pattern of NREM–REM sleep cycles, each cycle having a mean duration of about 100 minutes in a young adult. In a 6-month old infant about 55 percent of total sleep time (TST) is spent in NREM sleep (also called synchronized sleep or quiet sleep), while in 2-year olds, 80 percent of TST is NREM. In puberty and throughout adulthood, NREM sleep remains at about 80 percent of TST. NREM sleep is generally divided into four stages. Stage 1 is the transition from wake to very light sleep. Stage 2 is a deeper stage, which occupies the largest proportion of NREM. The deepest, quietest sleep stages, with the most regular respiration, are stages 3 and 4, also known as slow wave sleep (SWS). SWS, which occurs predominantly during the first half of the sleep period, shows huge interindividual variation (Bliwise and Bergmann, 1987) but on average occupies about 20 percent of TST in young adults.

REM sleep (also called dream sleep, paradoxical sleep, desynchronized sleep, or active sleep) decreases from about 50 percent to 25 percent of TST during the first two years of life, and occupies about 20 percent of TST from puberty through old age. REM sleep periods grow longer over the course of the night so that the greatest amount of REM sleep occurs during the early morning. The first REM period may last 5 to 15 minutes, whereas the latter ones may last as long as an hour. REM sleep has a circadian distribution that closely follows the body temperature cycle and is somewhat independent of when a person goes to sleep. REM sleep is often subdivided into *phasic* and *tonic* components. The phasic components consist of REM bursts, extraocular and middle ear muscle activity, muscle twitches, and short diaphragmatic pauses. In addition, the series of eye movements are sometimes associated with decreased muscle tone in the oropharyngeal muscles. When combined with inactivity of the diaphragm, this phasic inhibition may have dangerous consequences for subjects with impaired ventilation, obstructive or restrictive lung diseases (primary hypoventilation), or sleep-related breathing problems, such as sleep apnea syndrome (SAS) (Section 2). Of great importance is that this phasic REM phenomenon can supercede metabolic control of ventilation. As for tonic REM sleep (i.e., sleep during the time between bursts of eye movements), respiration is affected by the pervasive muscle atonia affecting the facial, respiratory accessory, and intercostal muscle groups. Because the latter facilitate air exchange and maintain shape of the thoracic cage, the atonia of tonic REM sleep measurably increases tonic workload. In infants, with a less rigid thorax, paradoxical breathing may occur, and a "caving in" of the chest may be observed rather easily.

2. Sleep Apnea Syndrome

The first description of SAS may have been Charles Dickens's 1837 description in *The Pickwick Papers* of an extremely fat boy named Joe who was persistently and pervasively sleepy. Later, medical writers coined the term *Pickwickian* to refer to such patients. Since that time great scientific strides have been made in understanding this condition, with the most significant work occurring in the last fifteen years. The reader is directed to several excellent sources (Guilleminault, 1982; Guilleminault and Dement, 1978; Lydic and Biebuyck, 1988; Kryger *et al.*, 1989; Saunders and Sullivan, 1984) for a more comprehensive description of the mechanisms, risk factors, and cardiovascular/pulmonary morbidity data for SAS. In this section, we will focus on a basic description of the syndrome as it is seen clinically, with an emphasis on the behavioral sequelae.

SAS is most common in men and postmenopausal women. Its prevalence increases with age. SAS is also positively associated with obesity and a history of chronic alcohol intake. Certain features of jaw and facial structure may predispose an individual to SAS. Complaints include daytime fatigue, tiredness, and somnolence that can be so severe that the subject will fall asleep not only in a quiet situation but also when driving an automobile or operating monotonous heavy machinery. Hypnagogic hallucinations and automatic behavior may accompany the daytime somnolence. Subjects frequently complain of moderate difficulty maintaining attention, clouded intellect, deterioration of memory and judgment, and confusion just after awakening. In rare cases, these symptoms are severe, and a brain tumor may be suspected, particularly when morning headaches also are reported. In such cases, the patient will report awakening with headaches, generally frontal but occasionally diffuse. These headaches usually disappear by late morning or early afternoon. Friends and family may report personality changes or outbursts of abnormal behavior such as depression, anxiety, or sudden episodes of jealousy or suspicion. Impotence may also occur. These daytime complaints occur in conjunction with abnormal sleep patterns. Bed partners report heavy snoring and restless sleep with unusual motor activity, including somnambulism, nocturnal disorientation, and confusion. Sometimes gasping for air is heard. Systemic hypertension and heart disease often occur in patients with severe SAS. This clinical picture may take years to develop. As the disease progresses, certain symptoms such as intellectual cloudiness and impotence may predominate and may be difficult to trace to the sleep-related breathing disorder. However, when nocturnal symptoms, particularly heavy repetitive snoring, are present it is appropriate to investigate the possibility of SAS (Section 4, below).

Personality changes associated with SAS include mild dysphoria and hostility. Such patients also tend to be somaticized and may have somewhat paranoid personality traits (Sink *et al.*, 1986). It is important to recognize that these characteristics are not a function of the somnolence per se because patients with *narcolepsy,* another disabling condition with profound sleepiness, show a somewhat different personality pattern, with more introverted and schizoid traits.

The intellectual deterioration accompanying SAS has been noted in children, middle-aged adults, and elderly individuals. In one study of the effects of surgical treatment of children 11- to 14-years-old with SAS, many of whom were performing poorly in the classroom, the number of arithmetic problems on the Wilkinson Addition Test answered correctly increased by nearly 50 percent after surgical treatment (Section 3) (Guilleminault *et al.,* 1982). A number of studies of neuropsychological function (for review, see Bliwise, 1989) in middle-aged patients have shown that a wide variety of mental functions, such as, psychomotor speed and sequencing, left-right spatial orientation, visuospatial reasoning, and immediate verbal memory may all be impaired in SAS.

We have shown some preliminary results also relating SAS to mental function in an aged population (Yesavage *et al.,* 1985). The subjects represented a heterogeneous sample from clinical and nonclinical sources; however, none was institutionalized. The measure of disturbed breathing was the respiratory disturbance index (RDI), i.e., the number of apneas and hypopneas per sleep hour. Fifty-eight men (mean age 68.1 $\pm$ 6.5) and 52 women (mean age 67.4 $\pm$ 7.5) underwent testing. Mean RDI for the men was 24.1 ($\pm$ 24.2) and for the women, 5.2 ($\pm$ 12.4). Each subject also took the following battery of cognitive performance tests: Raven Colored Progressive Matrices, Peabody Picture Vocabulary Test, the Digit Symbol subtest of the Wechsler Adult Intelligence Scale, the Benton Visual Retention Test, the Face–Hand Test, a Buschke list-learning task, Trailmaking A and B, the Stroop Test, and a reading comprehension paragraph. There were no significant relationships between cognitive performance and RDI in the female subjects, perhaps owing to the less severe sleep apnea in the women. The results for the males are shown in Table 1. They suggest that, even though SAS is correlated with neuropsychological impairment, the effect is far less when individuals with probable dementia (Mini-Mental State Exam score $\leq$ 26) are included. The results also imply that confounding factors, such as age, education, depression, and sleepiness may make the relationships between SAS and mental function more difficult to detect.

3. Treatments for Sleep Apnea Syndrome

Since the time of the original sleep laboratory description of SAS in the mid-1960s, over 25 different treatments have been subject to scientific study. Medications such as protriptyline, medroxyprogesterone, acetazolamide, almitrine, and theophylline have all been tried without uniform success. Various surgical procedures have been used with mixed results. The classic surgical

Table 1

Correlations between Sleep Apnea and Psychometrics[a,b]

Test	Nondemented MMSE[c] > 26 (N = 41)	Entire sample MMSE[c] > 12 (N = 58)
Raven Colored Progressive Matrices	−.55***	−.28*
Peabody Picture Vocabulary Test	−.36*	−.25
WAIS Digit Symbol	−.44**	−.25
Benton Visual Retention Test, correct	−.23	−.22
Benton Visual Retention Test, errors[d]	.31	.35**
Face–Hand Test errors[d]	.16	.16
Buschke list-learning task	−.05	−.04
Reading comprehension paragraph	−.09	.05
Stroop Test (C/B)[d]	.35*	−.25
Trailmaking A[d]	.24	.23
Trailmaking B[d]	.32*	.22

Note: Data based on Yesavage *et al.* (1985).
[a]Correlations partialed for age, education, depression, and sleepiness. Two-tailed probabilities are reported.   ***$p < .001$ **$p < .01$ *$p < .05$
[b]Sleep apnea defined as the Respiratory Disturbance (Apnea/Hypopnea) Index.
[c]MMSE = Mini-Mental State Exam.
[d]Higher scores indicate poorer performance.

treatment, tracheostomy (left open during sleep) is now seldom used, though it is effective in bypassing upper airway collapse in life-or-death situations. Other surgical procedures, such as, tonsillectomy, uvulopalatopharyngoplasty (removal of excess tissue in the mouth and throat), maxillofacial surgery (e.g., advancement of the lower jaw) are used in certain selected cases. By far the most common and uniformly successful treatment for SAS, however, is nasal continuous positive airway pressure (CPAP). Nasal CPAP introduces a small steady stream of room air through the nose through a light-weight mask. It is not an O_2 treatment. The mask is connected to an air blower that sits by the bed while the patient sleeps. The positive pressure through the mask essentially acts as pneumatic splint, preventing collapse of the airway during sleep. Nasal CPAP is almost uniformly successful in preventing sleep apnea, although some side effects (dry nose and mouth) can occur.

Can behavioral approaches be useful in treating SAS? There are several different ways to answer this question. Some researchers have shown that in normals, auditory signals presented during sleep can cue individuals to take a large breath (Badia *et al.,* 1984, 1985, 1986), and, in SAS patients, the duration —but not necessarily the number—of breathing disturbances may be reduced under such a paradigm (Badia *et al.,* 1988). Others (Josephson and Rosen, 1983) have described behavioral response-contingent awakening devices for treating the snoring associated with SAS. When snoring reaches a predetermined volume, a feedback tone sounds, which the subject switches off once he is aroused. Even subjects who initially had at least ten snoring episodes in excess of 60 db not only reduced their snoring levels, but also reduced the number of respiratory irregularities occurring during sleep, posttreatment. Related to these approaches are behavioral programs that attempt to control SAS by having individuals sleep on their sides rather than on their backs. Tennis balls placed in a sock attached to the back of pajamas are sometimes used, although more sophisticated position alarm sensors have recently been developed. It must be stressed that all of these behavioral approaches, if useful at all, are to be instituted in only the mildest cases. Severe SAS occurs regardless of the position of the sleeper.

Apart from such direct behavioral interventions, behavioral factors are of great importance in many types of treatments. Weight loss, for example, is often a successful treatment for SAS but often difficult to achieve without a highly structured behavior modification program. Other self-administered treatments such as the tongue-retaining device, dental appliances that advance the jaw slightly, and nasopharyngeal self-intubation are all highly dependent upon patients' willingness to undergo the procedure nightly. Compliance and self-regulation even enter into usage of nasal CPAP to some degree. Compliance estimates for CPAP vary between 65 and 83 percent (Nino-Murcia *et al.*, 1989), which are high but far from ideal. In addition, although instructed to use CPAP every night, one in three do not (Nino-Murcia *et al.*, 1989). Finally, a behavioral management perspective of SAS treatment would be incomplete without mention of the factors known to exacerbate the condition. Patients are typically told to avoid alcohol before bed as well as to avoid sedative-hypnotic medication, as these may increase or worsen preexisting sleep apnea. Obviously, behavioral control over the impediments to respiration in sleep is a key feature to any treatment plan.

4. Guidelines for Therapists

Patients experiencing the two main symptoms of daytime fatigue and a history of snoring (particularly loud, discontinuous snoring accompanied by gasping) should be considered for referral to a sleep disorders specialist. Additional risk factors (maleness, overweight, age 45 and above, history of alcohol intake, presence of pulmonary disease) should be viewed as additive, but not necessary, accessory symptoms to arouse suspicion of SAS. For example, a woman in her twenties who snores and falls asleep inappropriately is still a candidate for referral to a sleep specialist. In the United States, the American Sleep Disorders Association (with headquarters in Rochester, Minnesota) officially sanctions both individuals and clinics as specialists in this growing field.

Sleep disorders clinics exist in Japan, Australia, and Canada, and in most countries in Latin America and Western Europe, although the number of specialists is somewhat lower than in the United States.

The key diagnostic test used in most sleep clinics to make a definitive diagnosis of SAS is overnight laboratory *polysomnography,* i.e., the recording of multiple physiological parameters during sleep, including: electroencephalography, electro-oculography, surface chin electromyography, electrocardiography, chest and abdominal respiratory movement, nasal and oral airflow, and O_2 saturation. Sometimes other parameters are recorded, such as CO_2 concentration of the expired air or leg movement activity, to detect a sleep disorder called *nocturnal myoclonus* in which the legs jerk during sleep. All of these procedures are noninvasive. On occasion, invasive procedures such as insertion of an endo-esophageal balloon (to determine intrathoracic pressure) or esophageal pH electrodes (to study the overflow or reflux of stomach contents into the esophagus during sleep) are also performed. The tracings produced by an overnight study of such parameters are then interpreted by the sleep disorders specialist.

Laboratory polysomnography is expensive. In the United States a typical recording may cost between $800 and $1200. It is important for all health care professionals to understand that SAS cannot be diagnosed, nor should it ever be treated, on the basis of history alone. In recent years some experienced sleep disorders specialists have introduced the use of portable, ambulatory monitoring equipment, worn by subjects at home, to assist in the initial screening of suspected SAS patients (Ancoli-Israel, 1989; Nino-Murcia *et al.,* 1987). Although promising and obviously cost-effective at some level, such technologies are subject to a large number of difficulties (Nino-Murcia *et al.,* 1987), and fail to give a full appreciation of sleep architecture as does laboratory polysomnography. At present we recommend that no medically based intervention for SAS be undertaken until a diagnostic night of polysomnography has been performed within the sleep laboratory.

5. References

Ancoli-Israel, S. Ambulatory casette recording of sleep apnea. In J. Ebersole (Ed.), *Ambulatory EEG monitoring.* New York: Raven, 1989, pp. 299–315.

Badia, P., Harsh, J., Balkin, T., Cantrell, P., Klempert, A., O'Rourke, D., and Schoen, L. Behavioral control of respiration in sleep. *Psychophysiology,* 1984 *21,* 494–500.

Badia, P., Harsh, J., Balkin, T., O'Rourke, D., and Schoen, L. Behavioral control of respiration in sleep and sleepiness due to signal-induced sleep fragmentation. *Psychophysiology,* 1985, *22,* 517–524.

Badia, P., Harsh, J., and Balkin, T. Behavioral control over sleeping respiration in normals for ten consecutive nights. *Psychophysiology,* 1986, *23,* 409–411.

Badia, P., Harsh, J., Culpepper, J., and Shaffer, J. Behavioral control of abnormal breathing in sleep. *Journal of Behavioral Medicine,* 1988, *11,* 585–592.

Bliwise, D.L. Neuropsychological function and sleep. *Clinics in Geriatric Medicine,* 1989, *5,* 381–394.

Bliwise, D.L., and Bergmann, B.M. Individual differences in stages 3 and 4 sleep. *Psychophysiology,* 1987, *24,* 35–40.

Guilleminault, C. (Ed.), *Sleeping and waking disorders: Indications and techniques.* Menlo Park, California: Addison-Wesley, 1982.

Guilleminault, C., and Dement, W.C. (Eds.), *Sleep apnea syndromes.* New York: Alan R. Liss, 1978.

Guilleminault, C., Winkle, R., Korobkin, R., and Simmons, B. Children and nocturnal snoring: evaluation of the effects of sleep related respiratory resistive load and daytime functioning. *European Journal of Pediatrics,* 1982, *139,* 165–171.

Josephson, S.C., and Rosen, R.C. Response-contingent awakening in the modification of chronic snoring. *Sleep,* 1983, *6,* 121–129.

Kryger, M.H., Roth, T., and Dement, W.C. (Eds.), *Principles and practice of sleep disorders medicine.* Philadelphia: W.B. Saunders, 1989.

Lydic, R., and Biebuyck, J.F. (Eds.), *Clinical physiology of sleep.* Bethesda, Maryland: American Physiological Society, 1988.

Nino-Murcia, G., Bliwise, D.L., Keenan, S., and Dement, W.C. The assessment of a new technology for evaluating respiratory abnormalities in sleep: a comparison of the polysomnogram and an ambulatory microprocessor. *International Journal of Technology Assessment in Health Care,* 1987, *3,* 427–445.

Nino-Murcia, G., McCann, C.C., Bliwise, D.L., Guilleminault, C., and Dement, W.C. Compliance and side effects in sleep apnea patients treated with nasal continuous positive airway pressure. *Western Journal of Medicine* 1989, *150,* 165–169.

Orem, J., and Barnes, C.D. (Eds.), *Physiology in sleep.* New York: Academic Press, 1980.

Phillipson, E.A. Control of breathing during sleep. *American Review of Respiratory Disease,* 1978, *118,* 909–939.

Saunders, N.A., and Sullivan, C.E. (Eds.), *Sleep and breathing.* New York: Marcel Dekker, 1984.

Sink, J., Bliwise, D.L., and Dement, W.C. Self-reported excessive daytime somnolence and impaired respiration in sleep. *Chest,* 1986, *90,* 177–180.

Yesavage, J., Bliwise, D.L., Guilleminault, C., Carskadon, M., and Dement, W.C. Preliminary communication: intellectual deficit and sleep related respiratory disturbance in the elderly. *Sleep,* 1985, *8,* 30–33.

6. Further Reading

Guilleminault, C. and Dement, W.C. (Eds.), *Sleep apnea syndromes.* New York: Alan R. Liss, 1978.

Kryger, M.H., Roth, T., and Dement, W.C. (Eds.), *Principles and practice of sleep disorders medicine.* Philadelphia: W.B. Saunders, 1989.

Mendelson, W.B., *Human sleep: Research and clinical care.* New York: Plenum, 1987.

Orem, J., and Barnes, C.D. (Eds.), *Physiology in sleep.* New York: Academic, 1980.

Saunders, N.A., and Sullivan, C.E. (Eds.), *Sleep and breathing.* New York: Marcel Dekker, 1984.

Thorpy, M.J. (Ed.), *Handbook of sleep disorders.* New York: Marcel Dekker, 1990.

Williams, R.L., Karacan, I., Moore, C.A. (Eds.), *Sleep disorders: Diagnosis and treatment.* New York: Wiley, 1988.

Control of Breathing and Its Disorders

SHEILA JENNETT

1. Components of Normal Automatic Control

1.1. Brain Stem Neurons and Their Interconnections

The groups of nerve cells responsible for breathing are located in the brain stem (see Chapter 1). Their complex interconnections and the neural inputs they receive are the basis for rhythmic breathing and for selection of an ideal ratio of tidal volume to frequency, as well as regulation of the ventilation to meet continuously changing needs.

1.1.1. Respiration-Related Neuronal Activity

Earlier knowledge of the site of control of breathing was obtained from observations of the effects of damage of the brain stem at different sites. More recently, individual "respiratory" nerve cells in the brain stem of anesthetized animals have been located by exploration and recording from microelectrodes. In this way, cells have been found that fire in inspiration, in expiration, or at some part of either or both. Some of those that fire in inspiration are responsible for the initiation of each breath; they are the ones whose frequency of discharge must be increased if the depth of breathing is to be altered, the major factor in altering the effective overall ventilation of the lungs. Other nerve cells are more directly concerned with determining the frequency of breaths; the timing of their discharge pattern determines when inspiratory activity is stopped and started.

There are many nerve cells that fire in relation to the phases of breathing but

SHEILA JENNETT • Institute of Physiology, The University, Glasgow, G12 8QQ, Scotland.
Behavioral and Psychological Approaches to Breathing Disorders, edited by Beverly H. Timmons and Ronald Ley. Plenum Press, New York, 1994.

have functions not directly affecting the breathing itself. Neurons that mediate the rhythmic widening and narrowing of the larynx in the breathing cycle are an example.

1.1.2. Generation of the Breathing Rhythm

Inspiratory neurons fire at an accelerating rate and are intermittently switched off by the action of other neurons. They are switched on again after an appropriate interval, depending on input information to the brain stem.

Theoretically, this rhythmic activity could go on in the brain stem in the absence of input information from the rest of the body or from higher up in the brain. The respiratory neurons may be independent pacemakers, keeping the rhythm going even where there is nothing driving them, in the same way that the heart is capable of beating on its own. But normally, other neural influences continually modify both the strength and frequency of inspiratory activity.

1.2. Motor Pathways from Brain to Respiratory Muscles

1.2.1. From Brain to Spinal Motoneurons

The fiber of each inspiratory nerve cell reaches as far as either the cervical or the thoracic region of the spinal cord (Fig. 1). Each ends on the opposite side of the cord and makes a relaying connection (synapse) with a spinal motoneuron.

1.2.2. From Spinal Cord to Respiratory Muscles

The fibers of the spinal motoneurons leave the cord and the vertebral column to travel either in the phrenic nerve down through the neck and the thorax to the diaphragm, or in an intercostal nerve to the external intercostal muscles between the ribs. The process of neuromuscular transmission translates the impulses arriving at the end of each nerve fiber into electrical activation of one or more muscle fibers (which can be recorded by electromyography—EMG). This in turn leads to the mechanical event of contraction. The greater the drive to breathe, the more frequent are the nerve impulses within the period of each inspiration; the more frequent the impulses, the stronger the muscle contraction. When the muscle contracts more vigorously, the whole inspiratory effort is greater, and air is drawn into the lungs at a greater flow rate. Conversely, if the drive to breathe is decreased, the process is reversed; less frequent impulses produce weaker muscle contraction. So even though the time allowed for breathing *in* may be unchanged, the depth of the breath can be increased or decreased (Fig. 2). The force generated by the muscles is normally directly related to their neural activation, but if muscle becomes fatigued it may not respond fully.

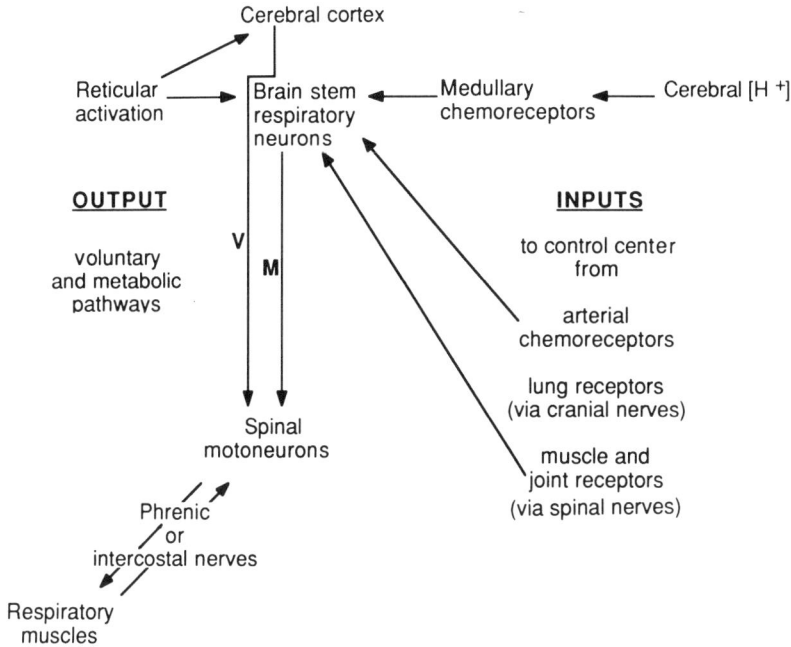

Figure 1. Outline of respiratory control. The influences upon the respiratory neurons are summarized on the right (inputs) and the efferent pathways on the left (output). The two-way arrows between respiratory muscles and spinal motoneurons signify the feedback from muscle receptors, which can influence the strength of contraction by a spinal reflex.

During normal resting breathing, the intermittent contraction of inspiratory muscles is all that is required since expiration occurs without effort each time the active expansion of the chest stops. When positive expiratory effort is needed, this is brought about by impulse traffic along different nerve fibers to expiratory muscles.

1.2.3. Spinal Integration

If it becomes more difficult to breathe—for instance, if the movement of the chest is restricted, the bronchial tubes are narrowed by an attack of asthma, or one is required to breathe through a narrow tube—the muscles have to work harder if they are to shift the same amount of air. Receptors in the muscles immediately detect this, and the signal along afferent fibers to the spinal cord leads to greater stimulation of the muscles (Fig. 1). Thus, although a normal awake person would perceive the increase in resistance, reflex readjustment occurs without reference to the conscious brain or even to the brain stem.

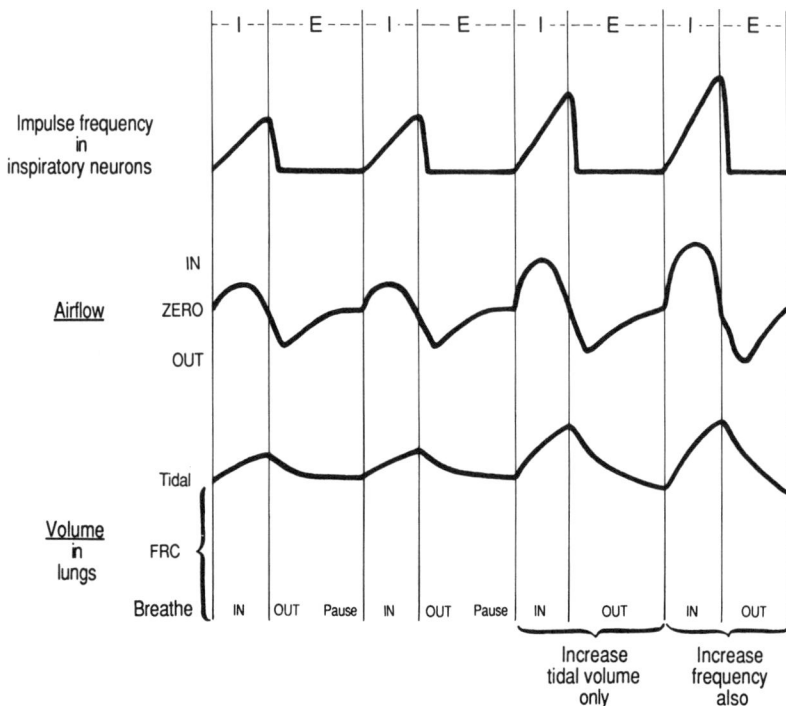

Figure 2. The pattern of breathing at rest (first two cycles) and the way in which ventilation can increase (third and fourth cycles). (Top) The output from medullary neurons, increasing throughout the inspiratory period. This "ramp" of activity is transmitted to spinal motoneurons and hence to inspiratory muscles. (Middle) The instantaneous rate of airflow during the respiratory cycle. Contraction of inspiratory muscles leads to inflow of air to the lungs; flow returns to zero at the end of inspiration; cessation of inspiratory activity leads to outflow, which slows to a pause (zero flow) before the next inspiration. (Bottom) Changes in lung volumes during the respiratory cycle. Note that moderate increases in tidal volume do not encroach on the functional residual capacity (FRC). An increase *only* in tidal volume (third breath) is achieved by a greater flow rate over an unchanged period. An increase in frequency of breathing (fourth breath) is achieved usually by cutting down the duration only of the expiratory phase: the pause disappears.

1.3. Inputs to the Brain Stem Complex

The neurons in the brain stem generate the rhythmic impulses that cause breathing, but the pattern and intensity of their output is continually modulated by a variety of information coming in.

This information comes from the lungs, the face and the upper respiratory passages, the thorax and its muscles, and from other muscles and joints, from the chemoreceptors that sense the state of the blood gases, from nearby in the brain stem where brain pH is sensed, and from many higher parts of the brain including the cerebral cortex (Fig. 1).

1.3.1. Influences from Higher Regions of the Brain

There is an involuntary cerebral stimulation of breathing when one is awake. This depends on reticular activation—the wakefulness influence originating from the brain stem. In sleep, ventilation decreases to a greater extent than does the metabolic rate, so that there is a relative degree of underventilation, with a rise of a few mm Hg in carbon dioxide tension (Pco_2).

In contrast, there appear to be "braking" influences from some parts of the brain on the brain stem centers—at least with respect to the frequency of breathing; this *increases* under many types of anesthesia and in some phases of sleep.

Breathing is, however, normally modulated quite independently of influences from the parts of the brain above the brain stem. (This is evident in the indefinitely prolonged survival in a "vegetative" state of patients whose higher brain function is effectively destroyed: the breathing continues and is regulated normally.)

1.3.2. Feedback Information

Several types of afferent input provide the control centers with a continual check on the effectiveness of their output. This is comparable to a heat-regulating thermostat. The sorts of information that the controller needs are:

1. Mechanical: How much inflation and deflation of the lungs has been achieved (and therefore how much air has been shifted)? This information comes from the stretch receptors in the lungs; the pattern of nerve impulses up the vagus nerve to the brain stem conveys a coded message about the lung volume at any instant, and about the rate and direction of change. And how much muscular effort has been involved? This information comes from the muscle spindles that sense the relation between the tension developed in the muscle and the actual shortening of its fibers. This in turn reflects the relation between the effort of breathing and the volume of air breathed; the nerve pathways in this case are spinal nerves.

2. Chemical: If the oxygen (O_2) and carbon dioxide (CO_2) tensions in the blood flowing through the lungs have been properly corrected, then the alveolar ventilation is appropriate. This information is obtained by the continual monitoring of arterial blood gas tensions by arterial chemoreceptors. If O_2 is lower, and CO_2 higher, than the normal level (because of even one small or prolonged breath), or if O_2 is high and CO_2 low (because of even one deep breath or sigh), there is immediate reflex adjustment in the next breath. If the requirement for

removal of CO_2 and intake of O_2 is suddenly and persistently increased (as it is when one runs or does any sort of muscular work), the ventilation is maintained at the correct increased level by this continual check on the arterial gas tensions; if they are not being kept normal, breathing increases.

1.3.3. Information from Somatic and Visceral Sensors

Information from contracting muscles and from moving joints signals that muscular activity is going on; this may contribute to the stimulation of breathing in work or exercise. But unlike the sensing of arterial blood gases, these inputs cannot determine the exact amount of ventilation to match the metabolic rate.

Virtually any sort of sensory stimulation can affect breathing: cold water immersion, water on the face, touch, and painful stimuli—including pain or discomfort from internal organs. While such stimulation tends to cause temporary interruptions to the normal pattern, they are corrected by the background regulatory system so that arterial blood gases are restored to normal.

1.3.4. Reflex Interruptions and Modifications of Breathing

The lungs have to be protected against entry of anything other than air. Reflexes originating around the mouth, nose, and throat ensure appropriate muscle action to close off the larynx when liquids or solids are swallowed or regurgitated; thus inspiration is inhibited, and inhalation of the material is avoided. When this defense does not quite succeed, and foreign material gains access to the respiratory tree, the cough reflex expels it—again inhibiting normal breathing and substituting explosive expiration.

2. Components of Normal Behavioral Control

2.1. Use of the Respiratory System for Purposes Other Than Breathing

We can talk only because we can interfere with the background rhythm of breathing. The complexities of speech are served not only by the coordination of muscles around the mouth and throat, but also by the close regulation of airflow rate, which entails a balance between inspiratory and expiratory muscle activity and resistance at the larynx.

Some thoracic and abdominal muscles that assist in breathing also take part in postural adjustments; there is an alteration in the breathing pattern when, for example, those muscles are in action lifting weights or pushing heavy objects. The breath may be held briefly so the diaphragm and chest wall can be fixed, allowing the muscles to work at the best mechanical advantage.

2.2. Deliberate Control of Breathing

2.2.1. The Direct Corticospinal Pathway

There is a motor pathway from cerebral cortex to spinal motoneurons that allows a direct voluntary influence on the respiratory muscles. Clearly, we can alter our breathing by voluntary action initiated in the cerebral cortex. Clinical and experimental evidence have both revealed that this influence is partly a direct one upon the spinal motoneurons—bypassing the brain stem control centers. The volitional prevention or alteration of breathing movements competes with, and can override, whatever signals are being received at the spinal level from the brain stem.

2.2.2. Breath Holding and Its Breakpoint

There is a limit to the voluntary *prevention* of breathing; the involuntary drives to spinal motoneuron activity build up and become overwhelming. These drives are both chemical and mechanical, arising from the asphyxial changes in blood gases and the absence of inflation of the lungs.

2.2.3. Deliberate Hyperventilation

There is a limit to a voluntary *increase* in breathing: deliberate hyperventilation is usually limited by the faintness it causes, due to cerebral vasoconstriction. Loss of consciousness can terminate the effort if it is excessive and persistent.

3. Goals of Normal Automatic Regulation and Effects of Failure

3.1. Maintaining Correct Volume of Ventilation for Gas Exchange Requirement (Metabolic Control)

3.1.1. Carbon Dioxide

When there are not other overriding drives affecting breathing, the neural control system acts to maintain a constant arterial P_{CO_2}. This must mean that the volume of CO_2 expired continually balances the volume produced by tissue metabolism. Measurements show that alveolar and arterial concentrations of CO_2 stay constant, which means that the volume of gas breathed out from the functional (alveolar) volume of the lungs must vary precisely with the rate of metabolic CO_2 production. In rest and activity, when the system is left to itself, it is so efficient that the matching occurs virtually breath-by-breath, even when metabolic activity is continually changing.

3.1.2. Oxygen

When alveolar PCO_2 is normal, there is automatically a normal alveolar concentration of O_2, if room air at sea level is being breathed. Therefore, there is full oxygenation of the blood. But if the inspired PO_2 is low because of high altitude, or if the arterial PO_2 is low because of impaired transfer in abnormal lungs, ventilation will be stimulated to increase by the *hypoxic drive* that can override the maintenance of normal PCO_2.

3.1.3. Homeostasis for the Brain

If for any reason ventilation is not adequate to maintain correct arterial blood gas levels, the arterial PCO_2 will rise and PO_2 will fall; these same changes will follow in the tissues, accompanied by a shift toward acidity. In any tissue, a change from the normal gas tension and pH environment can modify or impede cellular function. Neuronal function in the central nervous system (CNS) is particularly sensitive to such changes, but the brain is protected from them to an extent by the sensitive adjustment of its blood flow. If blood CO_2 rises and O_2 falls, brain blood flow increases; this increases the rate of removal of the brain's own metabolically produced CO_2 and the rate of supply of O_2. Thus the changes in brain tissue gas tensions are minimised.

3.2. Correction of Acid-Base State

A change in ventilation out of proportion to metabolic rate alters the CO_2 content of the body; just as diminished ventilation causes retention of CO_2 and acidity, so also excessive ventilation causes loss of CO_2 and alkalinity. These effects are physiologically utilized in the correction of any acid-base disturbance caused by ingestion or metabolism, in health or in disease. Acidity of the blood stimulates breathing causing greater excretion of CO_2, thus tending to correct the acidity; alkalinity of the blood depresses breathing causing retention of CO_2, thus tending to correct the alkalinity.

3.3. Pattern of Breathing for Minimal Work

Left to itself, the regulatory system appears to select very efficiently the best pattern of breathing for the least muscular effort (Fig. 3). When an increase is required in alveolar ventilation, an increase in tidal volume is much more effective than an increase in frequency; but very big tidal volumes are more demanding of muscular work. The conflict is resolved by CNS computation, resulting in correct alveolar ventilation with minimal work. Excessive work of breath-

Minimum work at resting
tidal volume and frequency

Work
of
breathing

Total work

Work against
elastic forces

Frictional work

Frequency increasing | Tidal volume increasing

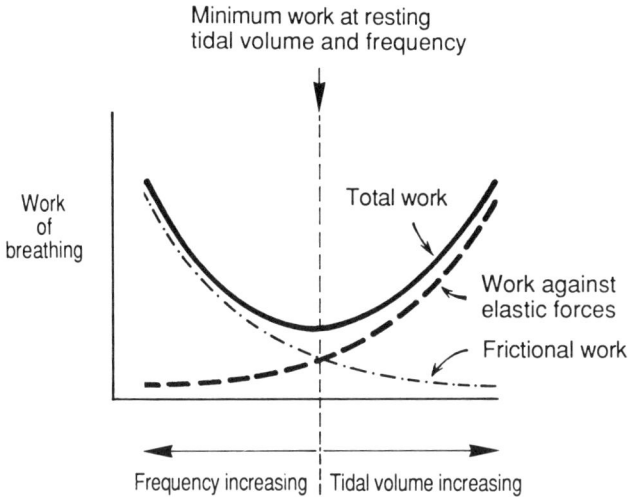

Figure 3. The work of breathing in relation to increase in tidal volume and to increase in frequency. At any given constant ventilation, decrease in tidal volume and increase in frequency (to left) increases frictional work and decreases elastic work; increase in tidal volume with decrease in frequency (to right) has the opposite effects.

ing may, however, occur due to abnormal lung mechanics or to the demands of very heavy exercise, causing the awareness of effort and discomfort known as dyspnea.

3.4. Correction following Reflex and Voluntary Interference

Left to itself, the normal regulatory system will restore the status quo promptly.

3.5. Summary

Normal regulatory mechanisms will maintain appropriate breathing with the least possible effort; ordinarily, the goal is normal arterial Pco_2 but the system will depart from this if other needs are overriding, namely, the correction of the acid-base state or of oxygenation. All this serves the crucial purpose of keeping the brain alive and well. If the brain is not fit to regulate breathing, it will itself suffer further from the disturbance of respiratory gas exchange; a vicious circle of the highest order can develop between lung dysfunction and brain dysfunction.

4. Disorders of Control

It is not possible to dissociate neural control from chemical control—an outdated classification that belonged to the era when it was thought that the respiratory neurons themselves were directly stimulated or depressed by the P_{CO_2} and P_{O_2} in arterial blood. The control by the central "computer" depends on all the neural inputs, including those stimulated or inhibited by information on the P_{CO_2} and P_{O_2} in the blood (arterial chemoreceptors), and the P_{CO_2} and acidity of the cerebral environment itself (medullary chemoreceptors), and possibly the chemical state within exercising muscles.

So, what can go wrong?

There may be

1. Failure to generate or to maintain a normal rhythmic pattern of breathing;
2. Failure to adjust the ventilation to balance metabolic requirements; or
3. Failure of voluntary intervention.

4.1. Disorders of the Pattern of Breathing

4.1.1. The Distinction between Normal and Abnormal Breathing

This is by no means always clear. First it is necessary to know the boundaries of normality in the pattern of breathing. Much of the older information on normal patterns of breathing requires updating now that accurate means of measurement are available without mouthpiece and noseclip (see Chapter 1). But it can be fairly stated that resting breathing shows some degree of fluctuation in both volume and timing, that it is normal to take a deep sighing breath once every minute or so, and that healthy people vary considerably in their own personal unconscious selection of the ratios of tidal volume to frequency and of thoracic to abdominal breathing. Also, the pattern may be, artificially, either irregular or excessively regular whenever there is awareness that breathing is being recorded or watched.

4.1.2. Abnormal Rhythmic Breathing

4.1.2a. Compensation for Mechanical Changes. Normal regulatory mechanisms cause adjustments that minimize muscular work or tend to prevent airway closure. For example, when, in bronchitis/emphysema, the resistance to airflow is increased, the breathing pattern alters. The details are not our concern here, but it is necessary to exclude mechanical disturbances of pulmonary function if any abnormality of regulation of breathing is suspected.

4.1.2b. Rapid Regular Breathing. This is a common feature of acute brain damage whether due to cerebrovascular accident (stroke) or to trauma. It is usually—but not necessarily—a true hyperventilation, with low P_{CO_2}. In some instances the pattern may be so rapid and shallow that a very high proportion of the volume turnover is dead space ventilation and thus does not lower the P_{CO_2}. This may occasionally be directly due to brain damage (central neurogenic ventilation) but more often relates to an abnormal drive to breathing, such as cerebral acidity.

4.1.3. Irregular Breathing Patterns

4.1.3a. Periodic Breathing. Perhaps the best-known breathing pattern abnormality is Cheyne–Stokes respiration, named after two physicians who drew attention to it in the nineteenth century (but Hippocrates had beaten them to it in the fourth century BC, when he described a patient whose breathing was "like that of a man recollecting himself, and rare, and large"). Typically, in this condition there is a smooth waxing and waning of breathing, mostly of tidal volume, with some seconds of apnea in each cycle. The occurrence of apnea qualifies the pattern to be called true Cheyne–Stokes breathing. There are lesser degrees of periodic breathing that do not feature complete apnea, and can occur in healthy people in certain circumstances: during transition from drowsiness to sleep, and between the stages of sleep, particularly in older people (see Chapter 3); during recovery from deliberate hyperventilation in some people, especially if they are drowsy; and in exposure to altitude hypoxia before acclimatization, especially during sleep.

These situations have in common a sudden change in drive to breathe and a gradual adjustment to a new P_{CO_2} (and hence a new pH). When falling asleep, the wakefulness drive to ventilation disappears, ventilation decreases, but this causes P_{CO_2} to rise and thus increase again the stimulus to breathe. Ventilation increases and brings P_{CO_2} back to normal—but in the absence of wakefulness the drive is insufficient and so the cycle continues until the control system settles at a new, higher P_{CO_2}. On exposure to hypoxia, the change is comparable, but in the opposite direction: there is an additional drive causing increased ventilation that decreases the P_{CO_2}. This in turn inhibits breathing and again the system oscillates until a regular pattern is established at a new, lower, P_{CO_2}. The periodicity is exaggerated in sleep, when the sensitivity to rising P_{CO_2} and decreasing P_{O_2} is diminished, so longer and larger swings are tolerated.

There are a variety of pathological situations in which periodic or true Cheyne–Stokes breathing occurs: in bilateral cerebral damage caused by stroke, or sometimes other sites of brain damage from vascular accident or trauma (especially if there is also hypoxia), and when blood circulation time is prolonged in cardiac failure. The periodicity is probably not often an abnormality of the respiratory control centers themselves, but rather a response to a particular pattern of alternate stimulation and inhibition. The effect of pathologically lengthened circulation time is explained in this way: as breathing wanes, the blood leaving the lungs has a progressively higher P_{CO_2} and lower P_{O_2}. But the blood takes a significant time to reach the sensors. The longer it takes, the more out of phase the stimulus will be with the effect on breathing. By the time an increasing stimulus is first sensed by the receptors, breathing may have stopped altogether. As blood continues to arrive at the sensors, it brings a stronger and stronger stimulus and breathing progressively increases. At the same time, because breathing has started again and is increasing, the state of the blood leaving the lungs is improving. When this blood reaches the sensors, the drive will diminish, and so on.

4.1.3b. Ataxic Breathing. Total disruption of the regular pattern occurs, rarely, when the brain stem itself is damaged in the region of the respiratory neurons or when the spinal metabolic motor pathway is damaged (see Section 4.2.1d). There is overall hypoventilation. To a lesser degree, healthy people show a disorganized pattern during REM sleep. These irregularities are associated with diminished responsiveness to P_{CO_2}.

4.2. Breathing Too Little or Too Much

4.2.1. Underventilation

4.2.1a. Adaptation to Excessive Work of Breathing. This is an adjustment, not an abnormality, of the control system. "Resetting" can occur, allowing arterial and alveolar P_{CO_2} to rise to higher levels. This means that CO_2 can be excreted from the body at a normal rate with less ventilation of the lungs: a smaller volume with a higher CO_2 concentration is expired per minute. The hypoventilation can be corrected only by relieving whatever is the mechanical problem in ventilating the lungs.

4.2.1b. Depression or Dysfunction of Brain Stem Neurons. The function of the respiratory neurons may be depressed or disordered:

1. By drugs. Many analgesic and hypnotic drugs are respiratory depressants, particularly the opiates and barbiturates. They decrease metabolic rate to some extent, so some of the decrease in ventilation is appropriate. Also, when given to anxious subjects or to those suffering from pain, they may partly restore breathing to normal from a state of hyperventilation. An apparent depression may be partly accounted for in these ways, but the drugs also truly depress the control mechanism and lead to a rise in P_{CO_2} and a fall in P_{O_2} in arterial blood.

2. By severe hypoxia and/or hypercapnia. As oxygen tension falls (hypoxia) the activity of respiratory neurons is depressed. Ventilation eventually decreases, despite stimulation of arterial chemoreceptors. If there is also a rising P_{CO_2} (hypercapnia) as in acute respiratory failure, this also becomes depressant at high levels. The same effect can result from deprivation of CNS blood supply (ischaemia) causing local accumulation of CO_2 and deprivation of oxygen.

3. By head trauma. Following severe head trauma, direct damage to the brain stem itself, or deprivation of blood supply resulting from the complication of raised intracranial pressure, can depress or stop breathing. Traumatic, vascular, or neoplastic damage to the medulla oblongata may cause grossly irregular breathing that is also depressed.

4.2.1c. Damage at the Spinal Level. If spinal motoneurons serving the respiratory muscles are damaged, or separated from the brain stem by severance of the connections, there is paralysis of respiratory muscles. Poliomyelitis was once not an uncommon cause of such damage. Traumatic transection of the spinal cord stops breathing entirely if the lesion is above the mid-cervical level. Low cervical and thoracic lesions leave diaphragmatic breathing intact while destroying all or some intercostal muscle activity.

4.2.1d. Loss of Metabolic Control: Ondine's Curse Syndrome. Severe depression of breathing may occur only during sleep. During wakefulness there is a drive to breathe regularly that is additional to the other controls. For example, most normal wide awake people recover gradually, without apnea, from deliberate hyperventilation, showing that their breathing is not ruled only by their blood gases. Breathing is ordinarily adjusted continually to maintain those gases at normal levels, but if the necessary sensors, nerve cells and motor nerve pathways for this automatic regulation are not all intact, there cannot be proper adjustment to metabolic demands. In such circumstances voluntary breathing can still occur because there is a separate motor pathway from cerebral cortex to spinal neurons (see Section 2.2.1); serious trouble arises when the conscious mind goes off duty during sleep, and sleep apnea ensues (Chapter 3). (This is referred to as *Ondine's Curse Syndrome.*) Still more severe, there can be apnea and hypopnea during the day whenever attention wanders.

Damage to both anterolateral columns of the spinal cord can produce the Ondine's curse syndrome because the motor pathways that serve automatic control are damaged but those serving voluntary control are preserved. The observation of sleep apnea in patients who had bilateral cordotomy, for the relief of pain, helped to establish the separateness of the two pathways.

4.2.1e. Peripheral Nerves and Respiratory Muscles. Disturbance of transmission along the motor nerves or across neuromuscular junctions, or muscular weakness itself, can cause respiratory paresis. Breathing suffers, along with all muscular activity, in the motoneuron diseases and those that primarily cause wasting of muscles.

4.2.2. Overventilation (See Chapter 10)

This may arise from central influences or because of excessive inputs from the various sensors, or it may be essentially behavioral, with no organic cause. Overventilation exists when the alveolar and arterial P_{CO_2} are lower than normal (hypocapnia). In this instance a normal CO_2 output per minute is maintained by breathing out a high volume with a low percentage of CO_2.

4.3. Inability to Exert Voluntary Control over Breathing

Following cerebrovascular accidents, some patients are unable to follow instructions to breathe deeply, to hold their breath, or to perform a vital capacity maneuver. This in a sense is the opposite situation from the Ondine's curse syndrome; the metabolic, automatic control of breathing continues, but the patients cannot voluntarily influence breathing any more than they could move a hemiplegic limb.

5. Summary

Normal automatic control of breathing achieves precise matching of the ventilation of the lungs to the needs of body metabolism, so the levels of O_2 and CO_2 in arterial blood hardly vary at all, whatever the rate of tissue usage. The pattern of breathing is organized for maximal efficiency with respect to the mechanical work it requires.

No part of the nervous system higher than the brain stem is required for this regulation. There is continual adjustment of the depth and frequency of breathing; this is in response to information carried back to the brain stem neurons from sensors that monitor the state of inflation of the lungs, the gas concentrations and pH in the arterial blood, and the pH in the brain. Reflex and voluntary influences and interruptions are superimposed on this background of automatic control, which rapidly restores the status quo when they are over.

Neurological breathing disorders comprise alterations and irregularities of breathing pattern, deviations from proper regulation of ventilation of the lungs to match metabolism, and partial or total paralysis of respiratory movements. Because the nerve pathways for automatic and voluntary control of breathing movements are separate, it is possible for either to be lost when the other is intact. The ideal state of affairs is to be virtually unaware of one's breathing; no voluntary intervention can improve upon its remarkable efficiency in a healthy person.

5

Breathing and the Psychology of Emotion, Cognition, and Behavior

RONALD LEY

Breathing is the only vital function that is under direct voluntary control as well as reflexive control. As such, it is a behavior that is subject to the psychological principles of both instrumental (*operant*) and Pavlovian (*respondent*) conditioning. While traditional approaches to the psychological study of emotion, cognition, and behavior have occasionally focused on changes in breathing as a consequence of some experimental manipulation, far less attention has been paid to the extent to which emotions, thoughts, and behaviors can be influenced by changes in breathing. The purpose of the this chapter is to bring attention to breathing as a behavioral act and to discuss its interactive effects with emotion, cognition, and behavior.

1. Conditioning, Behavior, Emotions, and Breathing

1.1. Conditioned Emotional Responses

The association between Pavlovian conditioning and the *drooling* dog is well established, but the association between Pavlovian conditioning and the *panting* dog is not. At about the same time that Pavlov published his first findings on "psychical secretions" (1897), C. S. Sherrington reported his discovery of conditioned "emotional anxiety" (1900). Although Sherrington's interest

RONALD LEY • Department of Psychology and Statistics, State University of New York, Albany, New York 12222.
Behavioral and Psychological Approaches to Breathing Disorders, edited by Beverly H. Timmons and Ronald Ley. Plenum Press, New York, 1994.

centered on vasomotor reflexes of the circulatory system, not digestive juices, he made the serendipitous observation that circulatory system responses (changes in heart rate and blood pressure) occurred during the warming up period following the onset of a noisy electric shock generator, but prior to delivery of the shock. Because the changes were those that might be expected if shock were anticipated, Sherrington called the response to the noise of the shock generator "emotional anxiety." Although Sherrington is not well remembered for this work, electric shock is now the most common unconditioned stimulus (UCS) used in the study of Pavlovian conditioning. The conditioning of fear is far more relevant to the study of human behavior than is the conditioning of salivation.

Perhaps it should be noted here that the term anxiety is often used to distinguish signaled fear (CR) from unsignaled fear (UCR). While the terms fear and anxiety are often used synonymously, the distinction between them is fundamental to an understanding of the importance of Pavlovian conditioning in human adaptation. Salter (1961) made a concise statement that incorporates Cannon's (1915) concept of a fight-flight response into a Pavlovian conditioning paradigm

> anxiety is thus basically anticipatory in nature and has great biological utility in that it adaptively motivates living organisms to deal with (prepare for or flee from) traumatic events in advance of their actual occurrence, thereby diminishing their harmful effects. (Salter, 1961, p. 221)

This statement illustrates how a liberalized interpretation of Pavlovian conditioning (e.g., Rescorla, 1988) unites the psychological concepts of emotion (anxiety), cognition (the *anticipation* of a threatening event), and behavior (preparation for encounter with, or flight from, the threatened event). The psychotherapeutic implications of a liberalized interpretation are discussed by Davey (1989).

2. The Effects of Breathing on Emotions and Behavior

Experimental studies of conditioned emotions and breathing (Anderson and Parmenter, 1941; Caldwell, 1946, 1986; Gantt, 1944; Goldman, 1939; Masserman, 1943; Minami *et al.*, 1943) make it clear that emotional arousal gives rise to conditionable changes in ventilation. The issue to be considered here centers on the effects of *voluntary* changes in ventilation on emotional arousal. It appears that the connection between emotions and breathing is a reciprocative relationship in which changes in one lead to corresponding changes in the other. For example, if you are angered, but wish to keep your feelings in tow, voluntary restriction of ventilation will help (i.e., keep your mouth shut and breathe slowly through the nose or pursed lips). If, on the other hand, you wish to increase your excitement and express vividly your emotions, breathe hard and fast, and shout at the top of your lungs. Brief periods of hyperventilation increase arousal, at least in the short run (long-term hyperventilation has the opposite effect). The adaptive advantage of the short-term hyperventilation that accompanies emotional arousal has been pointed to by Lum (1981)

> Thus moderate degrees of hyperventilation—classically in the "fight or flight" situation—cause increased motor excitability and also increased sensitivity to sensory stimuli: lights appear brighter, sounds louder; photophobia and hyperacusis are not uncommon. The survival value of this complex response is obvious: heightened sensory perception, the muscular system tense and alert, the reflexes quickened. (Lum, 1981, p. 3)

The oldest systematic nonscientific study of the effects of breathing on behavior or experience can be found in the yogic methods of meditation used in ancient Eastern religious practices. (For a concise review, see Chapter 15). Effective breathing exercises, free of mystical trappings, can be understood in terms of the basic principles underlying breathing retraining programs used by respiratory physical therapists in the treatment of chronic lung diseases (asthma, bronchitis, and emphysema), stress-related disorders, and panic disorder (Chapters 11 and 13). While relatively subjective assessments of such programs have, in the main, been favorable, a few studies have demonstrated *objective* indices of positive physical and psychological changes (e.g., Bonn et al., 1984).

Among those studies that have focused on the direct effect of controlled breathing on physiological and psychological measures of *experimentally induced emotional arousal* was one by McCaul et al. (1979); they found that voluntary retardation of breathing reduced physiological arousal (decreased electrodermal response and increased finger-pulse volume) and psychological arousal (reduced scores on self-reports of anxiety). In a related study (Cappo and Holmes, 1984), breathing was controlled by means of voluntary prolongation of the expiratory phase of the respiratory cycle relative to the inspiratory phase (i.e., brief inhalation and prolonged exhalation); this type of controlled breathing caused a reduction in physiological and psychological arousal induced by the threat of electric shock.

In a direct test of the connection between hyperventilation and emotional arousal, Thyer et al. (1984) measured Pco_2, finger temperature, and anxiety prior to a brief period of voluntary hyperventilation. Posttest measures revealed a significant drop in Pco_2, a significant drop in finger temperature, and a significant increase in anxiety—findings that demonstrate clearly the emotional arousal elicited by hyperventilation.

3. Breathing and Cognition

3.1. The Effects of Thoughts on Breathing

3.1.1. Polygraphy and Lie Detection

Attempts to study the effects of thoughts on breathing are illustrated in polygraphic lie detector tests (Ekman, 1985; Lykken, 1984) in which ventilation is routinely monitored (Podlesny and Raskin, 1980). Increases in the frequency and depth of breathing and/or changes in the mode of breathing (i.e., diaphragmatic to thoracic), along with changes in other physiological variables (e.g., electrodermal response, blood pressure), in response to salient information are interpreted as evidence that the subject may have knowledge related to the information and may be trying to conceal it. While lie detector tests may be far from reliable (Gale, 1988; Ginton et al., 1982), they do indicate a degree of sensitivity of breathing to emotional thoughts or emotion-eliciting thoughts.

3.1.2. The Think Test

Polygraphic monitoring of breathing for the purpose of detecting lies or concealment of knowledge has found broad application in criminal investigations, but the effects of emotional thoughts on breathing has only recently received attention in medical and psychological diagnoses, namely, the diagnoses of emotionally based cardiac complaints and related psychosomatic disorders (Freeman et al., 1986; Nixon and Freeman, 1987a,b; Nixon et al., 1987). The Think Test, a measure of the effect of emotionally charged thoughts on breathing, is based on Hardonk and Beumer's (1979) observation of symptom-related variability in the recovery of basal PCO_2 following voluntary hyperventilation. Following the establishment of baseline PCO_2, patients are instructed to hyperventilate for approximately three minutes. During the first three or four minutes of recovery following the forced voluntary hyperventilation, patients are required to close their eyes and *think* about the details of the emotional episode in which their cardiac symptoms were first experienced. If PCO_2 drops 10 mm Hg or more during this Think Test period, hyperventilation is indicated.

Although the Think Test was developed as a diagnostic tool for patients presenting with ischemic heart disease, hypertension, cardiac arrhythmia, chest pain, or blackouts, it holds the promise of a useful procedure for determining the significance of antecedent life experiences in panic disorder, hyperventilatory complaints, and general anxiety.

3.2. The Effects of the Expectation of Noxious Events on Breathing

Cognitive psychology is sometimes defined as the flow of information through the mind of the information processor (e.g., Broadbent, 1963; Neisser, 1967). While such a definition is rich with connotations, the *sine qua non* of cognitive theories that submit best to experimental research is the concept of expectancy. As Tolman (1959) put it:

> I would also assert that "thinking," as we know it in human beings, is in essence no more than an activated interplay among expectancies resulting from such previously acquired readinesses which result in new expectancies and resultant new means-end readinesses. (Tolman, 1959, pp. 113–114)

Throughout his career, Tolman emphasized the inherent significance of the construct of expectancy in the psychological lives of humans.

3.2.1. Expectancy and Panic Attacks

Initial panic attacks are the consequence of the interaction between hyperventilation and dyspneic-fear (Ley, 1985b, 1989). Given a constant metabolic production of CO_2, a sudden increase in ventilation will result in a sudden decrease in P_{CO_2} and corresponding increase in pH (acute respiratory alkalosis). If hypocapnea persists and the intensity of dyspnea is perceived to be out of control and life-threatening, dyspneic-fear and hypocapneic sensations—such as, tachycardia and dizziness—will be experienced, and a hyperventilatory panic attack will have occurred.

The quest for causal agents of panic attacks has led to a rash of studies, most of which report some success in provoking attacks in patients with histories of panic disorder. Purported "panicogenic" agents include lactate infusions (Ley, 1988a; Margraf *et al.*, 1986; Shear, 1986), bicarbonate (Grosz and Farmer, 1972), yohimbine (Charney *et al.*, 1984), caffeine (Charney *et al.*, 1985), and 5 percent CO_2 in air (Gorman *et al.*, 1984). A careful study of this research leads to one irrefutable conclusion: If panic patients *expect* that an agent can induce a panic attack, odds are that it will. What accounts for this effect?

3.2.2. Expectancy Is Not Enough

Although the search for chemical agents in the production of panic attacks has provided evidence for a psychological agent, expectancy is not a sufficient explanation. The observation of the effect cannot be an explanation for the effect. What is the explanation for the positive correlation between expectancy of a panic attack and the occurrence of an attack? A clue was given in a study that provided clear evidence of the expectancy effect, independent of any chemical agents, a study in which a panic disorder patient experienced a panic attack following *false* feedback indicating that the subject's heart rate suddenly increased (Margraf *et al.*, 1987).

The clue lies in the emotional effect that information of a sudden increase in heart rate might have on a person who suffers panic attacks. If this information elicits fear, then ventilation should increase. Furthermore, if the subject's bodily movements are restricted by the requirements of physiological monitoring, and increases in metabolic CO_2 are therefore limited, then any increase in ventilation would be hyperventilatory (Ley, 1988b). If this situation obtains, then the expectancy effect in the production of panic attacks could be explained by a hyperventilation theory (Ley, 1985a,b, 1987, 1989).

3.2.3. The Anatomy of a Hyperventilatory Panic Attack

Evidence that supports a hyperventilation explanation for the effect of expectancy in the production of panic attacks can be found in an unwitting portrait of a hyperventilatory panic attack reported by Sanderson *et al.* (1988), based on data from a subject in Sanderson's dissertation (1987). In this study, a panic disorder patient was required to breathe compressed air for five minutes prior to a scheduled 20 minute period during which she was led to believe she was breathing a gas that might produce a panic attack. After six minutes of inhalation of compressed air (the gas the patient believed could produce a panic attack), a panic attack was reported by the patient: (1) respiration rate increased, (2) end-tidal Pco_2 dropped sharply from 26 to 17 mm Hg, (3) electrodermal conductivity increased sharply, (4) heart rate increased from 86 to 105 b/min, and (5) self-rated anxiety increased sharply. The report of panic plus the accompanying physiological changes provide a classic portrait of a hyperventilatory panic attack (Ley, 1992).

3.3. The Effects of Breathing on Thoughts: Hyperventilation and Cognition

While prolonged hypoventilation (i.e., hypercapnia) affects consciousness and cognitive processes, the effects of hyperventilation (i.e., hypocapnea) are of greater psychological interest because they can be induced through voluntary overbreathing or reflexive overbreathing induced by emotional arousal and sympathetic nervous system excitation. The effects of voluntary hypoventilation (hypercapnea), on the other hand, can be induced only for brief periods, because the build up of excessive arterial CO_2 will stimulate the respiratory centers (Comroe, 1974) and drive breathing beyond the limits of voluntary efforts to inhibit breathing. The effects of hypercapnea on cognition and behavior are most often studied by requiring subjects to breathe air supplemented with varying amounts of CO_2 (Henning *et al.*, 1990; Ley, 1991b).

3.3.1. Hyperventilation Theory of Panic Attacks

A hyperventilation theory of panic attacks (Ley, 1985b, 1988a,b) begins with the assumption that prolonged stress-induced hyperventilation produces the hypocapneic effects of dyspnea, tachycardia, and the other symptoms of the DSM-III-R (American Psychiatric Association, 1980) list of complaints associated with initial primary panic attacks. Secondary panic attacks are subsequent attacks acquired as conditioned responses in which the hyperventilatory hypocapnea provides the UCS (Ley, 1987; Wolpe and Rowan, 1988). The fear experienced during a primary hyperventilatory panic attack is the consequence of extreme dyspnea (a harbinger of suffocation) experienced in a perceptual context in which sufferers believe they have no control over the dyspnea, i.e., dyspneic-fear (Ley, 1989). The strange thoughts and behaviors that often accompany panic attacks are attributed to the cerebral hypoxia produced by hyperventilation.

3.4. Hyperventilation and Cognitive Deficit

While some of the bizarre behaviors that occur during panic attacks can be acquired through negative reinforcement of dyspneic-fear reduction, others may be caused by the cerebral hypoxia that results from hyperventilation. A wide range of hypoxic cognitive deficits has been documented (see Wyke, 1963). Hyperventilation has been demonstrated to have deleterious effects on performance of pilots flying under conditions of emotional tension (Balke and Lillehei, 1956; Hall, 1952; Hinshaw et al., 1943; Rushmer and Bond, 1944). Other studies have shown that hyperventilation produces decrements in cognitive/perceptual motor tasks, word association tests (Gellhorn and Kraines, 1937), tests of intellectual function (Gellhorn and Joslyn, 1937), motor coordination tests (Hinshaw et al., 1943), balancing and pegboard tests (Rushmer et al., 1941), and tests of manual dexterity, choice reaction time, and multiplication time (Rahn et al., 1946).

3.4.1. Catastrophic Cognitions

The broad effects of hyperventilation on mental function make it clear that the cerebral hypoxia induced by hyperventilation may be a causal factor in the production of the catastrophic cognitions so frequently associated with panic attacks. It is important to note, in this connection, that some cognitive explanations of panic disorder (Beck, 1987) confuse the sequence of events in panic attacks and attribute the experience of fear to a catastrophic misinterpretation of innocuous bodily sensations. Such an interpretation runs contrary to the findings of Wolpe and Rowan (1988), who reported that fear antedates catastrophic cognitions, to the findings of Rachman et al. (1988), who reported that catastrophic cognitions do not occur in 27 percent of panic attacks, and to the fact that panic attacks occur during nondreaming periods of sleep (Ley, 1988c).

3.4.2. Hallucinations

Cognitive deficits induced by hyperventilation are not limited to decrements in mental abilities and perceptual motor skills. Allen and Agus (1968) demonstrated that hallucinations could be induced through voluntary hyperventilation. More recently, Belcher (1988) described an institutionalized psychiatric patient whose relaxation-induced hallucinations could be terminated by forced exercise (walking). The efficacy of exercise in the termination of hallucinations can be derived from the assumption of the hyperventilation theory that, in chronic hyperventilation, panic attacks are more probable under conditions of low metabolic production of CO_2, i.e., during relaxation (Ley, 1988a). If hyperventilation can induce hallucinations, then reducing hypocapnea (as in increasing metabolism through exercise) should terminate them.

Although the punishing aspects of exercise (an activity which the patient did not like) might inhibit behavior or oral expression of thoughts, hallucinations are involuntary cognitive events produced by biochemical processes in the brain, not behaviors shaped by contingencies of positive and negative reinforcers. Since Allen and Agus (1968) have provided an empirical demonstration of the induction of hallucinations and since it is clear that cerebral hypoxia induced by hyperventilation leads to gross cognitive deficits, a hyperventilatory interpretation of Belcher's treatment is tenable.

3.5. Test Anxiety and Hyperventilation

Test anxiety, or evaluation anxiety, is the most pervasive emotional complaint among school age children (Barrios et al., 1981; Miller, 1983). Eysenck and Rachman (1965) estimated that 20 percent of grade school and high school pupils suffer performance debilitation as a consequence of anxiety during testing; an even larger percentage of college students (25 percent) is affected by test anxiety (Suinn, 1969). If anxiety experienced during tests increases ventilation, then part of the decrement in performance observed among test-anxious students may result from the cognitive deficit associated with the cerebral hypoxia induced by hyperventilation.

Ley and Yelich (1991) have recently begun a program of research designed to investigate the relationship between hyperventilation and the effects of test anxiety. In the first study, seventh-, eighth-, and ninth-grade students identified as either high- or low-test-anxious, were given instructions designed to elicit anxiety immediately prior to a computation test and a word-recall test. The observed decrease in end-tidal CO_2 from baseline was greater for the high-anxious students than for the low-anxious, findings consistent with the hyperventilation interpretation of the effects of test anxiety. Additional evidence was found in the surprisingly strong positive correlation ($r = 0.83$) between the test anxiety scale and the Nijmegen Hyperventilation Questionnaire (Ley and Yelich, 1991).

4. Hyperventilation, Cognition, and Conditioned Emotions

The links that connect breathing with cognition and emotion have important implications for theory and practice. If hyperventilation accompanies strong emotions (i.e., fear, frustration, anger, and sadness), then some of the irrational and bizarre behaviors and cognitions associated with these emotions (e.g., hysteria) may, in part, be a consequence of an underlying cerebral hypoxia produced by hyperventilation (Lum, 1975, 1976; Wyke, 1963).

Since strong emotions give rise to heightened arousal, it seems reasonable to suppose that the thoughts and behavioral manifestations of the heightened arousal are also produced, to some extent, by the cognitive deficit of hyperventilation-induced cerebral hypoxia. This proposition has important implications for theory, research, and treatment. The efficacy of cognitive therapies would be attenuated when salient issues of therapy focused on strong emotions. If hyperventilation accompanies such emotions, then the resultant cognitive deficit might interfere with the patient's ability to process the information. The "in one ear and out the other" phenomenon is a common complaint among psychotherapists and clinicians in general. Perhaps a graduated approach such as Wolpe's (1982) systematic desensitization is effective in part because this approach requires relaxation-induced low arousal before fear-eliciting conditioned stimuli (CSs) are introduced. One of the heretofore unrecognized benefits of relaxation and hypnotherapy in psychotherapy may be the increased likelihood that the patient understands and remembers what it is the therapist says. Perhaps evaluations of therapeutic techniques should include a measure of the patient's memory and understanding of what is going on in the therapeutic session.

4.1. Frustration, Stress, and Hyperventilation

Frustration is often defined as the emotion that follows the nonoccurrence of an event for which expectations were high. Since the conduct of everyday living depends on myriad routines for which there are predictable outcomes with varying degrees of probability, frustration is an inevitable part of life. The intensity of frustration depends on the frequency of the occurrence of frustrating events and on the importance of expectations; vending machines that fail to deliver aren't as serious as cars that fail to start.

Although the increase in vigor of behavior that accompanies the negative emotion of frustration has been well documented in human behavior (Blixt and Ley, 1969; Ditkoff and Ley, 1974) as well as in animal behavior (Amsel, 1969; Brown and Farber, 1951; Daly, 1971; Marzocco, 1951), no physiological evidence of frustration had been demonstrated until Otis (1973) reported a positive correlation ($r = .74$) between the magnitude of the frustration response (force on a reset lever) and the amplitude of the electrodermal response (increase in conductivity of skin). The significance of this finding lies in the connection between the electrodermal response and hyperventilation (Kartsounis and Turpin, 1987). Sudden increases in electrodermal conductivity have been observed on the occasion of adventitious panic attacks in the laboratory during physiological assessment by Lader and Mathews (1970) and in a clear-cut demonstration of a hyperventilatory panic attack by Sanderson et al. (1988).

Direct evidence of the effects of frustration on breathing has been recently reported by Schleifer and Ley (1992). In a study of stress among full-time data entry video display terminal operators, Schleifer and Ley monitored respiration rate, Pco_2, and heart rate. During two 120-minute daily work periods over three consecutive days, consistent changes in breathing and heart rate were recorded. After a five-minute baseline period, in which subjects sat quietly with eyes closed, followed by a five-minute period of progressive muscle relaxation instructions, a 120-minute period of numerical data-entry work was examined. During relaxation period, respiration rate dropped and Pco_2 increased. During the work period following the relaxation period, respiration and heart rates increased while Pco_2 decreased, findings that indicate hyperventilation and increased arousal. This research has special relevance for applied psychology because it demonstrates the sensitivity of breathing to the positive effects of relaxation as well as to the negative effects of stress, in the context of the video display terminal work environment.

5. Concluding Remarks

The psychology of breathing is a study of the interactions of breathing with emotion, cognition, and behavior. Pertinent research within the domain of the psychology of breathing illustrates the centrality of Pavlovian conditioning as a unifying paradigm that can account for the distinction between the classic hyperventilation panic attack and the conditioned anticipatory panic attack (Ley, 1987, 1992; Wolpe and Rowan, 1988).

While it is commonly understood that changes in breathing follow changes in emotion, cognition, and behavior, current research points clearly to the less commonly understood fact that changes in breathing lead to changes in emotion, cognition, and behavior. The implications of this reciprocative relationship are important for the purposes of diagnosis and treatment in clinical practice. If breathing affects emotions, cognitions, and behavior, then diagnosis of psychological complaints should include attention to signs of dysfunctional breathing, especially breathing under stress. The Think Test is a promising diagnostic tool. Furthermore, if changes in emotion, cognition, and/or behavior induced by changes in breathing ameliorate complaints, then new treatments can be developed that focus on breathing-induced changes to counteract the complaints. Breathing retraining programs are an obvious example; counterconditioning techniques aimed at eliminating hyperventilatory conditioned responses are less so.

5.1. Clinicians, Research, and the Progress of Science

Research is often frustratingly slow and unrewarding. To undertake an experiment to test a hypothesis or ask a question does not mean that an answer is forthcoming. And often, when the findings of research are published, the research is flawed or the data are misinterpreted. When this happens, it leads to a lot of confusion and complications that take a long time to sort out (Ley, 1991a). Clinicians, and other consumers of research literature, need to be reminded that published research is not equivalent to the *truth*. In science, the possibility of error always exists. Furthermore, in a sense, every clinician is a scientist in so far as the administration of a treatment to a patient is an experimental trial. Much would be gained if clinicians kept extensive records on treatment outcomes and published their findings from time to time.

The psychology of breathing holds the promise of becoming an important area of study within the new biological discipline of respiratory psychophysiology. Breathing may well be the bridge between psychology and physiology.

6. References

Allen, T., and Agus, B. Hyperventilation leading to hallucinations. *American Journal of Psychiatry*, 1968, *125*, 84–89.

Diagnostic and statistical manual of mental disorders. 3rd ed. Washington, DC: American Psychiatric Association, 1980.

Amsel, A. The role of frustrative nonreward in noncontinuous reward situations. *Psychological Bulletin*, 1958, *55*, 102–119.

Anderson, O.D., and Parmenter, R.R. A long term study of the experimental neurosis in the sheep and dog. *Psychosomatic Medicine Monographs*, 1941, *2*, whole nos. 3 and 4.

Balke, B., and Lillehei, J. Effects of hyperventilation on performance. *Journal of Applied Physiology*, 1956, *9*, 371–374.

Barrios, B.A., Hartmann, D.B., and Shigetoni, C. Fears and anxieties in children. In E.J. Mash and L.G. Terdal (Eds.), *Behavioral assessment of childhood disorders*. New York: Guilford, 1981, pp. 259–304.

Beck, A. Cognitive approaches to panic disorder. In S. Rachman and J. Maser (Eds.), *Panic: Psychological perspectives*. Hillsdale, New Jersey: Erlbaum, 1987.

Belcher, T.L. Behavioral reduction of overt hallucinatory behavior in a chronic schizophrenic. *Journal of Behavior Therapy and Experimental Psychiatry*, 1988, *19*, 69–71.

Blixt, S., and Ley, R. Force-contingent reinforcement in instrumental conditioning and extinction in children: A test of the frustration-drive hypothesis. *Journal of Comparative and Physiological Psychology*, 1969, *69*, 267–272.

Bonn, J.A., Readhead, C.P.A. and Timmons, B.H. Enhanced adaptive behavioral response in agoraphobic patients pretreated with breathing retraining. *The Lancet*, 1984, 665–669.

Broadbent, D.E. Flow of information within the organism. *Journal of Verbal Learning and Verbal Behavior*, 1963, *2*, 34–39.

Brown, J.S., and Farber, I.E. Emotions conceptualized as intervening variable—with suggestions toward a theory of frustration. *Psychological Bulletin*, 1951, *48*, 465–495.

Caldwell, W.E. *Consequences of long continued and unvarying motor conditioning in the sheep.* Unpublished doctoral dissertation, Cornell University, 1946.

Caldwell, W.E. Conditioned hyperventilation as a factor in animal, infant, and adult apnea: A theoretical analysis of experimental and clinical data. *Genetic, Social and General Psychology Monographs*, 1986, *112*, 327–341.

Cannon, W.B. *Bodily changes in pain, hunger, fear and rage: An account of recent researches into the function of emotional excitement.* New York: Appleton-Century-Crofts, 1915.

Cappo, B.M., and Holmes, D.S. The utility of prolonged respiratory exhalation for reducing physiological and psychological arousal in non-threatening and threatening situations. *Journal of Psychosomatic Research*, 1984, *28*, 265–273.

Charney, D.S., Heninger, G.R., and Breier, A. Noradrenergic function in panic anxiety: Effects of yohimbine in healthy subjects and patients with agoraphobia and panic disorder. *Archives of General Psychiatry*, 1984, *41*, 751–763.

Charney, D.S., Heninger, G.R., and Jatlow, P.I. Increased anxiogenic effects of caffeine in panic disorders. *Archives of General Psychiatry*, 1985, *42*, 233–243.

Comroe, J.H., *Physiology of Respiration* (2nd edition), 1974, Yearbook Medical Publishers, Chicago, IL.

Daly, H.B. Evidence for frustration during discrimination learning. *Journal of Experimental Psychology*, 1971, *88*, 205–215.

Davey, G.C.L. UCS reevaluation and conditioning models of acquired fears. *Behaviour Research and Therapy*, 1989, *27*, 521–528.

Ditkoff, G., and Ley, R. Effects of positive and negative force-contingent reinforcement on the frustration effect in humans. *Journal of Experimental Psychology*, 1974, *102*, 818–823.

Ekman, P. *Telling lies: Clues to deceit in the marketplace, politics, and marriage.* New York: W.W. Norton, 1985.

Eysenck, H.J., and Rachman, S. *The causes and cures of neurosis.* San Diego, CA: Knapp, 1965.

Freeman, L.J., Conway, A., and Nixon, P.G.F. Physiological responses to psychological challenge under hypnosis in patients considered to have the hyperventilation syndrome: Implications for diagnosis and therapy. *Journal of the Royal Society of Medicine*, 1986, *79*, 76–83.

Gale, A. The polygraph test: Lies, truth and science. London: Sage Publications, 1988.

Gantt, W.H. Experimental basis for neurotic behavior. *Psychosomatic Monographs*, 1944, *3*, whole no. 7.

Gellhorn, E., and Joslyn, A. The influence of oxygen want, hyperpnea and carbon dioxide excess on psychic processes. *Journal of Psychology*, 1937, *3*, 161.

Gellhorn, E., and Kraines, S.H. Word associations as affected by deficient oxygen, excess carbon dioxide, and hyperpnea. *Archives of Neurological Psychiatry*, 1937, *38*, 491 (one page).

Ginton, A., Daie, N., Elaad, E., and Ben-Shakhar, G. A method for evaluating the use of the polygraph in a real-life situation. *Journal of Applied Psychology, 1982, 67*, 132.

Goldman, M.M. *An experimental investigation of the goat by the conditioned reflex method.* Unpublished Master's thesis, Cornell University, 1939.

Gorman, J., Askanazi, J., Liebowitz, M., Fyer, A., Stein, J., Kinney, J., and Klein, D. Response to hyperventilation in a group of patients with panic disorder. *American Journal of Psychiatry, 1984, 141*, 857–861.

Grosz, H., and Farmer, B. Pitts and McClure's lactate-anxiety study revisited. *British Journal of Psychiatry, 1972, 120*, 415–418.

Hall, A.L. *The effects of decompression on subjects repeatedly exposed to 43,000 feet while using standard pressure breathing equipment: Involuntary hyperventilation during pressure breathing at 43,000 feet.* U.S. Naval School of Aviation Medicine Report on Project No. NM001 059.21.01, 1952.

Hardonk, H.J., and Beumer, H.M. Hyperventilation syndrome. In P.J. Vinken and G.W. Bruyn (Eds.), *Handbook of clinical neurology: Neurological manifestations of systemic disease.* Vol. 38, part 1. Amsterdam: North Holland, 1979.

Henning, R., Sauter, S., Lanphier, E., and Reddan, W. Behavioral effects of increased CO_2 load in divers. *Undersea Biomedical Research, 1990, 17*, 109–120.

Hinshaw, H.C., Rushmer, R.F., and Boothby, W.M. The hyperventilation syndrome and its importance in aviation medicine. *Journal of Aviation Medicine, 1943 14*, 100–104.

Kartsounis, L., and Turpin, G. Effects of induced hyperventilation on electrodermal response habituation to agoraphobia-relevant stimuli. *Journal of Psychosomatic Research, 1987, 31*, 401–412.

Lader, M., and Mathews, A. Physiological changes during spontaneous panic attacks. *Journal of Psychosomatic Research, 1970, 14*, 377–382.

Ley, R. Agoraphobia, the panic attack, and the hyperventilation syndrome. *Behaviour Research and Therapy, 1985a, 23*, 79–81.

Ley, R. Blood, breath, and fears: A hyperventilation theory of panic attacks and agoraphobia. *Clinical Psychology Review, 1985b, 5*, 271–285.

Ley, R. Panic disorder and agoraphobia: Fear of fear or fear of the symptoms produced by hyperventilation? *Journal of Behavior Therapy and Experimental Psychiatry, 1987, 18*, 305–316.

Ley, R. Hyperventilation and lactate infusion in the production of panic attacks. *Clinical Psychology Review, 1988a, 8*, 1–18.

Ley, R. Panic attacks during relaxation and relaxation-induced anxiety: A hyperventilation interpretation. *Journal of Behavior Therapy and Experimental Psychiatry, 1988b, 19*, 253–259.

Ley, R. Panic attacks during sleep: A hyperventilation-probability model. *Journal of Behavior Therapy and Experimental Psychiatry, 1988c, 19*, 181–192.

Ley, R. Dyspneic-fear and catastrophic cognitions in hyperventilatory panic attacks. *Behaviour Research and Therapy, 1989, 27*, 549–554.

Ley, R. The efficacy of breathing retraining and the centrality of hyperventilation in panic disorder: A reinterpretation of experimental findings. *Behaviour Research and Therapy, 1991a, 29*, 301–304.

Ley, R. Ventilatory control of heart rate during inhalation of 5% CO_2 and types of panic attacks. *Journal of Behavior Therapy and Experimental Psychiatry, 1991b, 22*, 193–201.

Ley, R. The many faces of Pan: Psychological and physiological differences among three types of panic attacks. *Behaviour Research and Therapy, 1992, 30*, 347–357.

Ley, R., and Schleifer, L. End-tidal pCO2, respiratory frequency and cardiac interbeat interval during VDT data-entry work. *Supplement to Psychophysiology, 1992, 29*, 48.

Ley, R., and Yelich, G. End-tidal pCO2 as an index of test anxiety. *Supplement to Psychophysiology, 1991, 28*, 38.

Lum, L.C. Hyperventilation: The tip of the iceberg. *Journal of Psychosomatic Research,* 1975, *19,* 375–383.

Lum, L.C. The syndrome of habitual chronic hyperventilation. In O.W. Hill (Ed.), *Modern trends in psychosomatic medicine.* Vol. 3. London: Butterworth, 1976, pp. 196–230.

Lum, L.C. Hyperventilation and anxiety state. *Journal of the Royal Society of Medicine,* 1981, *74,* 1–4.

Lykken, D.T. Polygraphic interrogation. *Nature,* 1984, 681–684.

Margraf, J., Ehlers, A., and Roth, W. Sodium lactate infusions and panic attacks: A review and critique. *Psychosomatic Medicine,* 1986, *48,* 23–51.

Margraf, J., Ehlers, A., and Roth, W. Panic attack associated with perceived heart rate acceleration: A case report. *Behavior Therapy,* 1987, *18,* 84–89.

Marzocco, F.N. *Frustration effect as a function of drive level, habit strength and distribution of trials during extinction.* Unpublished doctoral dissertation, State University of Iowa, 1951.

Masserman, J.H. *Behavior and neurosis.* Chicago: University of Chicago Press, 1943.

McCaul, K.D., Solomon, S., and Holmes, D.S. Effects of paced respiration and expectations on physiological and psychological responses to threat. *Journal of Personality and Social Psychology,* 1979, *37,* 564–571.

Miller, L.C. Fears and anxiety in children. In C.E. Walker and M.C. Roberts (Eds.), *Handbook of clinical child psychology.* New York: Wiley, 1983, pp. 337–380.

Minami, H., Moore, A.V., and Liddell, H.S. *Experimental research carried out on sheep at the Cornell Behavior Farm.* Unpublished study, 1943.

Neisser, U. *Cognitive psychology.* New York: Appleton-Century-Crofts, 1967.

Nixon, P.G.F., and Freeman, L.J. The "think test": A further technique to elicit hyperventilation. *Journal of the Royal Society of Medicine,* 1987a, *81,* 277–279.

Nixon, P.G.F., and Freeman, L.J. (1987b). What is the meaning of angina pectoris today? *American Heart Journal,* 1987b, *114,* 1542–1546.

Nixon, P.G.F., Freeman, L.J., and King, J.C. Breathing and thinking: Unacknowledged coronary risk factors. *Holistic Medicine,* 1987, *2,* 133–136.

Otis, J. *The effects of response delay interval and instructions on the magnitude of force of response in a nonreinforcement induced frustration paradigm.* Unpublished doctoral dissertation, State University of New York at Albany, 1973.

Pavlov, I.P. Lectures on the work on the principal digestive glands. In B.P. Babkin. *Pavlov: A biography,* Chicago: University of Chicago Press, 1949.

Podlesny, J.A., and Raskin, D.C. Effectiveness of techniques and physiological measures in the detection of deception. *Psychophysiology,* 1980, *15,* 344–349.

Rachman, S., Lepatka, C., and Levitt, K. Experimental analysis of panic-II. Panic patients. *Behavior Research and Therapy,* 1988, *26,* 33–40.

Rahn, H., Otis, A.B., Hodge, M.A., Epstein, M.A., Hunter, S.W., and Fenn, W.O. The effects of hypocapnea on performance. *Journal of Aviation Medicine,* 1946, *17,* 164–172.

Rescorla, R.A. Pavlovian conditioning: It's not what you think it is. *American Psychologist,* 1988, *43,* 151–160.

Rushmer, R.F., and Bond, D.D. The hyperventilation syndrome in flying personnel. *War Medicine,* 1944, *5,* 302–303.

Rushmer, R.F., Boothby, W.M., and Hinshaw, H.C. Some effects of hyperventilation with special reference to aviation medicine. *Proceedings of the Staff Meeting of the Mayo Clinic,* 1941, *16,* 801–808.

Salter, A. *Conditioned reflex therapy.* New York: Capricorn Books, 1961.

Sanderson, W. The influence of perceived control on panic attacks induced via inhalation of 5% CO_2 enriched air, unpublished doctoral dissertation, State University of New York at Albany, 1987.

Sanderson, W., Rapee, R., and Barlow, D. Panic induction via inhalation of 5.5% CO_2 enriched air:

A single subject analysis of psychological and physiological effects. *Behaviour Research and Therapy,* 1988, *26,* 333–335.

Shear, M.K. Pathophysiology of panic: A review of pharmacologic provocation tests and naturalistic monitoring data. *Journal of Clinical Psychiatry,* 1986, *47,* 18–26.

Sherrington, C.S. Experiments on the value of vascular and visceral factors for the genesis of emotion. *Proceedings of the Royal Society,* 1900, *66,* 390–403.

Suinn, R.M. The STABS, a measure of test anxiety for behavior therapy: Normative data. *Behavior Research and Therapy,* 1969, *7,* 335–339.

Thyer, B., Papsdorf, J., and Wright, P. Physiological and psychological effects of acute intentional hyperventilation. *Behaviour Research and Therapy,* 1984, *22,* 587–590.

Tolman, E.C. Principles of purposive behavior. In S. Koch (Ed.) *Psychology: A study of a science.* Vol. 2. New York: McGraw-Hill, 1959, pp. 92–157.

Wolpe, J. *The practice of behavior therapy.* 3rd ed. New York: Pergamon, 1982.

Wolpe, J., and Rowan, V.C. Panic disorder: A product of classical conditioning. *Behaviour Research and Therapy,* 1988, *26,* 441–450.

Wyke, B. *Brain function and metabolic disorders: The neurological effects of hydrogen-ion concentration.* London: Butterworth, 1963.

II

Hyperventilation
Diagnosis and Therapy

Diagnosis and Organic Causes of Symptomatic Hyperventilation

WILLIAM N. GARDNER

1. Introduction

The term *hyperventilation syndrome* may be subject to variable interpretations, but hyperventilation and its hypocapnic sequelae exist as indisputable facts of respiratory psychophysiology. Hyperventilation implies an excessive stimulation to breathing, which can be due to a wide range of psychogenic, physiological, and organic disorders. Moreover, symptoms of organic disease may mimic those of hypocapnia, and hyperventilation may coexist with organic disease. It is therefore essential that full assessment for organic disease is performed in all patients with apparent hyperventilation. While Ley (Chapter 5) and Bass (Chapter 10) address directly the psychological and psychiatric aspects of hyperventilation, this chapter represents the approach of a physiologist and chest physician to this difficult and controversial subject.

2. Physiology and Definitions

2.1. Introduction

Some basic principles of respiratory physiology of relevance to this chapter will be reviewed here; for a more detailed discussion, see Naifeh (Chapter 1). Respiration is concerned with elimination of carbon dioxide (CO_2) produced by

WILLIAM N. GARDNER • Department of Thoracic Medicine, Kings College School of Medicine and Dentistry, London SE5 9PJ, England.
Behavioral and Psychological Approaches to Breathing Disorders, edited by Beverly H. Timmons and Ronald Ley. Plenum Press, New York, 1994.

A   B   C   D

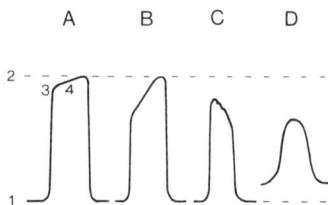

Figure 1. Examples of capnographic recordings for four breaths. The first breath is an acceptable trace. The second breath shows the increased plateau slope in exercise and lung disease. The third and fourth breaths show unacceptable profiles with failure to attain a plateau.

the muscles. CO_2 is delivered to the lungs in the venous system; some is eliminated to the atmosphere via the lungs and the remainder continues into the arterial circulation, determining the partial pressure of CO_2 in the arterial blood leaving the lungs ($Paco_2$). This is the same as the partial pressure in the lungs at the end of an expiration (end-tidal or alveolar Pco_2, $Paco_2$).

The volume of one breath is called the *tidal volume* and the total amount of air breathed in (or out) per minute is called *minute ventilation*. These can be easily measured with a spirometer. If the CO_2 production from the muscles remains constant, increase in ventilation will lead to increased elimination of CO_2 from the lungs and consequent reduction of residual Pco_2 in the alveolar air and arteries.

2.2. Alveolar and Dead-Space Volumes

Tidal volume can be divided into two components, the air in the lung (*alveolar volume*) and the air in the airways (*dead-space volume*). Only the alveolar volume is concerned with CO_2 elimination and therefore, ideally, $Paco_2$ is inversely related to alveolar volume rather than minute ventilation although the two usually behave in parallel. During expiration, dead-space gas with the same composition as inspired gas is exhaled first, followed by alveolar gas. The dead-space is about 200 ml, and the difference between alveolar volume and tidal volume is usually of academic interest except during very fast, shallow breathing, when most of the air breathed in merely fills the dead-space and only a small amount enters the lung. In this situation, tidal volume and ventilation can be high but alveolar volume low with a correspondingly high $PAco_2$ and $Paco_2$. In practical terms, this means that the patient can appear to be hyperventilating but yet have a normal or even raised $PAco_2$.

2.3. End-Tidal Pco_2

In subjects with normal lungs, arterial Pco_2 is very close to end-tidal Pco_2, which can be easily measured by continuous capnographic sampling from the nostril or mouth. Figure 1 shows examples of such tracings. 1A shows an ideal trace for one breath. The inspired value is denoted by (1), and, in the air-breathing situation, is close to zero. This is followed by a fast-rising phase as the dead-space gas is cleared and alveolar gas starts to reach the mouth, then the characteristic shoulder (3), and finally the alveolar plateau (4), which slowly rises to the end-tidal value (2) at the peak of the plateau. This denotes true alveolar gas with successful clearance of dead space, and in subjects with normal lungs is very close to arterial Pco_2. Figure 1B shows the steeper plateau characteristic of exercise and lung disease; end-tidal values need to be interpreted with caution and may overestimate $Paco_2$. Figure 1C and 1D show unacceptable traces. In Figure 1C, the volume expired has been insufficient to clear the dead-space and there is no alveolar plateau. In Figure 1D, the sample rate or the response time of the analyzer is too slow, as shown by the slurred up and down strokes and the failure to reach zero during inspiration.

2.4. Control of Breathing and CO_2

Normal tidal volume is about 0.5 liter, ventilation is about 5–8 liters/min, and $Paco_2$ is usually quoted as 4.7–6.0 kPa (35–45 mm Hg). As $Paco_2$ rises above this range, powerful arterial and intracranial chemoreflexes are stimulated, which increase breathing, eliminate more CO_2, and restore the $Paco_2$ to the normal range. Only in the terminal stages of lung disease is this mechanism overcome, allowing Pco_2 to rise above normal.

In contrast, the control of breathing in hypocapnia (i.e., below the normal range of $Paco_2$) is characterized by a paucity of evidence for reflexes to restore Pco_2 when it falls. Indeed, there is little evidence for any reflex-controlling mechanisms in this range. Breathing is probably controlled by a combination of the pacemaker in the medullary respiratory centers, and cortical influences; the latter can undoubtedly override any physiological mechanisms in this range. The lower limit for $Paco_2$ is therefore difficult to define and may be considerably lower than that quoted above. These facts are especially relevant to the present topic because they provide the necessary physiological basis for discussing the induction, maintenance and diagnosis of hyperventilation.

2.5. Definition of Hyperventilation

Hyperventilation has a strict physiological meaning of breathing in excess of metabolic requirements. This means that ventilation is too high in relation to the rate of CO_2 production, thus leading to a fall in Pco_2 below the normal range, i.e., arterial hypocapnia.

2.6. Symptoms of Hyperventilation

Hypocapnia may produce symptoms by two main mechanisms (Magarian, 1982). First, reduction of arterial Pco_2 causes respiratory alkalosis, with a decrease in the acidity of the blood and reduction of arterial bicarbonate. This causes increased neuronal irritability, with resulting symptoms such as tetany, muscle spasm, and paresthesia. Second, hypocapnia causes a reduction of blood flow to the brain, limbs, and heart, which can cause dizziness and light-headedness, cold extremities, and chest pain, respectively. Although etiological factors are uncertain and complex (Magarian, 1982), hyperventilation can be associated with, in addition to the chest pain, abnormalities on the electrocardiogram simulating cardiovascular disorders (Bass *et al.*, 1983, and Chapter 8).

3. Short Historical Survey

The effects of voluntary hyperventilation in normal subjects were first described by Haldane and Poulton (1908). The most specific symptom they described was tetany, or muscle spasm.

The first description of spontaneous symptomatic hyperventilation in patients was by Goldman (1922). Kerr *et al.* (1937) provided the first description of the hyperventilation syndrome, which was followed by a more detailed exposition by Ames (1955). These authors described the spontaneous occurrence of prolonged hyperventilation related to anxiety and stress in the absence of relevant organic disease. Presenting symptoms were more varied than those attributable to hypocapnia alone, presumably reflecting the additional clinical features of anxiety. Tetany was rare. They emphasized the difficulty of distinguishing the symptoms of hypocapnia from those of organic diseases. Subsequent authors (e.g., Lewis, 1954) described the additional anxiety that fear of organic disease may induce in the hyperventilating patient. Alkalosis and arterial hypocapnia were documented only to a limited extent in these early studies because of the technical difficulties in performing prolonged measurements of alveolar or arterial Pco_2.

There have been a few important advances since then, but there remains a paucity of controlled multidisciplinary studies in this difficult field, and there is increasing uncertainty about the usage of the term *hyperventilation syndrome* (Dent *et al.*, 1983). For example, undoubtedly, chronic hyperventilation can occur in the absence of manifest anxiety (Ames, 1955; Bass and Gardner, 1985; Lum, 1976). In other cases, anxiety may be secondary to the alarming symptoms of hypocapnia, rather than an initiating factor. In these cases, other etiological factors need to be invoked.

One suggested mechanism is that transient overbreathing may, once established, acquire the characteristics of a habit disorder (Lum, 1976). Large breaths are taken in an attempt to alleviate chest discomfort or the other unpleasant symptoms of hypocapnia.

Although there have been few descriptions of feedback control mechanisms in hypocapnia, there is indirect evidence that some form of active control may be operative in this range and may contribute to the maintenance of hyperventilation in these patients. Hypocapnia is very difficult to reverse once it has become established in both hyperventilating patients (Ames, 1955; Gardner and Bass, 1986) and normal controls (Okel and Hurst, 1961; Saltzman *et al.*, 1963). In chronic hyperventilation, prolonged CO_2 inhalation does not always produce restitution of $Paco_2$, and even during sleep $Paco_2$ returns to normal only after a few hours (Gardner and Bass, 1986). Folgering and Colla (1978) have described a negative feedback to CO_2 below the chemoreceptor threshold that may help to perpetuate hyperventilation.

Cognitive factors are probably important in the maintenance of hypocapnia (Salkovskis and Clark, 1986). The unpleasant and often alarming symptoms of hypocapnia are misattributed by the patient to serious disease, such as cancer, a stroke, or heart disease. If the correct diagnosis is not made at an early stage, anxiety exacerbates the hyperventilation; the consequent vicious circle soon leads to chronic invalidism and the thick folder syndrome (i.e., the patient attends a variety of doctors and clinics with progressively decreasing reward and increasing paranoia, secondary anxiety, and depression).

We have recently suggested that, because of the above uncertainties, the term *hyperventilation syndrome* should be abandoned and that hyperventilation should be regarded as a pathophysiological process for which a cause or causes should be sought (Gardner *et al.*, 1986). It has also been suggested that in many cases patients with chronic hyperventilation are really suffering from the more general disorder of *chronic somatization* (Bass and Murphy, 1990). Howell (1990) prefers the term *behavioral breathlessness* for a specific subgroup of these patients.

4. Diagnosis

Diagnostic criteria in current use are unsatisfactory. They are discussed below in order of increasing invasiveness and complexity.

4.1. Symptoms

Clinical features alone are often used to establish the diagnosis (e.g., Kraft and Hoogduin, 1984). Diagnosis is based on the report of an arbitrary number of presenting complaints drawn from long symptom checklists, often combined with the recognition of the major symptoms during a period of voluntary over-breathing. These techniques have shortcomings. With the exception of tetany, most quoted symptoms are nonspecific and subjective; they can only suggest the diagnosis. In addition, patients with severe chronic hyperventilation may have few symptoms. Recognition of symptoms during overbreathing can be helpful in some patients, but many are unable to complete this test; that in itself is a significant fact that can contribute to a positive diagnosis (Bonn *et al.*, 1984). Patients' descriptions of complaints may be unreliable, and interpretation depends on the subjective, and possibly biased, assessment of the administering therapist. Without a continuous measure of Pco_2, it is impossible to standardize the level of hypocapnia reached during the test. Finally, in the presence of established chronic hypocapnia, further attempts to overbreathe may produce meaningless results and may lead to a false negative diagnosis.

4.2. Signs (Features Found on Examination)

Hyperventilating patients do not always show obvious increase in chest wall movements. For example, we found that in patients with chronic hypocapnia, ventilation was only increased by about 10 percent compared to a matched control group. Repeated sighs are related to a sensation of inability to take a satisfying breath, or air hunger (Christie, 1935; Tucker, 1956). Although sighing is associated with abnormal chest wall movements, it may not necessarily be associated with hypocapnia, because the increase in tidal volume may be compensated for by a slowing of the respiratory rate. In panting, two mechanisms may operate to prevent hypocapnia: high respiratory rate may be compensated for by low tidal volume to prevent an increase in alveolar ventilation, and inadequate clearance of dead-space air may hinder the elimination of CO_2, as discussed above (Section 2.2).

4.3. Voluntary Overbreathing and Other Tests

Hardonk and Beumer (1979) have modified the voluntary overbreathing test by performing it with continuous measurement of end-tidal Pco_2 and by concentrating on the rate of recovery from hypocapnia. They claim that an abnormally slow return of Pco_2 to pretest levels is diagnostic of hyperventilation. However, both false positive and false negative responses to this test have been described (Wientjes *et al.*, 1984).

Others regard both voluntary overbreathing and exercise as forms of provocation that may provoke prolonged hypocapnia in certain situations (Ferguson *et al.*, 1969; Gardner and Bass, 1989). Another approach is provided by the Think Test (Nixon and Freeman, 1988), a technique designed to elicit hyperventilation through guided thoughts pertaining to relevant emotional episodes that preceded the onset of somatic complaints. *Breath-holding time* is often markedly reduced in these patients and can be measured easily in the clinic or at the bedside.

4.4. Measurement of Pco_2

Despite the clear physiological changes underlying hyperventilation, measurements of arterial or end-tidal Pco_2 have not been reported routinely. There are several reasons for this. In early studies, techniques for the continuous monitoring of expired breath were unavailable. Later, when rapid CO_2 analyzers and mass spectrometers provided for gas analysis, their high cost prohibited many clinicians from purchasing them for routine use. Moreover, it was usually assumed that brief, "spot," measurements were unreliable in detecting acute hyperventilatory attacks. We believe that such measurements, especially if combined with provocation tests, can be helpful in detecting chronic hyperventilation (Gardner *et al.*, 1986) and will provide a high positive yield when used for routine testing in a lung function laboratory (Gardner *et al.*, 1990). Recently, transcutaneous monitoring of PCO_2 combined with an ambulatory recording system has allowed prolonged recording of PCO_2 in patients with panic (Pilsbury and Hibbert, 1987), but interpretation is difficult because of the slow response time of the system.

5. Etiology of Hyperventilation

5.1. Introduction

Uncertainties about use of the term *hyperventilation syndrome* have been discussed above. There are undoubtedly etiological factors that remain to be identified, but clinical experience suggests that in many cases the etiology of hyperventilation often lies in the synergistic interaction between a range of physiological, organic, and psychological factors. It is helpful to distinguish initiating factors, which are responsible for the first acute episode of hyperventilation, from sustaining factors, which can keep $PaCO_2$ low and induce chronic hyperventilation (Lewis, 1954). Some of these factors have been discussed above. Usually, the interaction of a number of initiating factors is required to produce hypocapnia sufficiently profound to cause symptoms. For example, mild asthma combined with pyrexia, excessive talking, and anxiety may produce a sudden attack of chest pain, paresthesia, and tetany; this attack may be perceived as a life-threatening heart attack or stroke. If the true nature of the attack is not recognized by the attending physicians, fear of recurrent attacks and sudden death, combined with large breaths to relieve chest discomfort and physiological resetting, ensure that hypocapnia continues, resulting in the rapid onset of chronic invalidism. Hyperventilation without symptoms is of little consequence. Figure 2 shows a range of possible initiating factors on the left-hand side and a possible interaction of sustaining factors that could contribute to a feedback loop sustaining the hypocapnia, on the right.

Since the psychological causes of hyperventilation are addressed in several chapters in this book, the present discussion will be limited to organic factors. It must be borne in mind, however, that organic causes very often give rise to emotional factors that contribute to the positive feedback loop shown in Figure 2.

INITIATING FACTORS   SUSTAINING FACTORS

PSYCHIATRIC   - PERSONALITY
               - ANXIETY / PANIC
               - DEPRESSION
               - FACTITIOUS
LUNG DISEASE   - ASTHMA   SYMPTOMS OF DISEASE
               - BRONCHITIS   (EG, ASTHMA–TIGHT CHEST)
               - EMPHYSEMA
               - INTERSTITIAL
                 DISEASES   SYMPTOMS OF HYPOCAPNIA
               - EMBOLUS
               - HEART FAILURE   HABIT (BIG BREATHS)
PHYSIOLOGICAL - PYREXIA
               - ALTITUDE
               - TALKING   HYPER-   PHYSIOLOGICAL   MISATTRIBUTION
DRUGS   - CAFFEINE   VENTILATION   RESETTING   TO SERIOUS
               - NICOTINE   DISEASE
               - AMPHETAMINE
               - ASPIRIN
               - β BLOCKER
METABOLIC   - DIABETES
               - LIVER FAILURE
               - RENAL FAILURE   SECONDARY ANXIETY
ENDOCRINE   - PROGESTERONE
               - PREGNANCY
PAIN
CNS LESIONS
RESPIRATORY DYSKINESIAS
ANEMIA

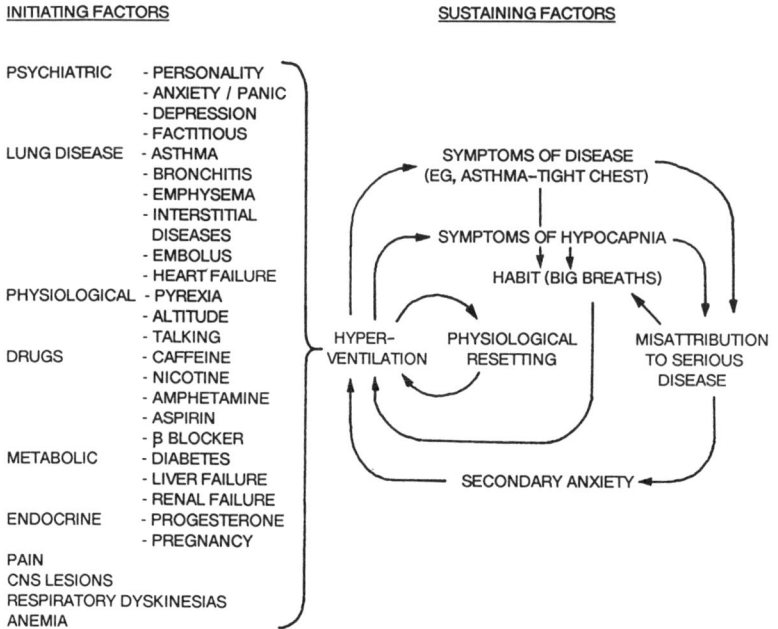

Figure 2. Etiological factors in hyperventilation.

5.2. Organic Causes of Hyperventilation

While respiratory disorders have the greatest influence on breathing, there are less specific reflexes, from most organs of the body, that can affect respiration. Most disorders affecting the lungs or airways can cause hyperventilation. This has been best documented for asthma and chronic bronchitis. McFadden and Lyons (1968) recorded values of $Paco_2$ as low as 2.8 kPa (21 mm Hg) during the incipient stages of asthma, and indeed profound and symptomatic hyperventilation may be a feature of the early stages of most respiratory disorders (Gardner *et al.*, 1990). The cause of this hyperventilation is uncertain but it may be due to stimulation of vagal receptors in the lungs and airways, stimulation of the chemoreceptors by hypoxia, or the mechanical effect of hyperinflation.

In some cases, severe symptomatic hyperventilation can occur when asthma is too mild to be detected by standard clinical investigations and lung function tests. Asthma as mild as this usually remains undiagnosed or is mislabeled as bronchitis or chestiness. There is often wheeziness or dyspnea during exertion, an association with hay fever or allergies, and a family history of asthma. Symptoms related to asthma are worse at night and early in the morning. Any childhood history of chestiness, bronchitis, wheeze, or persistent cough strongly suggests that asthma may be contributing to the present complaints.

Chronic bronchitis has a clinical picture that resembles asthma but it occurs almost entirely in smokers. It worsens progressively with age, and the airflow obstruction is less episodic and less responsive to bronchodilators than in asthma. There is usually "smokers cough" and early morning phlegm. Hypocapnia probably occurs in the early stages but has been less well documented. In *emphysema* there is both airflow obstruction and destruction of lung tissue parenchyma. Hypocapnia has been documented in early mild disease (Noehren, 1966).

Interstitial lung diseases are associated with progressive breathlessness and deterioration of lung function. Inflammation is followed by fibrosis of the lung tissue (parenchyma). In the early stages, lung washings taken during fiber optic bronchoscopy may show evidence of widespread lung inflammation even though chest x ray and lung function tests are normal. Hypocapnia may occur in this stage but has not been documented. In more severe disease, resting ventilation increases, but $Paco_2$ remains near normal until the terminal stages because of associated increase in dead-space volume; significant hypocapnia may, however, occur during exercise (Lourenco et al., 1965). Interstitial lung diseases include *cryptogenic fibrosing alveolitis, sarcoidosis, extrinsic allergic alveolitis,* and industrial *pneumoconioses.*

Pulmonary emboli are clots that detach from deep venous thrombi (attached clots) in the large veins of the arms or legs. If sufficiently large, they can lead to circulatory arrest and death; when small, they often multiply and produce progressive *infarction* (destruction) of discrete areas of the lung. Infarcts classically cause pleuritic chest pain of sudden onset, *hemoptysis* (bloody sputum), breathlessness, characteristic changes on the ECG, and a peripheral wedge-shaped shadow on the chest x ray. They can be very difficult to diagnose. The association of pulmonary embolism with hypocapnia has been repeatedly demonstrated (e.g., Szucs et al., 1971).

Severe *pulmonary edema* secondary to left ventricular failure may cause respiratory or metabolic acidosis with increase of $Paco_2$, but reduction of $Paco_2$, with respiratory alkalosis, has also been documented in some cases (Avery et al., 1970).

Physiological conditions such as *pyrexia, altitude* and excessive *talking,* and *chronic pain* (Glynn et al., 1981) are associated with documented hypocapnia, but this rarely causes symptoms of hypocapnia unless it is combined with other factors. The hyperventilation that results from fever (and other expressions of *hyperthermia*) could be regarded as being compensatory in that the heat loss through excessive ventilation decreases body temperature.

Among the most common drugs that cause hyperventilation are stimulants (e.g., caffeine, nicotine, amphetamine) and aspirin (Temple, 1981). Their effect on ventilation may be due to a direct effect on the brain—stimulation or chemoreceptors—or may be an indirect consequence of an increase in metabolism. *Beta-blocking drugs,* widely used to treat hypertension and anxiety, are a potent cause of asthma and can thus indirectly induce hyperventilation.

Metabolic disorders such as *diabetic acidosis, liver, and renal failure* cause severe hyperventilation (e.g., Vanamee *et al.,* 1956). Although usually obvious, in the presence of a psychiatrically disturbed patient they could be overlooked.

Progesterone stimulates breathing and causes a fall of $Paco_2$ in normal subjects (Skatrud *et al.,* 1978). Hypocapnia occurs during pregnancy and the luteal phase of menstruation, with a reduction in $Paco_2$ of 0.67–1.1 kPa (5–8 mm Hg). The $Paco_2$ falls from an average value of about 5 kPa (38 mm Hg) to about 4 kPa (30 mm Hg) by mid-pregnancy and remains at this level until term. Although hyperventilation sufficient to cause tetany has not been documented in normal pregnant patients, it is conceivable that in pregnant women with chronic hypocapnia for other reasons, symptomatic hyperventilation may be precipitated by the additional influence of progesterone.

In *anemia,* hyperventilation is a consequence of the hypoxia that results from insufficient hemoglobin in plasma. The hyperventilation that results from *hemorrhage* is a consequence of ischemia.

Thyrotoxicosis is usually quoted in reviews as a cause of hyperventilation (e.g., Hardonk and Beumer, 1979). Although dyspnea and muscle weakness are common and are often accompanied by increase in respiratory frequency, there is little evidence that thyrotoxicosis causes hypocapnia.

A range of disorders of the central nervous system can cause hyperventilation if focal lesions involve the respiratory centers in the brain stem. Global disorders such as *dementia* can also cause disturbances of respiratory rate and depth, as can *respiratory dyskinesia.*

6. Investigative Sequence

The stages in the diagnostic process will now be discussed in the order in which they should be approached by the physician or therapist faced with a patient with possible hyperventilation (Gardner and Bass, 1989). These are summarised in Table 1.

6.1. Investigation of Presenting Symptoms

Many of the symptoms of hyperventilation are nonspecific and could equally well be due to organic disease. Before hyperventilation is considered as a possible diagnosis, all other possible causes of the presenting symptoms must be excluded. For most symptoms, routine clinical assessment and simple investigations suffice. But for others, especially chest pain and neurological symptoms,

Table 1
Diagnostic Sequence

---

1. *Investigation of presenting symptoms*: cardiac, respiratory and neurological assessment.
2. *Diagnosis of hyperventilation*
    2.1. *Symptoms*: disproportionate breathlessness, air hunger, chest pain, paresthesia, tetany, dizziness, etc. Description of attacks by observer.
    2.2. *Signs found on examination*: sighing, panting, increased chest movement (may be absent).
    2.3. *Bedside tests*: respiration rate, breath-holding time, symptom reproduction by overbreathing.
    2.4. *Laboratory procedures*: end-tidal, arterial, or transcutaneous Pco_2 at rest, during and after exercise, and during recovery from three minutes of overbreathing.
3. *Assessment of cause(s) for overbreathing*: detailed history from patient of event initiating attacks, clinical assessment for relevant organic and psychogenic disease, exclusion of asthma.
4. *Treatment*: treatment of causes (if found), reassurance, empirical treatment for hyperventilation.

---

specialized investigations are usually required before either patient or physician is prepared to accept hyperventilation as a possible cause of the presenting complaints. This investigative sequence has often been completed before the patient is referred.

6.2. Diagnosis of Hyperventilation

The next step is to attempt to *prove* the existence of hyperventilation either at rest or after provocation. Sometimes, associates of the patient or casualty officers will give an unequivocal description of hyperventilation during an acute attack. Symptoms, signs and bedside tests have been discussed above. Actual documentation of arterial or end-tidal hypocapnia should always be attempted. Capnographs are now relatively inexpensive; ideally, they should be standard equipment in clinics dealing with these patients. If $Paco_2$ is not low at rest, a tendency to hyperventilate may be unmasked by provocations; these could include exercise (e.g., brisk walking for 5–10 minutes) and 1–3 minutes of voluntary overbreathing, to a level of end-tidal Pco_2 below 2.6 kPa (20 mm Hg). Overbreathing should be performed with caution if there is evidence of coronary artery disease or chest pain. Normal values for these tests should be established for each laboratory. Our criteria are that diagnosis is established if $Paco_2$ is below about 4 kPa (30 mm Hg) at rest or during or after exercise, or remains low 5 minutes after voluntary overbreathing. This protocol also allows assessment of the relationship of symptoms to hypocapnia. As discussed above, hyperventilation may be intermittent, and failure to demonstrate hypocapnia during these tests does not exclude hyperventilation at other times, but it reduces the likelihood that hypocapnia is responsible for the symptoms. These test results must always be used in conjunction with the clinical assessment.

6.3. Search for Organic Causes of Hyperventilation

The demonstration of hypocapnia indicates an additional and pathological drive to breathe, and the source of this excessive drive must be sought. A careful history should be taken of the events surrounding the first attack of hyperventilation to identify likely initiating factors, and of subsequent events, for evidence of the vicious circles in Figure 2. Smoking and occupational history should be documented. Blood biochemistry, blood count, erythrocyte sedimentation rate, thyroid function, and chest x ray should be ordered routinely, as should standard lung function tests (or peak flow measurements) before and after induced bronchodilation. Normal chest x ray and lung function tests do not necessarily exclude early respiratory disease, and other tests may be required. If asthma is suspected, a plastic peak flow meter can be given to the patients for home monitoring. An early morning value more than approximately 20 percent below the evening value, especially if reversible with bronchodilators, is highly suggestive. If the diagnosis is still in doubt, a treatment trial with twice daily inhaled beta-agonist drugs and inhaled steroids can be commenced. Histamine (Juniper et al., 1978) or other forms of bronchial challenge will provide definitive proof of asthma but are only available in specialist chest departments. Ventilation/perfusion scans are essential if pulmonary embolism is suspected; an abnormal scan may be difficult to interpret, but a normal scan will exclude both emboli and most respiratory disorders.

7. Treatment

There are three aspects of treatment: treatment of underlying organic disease, treatment of primary or secondary psychological disturbance, and direct treatment of hyperventilation if no underlying cause can be found. The latter two are described in more detail in Chapters 9–11 and 17.

If organic and/or psychological causes for the hyperventilation are discovered, specific treatment should be instituted before secondary psychological disturbances become established. Cessation of hyperventilation following treatment confirms the diagnosis.

In all cases, the underlying physiological disturbances and the etiological sequence of events should be carefully explained. This involves reattribution of symptoms, reassurance that hyperventilation is not life-threatening, and demonstration to the patient that there is no serious underlying organic disease to account for the symptoms. All unnecessary drugs should be stopped. These simple measures are often sufficient, although more sophisticated treatment will be needed in some cases.

8. Conclusion

The causes of symptomatic hyperventilation are often unknown but in many cases are due to the complex interaction of a number of psychological, organic, and physiological disorders. The symptoms of hypocapnia produced by hyperventilation may be the cause, as well as a consequence, of anxiety. Therefore, it is mandatory to perform a full range of basic investigations even in the presence of manifest psychological disorder. However, it is also essential to avoid an endless search for organic etiology and excessively expensive and invasive investigations. Clinical judgement should determine when the investigative process should cease.

9. References

Ames, F. The hyperventilation syndrome. *Journal of Mental Science,* 1955, *101,* 466–525.

Avery, W.G., Samet, P., and Sackner, M.A. The acidosis of pulmonary edema. *The American Journal of Medicine,* 1970, *48,* 320–324.

Bass, C., Cawley, R., Wade, C., Ryan, K.C., Gardner, W.N., Hutchison, D.C.S., and Jackson, G. Unexplained breathlessness and psychiatric morbidity in patients with normal and abnormal coronary arteries. *Lancet,* 1983, *i,* 605–609.

Bass, C., and Gardner, W.N. Respiratory and psychiatric abnormalities in chronic symptomatic hyperventilation. *British Medical Journal,* 1985, *i,* 1387–1390.

Bass, C., and Murphy, M.R. Somatisation disorder: Critique of the concept and suggestions for future research. In C. Bass (Ed.), *Somatisation: Physical symptoms and psychological illness.* Oxford: Blackwells, 1990.

Bonn, J.A., Readhead, C.P.A., and Timmons, B.H. Enhanced adaptive behavioural response in agoraphobic patients pretreated with breathing retraining. *Lancet,* 1984, *ii,* 665–669.

Christie, R.V. Some types of respiration in the neuroses. *Quarterly Journal of Medicine,* 1935, *16,* 427–434.

Dent, R., Yates, D., and Higgenbottom, T. Does the hyperventilation syndrome exist? *Thorax,* 1983, *38,* 223 (one page).

Ferguson, A., Addington, W.W., and Gaensler, E.A. Dyspnea and bronchospasm from inappropriate post exercise hyperventilation. *Annals of Internal Medicine,* 1969, *71,* 1063–1072.

Folgering, H., and Colla, P. Some anomalies in the control of PA_{CO_2} in patients with the hyperventilation syndrome. *Bulletin Europeen de Physiopathologie Respiratoire,* 1978, *14,* 503–512.

Gardner, W.N., and Bass, C. Hyperventilation in clinical practice. (A Review). *British Journal of Hospital Medicine,* 1989, *41,* 73–81.

Gardner, W.N., Green, S.E., and Ford, T.A. Measurement of end-tidal P_{CO_2} during lung function measurement. *American Review of Respiratory Diseases,* 1990, *141,* A308.

Gardner, W.N., Meah, M.S., and Bass, C. Controlled study of respiratory responses during prolonged measurement in patients with chronic hyperventilation. *Lancet,* 1986, *ii,* 826–830.

Glynn, C.J., Lloyd, J.W., and Folkhard, S. Ventilatory responses to intractable pain. *Pain,* 1981, *11,* 201–211.

Goldman, A. Clinical tetany by forced respiration. *Journal of the American Medical Association,* 1922, *78,* 1193–1195.

Haldane, J.S., and Poulton, E.P. The effects of want of oxygen on respiration. *Journal of Physiology*, 1908, *37*, 390–407.

Hardonk, H.J., and Beumer, H.M. Hyperventilation syndrome. In P.J. Vinken, and G.W. Bruyn (Eds.), *Handbook of neurology*. Vol. 38. Amsterdam: North Holland Biomedical Press, 1979.

Howell, J.B.L. Behavioural breathlessness. *Thorax*, 1990, *45*, 287–292.

Juniper, E.F., Frith, P.A., Dunnett, C., Cockcroft, D.W., and Hargreave, F.E. Reproducibility and comparison of responses to inhaled histamine and methacholine. *Thorax*, 1978, *33*, 705–710.

Kerr, W.J., Dalton, J.W., and Gliebe, P.A. Some physical phenomena associated with the anxiety states and their relation to hyperventilation. *Annals of Internal Medicine*, 1937, *11*, 961–992.

Kraft, A.R., and Hoogduin, C.A.L. The hyperventilation syndrome. A pilot study of the effectiveness of treatment. *British Journal of Psychiatry*, 1984, *145*, 534–542.

Lewis, B.I. Chronic hyperventilation syndrome. *Journal of the American Medical Association*, 1954, *155*, 1204–1208.

Lourenco, R.V., Turino, G.M., Davidson, L.A.G., and Fishman, A.P. The regulation of ventilation in diffuse pulmonary fibrosis. *American Journal of Medicine*, 1965, *38*, 199–216.

Lum, L.C. The syndromes of habitual chronic hyperventilation. In O.W. Hill (Ed.), *Modern trends in psychosomatic medicine*. Vol. 3. London: Butterworths, 1976.

McFadden, E.R., and Lyons, H.A. Arterial blood gas tension in asthma. *New England Journal of Medicine*, 1968, *278*, 1027–1032.

Magarian, G.J. Hyperventilation syndromes: Infrequently recognized common expressions of anxiety and stress. *Medicine* (Baltimore), 1982, *61*, 219–236.

Nixon, P.G.F., and Freeman, L. The "think test": A further technique to elicit hyperventilation. *Journal of Royal Society of Medicine*, 1988, *81*, 277–279.

Noehren, T.H. Hyperventilation syndrome and its relation to pulmonary emphysema. *Medicine* (New York), 1966, *66*, 1076–1080.

Okel, B.B., and Hurst, J.W. Prolonged hyperventilation in man. *Archives of Internal Medicine*, 1961, *108*, 757–762.

Pilsbury, D., and Hibbert, G. An ambulatory system for long term continuous monitoring of transcutaneous Pco_2. *Bulletin Europeen Physiopathologie Respiratoire*, 1987, *23*, 9–13.

Salkovskis, P.M., and Clark, D.M. Cognitive and physiological processes in the maintenance and treatment of panic attacks. In I. Hand and H.-V. Wittchen (Eds.), *Panic and phobias*. Heidelberg: Springer Verlag, 1986.

Saltzman, H.A., Heyman, A., and Sieker, H.D. Correlation of clinical and physiologic manifestations of sustained hyperventilation. *New England Journal of Medicine*, 1963, *268*, 1431–1436.

Skatrud, J.B., Dempsey, J.A., and Kaiser, D.G. Ventilatory responses to medroxyprogesterone acetate in normal subjects: Time course and mechanisms. *Journal of Applied Physiology*, 1978, *44*, 939–944.

Szucs, M.M., Brooks, H.L., Grossman, W., Banas, J.S., Meister, S.G., Dexter, L., and Dalen, J.E. Diagnostic sensitivity of laboratory findings in acute embolism. *Annals of Internal Medicine*, 1971, *74*, 161–166.

Temple, A.R. Acute and chronic effects of aspirin toxity and their treatment. *Archives of Internal Medicine*, 1981, *141*. 364–369.

Tucker, W.I. Diagnosis and treatment of the phobic reaction. *American Journal of Psychiatry*, 1956, *112*, 825–830.

Vanamee, P., Poppell, J.W., Glicksman, A.S., Randall, H.T., and Robert, K.E. Respiratory alkalosis in hepatic coma. *Archives of Internal Medicine*, 1956, *97*, 762–767.

Wientjes, C., Grossman, P., and Defares, P. Psychosomatic symptoms, anxiety and hyperventilation in normal subjects. *Bulletin Europeen Physiopathologie Respiratoire*, 1984, *20*, 90–91.

Hyperventilation Syndromes
Physiological Considerations in Clinical Management

L. C. LUM

1. Introduction

This study of Da Costa's syndrome and hyperventilation-based illness spans 25 years and 3500 patients. With the first 2000, clinical diagnosis was backed by laboratory control—spirometry, blood gases, and end-tidal P_{CO_2}; latterly, clinical criteria alone have been used. Measurements rarely enhance the evidence of the experienced eye (Lum, 1975, 1976, 1977, 1978, 1981, 1987).

The treatment regimen that is its central theme rests on its proven effectiveness. It is often criticized as an *uncontrolled* study. But the massive literature accumulated since the time of Da Costa, on uncorrected hyperventilation in its various guises, reveals that in adults, 75 percent persist or get worse; in children, 40 percent of cases still have symptoms in adult life. In contrast, correction of hyperventilation has consistently reversed this outcome: 75 percent completely recover; 90 percent return to normal life. This forms a close analogy with the "waiting list" control widely accepted in America, in which the fate of untreated patients on the waiting list is compared with the fate of those treated. Hyperventilators have waited 120 years for an effective treatment!

These disorders exhibit a profound derangement of mental, nervous, and psychological functions. A rational approach to treatment demands clear under-

L. C. LUM • Department of Chest Medicine (Emeritus), Papworth and Addenbrooke's Hospitals, Cambridge, England.
Behavioral and Psychological Approaches to Breathing Disorders, edited by Beverly H. Timmons and Ronald Ley. Plenum Press, New York, 1994.

standing of the disturbance in function of the central nervous system produced by variations in carbon dioxide. Here I acknowledge my great debt to Professor Barry Wyke, Director of Neurological Research at the Royal College of Surgeons of England, for much personal help (Wyke, 1963, 1969).

An extensive American literature, from 1922 to the 1960s, firmly established hyperventilation as the basis of "neurotic" illness. This was all ignored in England, where Wood's (1941) analysis of Da Costa's syndrome had decisively cast it in the role of psychiatric illness, and eliminated it from the diagnostic repertoire of English physicians. Moreover, the truly general physician was eliminated from the National Health Service by a hierarchic structure demanding early specialization. A watertight barrier separated psychiatry from general medicine, confining them, not only to separate disciplines, but also to separate institutions. Psychoanalytic theory further distanced "neurotic illness" from physiological thought.

Its reemergence (Lum, 1975, 1976; Evans and Lum, 1977) roused considerable resistance, even hostility. The cases presented had been evaluated in a laboratory specifically designed to study derangement of lung function. Nevertheless, it was suggested that we had misdiagnosed asthma, allergies, or merely "nondisease." Consequently, much recent work in England has been a reworking of ideas covered in the earlier American literature. Latterly, however, such objections have been largely discarded, and the central role of overbreathing in panic states, phobias, "nonorganic illness"—even acute schizoid reactions (Allen and Agus, 1968)—has been established. This wider perspective, however, means that it is no longer reasonable to speak simply of *the hyperventilation syndrome*. Rather, we should use the plural *hyperventilation syndromes* (HVS), to cover its diverse presentations. The extensive symptom profile in the Editor's Introduction is a checklist compiled from my own experience. Close questioning, with reference to the checklist, is needed to elicit the full inventory of symptoms.

The water was further muddied by some academics new to the concept, who insisted that a diagnosis of hyperventilation required that the Pco_2 should be consistently below an arbitrary 30 mm Hg. However a syndrome—by definition, a characteristic *combination* of symptoms—cannot be defined or denied by one single measurement. Hyperventilation is commonly episodic; any fall in blood CO_2 causes respiratory alkalosis, even when the Pco_2 remains normal. The overwhelming weight of opinion is that symptoms depend on *lowering* the Pco_2, not on the resting level (Magarian, 1982). An elderly man in chronic respiratory failure with a Pco_2 of 65 mm Hg felt panic when this fell to 55 mm Hg, and he became agoraphobic; all cleared up when he was taught not to overbreathe.

Physicians often fail to make the crucial distinction between hyperventilation and hyperpnea. *Hyperpnea* means obvious panting; hyperventilation—which means simply breathing in excess of metabolic need—is usually quite imperceptible. A short period of hyperventilation depletes body stores of CO_2; once established, hypocapnea can be maintained by apparently normal breathing, with an occasional deep breath or sigh.

2. Etiology

Physicians interpret symptoms in terms of current disease concepts; e.g., neurocirculatory asthenia, soldiers' heart, mitral valve prolapse, allergy, and postviral syndromes are among the many attributions. The lifelong ill health of Florence Nightingale and Charles Darwin was ascribed to heart disease from infections supposedly contracted in the Crimea and the Andes, respectively (Pickering, 1974). Their illnesses have classic features of Da Costa's syndrome, and they died, respectively, at ages 90 and 75! The virus theory (now resurrected as "ME") ignores the fact that bacterial infections, and any pyrexia, may equally well usher in the illness, as may childbirth, operations, anesthesia, acute lung conditions, accidents, or industrial injury. However, it is manifest that, over the years, the symptoms and illness have remained the same—only the attribution has changed.

A careful history usually suggests that the habit of overbreathing is established in early childhood. Eighty percent of the author's female patients give a history of defective bonding with one or both parents—more often the father. The parent may be unable to show physical affection, be overly strict, alcoholic, a wife beater, or just too busy to bond with the child. The child tries to attract affection, or avoid censure, by becoming perfectionist or overly meticulous. In the remaining 20 percent, a history of breathing troubles (asthma, bronchitis, emphysema) or life-threatening illness is often found in the patient's family. Similarly, there may have been loss of a parent by death or divorce. Insecurity tends to carry over into adult relationships. Women, no matter how successful or attractive, almost always have a basic insecurity. The habit is often passed from mother to daughter. Hyperventilating girls tend to be brought by hyperventilating mothers. Men differ. They are often achievers who set goals above their abilities or fail to adjust to changing work patterns, a state pithily described as *promotion depression.*

It needs to be emphasized that hyperventilation is a *normal* response to stress. None is immune. It becomes abnormal when it becomes habitual and when everyday stress produces an excessive and symptomatic response. Prolonged stress with hyperventilation is known to result in increasing responsiveness of the respiratory control system. Whether there is a genetic factor can only be speculative; what is certain is that the hyperventilation threshold can be lowered, and the response exaggerated, by antecedent stress, suggesting that conditioning is the major factor. In everyday terms, an emotional explosion is more likely when we are under prolonged stress than when we are content and relaxed.

Symptoms are clearly influenced by the prevailing emotional state; voluntary overbreathing rarely produces panic in the security of the doctor's office. Acute attacks usually erupt from antecedent and drawn-out stress. Phobic reactions are clearly preceded by anticipatory overbreathing, with sympathetic arousal sensitizing the patient to the feared situation.

Many studies have shown that more than one third of normals overreact to respiratory stimuli. Is it a coincidence that the same proportion of the population suffer from "neurotic" illness?

3. Factors Affecting Symptom Threshold

3.1. Climate, Weather, and Barometric Pressure

Heat and humidity stimulate hyperventilation. Humans as well as dogs pant to lose heat. A steep fall in barometric pressure can do the same. Many patients relate symptoms directly to changing weather patterns; some foretell approaching weather changes by their symptoms. A recent spell of violent storms caused many panic attacks, some requiring admission to hospital. Muscle pains are among the commonest symptoms—farmers predict weather changes from their "rheumatics." Normal breathers feel humid weather as airless and muggy, causing physical and mental lethargy. Fevers likewise directly stimulate the respiratory center.

3.2. Exacerbation of Symptoms at Rest

Overbreathing, if continued for hours or days, continues when the stressor is removed, since the control center becomes set to maintain the lower level of P_{CO_2}. There is a loss of fine tuning, so that breathing does not accurately follow changes in activity. In the evening, the breathing appropriate to daytime activity fails to adjust to the lower metabolic need of watching TV or sleeping. As a corollary, the commonest situation for panic attacks is driving a car (maximum stimulation with minimum exertion); next commonest are watching TV and in bed! Likewise, symptoms are often provoked or exacerbated on holiday. Hyperventilators seem to keep going while the pressure is on, and crack when it is lifted.

3.3. Menstruation

Progesterone, secreted during the postovulation phase, is a considerable respiratory stimulant. During the premenstrual week the Pa_{CO_2} can fall by as much as 25 percent. The symptoms of PMT—headache, lethargy, tension, irritability—are all common manifestations of overbreathing.

3.4. The Voice

Singers and actors (and wind instrumentalists) are particularly vulnerable. Hyperventilation has terminated many singing careers. Rosa Ponselle, one of the greatest dramatic sopranos, fainted outright on her audition, panicked on her Metropolitan debut with Caruso, and was so plagued with stage fright that she retired prematurely at the height of her career.

3.5. Blood Glucose

Blood glucose is of crucial importance and is considered below (Section 5.1.).

4. Perception of Internal and External Environment

The widespread symptoms (Rice, 1950; Lum, 1976), aptly described as a "welter of disturbing bodily sensations" are the more disturbing for lack of apparent cause, and even more so because of their alien nature. Sensations evoked by chemical stimulation of nerves and cortical neurons have no counterpart in everyday experience; hence, their bizarre quality, and the patient's difficulty in describing them—an imprecision that reinforces the idea that it is "all in the mind." Suicidal thoughts are common; some patients admit to having actively prepared for suicide. One patient had accumulated lethal doses of sedatives. She said, in effect, "My body no longer feels nor works like mine; I get unpleasant sensations I can't interpret, even my mind no longer seems the same. Life on this plane is not worth living." Hyperventilators have good reason for anxiety, depression, or both.

4.1. Hallucinations

Hallucinations are rarely volunteered without specific inquiry, but are occasionally admitted (Allen and Agus, 1968). They reinforce fear of madness.

4.2. Depersonalization and Unreality

Feelings of unreality and distortion of the body image are common and frightening, as are occasional out of the body sensations. Cerebral function during hyperventilation is impaired both by hypoxia (see Section 5.3.) and by a reduction in the activating drive from the brain stem reticular system.

The reticular system controls cortical arousal; consciousness, emotional drive, and autonomic tone depend on it. Primary sensory tracts, carrying light, sound, touch, bodily sensations, etc. by which we experience our body and the environment, pass through it on their way to the brain. Here, impulses may be blocked, amplified, and routed to cortical areas serving emotion, endocrine arousal, and short- or long-term memory. Primary sensation itself is uncolored by emotional affect or association. Reticular cells add color, warmth, and associations, via tracts that it sends to the cortex, limbic system, and hypothalamus (Wyke 1963).

The activity of these reticular cells is controlled directly by CO_2: increase stimulates, and hypocapnea depresses. Hence, as hypocapnea deepens, cortical arousal and affect diminish, perception of self and the environment dims; the landscape of the mind becomes drained of warmth and color, distant and unreal. The extreme is stupor progressing to coma. These changes in consciousness are mirrored in the EEG.

Thus hypocapnea exerts an all-pervasive influence on the nervous system: on consciousness and lucidity, on nerve transmission, and on the balance of autonomic activity. It profoundly affects perception of self and the environment, and adaptation of the internal response to environmental change.

5. Physiological Mechanisms

5.1. Blood Glucose

The cerebral effects of hypocapnea are well known. Their dependence on the blood glucose level is generally overlooked. Symptoms of hypoglycemia resemble those of hypocapnea. Faintness, weakness, cold sweats, and disturbance of consciousness are common to both, since the brain is fueled by glucose as well as by oxygen. It is not surprising, therefore, that the effects of hyperventilation on consciousness (and on the EEG) are greatly influenced by the blood sugar. They are aggravated by *coincident* hypoxia and hypoglycemia, and minimized when both Pao_2 and blood glucose are high. During overbreathing, both EEG and cortical function begin to deteriorate as glucose values fall below 100 mg%. The effect of 3 minutes of hyperventilation is slight when the blood sugar is in the 85–90 mg% range, but, with a blood sugar of 70–75 mg%, a similar period of overbreathing can produce gross disturbances of consciousness and of the EEG (Engel *et al.*, 1947). It should be noted that these values are well within the *normal range* of fasting blood sugar.

Clinically, a hypoglycemic effect is likely when symptoms cluster in late morning or late afternoon. By the same token it may be more difficult to elicit a positive provocation test if the patient has eaten an hour beforehand. Depersonalization and feelings of unreality are more likely when blood sugar is low, and these symptoms should direct inquiry to the diet.

Paradoxically, a high carbohydrate diet is *not* desirable. Carbohydrates tend to produce a rapid rise in glucose, followed by a sharp fall to fasting levels or below. Hypoglycemic symptoms are likely to occur during the fall, even when glucose is within the normal range. Proteins, on the other hand, cause a moderate and prolonged rise in blood sugar, lasting several hours. The ideal diet then, has a high protein intake spread evenly throughout the day. The blood glucose is particularly important in panic attacks and any form of seizure. Panic, and occasionally seizures, may occur only at times when this is low. In two cases, previously diagnosed as epileptic, diet and breathing control abolished all seizures.

5.2. Respiratory Alkalosis

Alkalosis alone cannot fully explain the symptoms. Altitude adaptation allows residents at high altitudes to remain well despite chronic respiratory alkalosis. In symptomatic hyperventilation, however, the PCO_2 fluctuates, often wildly, (Lum, 1981), causing a constantly changing pH in nerve cells and tissue fluid to which no adaptation is possible (Fig. 1).

5.3. Hypoxia

Cerebral vascular constriction is the first and most direct response to hyperventilation, reducing available oxygen by about half. Of all body tissues, the

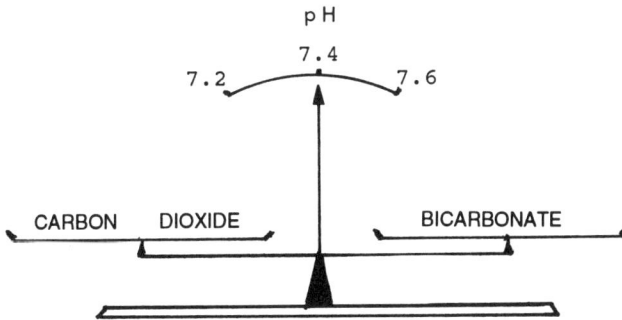

Figure 1. The interlocking relationship between pH, carbon dioxide, and bicarbonate. The blood is slightly alkaline, with a pH of approximately 7.4. This is maintained by the ratio of CO_2 to bicarbonate ion. Significant amounts of CO_2 can be lost in a few minutes of overbreathing, immediately causing respiratory alkalosis. Compensation, by excretion of bicarbonate, is relatively slow and may take hours or days.

cerebral cortex is the most vulnerable to hypoxia. Cortical activity is depressed, causing dizziness, vasomotor instability, and blurring of consciousness as well as vision. Loss of cortical inhibition commonly results in crying and emotional lability.

5.4. Loss of CO_2 from Neurons

During moderate hyperventilation, loss of CO_2 ions from neurons stimulates neuronal activity, causing increased sensory and motor discharges, muscular tension and spasm, speeding of spinal reflexes, heightened perception (photophobia, hyperacusis), and other sensory disturbances. More profound hypocapnea, however, increasingly depresses activity. Finally, the nerve cell becomes inert. This parallels the clinical state: initial alertness with increased activity, progressing through decreased alertness, to stupor and coma.

5.5. Tetany

Tetany has been traditionally ascribed to alkalosis, but its cause, as well as the role of increased calcium ions, is not fully understood. It is certainly secondary to the alkalosis. A Pco_2, of around 20 mm Hg—at which electrical discharges in experimental nerve preparations are at their greatest—is also about the point at which tetany appears in humans.

The muscles that maintain the "attack defense" posture—hunched shoulders, jutting head, clenched teeth, scowling—are those most prone to develop muscular spasm. Painful nodules are readily felt in the shoulder girdle, the nape of the neck, and the anterior chest. Temporal headache, from dull ache to classic migraine, centers on such nodules in the parietal region. Less common are general limb pains, particularly in the legs, with a tendency to spasm of whole muscle groups. The whole body expresses tension; patients do not know how to relax in any posture.

5.6. Sympathetic Dominance

Sympathetic dominance is evidenced by dilated pupils, dry mouth, sweaty palms, gut and digestive dysfunction, abdominal bloating, and tachycardia.

5.7. Allergies

Overbreathing increases circulating histamine (Kontos et al., 1972). There is a high incidence of allergies. Some patients report food intolerance during exacerbations, which disappear during good phases.

6. Pseudoallergy

Strong perfumes or other smells may trigger hyperventilation; dizziness, faintness, collapse, are then thought to be an allergic response. The total allergy syndrome (now discredited) postulated allergy to pollutants that are now universal (smoke, exhaust fumes, and all petrochemicals). In industry, outbreaks of dizziness, nausea, headache, and collapse often follow spillage of pungent, but harmless, chemicals. Drug reactions may also reflect hyperventilation; salbutamol (to which asthmatics are prone) facilitates overbreathing. Tremors, tachycardia, and headache can often be abolished by appropriate breathing instruction. Collapse following dental injections is often due to needle phobia rather than to the anesthetic agent (Lum, 1985).

7. Panic and Phobic States

Panic feelings are common, often associated with the misattribution of symptoms, to imply sudden threat to life or sanity. Of 701 cases of HVS seen over a six-year period, panic attacks occurred in 131 (19 percent) and phobic avoidance in 213 (30 percent). The remaining 51 percent had mainly somatic symptoms (Lum, 1987). As the initial diagnosese were made by general practitioners, these figures are probably representative of the incidence in the general population.

7.1. Sex Distribution

Among those with somatic symptoms only, there was a small preponderance of men (53 percent of total). However, twice as many women had panic attacks and four times as many, showed phobic avoidance tendencies.

8. Implications for Treatment

8.1. Breathing Retraining

Breathing retraining remains the core of treatment. The aim is to suppress thoracic breathing and restore slow, regular diaphragmatic breathing (Cluff, 1984). However, reattribution of symptoms to hyperventilation, and attention to the physiological factors discussed here, are imperative.

8.2. Diet

The blood sugar plays a significant role for the majority of patients; it may be the key factor in epileptiform seizures and in panic attacks. The importance of a high protein intake spread evenly throughout the day is certain. Frequent carbohydrate nibbling aggravates symptoms. Caffeine and other respiratory stimulants should clearly be avoided.

8.3. Education

Patients must learn to recognize situations and times (e.g., premenstrual) that make them more vulnerable. Parties, social occasions, and family reunions, with much talking, can be disastrous. Most overbreathers are fast and breathless talkers and must learn to modify speech patterns. Moving house and building alterations rank with work stress and marital discord as precipitants of overbreathing.

8.4. Relaxation

Hyperventilators live in a state of unremitting tension, which shows in every attitude and movement: sitting, standing, walking, driving a car, or even holding a pen. They must learn to express the body language of relaxation in all these situations. Walking with a relaxed, limber gait, is important in the relief of painful back muscles.

8.5. Hypnotherapy

Hypnosis is a powerful tool in deconditioning phobics. Self-hypnosis is often helpful in panic and free-floating anxiety.

8.6. Self-Understanding

It is essential that patients recognize their own weaknesses. They must resist those inner drives which impel them to take on more than they can handle. Often this translates into learning to say "no." A gain in assertiveness often signals a turning point in treatment.

9. Summary

The good doctor, like a good judge, bases his judgment on a balance of probabilities. The physician faced with a sick patient cannot be confined by overstrict diagnostic criteria appropriate to research. He will not withhold treatment of proven effectiveness because of academic quibbling. He is well aware that, even in the presence of organic disease, relaxation and breathing exercises can alleviate symptoms of stress. Alleviation will not cause him to ignore the possibility of underlying pathology.

This paper discusses aspects of hyperventilation generally unfamiliar to workers in this field. It places breathing retraining in the context of environmental, occupational, dietary, and other factors usually ignored. Space dictates a highly selective treatment of physiology and the omission of many important topics (e.g., the provocation test). These are adequately treated elsewhere (Lum, 1981, 1987).

10. References

Allen, T.E., and Agus, B. Hyperventilation leading to hallucinations. *American Journal of Psychiatry* 1968, *125*, 632–637.

Beumer, H.J., and Hardonk, H.K. Hyperventilation syndrome. In P.J. Vinken and D.W. Bruyn (Eds.), *Handbook of clinical neurology. Vol. 38*. Amsterdam: North-Holland Publishing Company, 1979, pp. 309–360.

Cluff, R.C. Chronic hyperventilation and its treatment by physiotherapy. *Journal of the Royal Society of Medicine*, 1984, *77*, 855–862.

Engel, G.L., Ferris, E.B., and Logan, M. Hyperventilation: Analysis of clinical symptomatology. *Annals of Internal Medicine*, 1947, *27*, 683–704.

Evans, D.W., and Lum, L.C. Hyperventilation: An important cause of pseudoangina. *Lancet*, 1977, pp. 155–157.

Kontos, H.A., Richardson, D.W., Raper, A.J., Zubair-ul-Hassan, and Patterson, J.L. Mechanism of action of hypocapnic alkalosis on limb blood vessels in man and dog. *American Journal of Physiology*, 1972, *223*, 1296–1307.

Lum, L.C. Hyperventilation: the tip and the iceberg. *Journal of Psychosomatic Research*, 1975, *19*, 375–383.

Lum, L.C. The syndrome of habitual chronic hyperventilation. In O. Hill (Ed.), *Modern Trends in Psychosomatic Medicine. Vol. 3*. London: Butterworths, 1976, pp. 196–230.

Lum, L.C. Breathing exercises in the treatment of hyperventilation and chronic anxiety states. *Chest Heart and Stroke Journal*, Spring, 1977, *2*, 6–11.

Lum, L.C. Respiratory alkalosis and hypocarbia. The role of carbon dioxide in the body economy. *Chest Heart and Stroke Journal*, Winter, 1978/79, *3*, 31–34.

Lum, L.C. Hyperventilation and anxiety state. *Journal of the Royal Society of Medicine*, 1981, *74*, 1–4.

Lum, L.C. Hyperventilation and pseudo-allergic reactions. In P. Dukor, P. Kallos, H.D. Schlumberger, and G.B. West (Eds.), *Pseudo-allergic reactions. 4*. Basel: Karger, 1985, pp. 106–118.

Lum, L.C. Hyperventilation syndromes in medicine and psychiatry: A review. *Journal of the Royal Society of Medicine*, 1987, *80*, 229–231.

Magarian, G. Hyperventilation syndromes: Infrequently recognized common expressions of anxiety and stress. *Medicine*, 1982, *61*, 219–236.

Pickering, Sir G. *Creative malady*. London: Allen and Unwin, 1974.

Rice, R.L. Symptom patterns of the hyperventilation syndrome. *American Journal of Medicine*, 1950, *8*, 691–700.

Wood, P. Aetiology of DaCosta's syndrome. *British Medical Journal*, 1941, *1*, 845–851.

Wyke, B. *Brain function and metabolic disorders*. London: Butterworths, 1963.

Wyke, B. *Principles of general neurology*. London: Elsevier, 1969.

8

Psychiatric and Respiratory Aspects of Functional Cardiovascular Syndromes

CHRISTOPHER BASS, WILLIAM N. GARDNER, AND GRAHAM JACKSON

1. Introduction

Patients who exhibit morbid concern about their heart yet do not present symptoms suggestive of heart disease are more likely to be referred to the psychiatrist than to the cardiologist. The fear may range from phobic concern, hypochondriacal preoccupation, to delusional conviction.

A much larger group of patients complain of symptoms referred to the heart or suggestive of heart disease, but have no evidence of it. Patients with these *functional cardiovascular syndromes* (FCSs) report a characteristic array of symptoms, and in most published accounts breathlessness is one of the most frequently reported complaints (Wood, 1968). Indeed, Cohen and White (1947) remarked that, "respiratory symptoms constituted a characteristic and therefore diagnostic feature of *neurocirculatory asthenia* (NA), a term used by American authors to describe patients with FCSs. Thus FCS is a term that encompasses a heterogeneous group of disorders that comprise psychological, cardiovascular, and respiratory symptoms in varying proportions. These essentially *polysymptomatic* disorders are the subject of this chapter.

CHRISTOPHER BASS • Department of Psychological Medicine, John Radcliffe Hospital, Headington, Oxford OX3 9D4, England.   *WILLIAM N. GARDNER* • Department of Thoracic Medicine, Kings College School of Medicine and Dentistry, London SE5 9PJ, England. *GRAHAM JACKSON* • Cardiac Department, Guy's Hospital, London SE1 9RT, England.
Behavioral and Psychological Approaches to Breathing Disorders, edited by Beverly H. Timmons and Ronald Ley. Plenum Press, New York, 1994.

2. Psychiatric Aspects

Freud (1962) was among the first to realize that anxiety could present in the guise of somatic symptoms, or "anxiety equivalents." His views were not universally accepted, however, possibly because much of the subsequent work on patients with FCSs was conducted by physicians, who considered an organic etiology most likely. There were many reports of the cardiovascular manifestations of anxiety published before the Second World War. This literature was recently reviewed by Skerritt (1983).

In a collaborative study with the psychiatrists Maxwell Jones and Aubrey Lewis, the cardiologist Paul Wood eventually established the importance of psychological factors in the etiology of these disorders (Wood, 1941a–c). They found that these patients could be assigned a variety of psychiatric diagnoses, notably, anxiety neurosis, depression, psychopathic personality, and hysteria (Jones and Lewis, 1941).

In an attempt to clarify the terminology in this field, Wood suggested that the eponym *Da Costa's syndrome* was the most appropriate term for FCSs, giving credit to the eminent American physician who published the original description of the disorder 70 years previously (Da Costa, 1871). Surprisingly, the term Da Costa's syndrome has been retained by most British (but not American) physicians and modern textbooks of medicine (Somerville, 1983) to describe patients with FCSs.

The psychoanalyst Erik Wittkower and his colleagues were among the first to point out the important relationship between a *phobic* tendency and *breathlessness* in patients with FCSs (Wittkower *et al.*, 1941). In certain situations such as crowds and confined spaces, phobic patients became anxious and developed breathlessness and chest tightness that mimicked angina. This important association between *situational* factors and somatic symptoms of anxiety in patients with FCSs will be referred to later.

Marks and Lader (1973) remarked that the numerous names given to conditions characterized by emotional and cardiovascular symptoms were indistinguishable from anxiety states. They estimated that the prevalence of anxiety states in a normal population was 2.0–4.7 percent in Britain and the United States, and that these disorders accounted for 10–14 percent of patients in cardiology practices in those countries. Similar views were expressed by the American psychiatrist Lipowski (1980), who noted that most psychiatrists viewed NA as a clinical variant of anxiety disorder.

More recently, American psychiatrists have suggested that the symptomatology in patients with FCSs is embodied in the DSM-III-R (American Psychiatric Association, 1987) description of *panic disorder*. This is characterized by anxiety that is particularly severe (panic), situational, somatic, and accompanied by a variety of other physical symptoms, such as breathlessness and chest pain. If panic symptoms persist, the syndrome is said to lead to phobic avoidance.

The British psychiatrist, Tyrer (1985), has criticized this tendency in DSM-III-R to separate a specific "medical model" panic syndrome from the main body of anxiety disorders. Psychiatric nosology has always found it difficult to accommodate the diverse modes of presentation of anxiety, especially when the anxiety is accompanied by multiple somatic complaints. The shortcomings of psychiatric classification are reflected in the numerous synonyms that have been used to characterize these patients since 1864 (Table 1).

Tyrer (1976a) has discussed why so many of these conditions have been described as though they were separate entities. He pointed out that there are two parts to each condition, a disorder of cardiac function with appropriate symptoms and signs, and a diffuse mixture of nonspecific symptoms attributable to anxiety. The latter include palpitations, dyspnea, dizziness, weakness, lability of mood,

Table 1
Da Costa's Syndrome Synonyms: 1869–1980[a]

Year	Description	Author
1864	Muscular exhaustion of heart	Hartshorne
1869	Neurasthenia	Beard
1871	Irritable heart	Da Costa
1873	Cerebrocardiac neuropathia	Krishaber
1894	Anxiety neurosis	Freud
1901	Cardiac neurosis	Herrick
1914–18	Soldier's heart	British Army
	Disordered action of the heart (DAH)	
1917	Effort syndrome	T. Lewis
1918	Neurocirculatory asthenia	Oppenheimer *et al.*
1938	Hyperventilation syndrome	Soley and Shock
1939	Cardiovascular neurosis	Caughey
1941	Da Costa's syndrome	Wood
1952	Psychophysiologic cardiovascular reaction	DSM-I
?	Vasomotor neurosis	Friedman
1957	Vasoregulatory asthenia	Holmgren
1962	Hyperkinetic heart syndrome	Gorlin
1966	Hyperdynamic beta-adrenergic circulatory state	Frohlich
1968	Psychophysiologic cardiovascular disorder	DSM-II
1968	Nervous heart complaint	Nordenfelt
1971	Autonomically mediated cardiovascular functional disorder	Marsden
1980	Psychogenic cardiac nondisease	Lipowski
1980	Panic disorder	DSM-III

[a]Adapted (and extended) from Cohen and White (1951).

and *hyperventilation*. Relative preponderance of one or more of these symptoms accounts for the variation in adjectives used to describe these disorders. Another reason for the plethora of synonyms is that these patients consult various hospital specialists, who each perceives the array of symptoms from the viewpoint of the symptoms relevant to his or her own speciality. Hence, psychiatrists ascribe the cardiovascular manifestations to anxiety (Marks and Lader, 1973), cardiologists invoke augmented adrenergic activity (Frohlich *et al.*, 1966), and chest physicians perceive the symptoms as consequences of hyperventilation (Lum, 1976). The etiologic significance of hyperventilation will be discussed in later sections.

In summary, at least one in ten patients who attend cardiac clinics have FCS: a substantial number of these report phobic symptoms or have phobic neuroses (Bass and Wade, 1984; Cohen and White, 1951; Wood, 1941). These neurotic symptoms frequently antedate the onset of cardiovascular symptoms and should always be inquired after. Of the multiple somatic symptoms reported by these patients, breathlessness and chest pain are the most common, and these complaints often have a marked situational component. The problem is complicated by the fact that a proportion of patients with multiple somatic complaints may deny or minimize psychological problems (Bass and Gardner, 1985; Tyrer, 1976a). These patients who habitually somatize psychological conflict or distress may be more difficult to treat than patients who both acknowledge and report symptoms of anxiety (see Sections 4 and 5).

3. Respiratory Aspects

3.1. Breathlessness in FCSs

We have already emphasized that breathlessness is one of the cardinal complaints in patients with FCSs. This may be expressed by the patient as an inability to take a satisfactory breath, "air hunger," or feelings of suffocation or breathlessness provoked by trivial physical exertion or change in posture (Cohen and White, 1947; Wittkower *et al.*, 1941). These complaints may be accompanied by the clinical sign of sighing or gasping, which, in severe cases, may be audible.

Studies of respiratory variables in patients with FCSs have revealed a number of consistent findings. These patients are more likely to have sighing or "suspirious" respirations (White and Hahn, 1929) and significantly higher resting respiratory rates, with smaller tidal volume and shorter breath-holding times, than controls (Jones and Skarisbrick, 1941). In addition, there is a more marked increase in minute volume *after* exercise in patients compared with controls (Cohen and White, 1947). The latter authors speculated that high blood lactate concentration during and after exercise in these patients may act as a stimulus to augmented ventilation. The hypothesis advanced by Pitts and McClure (1967) that elevating the serum lactate (by infusion) in anxiety neurotics at rest could *cause* anxiety symptoms was based on this observation.

More recently, Bass *et al.* (1983) found that complaints of gasping and sighing at rest and "air hunger" were reported by three-quarters of patients with chest pain resembling angina pectoris but with normal coronary arteries. There was an association between complaints of breathlessness and psychiatric problems in these patients, all of whom had normal lung function. Mean end-tidal Pco_2 was significantly lower in these patients than in a control group with obstructive coronary lesions. Because one-quarter of the breathless patients without significant coronary lesions had resting end-tidal Pco_2 within the normal range (35–45 mm Hg), it was suggested that hyperventilation (or hypocapnia) may not always accompany subjective complaints of breathlessness. Alternatively, hyperventilation may occur at times other than during laboratory measurement. The role of hyperventilation as an etiological factor in FCSs merits further discussion.

3.2. Hyperventilation as an Etiological Factor in FCSs

There is a current tendency to regard the hyperventilation syndrome (HVS) and functional heart disease as synonymous (Hardonk and Beumer, 1979; Magarian, 1982). In our view this is unjustified; the psychopathology in these functional syndromes is diverse, and the varied symptomatology is not the result of a single pathophysiological mechanism.

The reproduction of chest pain during a period of forced overbreathing is often accepted as evidence that HV is the most likely etiologic factor. But of the diverse somatic symptoms that can occur in symptomatic HV, chest pain is probably the least reproducible following provocation. Thus in most studies of patients with FCSs whose symptoms are ascribed to HV, less than half are reported to experience chest pain during provocation.

For example, Evans and Lum (1977) studied 50 patients who had been referred to a respiratory physiology laboratory for further investigations of angina pectoris, which the cardiologist considered likely to be of a hyperventilatory origin. In 37 patients there was no evidence of organic heart disease. They termed the chest pain in these patients *pseudoangina,* since it possessed characteristics that were both typical and atypical of angina pectoris, and concluded that HV was responsible for the symptoms in all of the 50 cases. Laboratory diagnosis was based on a typical spirometric pattern, low or low-normal resting Pco_2, and/or on the reproduction of chest pain by voluntary overbreathing. Half the patients with hyperventilation had end-tidal Pco_2 within the normal range (≥ 35

mm Hg), and precordial pain was reproduced in half the 50 patients after 2–3 minutes of forced breathing. This study highlights the difficulties in establishing the diagnosis of HVS (see Chapter 6).

In a more recent study, Bass et al. (1990) found that chest pain complaints were reproduced in only 39 percent of patients with chest pain but negative treadmill exercise tests. These patients had lower resting end-tidal Pco_2 and shorter breath-holding times than those in whom chest pain was not reproduced. In this study chest pain was reproduced in five patients simply by asking the patient to breath-hold (Chambers et al., 1988). Mechanical factors are clearly involved in the production of this type of pain (see Section 3.3).

These findings suggest that (1) FCSs are not synonymous with HVS (2) subjective reports of breathlessness do not necessarily imply that the patient is hypocapnic and (3) even when the diagnosis of HVS is made (and this is a contentious issue—Chapter 6), voluntary hyperventilation (VHV) fails to reproduce chest pain in about half the subjects in whom it is attempted. Nevertheless, patients with FCSs in whom breathlessness is a prominent symptom should be subjected to both a breath-holding test and VHV because these may yield information that may be of important practical use to the therapist; both procedures may reproduce chest pain and demonstrate the true etiology of the pain to the patient. However, these tests may be potentially dangerous in patients with compromised coronary circulations (see Sections 3.4 and 4.2). The nature and origin of the chest pain in patients with functional heart disease has been the subject of numerous investigations, and calls for some discussion.

3.3. The Etiology of Chest Pain in Functional Heart Disorders

It is often assumed that the chest pain in patients with symptomatic hyperventilation is "psychogenic." This is not the case. Overbreathers have real, chest-localized sensations of varying intensity, which may or may not be painful. The mechanisms by which these chest sensations arise following overbreathing include intercostal muscle tension or spasm and intercostal muscle fatigue.

Friedman (1945) was one of the first to demonstrate that chest pain in patients with FCSs and exaggerated thoracic breathing was of musculoskeletal origin. He conducted a study, which is unlikely to be repeated, in which patients with NA had their upper chest walls immobilized with tight strapping for six days. After two days the chest pain was abolished in all patients, but it reappeared when the adhesive tape was removed. Friedman also demonstrated that healthy volunteers developed considerable tachypnea and dyspnea during exercise when they were forced to breathe almost exclusively from the upper third of the chest (he immobilized the lower third of the chest and upper abdomen with tight strapping). Nine of these ten subjects subsequently developed precordial pain after exercise, and the pain disappeared after the adhesive tape restraints were removed. This musculoskeletal pain appears to be independent of respiratory alkalosis, and it is not related to absolute levels of arterial Pco_2 (Hibbert and Pilsbury, 1989).

Other suggested causes of chest pain in patients with symptomatic HV are pressure on the diaphragm by a distended stomach (a consequence of aerophagy), spasm of the diaphragm, and coronary artery vasoconstriction (Magarian, 1982). The latter will be considered in the next section.

Psychological factors are also important. Tyrer *et al.* (1980) demonstrated that in anxious and hypochondriacal patients with predominantly cardiac symptoms, much of the patients' somatic preoccupation was explained by *heightened levels of cardiac awareness*. These patients were troubled by symptoms from essentially normal physiological activity, and the reason for their sensitive awareness of bodily function was in turn probably related to personality, attributional factors (the pain may be maintained and aggravated by the belief that it arises in the heart), and iatrogenic factors.

Thus, the chest pain in patients with FCSs may be a consequence of diverse etiological factors, some of which may act concurrently. In patients with symptomatic HV in whom chest pain is reproduced by VHV, the symptom is invariably musculoskeletal in origin (and often accompanied by chest wall tenderness). In the absence of demonstrable HV, chest-localized sensations produced by palpitations may become a focus for somatic preoccupation. In addition, anxious patients often become hypervigilant, which leads them to examine their bodily sensations more closely than they normally would.

3.4. Effects of Hyperventilation on Cardiovascular Function

Hyperventilation can induce marked constriction of coronary arterioles, while inhibiting transfer of oxygen from hemoglobin to tissue cells (Bohr effect). In addition, hyperventilation induces increased heart rate and cardiac output, constriction of skin blood vessels, and dilatation of muscle and splanchnic vessels among normal individuals, as well as inhibiting the carotid baroreflex and shifting the blood acid balance toward alkalosis (Magarian, 1982).

A number of ECG abnormalities commonly occur during hyperventilation in both normal subjects and patients with chest pain and normal coronary arteries (Lary and Goldschlager, 1974). These include T wave flattening, S-T segment depression, prolonged Q-T periods, and sinus tachycardia.

This ECG evidence of ischemia may reflect metabolic myocardial abnormalities. Hyperventilation leads to a progressive fall in CO_2, and lactic acid is produced as a result of myocardial hypoxia. Sympathetic nervous activity becomes dominant, increasing myocardial demand for oxygen at a time of lactic acidosis. As a result, the myocardium may become more ischemic, and ECG abnormalities may occur as a consequence of this hyperventilation-induced metabolic lactic acidosis.

It is conceivable that hypocapnic alkalosis resulting from hyperventilation may produce vasospasm with ischemic ECG changes and chest pain in patients with normal coronary arteries. Such a series of events was recently suggested by Freeman and Nixon (1985) as a possible pathophysiological mechanism in a 62-year-old man with normal coronary arteries and repeated episodes of chest pain. Symptomatic hyperventilation was confirmed in this patient by a demonstration of profound arterial hypocapnia during a spontaneous episode of chest pain with S-T segment elevation. Although his resting end-tidal P_{CO_2} was normal, it was possible to reproduce chest pain and S-T elevation, in those leads in which the elevation occurred in the spontaneous attack, by asking him to hyperventilate.

In summary, hyperventilation can produce (1) pseudoischaemic ECG changes in normal subjects, and (2) can precipitate myocardial infarction in patients with obstructive coronary lesions (Lisker and Leff, 1983). Because of this, concurrent ECG monitoring should be mandatory in patients with established or suspected heart disease who are subjected to VHV.

4. Assessment

Both noncardiac causes of chest pain (such as disorders of the esophagus and thoracic spine) and cardiac causes should be excluded before a patient is assigned a diagnosis of functional chest pain (Areskog and Tibbling, 1981). In this section we will review the investigative sequence that should be undertaken to differentiate between these various causes of chest pain.

4.1. Cardiac Assessment

Characteristics of the chest pain and associated clinical features are of limited value in discriminating between cardiac and noncardiac sources of pain (Areskog and Tibbling, 1981). Bass (1984) used discriminant function analysis in an attempt to predict which patients undergoing coronary angiography had significant coronary heart disease. He found that the following four clinical features predicted the *absence* of significant coronary obstruction: (1) complaints of the need to sigh and gasp at rest; (2) situational breathlessness, i.e., subjective sensation of breathlessness in situations such as crowds or confined spaces; (3) duration of chest pain in excess of five months; and (4) being a psychiatric "case." Pain that was consistently related to physical exertion, precipitated by cold, and relieved with five minutes by glyceryl trinitrate predicted significant coronary obstruction. Surprisingly, pain that was described as tight or gripping, precipitated by emotion, or awakening the patient from sleep had no discriminatory power.

The resting ECG is of limited use, as there are no characteristic ECG changes in patients with FCSs. It may also be normal in the presence of advanced coronary disease.

A treadmill exercise test is obligatory but there are problems with both performance and interpretation. Anxious patients may not be able to complete the test. The exercise may induce hyperventilation with its associated pseudoischemic ECG changes (Bass et al., 1988). Perceptive cardiologists may observe hyperventilation during the test, and a method of measuring end-tidal PCO_2 during the treadmill test has been described by Chambers et al. (1988). Patients identified at this time should receive the appropriate treatment rather than undergo further investigations such as coronary angiography.

The dramatic and persistent nature of cardiovascular complaints in these patients often influences the decision to investigate the patient further with a coronary angiogram. Demonstration of patent coronary arteries will reassure both patient and physician and encourage the search for other possible etiologies. These include disorders of the esophagus, thoracic spine musculoskeletal pain, and hyperventilation with all its various causes.

The main focus of this chapter is on respiratory and psychiatric factors. Esophageal disorders may be present (e.g., diffuse esophageal spasm or *nutcracker esophagus*), although the relevance of these findings to complaints of chest pain is unclear; in some patients they are epiphenomena (Richter et al., 1989).

4.2. Assessment for Evidence of Hyperventilation

Procedures to establish the diagnosis of hyperventilation are described by Gardner in Chapter 6. Hyperventilation and chest pain may be directly related, as described above (Section 3.3), but they may also be unrelated or only indirectly related. As an example of the latter, the sensations of bronchial irritation induced by asthma may be perceived as chest pain by a patient whose asthma has remained undiagnosed. These patients may also have hyperventilation as a direct consequence of their asthma.

A sequence of tests can be performed in a respiratory laboratory to determine whether chest pain is or is not related to respiratory factors. They may also discriminate between pain that is a consequence of coronary spasm (induced by hypocapnia) and mechanical pain that results from excessive chest wall movements. The latter may be associated with evidence of chest wall tenderness (Epstein et al., 1979), which should always be documented.

Once the diagnosis of hyperventilation has been established, the investigations described in Chapter 6 should be performed to exclude possible organic etiologies.

4.3. Psychiatric Assessment

Psychiatric assessment should include inquiry about antecedent life events, personality factors (is the patient habitually anxious), the circumstances in which the symptoms first arose, the duration of the main complaints, and current life stress (chronic social difficulties are likely to be illness-sustaining). Assessment of the mental state may reveal evidence of *anxiety* and *phobic symptoms* (the latter may have antedated the onset of somatic complaints), extreme degrees of *fatigue, somatic preoccupation,* and *depersonalization.* If apprehension or panic accompany the physical symptoms, what fears are entertained during an attack? Many of these patients fear heart disease, and may have either a family history of premature coronary disease or recently suffered a loss of a relative or friend by sudden cardiac death. Some patients, who habitually somatize psychological distress, may have a past history of multiple unexplained physical symptoms involving different organ systems.

It is especially important to elicit the patient's *attribution* of his physical symptoms, as this may have an important bearing on prognosis. For example, patients with a hypochondriacal disposition who retain a belief that their symptoms have an organic basis, despite evidence to the contrary, tend to have a worse prognosis (Greer and Cawley, 1966).

5. Management

5.1. Excluding Organic Disease

This is important (see Section 4) because patients will often not accept reassurance until basic investigations have been completed.

5.2. Explanation and Reassurance

The second phase involves explanation and reassurance that the patient has a genuine disorder to account for the symptoms, and that this disorder has a good prognosis. In some patients explanation and reassurance may be all that is required.

5.3. Cognitive–Behavioral Treatment

This treatment, which is described more fully in Chapter 10, has been shown to be effective in patients with atypical chest pain (Klimes *et al.,* 1990). The treatment can be carried out by psychologists, nurse therapists, or physiotherapists, and often includes breathing exercises such as those described by Innocenti (1987) and De Guire *et al.* (1992). These exercises are aimed at converting the patient from a predominantly thoracic pattern of breathing to a pattern characterized by slow (8–12 breaths per minute), regular diaphragmatic breathing. Although the cognitive component of treatment has been shown to be effective it is less clear whether the breathing retraining adds to the effects of this treatment (see Chapter 10).

5.4. Psychotropic Drugs

We try to avoid prescribing benzodiazepines because of the risk of dependence. Sympathetically mediated symptoms such as palpitations, trembling, and sweating may well respond to beta-blockers (Tyrer, 1976a), which have also been shown to raise Pco_2 in patients who are overbreathing (Folgering and Cox, 1981). If depressive symptoms accompany the somatic complaints, then treatment with tricyclic antidepressants may be required. Monoamine oxidase inhibitors may be indicated in patients with clinical features that include hypochondriacal and phobic symptoms (Tyrer, 1976b). These drugs should be reversed for the more severe and intractable cases.

It is important to retain a *flexible* approach to management (Bass, 1990). For example, for patients with many cardiovascular and respiratory symptoms who deny the psychological aspects of their condition, a somatically-based treatment approach combining beta-blockers and breathing exercises may be indicated. When discrete episodes of hyperventilation-induced panic accompany the cardiovascular, and other, complaints, Salkovskis *et al.* (1986) have shown that a treatment package that combines cognitive therapy and breathing retraining is effective in reducing panic attack frequency. Inpatient admission is recommended for patients whose symptoms are associated with profound hypocapnia (resting end-tidal $Pco_2 < 25$ mm Hg), and for those whose hyperventilation has led to either multiple emergency room admissions or severe functional disability. Admission should be to an appropriate liaison psychiatry bed on a general medical ward, rather than to an inpatient psychiatric unit.

6. Conclusions

Functional cardiovascular syndromes comprise a common and complex group of disorders characterized by psychiatric, cardiovascular, and respiratory symptoms. Because the symptomatology is so diverse, an *interdisciplinary approach* is called for in both the investigation and the management of these patients, a task that is best achieved when there is collaboration between departments of psychiatry, cardiology, and thoracic medicine within the general hospital. Psychiatrists have found it difficult to classify these disorders because (1) the symptoms are so diverse, and (2) there may be no conspicuous psychiatric disturbance. Hyperventilation certainly contributes to, and aggravates, symptoms in a proportion of cases; the frequency with which it is diagnosed depends on the age, sex, and characteristics of the sample studied, as well as the criteria used to establish the diagnosis.

One consistent finding from studies of patients with FCSs is the high incidence of phobic complaints and/or panic anxiety: some of these patients may benefit from a cognitive or behavioral approach to treatment (Klimes *et al.*, 1990). Another important practical point in the management of these patients is that their capacity to respond to the treatment depends to a large extent on their attribution of the somatic complaints and their psychological-mindedness. Patients who continue to attribute the symptoms to a physical disease, despite evidence to the contrary, may prove more refractory to treatment.

7. References

American Psychiatric Association. *Diagnostic and Statistical Manual of Mental Disorders.* 3rd ed., revised. Washington, D.C.: A.P.A., 1987.

Areskog, N.H., and Tibbling, L. Differential diagnostic aspects of chest pain. *Acta Medica Scandinavica, (Suppl.)* 1981, *27,* 664–672.

Bass, C. Unexplained chest pain: Clinical and psychological studies in patients with presumptive angina. Unpublished M.D. dissertation, University of London, 1984.

Bass, C. Functional Cardiorespiratory Syndromes. In C. Bass (Ed.), *Somatization: Physical symptoms and psychological illness.* Oxford: Blackwells, 1990.

Bass, C., and Gardner, W.N. Respiratory and psychiatric abnormalities in chronic symptomatic hyperventilation. *British Medical Journal,* 1985, *290,* 1387–1390.

Bass, C., and Wade, C. Chest pain with normal coronary arteries: A comparative study of psychiatric and social morbidity. *Psychological Medicine,* 1984, *14,* 41–51.

Bass, C., Cawley, R.H., Wade, C., Gardner, W.N., Hutchison, D.C., Ryan, K., and Jackson, G. Unexplained breathlessness and psychiatric morbidity in patients with normal and abnormal coronary arteries. *Lancet,* 1983, *1,* 605–609.

Bass, C., Chambers, J.B., and Gardner, W.N. Hyperventilation provocation in patients with chest pain and a negative treadmill exercise test. *Journal of Psychosomatic Research,* 1990, *35,* 83–89.

Bass, C., Chambers, J.B., Kiff, P.J., Cooper, D., and Gardner, W.N. Panic anxiety and hyperventilation in patients with chest pain: A controlled study. *Quarterly Journal of Medicine,* 1988, *69,* 949–959.

Chambers, J.B., Kiff, P.J., Gardner, W.N., Jackson, G., and Bass, C. Value of measuring end-tidal partial pressure of carbon dioxide as an adjunct to treadmill exercise testing. *British Medical Journal,* 1988, *296,* 1281–1285.

Cohen, M.E., and White, P.D. Studies of breathing, pulmonary ventilation and subjective awareness of shortness of breath (dyspnoea) in neurocirculatory asthenia, effort syndrome, anxiety neurosis. *Journal of Clinical Investigation,* 1947, *26,* 520–529.

Cohen, M.E., and White, P.D. Life situations, emotions, and neurocirculatory asthenia (anxiety neurosis, neurasthenia, effort syndrome). *Psychosomatic Medicine,* 1951, *13,* 335–357.

Da Costa, J.M. On irritable heart: A clinical study of a form of functional cardiac disorder and its consequences. *American Journal of Medical Sciences,* 1871, *61,* 17–52.

De Guire, S., Gevirtz, R., Kawahara, Y., and Maguire, W. Hyperventilation syndrome and the assessment of treatment for functional cardiac symptoms. *American Journal of Cardiology,* 1992, *70,* 673–677.

Epstein, S.E., Gerber, L.H., and Borer, J.S. Chest wall syndrome: A common cause of unexplained cardiac pain. *Journal of the American Medical Association,* 1979, *241,* 2793–2797.

Evans, D.W., and Lum, L.C. Hyperventilation: An important cause of pseudoangina. *Lancet,* 1977, *1,* 155–157.

Folgering, H., and Cox, A. Beta-blocker therapy with metoprolol in the hyperventilation syndrome. *Respiration,* 1981, *41,* 33–39.

Freeman, L., and Nixon, P.G.F. Are coronary artery spasm and progressive damage to the heart associated with the hyperventilation syndrome? *British Medical Journal,* 1985, *291,* 851–852.

Freud, S. On the grounds for detaching a particular syndrome from neurasthenia under the description "anxiety neurosis." In the standard edition of *The Complete Psychological Works of Sigmund Freud.* Vol. III. London: Hogarth Press, 1962 (originally published in 1894).

Friedman, M. Studies concerning the aetiology and pathogenesis of neurocirculatory asthenia: IV. The respiratory manifestations of neurocirculatory asthenia. *American Heart Journal,* 1945, *30,* 557–566.

Frohlich, E.G., Dunstan, H.P., and Page, I.H. Hyperdynamic beta-adrenergic circulatory state. *Archives of Internal Medicine,* 1966, *117,* 614–619.

Greer, S., and Cawley, R.H. Some observations on the natural history of neurotic illness. *Archdall Medical Monograph No. 3.* Sydney: Australia Publishing Company, 1966.

Hardonk, H.J., and Beumer, H.M. Hyperventilation syndrome. In P.J. Vinkin, and G.W. Bruhn (Eds.), *Handbook of Neurology.* Vol. 38. Elsevier/N. Holland: Medical Press, 1979, pp. 309–360.

Hibbert, G.A., and Pilsbury, D. Hyperventilation: Is it a cause of panic attacks? *British Journal of Psychiatry,* 1989, *155,* 805–809.

Innocenti, D.M. Chronic hyperventilation syndrome. In P.A. Downie (Ed.), *Cash's Textbook of Chest, Heart and Vascular Disorders for Physiotherapists.* 4th ed. London: Faber and Faber, 1987.

Jones, M., and Lewis, A. Effort syndrome. *Lancet,* 1941, *1,* 813–818.

Jones, M.S., and Skarisbrick, R. A comparison of the respiration in patients with effort syndrome and in normal subjects. *Proceedings of the Royal Society of Medicine,* 1941, *34,* 549–554.

Klimes, I., Mayou, R.A., Pearce, M.J., Coles, L., and Fagg, J.R. Psychological treatment for atypical chest pain: A controlled evaluation. *Psychological Medicine,* 1990, *20,* 605–611.

Lary, D., and Goldschlager, N. Electrocardiographic changes during hyperventilation resembling myocardial ischaemia in patients with normal coronary arteries. *American Heart Journal,* 1974, *87,* 383–390.

Lipowski, Z.J. Cardiovascular disorders. In H.I. Kaplan, A.M. Freedman, and B.J. Sadock (Eds.), *Comprehensive Textbook of Psychiatry.* Baltimore: William and Wilkins, 1980, pp. 1891–1907.

Lisker, B.H., and Leff, S.E. Transmural ischaemia during pre-exercise hyperventilation. *American Journal of Cardiology,* 1983, *51,* 613–614.

Lum, L.C. The syndrome of habitual chronic hyperventilation. In O. Hill (Ed.), *Modern Trends in Psychosomatic Medicine.* London: Butterworth, 1976.

Magarian, G.J. Hyperventilation syndromes: Infrequently recognised common expressions of anxiety and stress. *Medicine* 1982, *61,* 219–236.

Marks, I., and Lader, M. Anxiety states (anxiety neurosis): A review. *Journal of Nervous and Mental Diseases,* 1973, *156,* 3–18.

Pitts, F.N., and McClure, J.N. Lactate metabolism in anxiety neurosis. *New England Journal of Medicine,* 1967, *277,* 1329–1336.

Richter, J.E., Bradley, L.A., and Castell, D.O. Esophageal chest pain: Current controversies in pathogenesis, diagnosis, and therapy. *Annals of Internal Medicine,* 1989, *110,* 66–78.

Salkovskis, P.M., Jones, D.R.O., and Clark, D.M. Respiratory control in the treatment of panic attacks: Replication and extension with concurrent measurement of behaviour and pCO_2. *British Journal of Psychiatry,* 1986, *148,* 526–532.

Skerritt, P.W. Anxiety and the heart—A historical review. *Psychological Medicine,* 1983, *13,* 17–25.

Somerville, W. Da Costa's syndrome. In D.J. Weatherall, J.G. Ledingham, and D.A. Warrell (Eds.), *Oxford Textbook of Medicine.* Vol. 2. Oxford: Oxford University Press, 1983, pp. 194–195.

Tyrer, P. *The Role of Bodily Feelings in Anxiety.* London: Oxford University Press, 1976a.

Tyrer, P. Towards rational therapy with monoamine oxidase inhibitors. *British Journal of Psychiatry* 1976b, *128,* 354–360.

Tyrer, P. Neurosis divisible? *Lancet,* 1985, *1,* 685–688.

Tyrer, P., Lee, I., and Alexander, J. Awareness of cardiac function in anxious, phobic and hypochondriacal patients. *Psychological Medicine,* 1980, *10,* 171–174.

White, P.D., and Hahn, R.G. The symptom of sighing in cardiovascular diagnosis: With spirographic observations. *American Journal of Medical Sciences,* 1929, *177,* 179–188.

Wittkower, E., Rodger, T.F. and Macbeth Wilson, A.T. Effort syndrome. *Lancet,* 1941, *1,* 531–535.

Wood, P. Da Costa's syndrome (or effort syndrome). *British Medical Journal,* 1941a, *1,* 767–772.

Wood, P. Da Costa's syndrome (or effort syndrome). The mechanism of the somatic manifestations. *British Medical Journal,* 1941b, *1,* 805–811.

Wood, P. Aetiology of Da Costa's syndrome. *British Medical Journal,* 1941c, *1,* 845–851.

Wood, P. Cardiovascular disorders associated with psychiatric states. In P. Wood (Ed.), *Diseases of the Heart and Circulation.* London: Eyre and Spottiswoode, 1968.

Hyperventilation and Psychopathology
A Clinical Perspective

HERBERT FENSTERHEIM

1. Introduction

Hyperventilation often plays an important role in the clinical diagnosis and treatment of psychological disorders. Given the high frequency of incorrect breathing patterns in the adult population (Lum, 1976), attention to the symptoms of hyperventilation should be a routine part of every psychological examination, regardless of the specific presenting complaints. Faulty breathing patterns affect patients differently. They may be the central problem, directly bringing on the pathological symptoms; they may magnify, exacerbate, or maintain symptoms brought on by other causes; or they may be involved in peripheral problems that must be ameliorated before psychotherapeutic access is gained to the core treatment targets. Their manifestations may be direct and obvious, as when overbreathing leads to a panic attack, or they may initiate or maintain subtle symptoms that perpetuate an entire personality disorder. Diagnosis of hyperventilatory conditions is crucial.

2. Diagnostic Criteria

The diagnostic goals of the clinical researcher and of the working clinician must be quite different. The researcher is primarily (although not exclusively)

HERBERT FENSTERHEIM • Department of Psychiatry, Cornell University Medical College, New York, New York 10021.
Behavioral and Psychological Approaches to Breathing Disorders, edited by Beverly H. Timmons and Ronald Ley. Plenum Press, New York, 1994.

concerned with gaining hard data about the characteristics, the processes, and the treatment of the hyperventilation conditions. Thus, in diagnosis, it is most important to avoid the type I error, that is, to minimize false positives. Should non-hyperventilators be included in the hyperventilator subject group, important findings may be masked or distorted. Hence, researchers should use the most rigorous diagnostic criteria available. Also, much of their work is in clinical areas such as panic reactions or pseudoangina, where there is a strong probability of finding large numbers of true hyperventilators.

The working clinician, on the other hand, is primarily concerned with avoiding the type II error, i.e., the failure to diagnose hyperventilation when it is truly present—the false negative. The clinician should be aware of the fact that the critical diagnostic test in this area has not yet been devised, that available tests are suggestive rather than conclusive, and that there is yet "no satisfactory or widely accepted definition of hyperventilation syndrome" (Bass and Gardner, 1985, and see Chapter 6). However, even if hyperventilation is a misdiagnosis, aside from possibly wasted time and increased costs, no deleterious effects are expected from the treatment that follows. Indeed, even when based on misdiagnosis, the breathing retraining and the relaxation treatment may still provide beneficial results to the patient. Unlike the situation for the researcher, it is far better for the clinician to make the diagnosis of hyperventilation when it is not present than to fail to diagnose hyperventilation when it is. Thus, the clinician must work with low probabilities and with minimal supporting evidence. No single test (such as failing to respond to provocation) can rule out the diagnosis.

3. The Secondary Reactions

Much attention is paid to the direct impact of hyperventilation on patients. There is increasing evidence of the interactions between hyperventilation and panic disorder (Gorman et al., 1988; Hibbert, 1984; Ley, 1989; Wolpe and Rowan, 1988), as well as between hyperventilation and cardiac disorders (Freeman and Nixon, 1985; King and Nixon, 1988). Among other conditions, hyperventilation has been implicated in sleep disorders (Ley, 1988), affective disorders (Gibson, 1978), and migraine and epilepsy (Fried, 1987). It has long been known that hyperventilation can be expressed in forms resembling many different physical illnesses (Kerr et al., 1937), and Lum (1981) has noted that it has replaced syphilis as the "great mimic." As with physical symptoms, the psychological manifestations of hyperventilation may also imitate many different disorders. Compernolle et al. (1979), for example, report the symptoms of hyperventilation being misdiagnosed as anything from hysteria, to conduct disorders with outbursts of violence, to schizophrenia with depersonalization. All these findings deal with the direct impact of hyperventilation on the person.

Researchers have also paid much attention to the patient's direct reaction to the primary effects of hyperventilation. In the area of panic they have studied the effects of cognitions on the development and maintenance of panic reactions (Beck and Emery, 1985; Clark, 1986). Despite some criticism of this work (Ley, 1987), it is important in the treatment of panic disorders because it leads to corrective information and education as an effective part of the therapy for this disorder (Sanderson and Beck, 1989). Another important direct reaction to the primary effects of hyperventilation is described by Lum (1975, 1976). This is the hyperventilation–anxiety–increased hyperventilation spiral, in which the anxiety and the hyperventilation feed into each other, raising disturbances and symptoms to ever higher levels. Thus, small, easily coped with, disturbances of any kind may rapidly escalate to levels at which they become uncontrollable and over- whelming. However, these reactions are not necessarily simple ones. Garssen *et al.* (1983), who report on how cognitive variables may influence the develop- ment of an agoraphobic condition, recognize that there is no question of a simple cause/effect relationship. Indeed, clinical observation suggests that the effects of the direct reactions may be subtle and complex, and may have many conse- quences that reach far beyond the primary symptoms themselves.

One such subtle effect may be illustrated by citing a recent therapeutic experience. The patient, a woman in her early fifties, was in long-term psycho- dynamic treatment. In one area of major concern, her relations with men, she had great difficulty in eliciting useful associations, and all attempts to analyze this resistance failed. The therapist then tried, unsuccessfully, to have the patient associate under hypnosis. After entering into a trance, the patient would begin to associate, but then would suddenly snap out of the trance. At this point the patient was referred to me to see what could be "done with the resistance."

Examination showed the patient to be a moderately severe chronic hyper- ventilator. Observation further revealed that whenever she thought or spoke of men, whether or not she was in a trance state, there would be a definite and marked increase in hyperventilation (see Conway *et al.,* 1988). A working hy- pothesis was then formulated in terms of the hyperventilation–anxiety spiral. When thinking of men, her anxiety level would increase. This, in turn, would increase the primary hyperventilation disturbances. To avoid this increased dis- turbance, she would avoid thinking of men and so the "resistance" developed. Breathing retraining along with practice in maintaining correct breathing while thinking of men solved the avoidance problem. In her psychodynamic therapy she became able to remain in the trance state and thereby produce more useful associations about men. Thus, what superficially appeared to be a complex psychodynamic problem turned out to be a simple problem of avoidance of hyperventilation symptoms.

Three aspects of the secondary reactions to hyperventilation will be consid- ered: (1) the interaction between hyperventilation and the temperamental characteristics of the patient; (2) the development of secondary symptoms; and, probably most important, (3) the impact of hyperventilation on the psychological organization of the patient, to the point at which the hyperventilation may influence an entire lifestyle. A consideration of the report of Lazarus and Kostan (1969) may serve to illustrate these features.

Lazarus and Kostan (1969) state that fears of death are so prevalent among people who hyperventilate, that whenever hyperventilation is noted the patient should be questioned about such fears. They identify three categories of these fears. The first is a feeling of doom and imminent death. The second consists of medical phobias, such as the fear of cancer or the fear of a heart attack. The third is the fear of the death of a significant person. Lazarus and Kostan hypothesize that it is these fears that bring on the hyperventilation, and that it is the fears, not the hyperventilation, that should be the treatment target. In light of our current understanding that such fears may be the product of habits of incorrect breathing, rather than the cause (Lum, 1976), the fears may be reinterpreted.

The feeling of doom may well be a manifestation of the interaction between the physiological consequences of overbreathing and the patient's temperament. One physiological change occurring during hyperventilation is increased dominance of the sympathetic nervous system (Lum, 1978/1979). This often elicits a series of physical symptoms, but also produces subjective sensations that are usually experienced as anxiety, fear, and/or panic. However, individuals experience these subjective sensations differently (Eysenck, 1970; Fensterheim, 1983); one form this experience may take is the sense of depression or of doom. Wolpe (1979), for example, reports that depression may be viewed as a conditioned anxiety reaction, and thereby would be responsive to treatment by systematic desensitization. In sum, feelings associated with death may stem from the direct impact of overbreathing on the autonomic nervous system.

It should be noted that hyperventilation may bring on depressive feelings in more indirect and complicated ways. For one, if an obsessive tendency is present, the tension mechanically induced by overbreathing might exacerbate the obsessions. Since feelings of depression are often a consequence of increased obsessiveness, hyperventilation may be the root cause of such depression. A second possibility concerns the screening effect of the overbreathing-induced tension. As anxiety can screen out the positive impact of natural sexual stimuli (Masters and Johnson, 1970), so can it screen out the impact of other positive experiences. In this manner, the patient becomes increasingly insensitive to the positive reinforcers of life. Such decreases in positive reinforcement may lead to increases in depression, which, in turn, may be characterized as feelings of doom. Other such links between hyperventilation and depressive affect (which often includes feelings of doom and fears of death) might be formulated, but these examples make the point.

The second category, the fears of dying of cancer or of a heart attack, may also be understood as an outcome of hyperventilation. We already noted the fact that physical symptoms of hyperventilation may imitate other somatic disorders. Hence, they are frequently misdiagnosed. Lum (1976) has added to our diagnostic vocabulary the British term "fat folder syndrome." This is a situation in which the patient has symptoms from an undiagnosed hyperventilation condition, and he/she goes from medical specialist to medical specialist without successful treatment; the folder grows fatter and fatter, but the patient receives no help. The consequence is a patient with a serious-looking or painful set of symptoms that puzzles the medical profession. Of course the patient is concerned and worried; this, in turn, brings on increased attention to the symptoms and increased hyperventilation. These, in their turn, maintain or increase the symptoms. Given the generally aroused state of the sympathetic nervous system brought on by hyperventilation, it is not surprising that phobic reactions to the symptoms, or to thoughts of the symptoms, develop. Once developed, these phobias would become self-sustaining through the hyperventilation–anxiety spiral. Further, should there be a temperamental predisposition towards obsessiveness, an additional obsessive overlay to the phobic reaction may come about. All this would be further maintained and exacerbated by such cognitive variables as the patient's self-labeling of being seriously, perhaps fatally, ill. Thus, the fear of death is prominent.

The third category, the fear of the death of a significant person, is often seen when a pattern of agoraphobic avoidance develops. Indeed, this fear is so common that there is discussion as to whether all agoraphobic patients suffer from separation anxiety (the infantile anxiety concerned with the absence of a caring person, usually the mother) and/or have very strong dependency needs. These attributes are thought to bring about the death fears. Others argue that the fear stems from the helplessness that is allied with panic attacks and the great fear of having an attack when no one is there to help. As there are few "safe people" in the patient's life, the loss of any one of them is a major threat. It is from this background that the fear of the death of a significant person emerges. Note that the discussion is about the roots of the fear; there is the general acceptance that the fear itself is common.

Although most clearly seen when there is an agoraphobic pattern, the fear of the death of a significant person is not limited to the presence of such a pattern. It may be present whenever there are strong anticipatory anxieties and fears of potential helplessness associated with the panic attacks. Further, it probably may also be present regardless of what initiates or maintains the attacks. Indeed, from the subjective descriptions of panic, one cannot differentiate clearly between those attacks in which hyperventilation is involved and those in which it isn't. Garssen *et al.* (1983) attempted to do so on the basis of somatic symptoms present during an attack. However, according to the DSM-III-R (American Psychiatric Association, 1987) definition, most of the symptoms that identify a panic are somatic sensations, regardless of the basis for the panic. Further, even nonhyperventilation-induced panic may have hyperventilation superimposed on it (i.e., the panic induces the hyperventilation, which then exacerbates the panic), the hyperventilation being secondary to the panic. Clinically, even when the patient shows a positive response to the provocation test the presence of a primary nonhyperventilation panic cannot be ruled out.

The clinical diagnosis of the cause of the panic usually cannot be made with great certainty during the early part of treatment. This writer has seen several patients who were true and severe hyperventilators by any standard. With breathing retraining they became able to abort incipient panics, and these attacks soon disappeared completely. However, after brief periods the panics would return, and at those times, so far as could be determined, hyperventilation was not at all involved. These new attacks readily responded to the customary *in vivo* exposure treatments. Even initial response to treatment may not distinguish between the different panics (Bonn *et al.*, 1984). Thus, with the great similarity in the subjective experiences of the differently induced panics, with the feelings of helplessness and hence the need for a caring person, it is not surprising that many times we find the patient fears the death of a caring person.

From this discussion of hyperventilation and the fear of death in various forms, several points emerge. Hyperventilation in some patients can produce depression-like feelings. The patient then becomes labeled by self and others as being depressed, is treated as such, and adopts a generally depressive life-style. The patient may develop a phobic reaction to the somatic sensations of hyperventilation, and have an automatic fear-of-dying reaction to those sensations or to the thoughts of them. This usually brings on "hypochondriacal" behavior, constant contact with physicians, and disruption of close personal relationships. Often, for example, it brings great tension and conflict to a marriage. Also, hyperventilation may lead to an agoraphobic life-style, with increasing avoidance, narrowing life space, and morbid dependency on certain people. These secondary reactions may have an impact on the person that is as large as, or even larger than, that of the obvious primary hyperventilation symptoms.

4. Problems in Formulation and Treatment

Unfortunately, in a clinical practice many patients do not present with clearcut problems indicating hyperventilation. In the example concerning "hypochondriacal" behavior cited above, the impact of hyperventilation on family life may be so great that the core problem of hyperventilation would be difficult to identify. The descriptions of irrational fights, of angers and withdrawals, of sexual difficulties, may be so preeminent that hyperventilation is not even considered. Even a careful history may not reveal the importance of the hyperventilation. The history may show that the core of the problems now manifested had always been present; it does not reveal that the tensions secondary to hyperventilation exacerbated what had previously been a controlled problem.

There are several factors that disguise the role, or even the presence, of hyperventilation in subtle and complex psychopathologies. The hyperventilation symptoms may be minimal or atypical, yet still be the key in maintaining an entire pathological structure. The hyperventilation may be masked by more severe signs of other pathology. There may be an obvious formulation of the pathology so that hyperventilation is not even considered. Fensterheim (1981) reports one such instance where the obvious formulation was "the fear of success combined with compulsive gambling," and where long and varied treatment had been completely unsuccessful. Examination revealed severe chronic hyperventilation; panics were triggered by enthusiasm-induced overbreathing when near success. Gambling-and-losing was a conditioned operant behavior leading to depression, which, in turn, changed the breathing pattern and reduced the panic. Breathing retraining did away with the entire pattern.

Both the direct and the magnifying effects of hyperventilation may have a particularly pervasive and disguised impact in the area of social phobias. A hyperventilation-prone person may breathe incorrectly while speaking, feel anxious, label self as a social phobic, and act accordingly (i.e., withdrawal, avoidance, and lowered self-esteem). Or, a true social phobia may be present but be so magnified by hyperventilation that the person cannot cope with the fear; thus, avoidance is the only available solution. The avoidance may generalize and become so widespread that the person now meets the DSM-III-R (American Psychiatric Association, 1987) criteria for avoidant-personality disorder. In this manner, hyperventilation may be the core of a complex neurotic structure, it may play a magnifying role in a structure that exists independently, or it may play a peripheral or an unimportant role—or no role at all—in such a structure. Therefore, the diagnosis of hyperventilation by itself is not sufficient. Once diagnosed, the relation between hyperventilation and other aspects of the patient's complaints must be formulated. The manner in which the hyperventilation reinforces, inhibits, distorts, or otherwise changes other behaviors, feelings, thoughts, and motives—and the manner in which it influences the patient's psychological organization—must be hypothesized (Fensterheim, 1983). Such a formulation would indicate whether or not the hyperventilation should be treated, and, if so, at what point in treatment breathing retraining should be introduced.

Hyperventilation may also interfere with treatment. Certain forms of systematic desensitization require a state of deep relaxation, and hyperventilation may keep the patient from attaining the level of relaxation necessary for that procedure. Flooding or satiation in imagery, when accompanied by excessive overbreathing, may lead to such side effects as headaches or prolonged experience of disturbance after the procedure is terminated. Anticipatory anxieties heightened by hyperventilation may prevent patients from experiencing in vivo exposure to phobic situations or from performing assigned assertiveness tasks. In many such instances, breathing retraining is necessary before the therapeutic procedures can be carried out. Also note that there are times when the therapeutic procedures can be successfully used, but when treatment of the hyperventilation is important for preventing relapse (Bonn et al., 1984).

To further complicate the entire picture, it must be noted that hyperventilation can also be either a derived or a reinforced condition. A set of amusing responses to voluntary hyperventilation may illustrate this possibility. While far from invariable, such overbreathing often elicits recognizable symptoms of panic (Folgering, 1988). However, there are obvious hyperventilators who report strong feelings of relaxation with voluntary overbreathing. Careful questioning yields a reasonable answer to this very unexpected reaction. Overbreathing elicits the not-uncommon feelings of exhaustion and fatigue, but these otherwise extremely tense and anxious patients interpret the feeling as relaxation with a pleasant hedonic tone. Although there are no indications that these patients deliberately hyperventilate in everyday situations in order to achieve this pleasant "state of relaxation," it is conceivable that some patients do.

5. Summary

The clinical psychotherapist must avoid failing to diagnose hyperventilation when it is present. Hence, given the current state of the art, the therapist will often have to make this diagnosis with only minimal evidence. The manifestations of hyperventilation vary widely, and many times take on subtle and disguised forms. They vary according to their interaction with the patient's temperament, with the patient's reaction to their effects, and with their impact on the patient's psychological organization. They may be involved in complex behavioral patterns, sometimes as the key and sometimes in the most peripheral role. They may also interfere with certain treatment procedures. Investigation of hyperventilation should be a routine part of every psychological examination. However, the decision of when to treat, or even of whether to treat, must be based on an overall therapeutic formulation.

6. References

American Psychiatric Association. Diagnostic and statistical manual of mental disorders. 3rd ed., revised. Washington, D.C.: A.P.A., 1987.
Bass, C., and Gardner, W. Diagnostic issues in the hyperventilation syndrome. British Journal of Psychiatry, 1985, 146, 101–102.

Beck, A., and Emery, G. *Anxiety disorders and phobias.* New York: Basic Books, 1985.

Bonn, J.A., Readhead, P.A., and Timmons, B.H. Enhanced adaptive behavioural response in agoraphobic patients pretreated with breathing retraining. *Lancet,* 1984, *2,* 665–669.

Clark, D. A cognitive approach to panic. *Behaviour Research and Therapy,* 1986, *24,* 461–470.

Compernolle, T., Hoogduin, K., and Joele, L. Diagnosis and treatment of the hyperventilation syndrome. *Psychosomatics,* 1979, *19,* 612–625.

Conway, A., Freeman, L., and Nixon, P.G.F. Hypnotic examination of trigger factors in the hyperventilation syndrome. *American Journal of Clinical Hypnosis,* 1988, *30,* 296–304.

Eysenck, H.J. The classification of depressive illness. *British Journal of Psychiatry,* 1970, *117,* 241–250.

Fensterheim, H. Clinical behavior therapy for depression. In J.F. Clarkin and H.I. Glazer (Eds.), *Depression: Behavioral and directive intervention strategies.* New York: Garland Press, 1981.

Fensterheim, H. The behavioral psychotherapy model of phobias. In H. Fensterheim and H.I. Glazer (Eds.), *Behavioral Psychotherapy: Basic Principles and Case Studies in an Integrative Clinical Model,* New York: Brunner/Mazel, 1983.

Folgering, H. Diagnostic criteria for the hyperventilation syndrome. In C. von Euler and M. Katz-Salamon (Eds.), *Respiratory Psychophysiology,* New York: Stockton Press, 1988.

Freeman, L.J., and Nixon, P.G.F. Dynamic causes of angina pectoris, *American Heart Journal,* 1985, *11,* 1087–1092.

Fried, R. *The Hyperventilation Syndrome.* Baltimore: Johns Hopkins University Press, 1987.

Garssen, B., van Veenendaal, W., and Bloemink, R. Agoraphobia and the hyperventilation syndrome. *Behaviour Research and Therapy,* 1983, *21,* 643–649.

Gibson, H.B. A form of behavior therapy for some states diagnosed as "affective disorder." *Behaviour Research and Therapy,* 1978, *16,* 191–195.

Gorman, J., Goetz, R., Uy, J., Ross, D., Martinez, J., Fyer, A., Liebowitz, M., and Klein, D. Hyperventilation occurs during lactate-induced panic. *Journal of Anxiety Disorders,* 1988, *2,* 193–202.

Hibbert, G.A. Hyperventilation as a cause of panic attacks. *British Medical Journal,* 1984, *288,* 263–264.

Kerr, W.J., Dalton, J.W., and Gliebe, P.A. Some physical phenomena associated with anxiety states and their relation to hyperventilation. *Annals of Internal Medicine,* 1937, *11,* 961–992.

King, J.C., and Nixon, P.G.F. A system of cardiac rehabilitation: Psychophysiological basis and practice. *British Journal of Occupational Therapy,* 1988, *51,* 376–384.

Lazarus, H.R., and Kostan, J.J. Psychogenic hyperventilation and death anxiety. *Psychosomatics,* 1969, *10,* 14–22.

Ley, R. Panic disorder and agoraphobia: Fear of fear or fear of the symptoms produced by hyperventilation?, *Journal of Behavior Therapy and Experimental Psychiatry,* 1987, *18,* 305–316.

Ley, R. Panic attacks during sleep: A hyperventilation-probability model, *Journal of Behavior Therapy and Experimental Psychiatry,* 1988, *19,* 181–192.

Ley, R. Dyspneic–Fear and catastrophic conditions in hyperventilatory panic attacks. *Behaviour Research and Therapy,* 1989, *27,* 549–554.

Lum, L.C. Hyperventilation: The tip and the iceberg. *Journal of Psychosomatic Research,* 1975, *19,* 375–383.

Lum, L.C. The syndrome of habitual chronic hyperventilation. In O. Hill (Ed.), *Modern trends in psychosomatic medicine.* Vol. 3. Boston: Butterworth, 1976.

Lum, L.C. Respiratory alkalosis and hypocarbia. *The Chest, Heart and Stroke Journal,* 1978/79, *3,* 31–34.

Lum, L.C. Hyperventilation and anxiety state. *Journal of the Royal Society of Medicine,* 1981, *74,* 1–4.

Masters, W.H., and Johnson, V.E. *Human sexual inadequacy.* Boston: Little, Brown, 1970.

Mathews, A.M., Gelder, M.G., and Johnston, D.W. *Agoraphobia: Nature and treatment*. New York: Guilford Press, 1981.

Sanderson, W.C., and Beck, A.T. Classical conditioning model of panic disorder: Response to Wolpe and Rowan. *Behaviour Research and Therapy*, 1989, *27*, 581–582.

Wolpe, J. The experimental model and treatment of neurotic depression. *Behaviour Research and Therapy*, 1979, *17*, 555–565.

Wolpe, J., and Rowan, V. Panic disorder: A product of classical conditioning. *Behaviour Research and Therapy*, 1988, *26*, 441–450.

Management of Patients with Hyperventilation-Related Disorders

CHRISTOPHER BASS

1. Introduction

Recent comprehensive reviews of hyperventilation (Cowley and Roy-Byrne, 1987; Gardner and Bass, 1989; Garssen and Rijken, 1986; Magarian, 1982) reflect the magnitude of current interest in the subject. In part, this was stimulated by the publication of DMS-III-R in 1980 (American Psychiatric Association, 1980), when panic disorder was proposed as a separate diagnostic entity. That panic disorder and hyperventilation share common features is not disputed. The main area of controversy concerns the nature of the relationship between them.

2. Disorders Associated with Hyperventilation

Hyperventilation occurs commonly in panic and other anxiety-related disorders. The consensus from many studies is that approximately two-thirds of patients with agoraphobia with panic recognize the similarity between symptoms of voluntary hyperventilation and those of their usual panic attacks (Bass *et al.*, 1989; de Ruiter *et al.*, 1989; Garssen *et al.*, 1983; Hibbert and Chan, 1989). The direction of the relationship between hyperventilation and panic is less clear-cut: a recent study has suggested that hyperventilation may be a consequence of,

CHRISTOPHER BASS • Department of Psychological Medicine, John Radcliffe Hospital, Headington, Oxford OX3 9DU, England.
Behavioral and Psychological Approaches to Breathing Disorders, edited by Beverly H. Timmons and Ronald Ley. Plenum Press, New York, 1994.

rather than a cause of or major contributor to, the severity of panics (Hibbert and Pilsbury, 1989).

Hyperventilation can also occur in depression (Damas-Mora *et al.*, 1976), and as a complication of organic lung disease—especially chronic obstructive airways disease and asthma (Burns and Howell, 1969; McFadden and Lyons, 1968; see Chapter 6). In patients with lung disease and hyperventilation, the symptoms of breathlessness are often disproportionate to the organic findings (Howell, 1990).

3. Treatments

The three major treatments in hyperventilation-related disorders are drugs, respiratory retraining (physiotherapy or controlled-breathing training), and psychological treatments. These will be discussed in turn.

3.1. Physical Treatments

Many drugs are potentially useful in patients with hyperventilation-related symptoms. Whenever hyperventilation occurs as part of a panic syndrome it should be amenable to pharmacological treatment. The three most effective treatments for panic patients are tricyclic antidepressants (e.g., imipramine), monoamine oxidase inhibitors (e.g., phenelzine), and triazolobenzodiazepines (e.g., alprazolam). Only the former two classes of drugs are available in the United Kingdom.

Both imipramine and phenelzine have been shown to benefit patients with panic–hyperventilation syndromes, in randomized, placebo-controlled studies. However, these drugs are not without risks, and some patients with panic–hyperventilation symptoms are extremely sensitive to their side effects. The drugs should be prescribed for 6–9 months and then tapered gradually. There is a risk of relapse in 30–60 percent of patients, and some patients on phenelzine develop an increase in symptoms after withdrawal (Fyer, 1988).

Other drugs shown to be effective in patients with hyperventilation-related complaints are beta-blockers (e.g., metoprolol) and a tricyclic antidepressant that enhances the activity of cerebral serotinergic neurons (clomipramine).

In a double-blind crossover trial, Folgering and Cox (1981) found that the beta-blocker metoprolol (100 mg for 4 weeks) increased end-tidal Pco_2 in patients, most of whom had fewer somatic complaints than did the patients given a placebo. Although these results appear promising, this author has found beta-blockers to be of little value in patients with hyperventilation-related disorders, especially when it occurs with panics.

In an uncontrolled study of six patients with hyperventilation syndrome who had not responded to anxiolytics or behavior therapy, Hoes *et al.* (1980) found clomipramine to be beneficial. They suggested that clomipramine pharmacologically immobilized the startle response, by enhancing serotonin transmission.

Drug treatments of panic–hyperventilation disorders can be used either alone or in combination with psychological treatments, such as exposure, cognitive therapy, or breathing retraining.

3.2. Breathing Retraining (Physiotherapy or Controlled Breathing)

There is now a considerable amount of evidence to suggest that voluntary control of certain respiratory variables can modify the level of subjective anxiety experienced under a variety of different circumstances. That these respiratory variables are susceptible to voluntary control is not disputed. An important demonstration of this phenomenon was reported by Stanescu *et al.* (1981), who studied patterns of breathing and ventilatory responses to CO_2 in subjects practicing hatha yoga and in a control group matched for age, sex, and height. The practice of yoga involves control of posture and manipulation of breathing, including slow, near vital capacity maneuvers accompanied by apnea at the end of inspiration and expiration. The yoga subjects had lower respiratory rate and minute volume, but higher tidal volume and end-tidal Pco_2, than controls. All these differences were significant; in addition, ventilatory response to CO_2 was significantly lower in the yoga group. The authors speculated that particular patterns of breathing repeated almost daily for years become automatic by a process of conditioning or learning (see Chapter 15).

Investigations concerned with the question of whether alterations in respiratory variables can modify measures of psychological distress have generally sought to pace the rate of breathing while subjects are under anxiety-provoking conditions (see Chapter 13). McCaul *et al.* (1979) demonstrated that voluntary slowing of the respiratory rate of subjects under stressful conditions reduced physiological arousal, as measured by skin resistance and finger pulse volume, and reduced self-report of anxiety. Subsequent studies from the same laboratory provided evidence to support claims by yoga masters that a specific form of slowed respiration—that is, rapid inhalation followed by slow exhalation at a reduced respiratory rate—is an effective technique for reducing physiological arousal when one is anticipating and confronting a threat (Cappo and Holmes, 1984).

These observations have important implications for treatment, and suggest that techniques aimed at enhancing voluntary control of breathing should have therapeutic application in patients with symptomatic hyperventilation. A summary of the studies that have used breathing retraining or physiotherapy will now be described.

3.3. Psychological Treatments

Many studies that have used breathing retraining have also included psychological techniques, especially cognitive behavioral treatment. Broadly speaking, psychological treatment involves four components:

1. *Replication experiments.* Voluntary hyperventilation (VH) is used to reproduce symptoms that occur in real life.
2. *Reattribution.* This involves reattribution of symptoms that occur during panic attacks to hyperventilation, and explanation about the causes and maintenance of panic attacks.
3. *Coping strategies,* such as breathing retraining (slow, regular, diaphragmatic breathing).
4. *Graded exposure* to avoided situations.

In the last decade there have been many studies of the efficacy of these treatments, most commonly in patients with anxiety disorders. In one study, Bonn *et al.* (1984) found that pretreatment of agoraphobic patients with respiratory control had a more enduring effect than behavioral exposure alone. That is to say, six months after treatment, patients who had received the exposure plus breathing retraining demonstrated significantly more improvement on mean resting breathing rate, global phobia score, somatic symptom score, and panic frequency, than did those who received exposure alone.

Similar findings were reported by Salkovskis *et al.* (1986). These authors made the important observation that the more the patients perceived the effects of overbreathing (during VH) to be similar to their panic attacks, the better the response to treatment. Further evidence for the efficacy of breathing therapy was advanced by Grossman *et al.* (1985). These authors assigned 47 patients with positive VH tests (i.e., symptoms reproduced by overbreathing) to either ventilatory training (slow, paced breathing) or a comparison group. Both groups had home assignment sessions. The group who received paced breathing showed significant improvement on hyperventilation complaints and on trait and state anxiety. Furthermore, alterations in resting Pco_2 and rate of recovery of Pco_2 following VH were positively associated with changes in each of the self-report variables. A more recent study also confirmed the efficacy of breathing retraining in patients with functional cardiac symptoms (De Guire *et al.*, 1992). These findings suggest that breathing therapy brings about long-term changes in the central control of respiration.

3.4. Breathing Control without the Cognitive Element May Be Ineffective

These encouraging findings, broadly in support of the efficacy of breathing retraining in patients with anxiety disorders, have been questioned by Salkovskis

(1988) and a recent publication that suggests that breathing retraining has limited effectiveness in patients with panic (de Ruiter *et al.*, 1989). This study suggests that the cognitive element appears to be necessary for the successful treatment using respiratory control. Importantly, this and a more recent study (van den Hout *et al.*, 1992) suggest a less important role for hyperventilation in panic than do earlier studies. Indeed, they suggest that hyperventilation may be an epi-phenomenon of panic, rather than one of the primary causal factors. However, these conclusions have been challenged by Ley (1991), who has pointed out that the group that received breathing retraining showed a reduction in frequency of panic attacks while the other two groups did not.

In another study that questioned the efficacy of respiratory control in pa-tients with panic, Hibbert and Chan (1989) divided 40 panic patients into hyper-ventilators and nonhyperventilators on the basis of a conventional provocation test. All patients were treated for two weeks with either training in controlled breathing or a placebo treatment. Subsequently, both groups received a limited period of conventional anxiety treatments—most commonly, *in vivo* exposure. Although observer ratings of anxiety showed a greater improvement for the group that received breathing retraining, there was no evidence that hyperventila-tors benefited more from respiratory retraining than nonhyperventilators. Self-report measures of anxiety, avoidance, and depression/dysphoria showed no difference between treatments. The authors concluded that training in respiratory control was of no specific benefit in patients identified as hyperventilators by VH, although it may have a nonspecific effect in the treatment of patients with panic attacks.

To conclude, both studies, by de Ruiter *et al.* (1989) and Hibbert and Chan (1989), suggest that the cognitive component of treatment—i.e., replication of symptoms, reattribution, and reassurance—is effective. The contribution of res-piratory training, *in pure form*, remains controversial. Clearly, further studies are required to clarify this issue.

4. Concluding Remarks

What is the therapist to do if the patient is referred with hyperventilation syndrome or hyperventilation-related symptoms? There seems little doubt that the cognitive component of therapy is effective: explaining the cause of frighten-ing somatic symptoms, and reassuring the patient that they are a consequence of hyperventilation, which can be mastered and controlled, often has a potent anxiety-reducing effect. Many patients with hyperventilation-related symptoms have seen other physicians who may have carried out investigations to exclude an organic cause for the symptoms. In all probability, the patient will have been told that there is nothing seriously wrong. Regrettably, this will be of little benefit if the symptoms continue to cause anxiety. The crucial therapeutic element for patients with such complaints is to provide a *suitable alternative explanation* for the symptoms, an explanation that is congruent with the patients' culture and intelligence. All but those with very abnormal illness beliefs, a strong investment in illness, or an inability to make links between life situations, emotional upsets, and bodily complaints are likely to benefit from this procedure.

Thus the cognitive component of treatment (replication, reattribution, explanation and reassurance), if carried out carefully, will almost certainly be of therapeutic benefit. These general principles of treatment can be applied by physiotherapists, nurse therapists, psychologists, and clinicians who deal with patients with panic–hyperventilation symptoms.

It is also worth noting that it is possible to make patients worse with breathing exercises, at least in the initial phase of treatment. Efforts to reduce ventilation through exclusive attention to a reduction in respiratory frequency may produce an *increase* in ventilation, an effect opposite to the express purpose of breathing retraining (Ley, 1991). Much more research on the efficacy of breathing retraining needs to be carried out before it becomes widely accepted as an essential component of treatment in patients with hyperventilation-related syndromes.

5. References

American Psychiatric Association. *Diagnostic and statistical manual of mental disorders.* 3rd ed., revised. APA, Washington, D.C.: A.P.A., 1980.

Bass, C., Lelliott, P., and Marks, I. Fear talk versus voluntary hyperventilation in agrophobics and normals: A controlled study. *Psychological Medicine,* 1989, *19,* 669–676.

Bonn, J.A., Readhead, C.P.A., and Timmons, B.H. Enhanced adaptive behavioural response in agoraphobic patients pretreated with breathing retraining. *Lancet,* 1984, *2,* 665–669.

Burns, B., and Howell, J.B. Disproportionately severe breathlessness in chronic bronchitis. *Quarterly Journal of Medicine,* 1969, *38,* 277–294.

Cappo, B.M., and Holmes, D.S. The utility of prolonged respiratory exhalation for reducing physiological and psychological arousal in non-threatening and threatening situations. *Journal of Psychosomatic Research,* 1984, *28,* 265–273.

Cowley, D.S., and Roy-Byrne, P.R. Hyperventilation and panic disorder. *American Journal of Medicine,* 1987, *83,* 929–937.

Damas-Mora, J., Grant, L., Kenyon, P., Patel, M.K., and Jenner, F.A. Respiratory ventilation and carbon dioxide levels in syndromes of depression. *British Journal of Psychiatry,* 1976, *129,* 457–464.

De Guire, S., Gevirtz, R., Kawahara, Y., and Maguire, W. Hyperventilation syndrome and the assessment and treatment for functional cardiac symptoms. *American Journal of Cardiology,* 1992, *70,* 673–677.

de Ruiter, C., Rijken, H., Garssen, B., and Kraaimaat, F. Breathing retraining, exposure and a combination of both, in the treatment of panic disorder and agoraphobia. *Behaviour Research and Therapy,* 1989, *27,* 647–655.

Folgering, H., and Cox, A. Beta blocker therapy with metroprolol in the hyperventilation syndrome. *Respiration,* 1981, *41,* 33–37.

Fyer, A.J. Effects of discontinuation of antipanic medication. In I. Hand, and H.-J. Wittchen (Eds.), *Panic and Phobias.* Vol. 2. Berlin: Springer Verlag, 1988.

Gardner, W.N., and Bass, C. Hyperventilation in clinical practice. *British Journal of Hospital Medicine,* 1989, *41,* 73–81.

Garssen, B., and Rijken, H. Clinical aspects and treatment of the hyperventilation syndrome. *Behavioural Psychotherapy,* 1986, *14,* 46–68.

Garssen, B., Van Weenendaal, W., and Bloemink, R. Agoraphobia and the hyperventilation syndrome. *Behaviour Research and Therapy,* 1983, *21,* 643–649.

Grossman, P., de Swart, J.C., and Defares, B.B. A controlled study of a breathing therapy for treatment of hyperventilation syndrome. *Journal of Psychosomatic Research,* 1985, *29,* 49–58.

Hibbert, G.A., and Chan, M. Respiratory control: Its contribution to the treatment of panic attacks. *British Journal of Psychiatry,* 1989, *154,* 232–236.

Hibbert, G.A., and Pilsbury, D. Hyperventilation: Is it a cause of panic attacks? *British Journal of Psychiatry,* 1989, *155,* 805–809.

Hoes, M.J., Colla, P., and Folgering, H. Clomipramine treatment of hyperventilation syndrome. *Pharmakopsychiatry,* 1980, *13,* 25–28.

Howell, J.B. Behavioural breathlessness. *Thorax,* 1990, *45,* 287–292.

Ley, R. The efficacy of breathing retraining and the centrality of hyperventilation in panic disorder: a reinterpretation of experimental findings. *Behavior Research and Therapy,* 1991, *29,* 301–304.

Magarian, G.J. Hyperventilation syndromes: Infrequently recognised common expressions of anxiety and stress. *Medicine,* 1982, *61,* 219–236.

McCaul, K.D., Solomon, S., and Holmes, D.S. Effects of paced respiration and expectations on physical and psychological responses to threat. *Journal of Personality and Social Psychology,* 1979, *37,* 564–571.

McFadden, E.R., and Lyons, H.A. Arterial blood gas tension in asthma. *New England Journal of Medicine,* 1968, *278,* 1027–1032.

Salkovskis, P.M. Hyperventilation and anxiety. *Current Opinion in Psychiatry,* 1988, *1,* 76–82.

Salkovskis, P.M., Jones, D.R., and Clark, D.M. Respiratory control in the treatment of panic attacks: Replication and extension with concurrent measurement of pCO_2. *British Journal of Psychiatry,* 1986, *148,* 526–532.

Stanescu, D.C., Nemery, B., Veriter, C., and Marechal, C. Pattern of breathing and ventilatory response to CO_2 in subjects practising Hatha-Yoga. *Journal of Applied Physiology,* 1981, *51,* 1625–1629.

van den Hout, M.A., Hoekstra, R., Arntz, A., Cristiaanse, M., Ranschaert, W., and Schouten, E. Hyperventilation is not diagnostically specific to panic patients. *Psychosomatic Medicine,* 1992, *53,* 182–191.

11

The Role of the Physiotherapist in the Treatment of Hyperventilation

ELIZABETH A. HOLLOWAY

1. Introduction

I have been using the treatment techniques described here almost daily since 1979. They are largely based on the methods developed and used by the consultant chest physician Dr. L.C. Lum (1977) and physiotherapists Diana Innocenti (1987) and Rosemary Cluff (1984), all at Papworth Hospital, Cambridgeshire. The treatment consists of carefully assessing hyperventilators, educating them into an awareness of the problem, encouraging them to observe present erratic breathing patterns and to consciously convert to a slow, rhythmic, abdominal pattern that eventually becomes automatic. The aim is to reduce the volume of air moved in and out of the lungs so that it is appropriate for the metabolic rate at that time, thus enabling a normal Pco_2 to be maintained. Finally, patients are taught to recognize unnecessary stress and tension in the body and mind, and to learn to remedy this by using simple relaxation methods, both general and specific.

Before describing the method, I will compare the normal breathing patterns that we hope to restore and the disturbed patterns that hyperventilating patients present.

ELIZABETH A. HOLLOWAY • Knebworth Physiotherapy Clinic, Knebworth, Hertfordshire SG3 6HG, England.
Behavioral and Psychological Approaches to Breathing Disorders, edited by Beverly H. Timmons and Ronald Ley. Plenum Press, New York, 1994.

1.1. Normal Breathing

A normal, resting breathing rate is 8–14 breaths per minute. During inspiration, the active phase of breathing, movement of the diaphragm together with movement of the upper abdominal wall take place, and there is virtually no movement of the upper thorax or accessory muscles of respiration, i.e., the neck and upper trunk muscles. Expiration involves no effort and is a downward relaxation of the respiratory muscles, *excluding* the diaphragm. During inspiration the upper abdominal wall swells and during expiration it relaxes with a slight pause before inspiration occurs again. Normal breathing is quiet and effortless. At rest and during relaxed activities, this slow, easy abdominal excursion occurs, with negligible movement of the accessory muscles and minimal sternal movement. These patterns will fluctuate in response to varying physical and emotional stimuli experienced by the individual.

1.2. Hyperventilators' Breathing Patterns

Short periods of overbreathing are perfectly normal reactions to stress; note the fight-or-flight response. However, when it occurs for prolonged periods, then overbreathing is abnormal and provokes the "welter of bodily symptoms" (Chapter 7). Some individuals overbreathe inappropriately for short periods and may suffer from intermittent symptoms, especially in the early stage. If adequate treatment is given at this point, patients will not progress into the later, chronic stage of the condition.

A hyperventilator's rate of breathing may fluctuate considerably, often above 15 breaths per minute, sometimes reaching more than 30. The pattern is erratic, often punctuated by yawns, sighs, small coughs or sniffs. Breathing is occasionally noisy, usually on expiration but sometimes on inspiration. The overbreather rarely uses the diaphragm and tends to breathe continuously with the upper chest: "effortless heaving of the sternum." Occasionally, the neck muscles, clavicle, and shoulders may be seen moving up and down, often gently but sometimes vigorously. To the careful observer there are a variety of patterns that may ultimately cause problems. One not uncommon habit is that of splinting; that is, tightly contracting the abdominal muscles. Many middle-aged women were told when young to "stand up straight, pull your tummy in, tuck your seat in, and pull your shoulders back." Such habits become second nature and patients have great difficulty in becoming aware of relaxation of their abdominal muscles as well as other areas of the body. Animals at rest (cats are good examples) move only their abdomens. Patients must learn to relax, drop their shoulders and upper chest, and breathe easily and rhythmically with the abdomen.

Although overbreathing is the most frequently described abnormal pattern, I have noted that quiet breath-holding, or apneas, combined with irregular breathing is a pattern associated with just as many problems as the obvious hyperventilation pattern. Patients with these irregular apneic patterns respond equally well to the treatment described here. I would estimate that they make up approximately 20–30 percent of our caseload, and they surely deserve more attention from researchers.

2. Initial Assessment

2.1. Source of Referral

A hyperventilator will often have been referred after diagnosis by a GP or consultant physician. In some cases, the doctor will have given the patient considerable insight into the condition, after noting there is a fat folder, taking a list of symptoms, observing the breathing pattern, and—in noncardiac cases—performing an overbreathing test (voluntary hyperventilation). Other tests may also be performed (Chapter 6). In other cases, only a provisional diagnosis has been made, and the patient is recommended to the physiotherapist with little or no explanation given and no tests or symptomology recorded. In addition, it is not unusual for the therapist to recognize this condition and identify it in patients referred with other diagnoses, e.g., back pain, fibrositis, migraine, sinusitis, etc. With self-referral to chartered physiotherapists now permitted in Britain, and more publicity in the general press, patients are also beginning to come directly for assessment and treatment. "Cured" patients may encourage friends and colleagues to come for advice. Health visitors, midwives, and psychologists also refer patients.

2.2. Observation

On the first encounter many points may be observed. Some patients like to shake hands, and damp, cold, warm, clammy, firm, or weak grasps may be noted. The hyperventilator's demeanor may be one of weariness, tiredness, apathy, or exhaustion; conversely, it may be tense, excitable, "high," or over-alert, with wide-open eyes, hunched shoulders, crossed legs and arms, etc. Quick arm and hand movements may occur during speech, or frequent shifting in the chair and fidgeting, finger and foot-tapping, or jaw-twitching. Quality and speed of speech are important; also its variability when the patient is discussing trigger factors (see Section 2.5), emotions (Chapter 17), and other problems. Areas of breathing, i.e., apical or abdominal or a mixture, and rate and regularity, are of fundamental importance and must be recorded. Sighs, yawns, sniffs, coughs, and "emotional" breathing are significant, tell tale signs.

These may even be noted when the patient makes an appointment over the telephone.

2.3. History

Notes from the referring physician and hospital records will have been scrutinized before the patient's first visit. Then, as is the usual practice in physiotherapy, a careful history is taken regarding medication, previous surgical procedures, especially those related to abdominal and nasal problems and accidents, previous treatments, etc. This may be an education in itself for the therapist. Some unfortunate, long-term sufferers have undertaken many strange remedies!

It must always be borne in mind that other conditions may present themselves or arise later. One should not be complacent and attribute every symptom to hyperventilation. A therapist has time to listen and evaluate; if there is any doubt at all, the patient should be referred back to the medical practitioner for an opinion. In some cases, further investigations are carried out. I have been sent patients diagnosed as hyperventilators who, after the initial subjective examination, have had to be referred back for help with such problems as asthma, anemia, thyroid disorders, etc. Some patients will have already been checked for such problems, but the therapist must always be vigilant. Furthermore, when the accompanying problems are under medical control, the patient can gain a great deal more from relaxation and breathing reeducation.

Clearly, cooperation between the medical practitioner and the therapist is essential. When advisers are not *au fait* with hyperventilation or are not prepared to talk with the patient about the condition, treatment is more difficult. When medical backing is poor, the patient remains skeptical rather than whole heartedly involved. If it is confirmed by the doctor that there are no additional problems, then encouragement is given to practice the breathing and relaxation regularly. Patients will return to the therapist confident and motivated. They have been taken seriously and have not been told they are neurotic. Best of all, there is something they can do to help themselves.

A number of hyperventilators will have musculoskeletal, nasal or other conditions. After checking with the medical practitioner, a physiotherapist may be able to deal with some of these disorders using other skills, e.g., manipulation, massage, electrical treatments, or exercise advice. As the treatment for hyperventilation progresses, many of the accompanying problems may be resolved.

2.4. Symptoms

It is important to obtain a *full* list of all the symptoms experienced. Most patients need no encouragement to itemize these: their friends, families, and GPs are heartily sick of listening to their many complaints. There are, though, a small number of withdrawn persons who do need to be encouraged to identify problems. During the first session, a rapport should be built between the therapist and patient. Initially, patients should be encouraged to talk. I find that if they can get most concerns "off their chests," they will be more receptive to treatment and advice later on. Sometimes a patient will confide a problem not previously discussed with the medical practitioner—for example, agoraphobia, visual problems, marital conflict, sleep disorders, loss of weight, etc. Experience in treating hyperventilation, knowledge of the physiology of the condition, and assessment of the patient's personality are therefore all important. Access to the medical practitioner by the therapist is sometimes necessary for discussion and medical guidance.

A comprehensive list is also important because, when checking back at a later date, the patient will have forgotten many of his or her problems, and both therapist and patient may not appreciate the progress made. Some therapists use itemized questionnaires. I often encourage diary-keeping (see Section 3.2.2), and sometimes find that patients have already started to do this as an outlet for their feelings. They are told that the diary will be for their own use and for no one else's perusal. When they complain of feeling ill in a few months' time and then refer back to their diaries, they will appreciate how ill they previously felt. The therapist should also record any advice given, for future reference.

2.5. Identification of Trigger Factors

During the history taking, a trigger point may emerge, from which time all the problems appear to have developed. This may have been a period of physical or emotional stress such as after a surgical procedure. For example, if an abdominal incision has been made, there may be inhibition of the abdominal muscles and diaphragm, with greater rib cage excursion occurring at rest. Any pain, especially abdominal, can cause splinting and rigidity of abdominal muscles, which may persist and become habitual. This problem must be recognized and corrected as soon as possible.

The death or illness of a close family member may have triggered the problem (Chapter 17). Stress or life events scales may be useful here, for evaluating the levels of stress.

Interestingly, some patients report ear, nose, and throat problems (Chapter 2). Some have had surgery for removal of polyps, or other ENT procedures. Some have nasal drip and develop a habit of frequent sniffing. I think these subjects deserve further research.

2.6. Allergies

Some patients referred to me have attended various allergy clinics. Other patients report allergies, and I find it useful to note these. With hyperventilation there is an increase in histamine produced; the high levels of histamine might cause the allergy problems to manifest themselves (Chapter 7). Very gradually, as patients become proficient in their breathing and relaxation, they report that they can eat or drink many of the offending substances without symptoms.

2.7. Other Types of Breathing Training

When difficulty with breathing, or air-hunger, is experienced, people will frequently revert to a breathing exercise that they have learned in keep-fit, yoga, or antenatal classes. Unfortunately, this usually means filling the lungs, using the entire rib cage, and taking deep breaths—often holding the inspired air and then breathing out completely with emphasis on exhalation. *These practices will perpetuate hyperventilation symptoms or increase their severity, and must be discouraged immediately.* It is useful to find out what type of breathing exercise the patient has been performing and to ask for a demonstration. This may develop into an unintentional overbreathing test! It should be explained that different types of breathing are used, depending on the function required. For opera singing or cross-channel swimming, the required lung and muscle function of the chest is quite different from that during sedentary tasks. The exchange of gases and metabolic rate must be appropriate to the activity—or lack of it!

2.8. Voluntary Hyperventilation

This test depends partly on the facilities available to the therapist, and partly on the therapist's medical knowledge. Its aim is to provoke symptoms by overbreathing. Various authorities recommend different rates and durations for exacerbating problems. The test is not always effective; for example, chest pain symptoms are not easily reproduced. It should always be remembered that problems such as cardiac ischemia may occur. Resuscitation facilities and experienced staff should be at hand. Patients who experience therapy as anxiety-provoking may spontaneously overbreathe quite violently, thus eliciting mild or severe symptoms. One new patient awaiting her first treatment collapsed on the waiting room floor, and pulses were impossible to find. She required emergency transport to hospital. Later I learned this was a regular occurrence for her.

Voluntary hyperventilation is not only a diagnostic indicator but also a method for building confidence when used in a controlled manner later in treatment (see Section 3.16).

2.9. Panic Attacks

A disordered breathing pattern is typical in patients with panic attacks. Many factors may affect and complicate treatment. Diazepam initially slows the breathing rate, then sometimes there is a rebound tightening of muscle groups.

Varying levels of natural and administered hormones may trigger panic attacks at premenstrual times and at the menopause. Certain illnesses have an effect on the respiratory centers, provoking abnormal breathing patterns and causing a tendency to have attacks.

With patients who are familiar to the therapist, it is possible to discern an irregular breathing pattern developing. If the therapist has a good rapport with the patient, the attack may be averted. I have been able to do this, occasionally, over the telephone. Also, if the patient has an element of asthma as well as disordered breathing, it may be possible to avert the attack, and it is nearly always possible to help lessen its severity.

3. Reeducation of Breathing Patterns

3.1. Explanation and Demonstration

After greeting the patient and making him or her comfortable (preferably in an arm chair), and having taken the history, the therapist gives an introduction to the physiology and mechanisms of overbreathing. Attention is drawn to the relationship of symptoms and erratic breathing patterns. This link will be obvious if voluntary hyperventilation is, or has been, performed. It is important initially that the patient appreciates the basic mechanisms, the level of explanation depending on the patient's background, intelligence, interests, and personality. For a simple explanation of hyperventilation, I use the analogy of a motor car, which, although in perfect mechanical condition, is unable to run efficiently when filled with contaminated fuel. The human body works in a similar way. There is nothing wrong with the organs and systems but if the blood reaching them to feed them and make them work is the wrong mixture, then they will not function efficiently. Since the blood supplies all areas of the body, this can account for malfunction of different areas and systems. This analogy is particularly helpful for patients with multiple symptoms, although perhaps not quite accurate with regard to the car!

History and symptoms having been recorded and a possible trigger factor ascertained, it is also helpful to give patients a brief description of the mechanism of the fight-or-flight response with application to their everyday lives. Particular attention is drawn to the change in respiratory rate, muscle contraction, and tension. Frequently, patients have been given the impression that they are neurotic and hypochondriacal, and there is no physical element in their condition. They are consequently very relieved when they learn that there is something that they themselves can do to effect an improvement. If appropriate, I show the patient a simplified diagram of the vicious circle (Chapter 6) and explain how we are attempting to break it at two points: first, by changing the breathing pattern and hence the CO_2 deficit; and second, by increasing awareness through reassurance and education.

It is sometimes useful during the first treatment, or part of it, to have a spouse or close friend present. The patient's concentration and memory may be poor, and reinforcement of the above explanation is useful, particularly at a later date. On the other hand, having an unsuitable person present is likely to cause added stress. Here, the physiotherapist must decide which is best.

3.2. Preparation

By the end of the first session, a picture of the patient's background and difficulties has been constructed. A rapport has begun to be built up. Patients often ask what they can do to help themselves before they come for their next visit. This depends upon the patient and circumstances, but the following may need to be taught and discussed over the first few sessions.

3.2.1. Rebreathing

If panic attacks are severe, patients are shown how to rebreathe into a paper bag. This is an emergency or first aid measure. It must initially be practiced under supervision, as it is often done incorrectly (see below).

3.2.2. Handouts and Diaries

It is useful to give printed handouts for reinforcement. It must be appreciated that some of the chronically ill patients find concentration difficult. They are stressed by their first treatment session and often do not absorb all that is said to them (Chapter 5). It is helpful to encourage questions and mention that explanations will be repeated if the patient asks for them at a later date. Every teacher will know how necessary it is to repeat explanations.

The diary should perhaps not be filled in daily in detail, as the habit of dwelling on symptoms and feelings may become obsessive. However, a scale rated each evening regarding physical and mental symptoms can be useful. During the course of treatment, the diary may then be used as a basis of discussion with the patient.

3.2.3. Habits

Patients are encouraged to note and suppress coughs, sighs, sniffs, and yawns. Sighs and yawns may be controlled by either swallowing or holding the breath to a count of five, breathing out slowly, holding to five again, and then resuming easy abdominal breathing.

3.2.4. Books

Suitable books are often recommended, and a few of these are listed below (see Section 8). The first book on the hyperventilation syndrome written especially for patients is by a physiotherapist, Bradley (1991), and it can be recommended as both helpful and comprehensive.

3.2.5. Stress

At this stage patients should not invite extra stress and should start to practice saying "no" to further commitments! Phobics should avoid stressful situations until they have mastered the breathing and relaxation techniques.

3.3. Retraining Method

It is important to make sure that the patient's body is correctly supported during the treatment. A half-lying position may be adopted during the first few sessions. The patient's back is supported by pillows, and another pillow is placed under the knees to relax the abdominal muscles. A book may be placed on the abdomen to encourage abdominal movement and to provide resistance in the early treatments.

It should be noted that, contrary to many methods of breathing exercise, *inspiration* is the active phase. Expiration is passive and relaxed, and a pause should occur at the end of expiration. There should be no sound or effort involved. In order to become aware of the breathing process, the patient may place one hand over the sternum and the other over the upper abdominal wall. The lower hand, on the abdomen, rises during inspiration and falls gently during quiet, relaxed expiration. The upper hand should remain still, with the upper chest relaxed downwards. At first the therapist's hands may be placed over or under the patient's hands; then the patient practices with his or her hands only. There must be no holding of inspired air as is taught in some other breathing methods. I have found that the latter practice exacerbates some symptoms, particularly cardiac arhythmias and chest pains. The inspiratory phase should flow naturally into the relaxed expiratory phase. At a later stage, the patient is encouraged to relax more deeply and "let go" during the expiration. A pause is encouraged after expiration. During the early stages this is often found difficult. Later, with practice, longer pauses become easier and are encouraged. Exercises to prolong the pause may be practiced greatly.

In the early stages a muscular movement of the abdomen may appear with no reference to or coordination with the breathing pattern. This reflex movement or "bounce" occurring after expiration is easy to recognize but difficult to describe. "Air hunger" may also occur initially when a patient endeavors to control the breathing pattern too conscientiously and starts gasping for air. It may be followed by a contraction of the abdominal muscles, which can make the situation worse. These reactions may cause distress and frustration and should be dealt with in the early stages.

Physiotherapists should take careful note of breathing rhythms; any abdominal testing, noisy breathing, etc. should be corrected as early as possible. This is a reason for early frequent checks and later occasional ones, to avoid bad habits. Later, when slow breathing is being maintained for some minutes and the patient is praised for progress, he or she may "swell with pride" and give a "sigh of relief." Attention should be drawn to this bad habit!

In early stages of treatment, premenstrual women may find it difficult to achieve an easy abdominal excursion—there is an observable tightness and tension. This no longer happens once a good abdominal breathing rhythm becomes habitual.

The patient should be made aware of yawns and sighs and learn to suppress them. If there is early awareness of a yawn or sigh developing, a swallow will stifle it. If awareness occurs later, when the intake of air is greater and the shoulders rise, then a useful procedure is to (1) hold to the count of five, (2) very slowly exhale, (3) hold to the count of five, and (4) resume correct abdominal breathing. This may be practiced, and a printed card may be given for reference at home.

The patient is encouraged to count slowly and silently while practicing breathing exercises, aiming for a rate of 6–8 breaths per minute.

A full-length mirror or a smaller, hand-held mirror will help the patient observe areas of movement while breathing. Attention may be drawn to sternomastoid tensing and movement of the sternum and clavicles. Awareness of correct and incorrect breathing patterns should develop; emotional breathing, abdominal splinting, stress responses, and irregular patterns with regard to areas and rates of movement should be discussed and corrected. Patients are encouraged to note these patterns not only during practice sessions but also while performing daily living activities. *Breathing patterns are under voluntary control and will respond to conscious correction.* Within the optimum range of 6–8 breaths per minute, with shoulders dropped and upper chest relaxed, there are many possible variations in normal patterns. As treatment progresses, a comfortable, individual pattern will emerge.

3.4. Frequency of Sessions

When possible, patients are treated individually, once weekly for approximately 45 minutes to one hour; as they progress, once every two weeks, then once every three weeks, etc., until they are given appointments monthly. They may cancel an appointment the previous week if progressing well, and make another for the following month. Patients are discharged with the understanding that they can return if they have any problems. As treatment progresses they are told they may telephone if they require reassurance or help with the breathing and relaxation techniques. I sometimes ask them to telephone weekly for a report of progress.

3.5. Group Instruction

I treat hyperventilating patients individually and then, if they are agreeable and compatible, sometimes assemble them in a group. Classes are suitable when a good breathing rhythm has begun to be established individually and general relaxation techniques are understood. I tend to have two to five people together, and no more. Such groups can be very rewarding but large classes are inadvisable. Breathing rhythms and relaxation are difficult to check, and personal difficulties are not broached so easily. Problems arise in classes if the leader issues instructions for inspiration, expiration, and pauses to be performed by everyone at the same time. This should be avoided, and only general instructions should be given.

3.6. Hospitalization

Patients, I find, often require more than once-weekly treatments, but in many practices and for many patients this is not possible. There is also a case for people severely affected by hyperventilation benefiting from being taken out of a stressful environment for a short period. This gives them time to readjust and rethink their lives' priorities and values while being treated at least twice a day with breathing reeducation and relaxation training. This regime was instigated with remarkable success by Dr. Lum and his staff at Papworth Hospital. City hospitals with their noise, bustle, and general tension are not ideal for this type of reeducation, as compared to those in country environs such as Cambridgeshire. Treatment areas should be quiet, tranquil, and comfortable as far as possible. Ideally, treatment adjuncts such as music, art therapy, and gentle destressing massage should be available to help restore the individual's homeostasis. Inevitably patients have to reenter their own environment but are strengthened physically and mentally, and motivated to be in charge of their own lives. At the same time their bodies will have been trained to accept the new higher Pco_2 levels, and their relaxation training and bodily awareness enhanced.

3.7. Medication

The use of medication is fraught with problems and is continually changing (for example, regarding prescription of tranquilizers). British physiotherapists, through their hospital and other experience, gain knowledge of, but are not examined in the action of, pharmacological drugs. It is important, as has already been stressed, to have close liaison with the medical practitioner. With the latter's consent and the patient's cooperation, it is satisfying to see patients gradually reducing their medication, slowly coming off benzodiazepines and sometimes beta-blockers. It is generally up to the therapist to caution patients to withdraw very slowly over a long period, but the initiative comes from the patient who is usually very well motivated to reduce drug intake. There are also self-help groups that can sometimes give good advice and support.

3.8. Progress

During the course of treatment an assessment of the patient's behavior and characteristics will be taking place. Patients may be told that the degree of relief of symptoms is proportional to the amount of time expended on practicing the correct breathing and relaxation techniques! Patients must appreciate that the improved quality of life is due to their own perseverance and frequent practice of the treatment regimen. As patients progress in treatment, they often report less irritability with family and colleagues, an easing off in obsessiveness, and increased clarity of thought. Panic attacks are first controlled and then cease; coping ability improves; emotions may not have quite such extreme highs and lows; and a sense of humor reemerges.

All positive signs of improvement should be noted and praised. It must be borne in mind, however, that in the early stages, when patients may be tense and do their home exercises too intensely, they become *more* stressed. If they recognize this fact they should give up the session, not feel guilty, and come back to practice later. Patients at this stage should be encouraged to telephone for advice and reassurance.

3.9. Exacerbation of Symptoms

Many patients will have difficulty using their abdomen and diaphragm at first. As they begin to do so, they may not be able to suppress the upper thoracic excursion, and their rate may not yet have slowed to 6–8 per minute. Ventilation is thereby increased, and an exacerbation of symptoms may occur. Preliminary warnings of this occurrence may be given, and the patient may be provided with notes on coping techniques (see Section 3.15). Simple explanations and a good deal of encouragement may be required at this stage; supervision will need to be particularly supportive.

There is a danger when well-meaning patients (or therapists) draw attention to hyperventilation in friends. If breathing correction is not supervised, these people may experience more symptoms by resorting to previously learned incorrect breathing exercises.

3.10. Posture

When an easy, rhythmical pattern can be maintained for a period in a relaxed position, other postures may be used: sitting more upright, standing but leaning against a wall, standing, slow and fast walking, etc. It should be noted that in the standing position there is far less abdominal excursion. This is quite normal, and reassurance may be necessary. Any tightening of the abdominal muscles should be discouraged. Once they are improving and symptoms are diminishing, patients may then complain of lack of tone in the abdominal muscles. I often devote one session at a later stage to teaching a few simple exercises because of the importance of toning up these muscles. However, some of the most commonly performed abdominal exercises can exacerbate back problems. An experienced physiotherapist's advice should be sought so that the exercises are appropriate to the patient's ability, age, general condition, and medical history. Exercises should be supervised initially, as breath-holding may easily occur.

3.11. Matching Breathing Patterns to Activities

Obviously, as activities speed up there will be shorter pauses and faster, larger movement of the thorax with the accessory muscles coming into play. The breathing excursion must be compatible with the activity at that time. There is a tendency for hyperventilators to prolong the use of accessory muscles and to breathe at a fast rate after physical activities have ceased. Running on the spot or exercising may be practiced during treatment sessions, with encouragement of an earlier resumption of a slower, easy abdominal pattern. A good deal of practice standing and walking may be required before breathing control becomes satisfactory. As treatment progresses, breathing control should be maintained throughout the relaxation session until it becomes easy and natural. This may be slow, and a great deal of patience and encouragement is sometimes needed.

3.12. Speech

Teachers, singers, and others involved in using their voices frequently may be encouraged to read aloud, lowering the register, speaking more slowly and smoothly, and relaxing the jaw, shoulder muscles, etc. Hyperventilators should be discouraged from talking continuously in a steady stream, using long sentences, and then gasping and taking a sudden inhalation before setting off again! The aim is to encourage short, concise sentences in a low register most of the time. Periods of breath-holding may be practiced, using a watch with a seconds hand for timing, and avoiding gasping at the end of the period.

3.13. Clothing

Tight trousers or jeans, corsets, panty girdles, and belts should be avoided at all times. They inhibit abdominal movement and encourage upper chest movement, and thus act like an abdominal splint. It can be a real problem to wean patients off tight clothes!

3.14. Practice

Patients are told that with a minimum of two practice sessions per day, constant brief checks, and vigilance, the respiratory center will eventually adapt to the higher Pco_2 level, recognize it as normal, and maintain it involuntarily. Gradually normal breathing will become comfortable as the brain accepts the new pattern, but a great deal of practice is often necessary before the "automatic pilot" takes over. Many patients practice up to four times per day. They are often pleased to report that when they first awake in the morning, they are aware of abdominal movement occurring automatically.

3.15. Emergency or Coping Measures (when Pco_2 Is Likely to Fall)

At an early stage patients should report or should become aware of quickening or development of incorrect breathing in a stressful situation, or even when they only *think* of problems (Nixon and Freeman, 1988). Phobics should note when their breathing pattern variations occur. They should learn to anticipate these problem areas and employ emergency procedures as follows:

- Drop shoulders and relax personal areas of tension—say "let go" to the areas of tightness and tension.
- Slow the breathing rate as much as possible.
- Ensure that the abdomen is moving and not tightly held ("splinted") in anticipation of trouble.
- Use a paper bag (rebreathing) when other methods are not achieving success. The bag may be kept in a handbag or wallet but can only really be used in private or in a dire emergency! It is placed over the nose *and* mouth, where a seal is made by the fingers and thumbs of both hands. Six to twelve easy, natural breaths are then taken and the rebreathed gases will temporarily raise the Pco_2. The bag is then removed and abdominal breathing continued. If the latter is still not possible after a few seconds the bag may be used again. However, patients should not be encouraged

to use rebreathing as an easy way out. (N.B.: plastic bags should not be used because of the danger of a patient inhaling the bag if startled.)
• Rationalize the situation—in five years time will it matter? etc.

Use avoidance tactics in the early stages: do not go into stress-provoking situations. When there is some control of breathing and relaxation in everyday situations, small excursions into stressful areas may be made using the new skills under supervision. It is interesting to note that after a stressful occurrence, some patients report hyperventilation symptoms appearing immediately, whereas others do not report the onset of symptoms until some hours or even days later. Perhaps the lability and daily rhythms of Pco_2 levels vary in individuals.

3.16. Challenge

When patients gain confidence and are making progress, they are encouraged to overbreathe during one of the sessions. As soon as symptoms begin, they are instructed to resume the slow, abdominal pattern and chase away the symptoms. This may be performed two or three times to give confidence.

4. Relaxation

Relaxation techniques may be applied either to a general physical or mental state or to specific tensions. Patients' understanding of the fight-or-flight response can be related to their own tight, tense muscles and overactive minds. There are many techniques that have been and are being evolved for teaching relaxation. A simple method, which may be modified and adapted for individual patients, is used for hyperventilators.

4.1. General Physical Relaxation

Recognition of unnecessary tension in muscle groups is important. To encourage awareness and control of various areas of the body, the *contrast* method is therefore often used for the first few sessions. The patient is told to tighten, and then let go and relax, the toes and then feet three times. The method is used systematically, moving up slowly through the muscle groups of the body. The patient is encouraged to move abdominal muscles slowly and easily throughout, although this will probably be impossible in the early stages. The body is worked through twice, and the patient requested to repeat this sequence in home practice sessions. The difference between a hard, tense muscle group and a soft, flabby, relaxed group must be appreciated. The usual test of lifting and letting a limb drop may be helpful.

Later, physical relaxation is encouraged by starting at the feet and working up through the body *without* tensing of muscle groups. Using a calm, monotonous voice, the therapist directs suitable words and phrases to areas of the body. The patient is encouraged and expected to "let go," "feel heaviness," "feel warmth," etc., without a contraction. Patients are asked to close their eyes when they feel it comfortable to do so, to reduce external stimuli. Relaxation techniques may also be practiced if there is difficulty sleeping, combining slow, rhythmical breathing with relaxation.

4.2. Mental Relaxation

Patients often complain of their brains "whirling round" with problems and worries, and of being unable to still their thoughts. The fact that physical and mental relaxation are directly related, and reinforce one another, should be explained. Conscious relaxation of muscle groups and slow breathing will help the thinking processes to get into a lower gear. Relaxing mentally using the visualization method, listening to certain music, etc., reinforces physical relaxation of muscles. With eyes closed and having completed the physical relaxation procedure, the patient may be asked to visualize a garden or beach and use all the senses to appreciate the scene: sight (green grass and flowers); smell (perfume of the flowers); sound (birds singing); sensation (feeling of a gentle, warm breeze). Suggestions of comfort, tranquility, serenity, etc., may be introduced.

Visualization is not always appropriate, the patient's condition and progress should first be assessed. Patients' suggestions and modifications should be considered and discussed, and the visualization tailored to individual needs. Speed, tone of voice, etc., must be varied depending on the patient's breathing pattern and level of arousal.

Some patients experience discomfort, other unpleasant feelings, or even panic when they begin to relax (Chapter 13). Therapists must be vigilant and aware of these problems and rethink their treatment techniques. It may be necessary to curtail the relaxation aspect of treatment and use modified methods later. Experience is required, and consultation with colleagues advisable.

On the other hand, some patients are so exhausted when they come for treatment that they fall asleep as the relaxation session progresses. Sleeping should be discouraged, and a pleasant state between sleep and alertness encouraged. When relaxing well, a pleasant, floating feeling or calm, peaceful feeling may be experienced. This is encouraged and praised, as is warming of feet and hands when peripheral vessels dilate. This calm, relaxed state should be maintained as long as possible after the treatment practice session.

4.3. Tape-Recorded Instruction

Counting or monotonous commands are of help to reinforce the new habit of breathing, e.g., slowly in, slowly out, and rest, or in, two, three, out, two, three, rest, two three. An instruction card may be given for reference at home. There are many variations but it is important to be sensitive to each individual's pattern of breathing, which will slowly emerge.

An audio tape is a useful adjunct to remind the patient of, and reinforce, the relaxation sequence. At present I make a tape during a treatment session for use at home so that it is individually tailored to the patient's requirements. The amount of breathing reminders given depends on the stage of progress. Individual tapes made for each patient can be a great help but they must be reviewed and revised as treatment progresses. Patients usually find their home practice sessions even more helpful. The tape may also be used to avert panic situations if practiced in time. Patients should not, however, become dependent on the recording and should sometimes practice without it. It should be remembered that there is no point in making a standard tape for breathing patterns. Some commercial tapes give commands, assuming there is a universal pattern rather than individual variations.

4.4. Specific Tensions

Most people have specific areas of tension. The old wives' tale that trouble goes to the weakest part seems to be borne out! Many hyperventilators complain of cervical and trapezius aches or lumbar pain. As they become more proficient in breathing and relaxation and the P_{CO_2} rises, many of these aches will disappear.

Four common areas of tension to be discussed with and demonstrated to the patient are shoulders, hands, abdomen and jaw. Patients are encouraged to report on the personal areas of tension they have become aware of during everyday life. Note should be made if the abdomen tightens and the easy breathing rhythm is lost during telephone conversations, when admonishing juniors, when children are demanding, when one is being criticized, etc. Discussions of which gentle, rhythmical exercises or other methods can be used to diminish this tension are helpful.

5. Guidelines for Therapists

Successful treatment depends a good deal on the characteristics of the therapist. The therapist must be able to breathe in the desired manner and to exhibit a certain amount of relaxation during treatment. Particularly when speaking to the patient over the telephone, the voice should be low and able to convey calm confidence. The therapist who has practiced and, hopefully, mastered the technique of quiet breathing during stressful events will convey a good deal of conviction. Unfortunately, many therapists have a tendency to overbreathe!

It is very satisfying to receive early referrals before habitual hyperventilation has become established; a few treatments will usually suffice. The irregular breathing pattern is comparatively easy to abolish and the original, normal pattern reemerges; symptoms quickly disappear. Chronic hyperventilators, however, often require long-term supervision. Rapport must be built up over the period of treatment. Time is also of prime importance and must be suitably allocated for treatment sessions. Unless there is commitment and the possibility of continuing over sometimes quite a long period, it is debatable whether treatment should even be started.

Occasionally patients are initially aggressive; then firm, calm handling is important. Great patience is required to support some chronic hyperventilators. Nevertheless, if treated with sensitivity and understanding, hyperventilators are rewarding to treat and generally are extremely appreciative and grateful.

6. Conclusion

Eventually most patients maintain normal diaphragmatic breathing together with a degree of relaxation throughout most of the day. Hyperventilation symptoms are abolished or very greatly diminished. Instead of being governed physically, and sometimes mentally and emotionally "taken over" by the "welter of bodily symptoms," patients are now able to manage and be comfortable and at peace with body and mind. They should have acquired a certain amount of skill in avoiding or managing stress in the long and short term, both physically and emotionally.

7. References

Bradley, D. *Hyperventilation syndrome.* Auckland, New Zealand: Tandem, 1991; and Berkeley: Ten Speed Press, 1992.
Cluff, R.A. Chronic hyperventilation and its treatment by physiotherapy: Discussion paper. *Journal of the Royal Society of Medicine,* 1984, *77,* 855–862.
Innocenti, D.M. Chronic hyperventilation syndrome. In P.A. Downie, (Ed.), *Cash's textbook of chest, heart and vascular disorders for physiotherapists.* 4th Ed. London: Faber and Faber, 1987.
Lum, L.C. Breathing exercises in the treatment of hyperventilation and chronic anxiety states. *Chest, Heart, and Stroke Journal,* 1977, *2,* 6–11.

Nixon, P.G.F., and Freeman, L.J. The "think test": A further technique to elicit hyperventilation. *Journal of the Royal Society of Medicine,* 1988, *81,* 277–279.

8. Further Reading

Bradley, D. *Hyperventilation syndrome.* Auckland, New Zealand: Tandem, 1991; and Berkeley: Ten Speed Press, 1992.

Madders, J. *Stress and relaxation: Self-help techniques for everyone.* London: Macdonald Optima, 1988.

Patel, C. *The complete guide to stress management.* London: Macdonald Optima, 1989; and New York: Plenum Press, 1991.

Relaxation for Living (a registered charity), 29 Burwood Park Road, Walton on Thames, Surrey, England KT12 5LH (booklets, newsletters, classes).

III

Other Therapeutic Approaches to Breathing Disorders

12

Breathing and Vocal Dysfunction

DAPHNE J. PEARCE

1. Introduction

Speech is the culmination of two essential human functions: breathing and communication. Every aspect of speech can be scientifically analyzed in neurological and physiological terms, but as a function, the essence is the interaction of the processes involved. The complexity of this interaction is exemplified in phonation, or voice, the medium of human utterance and expression (Fig. 1). The physical apparatus, the *larynx* (Fig. 2), is one unit of the mechanism that includes breathing and the supralaryngeal structures (i.e., the structures above the larynx: the oropharynx and nasopharynx, the oral and nasal cavities). The larynx can be affected by external factors, such as dust and fumes, and by the most powerful internal force—emotion. From the infant's screams, to the quavering of senescence, the voice reflects feelings and well being; it betrays fears and doubts, and proclaims intentions. Professionals working with voice problems must consider all the factors in relation to one another; a disturbance in one area will upset the balance necessary to maintain healthy phonation appropriate to the speaker and acceptable to the audience.

2. Larynx

The larynx is a cartilagenous framework, lying at the base of the neck (at the level of the third to sixth cervical vertebrae), inferiorly attached to the trachea

DAPHNE J. PEARCE • Speech Therapy Department, St. Bartholomew's Hospital, London EC1A 7BE, England.
Behavioral and Psychological Approaches to Breathing Disorders, edited by Beverly H. Timmons and Ronald Ley. Plenum Press, New York, 1994.

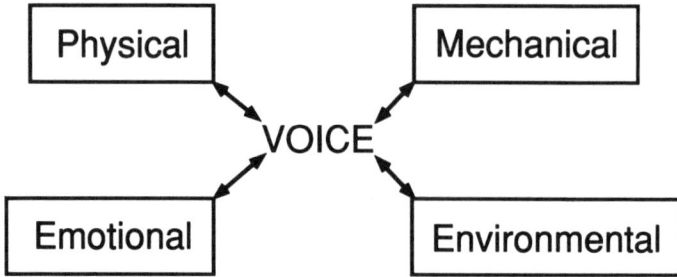

Figure 1. The interaction between the voice and other factors.

and superiorly opening into the pharynx. It houses the two vocal folds (formerly known as cords) composed of muscle and ligament with a covering of mucous membrane. The vibration of these vocal folds generates sound. It is indeed remarkable that they can effect such a range of pitch, loudness, and qualities of phonation.

The primary function of the larynx is not as a sound-generating organ, but as a valve to seal off the airway, preventing foreign substances from entering the

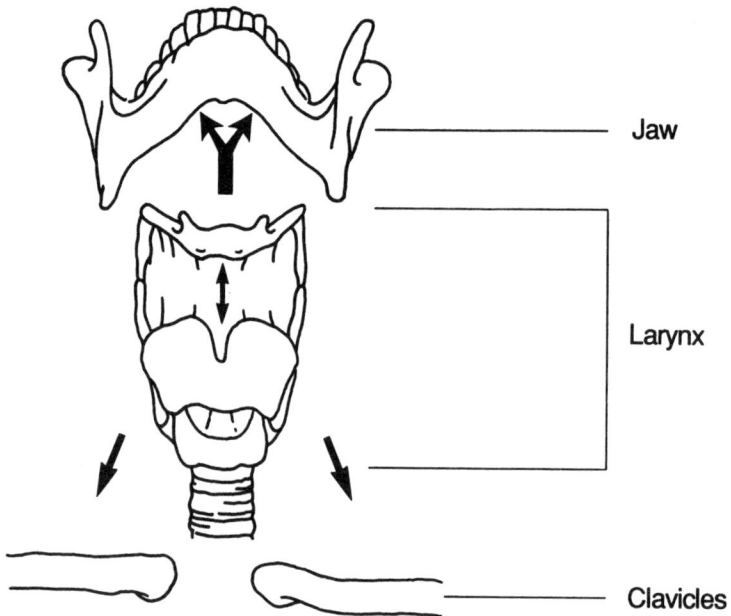

Figure 2. The dynamic relationship of the larynx.

respiratory tract. Its other functions are to ensure free passage of air into and out of the lungs; to prevent air escape during effortful activities, by creating a seal; and to produce sound. (For a detailed description of the larynx and its functions, see Aronson, 1980.)

3. Resonators

Phonation is a dynamic process, the size and shape of the resonators being altered by movement. The larynx will be both elevated and depressed to modify the pharyngeal cavity (Fig. 2). The fundamental vibration is fairly weak, as with any musical instrument, and needs a resonating body to amplify it. This is provided by the supralaryngeal structures that extend from the pharynx to the oral and nasal cavities (Fig. 2). The soft palate influences nasal resonance and the tongue modifies the oropharynx and the oral cavity. Finally, the movement of the lower jaw expands the oral cavity, allowing that free flowing projection most usually associated with the rich tones of accomplished singers. The sinuses, contrary to popular belief, do not function as resonators. Their structure, with the sound-absorbing mucous membrane lining and the small openings, is ineffective. Bunch (1982) explains the role of the sinuses in terms of the singer's perceptions, as opposed to the listener's perceptions.

4. Breathing

The energy source of vocal fold activity is the expired air stream generated by the respiratory system, the functions of the larynx and the breathing mechanism being physiologically fuscd. This is apparent in such spontaneous activities as laughing, yawning and sobbing. However, these activities are by nature void of control, and it is control of the flow and pressure of the expired air that is the crucial factor, providing breath support for voice and speech.

A disturbance of the breathing pattern is responsible for, or contributes to, many voice problems, provoking inappropriate modification of the mechanism, to compensate for the loss of sustained air pressure. It is only when a problem such as nasal congestion arises that many people are alcrted to the way in which they breathe.

Speech therapists advocate intercostal diaphragmatic breathing as described in Chapter 11. The adult breathing rate is about 14 breaths per minute, and the average volume of tidal air, 500 cc (vital capacity of the average male, 4000 cc). Normal conversational speech is undertaken at 40–60 percent of vital capacity. Voice production is the result of the interaction of the airstream with the vocal folds (see Boone, 1977, for a useful summary of the breathing mechanism).

5. Singing

No one appreciates the relationship between breathing and voice production, a subject in its own right, more than the singer does. Trained singers have a greater than average vital capacity, which they are capable of utilizing in sound production while expending less than average energy to sustain the voice performance. The trained singer utilizes the abdominal musculature in a way that suggests that these muscles are involved in producing and maintaining subglottal pressure for voice production. Sundberg *et al.* (1986) reported that subjects given visual feedback of transdiaphragmatic pressure were able to bring diaphragmatic activity under conscious control, refuting the previously held belief that this was not possible and opening new horizons for both respiratory and voice training.

In referring to the skilled breath control of the singer, the author specified "trained." Many popular singers do not have training, and consequently experience problems such as hyperventilation for a variety of reasons. The popular music industry is highly competitive, which in itself is stressful, creating tension patterns and habits that readily induce or contribute to a disturbance of the breathing mechanism. Singers frequently perform without adequate rehearsal in unsuitable environments. Driven by the desire to succeed, they may emulate the style of a star by, for example, adopting awkward postures. Without adequate and precise control of breathing vital to support the voice, they endeavor to adapt the laryngeal and articulatory mechanisms to sustain the performance, inevitably stressing the system.

6. Influences on Breathing and Phonation

The mechanisms of breathing and phonation are vulnerable to both internal and external influences, and breathing patterns are affected not only by general health, respiratory health, sex, and age but also by factors such as the individual's spoken language characteristics and stress. Speech is a learned skill bound by linguistic rules and conventions; often these, rather than physiological need, direct the breathing pattern. This is most conspicuous when subjects, while reading aloud, can be seen to delay replenishing their air supply until they reach a grammatically imposed, acceptable pause. The same strategies may also be applied in conversation, compounded by eagerness or anxiety to finish what they intended to say. Articulatory patterns not only influence the resonance as previously indicated, but also provoke the development of muscle tensions.

Society has become very aware of stress; it is useful to look briefly at some causes of stress and the reactions they provoke in relation to vocal function.

1. Vocal changes during puberty are usually affected innocuously but can be traumatic. The adolescent who finds his voice unpredictable, with erratic pitch breaks, becomes apprehensive of himself and of his listeners' reactions.

2. Voice is inextricably linked with personality, and specific vocal quality has been related to it (Moses, 1954). The development of contact ulcers has been attributed to the mode of phonation demonstrated in certain personality types, characteristically tense and intense, and exposed to stress (Aronson, 1980).

3. The voice portrays emotion. An abundance of studies regarding voice and emotion is succinctly summarized in Aronson (1980). One effect of emotion widely recognized in the medical field is the cardiac response to stress. Many people experience anxiety when speaking in public. Taggart et al. (1989) found that the heart rate increases from a normal average of 70 to 120 per minute, five minutes before a subject is due to give a presentation. It rises to 170 at the time of speaking and subsides to 90 at the conclusion.

Speakers may experience dryness in the mouth and altered perception of their own voice, and may lose the natural rhythm of their breathing pattern. There is an interplay between the rate of utterance and breathing. An increased rate of utterance urges the speaker to keep going; the absence of suitable pauses in their delivery compels them to maintain the verbal output and resort to gasps to "top up."

The significance of the precise balance of the interacting functions cannot be overemphasized—the importance of maintaining appropriate muscle tone throughout the system, enabling the apparatus to function like a correctly tuned engine. This gives positive feedback of both sensation and auditory perception.

4. Hyperventilation, in contrast, generates disturbed sensation. The strategies adopted in an attempt to overcome this further provoke the problem. Since the function of the vocal apparatus is disturbed, the physiological parameters are yet again adjusted to attempt to produce the intended output. It inevitably falters, giving another set of negative signals to disturb the speaker's reaction and self-esteem (Fig. 3).

7. Smoking

Many are aware of their own response to stress and seek solace in smoking. The problem is not only that carbon monoxide affects the cardiorespiratory system, but also that smokers modify their articulatory musculature and breathing patterns. The cigarette smoker is inclined to tense the lip posture and make an ingressive sucking action, predisposing breathing to a shallow, upper thoracic or clavicular breathing pattern. Smoking can be a sensitive subject, and patients must feel that the therapist is understanding and will support their effort to break the habit.

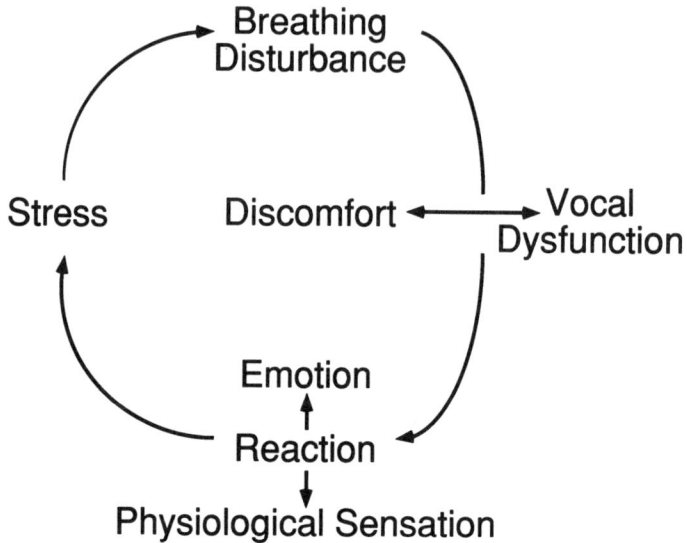

Figure 3. The chain reaction.

8. Posture

Gould (1971) proposes that voice production is secondary to the postural mechanism that influences and affects respiratory activity. He defines posture as

> the totality of dynamic inter-relationships between neural, muscular and skeletal elements involved in determining, maintaining and changing not only postural attitudes, but also the rate and volume of respiration in regard to the demand of the body's need which includes voice production.

The work of Alexander (Barlow, 1973) has contributed much to the awareness of posture and has demonstrated the importance of establishing balance throughout the body. While it is generally known that the shoulders should not be elevated when one is taking a breath, the instruction to keep the shoulders down will not in itself facilitate deep breathing. Instead, the shoulders will be brought forward, creating a curving of the spine and a concave chest in an attempt to use the residual air. Such a posture may be observed in people suffering from asthma.

9. Vocal Use and Abuse

The voice must fulfill certain requirements for any individual, in terms of loudness, pitch, and endurance. It must also be appropriate to the speaker. The voice is used to project a chosen image and thereby to elicit a desired response from the audience. It is therefore a tool, to control oneself as well as the environment. However, the mechanism must function correctly and the key to understanding the cause of problems is being able to identify the use, misuse, or abuse of the voice. It may also determine the individual's attitude or reaction to a voice problem. Professional voice users seek immediate help since they depend on the voice as the tool of their trade. Others delay for many reasons, including fear that there is something seriously wrong, indifference, or secondary gain. Many make demands on their voices without having prepared it for the job they want it to do, unwittingly causing vocal abuse.

Such abuse, including the effects of smoking and alcohol, contributes to chronic laryngitis (edema and vasodilation of the folds) with resulting dysphonia. Vocal nodules are the result of friction creating a tissue reaction manifest as a protuberance on the margin of the fold. In children they have been found to be associated with velopharyngeal incompetence, correlated with insufficient intra-oral pressure, as well as with personality types.

The onset of a voice problem may follow infection. Patients develop compensatory habits to enable them to speak when an irritated larynx should have been rested. A detailed case history is important and revealing. Although in many cases there is no visible cause, it is essential that the larynx be examined by a specialist to identify, or exclude the presence of, any pathology. The conventional terms of reference of voice disorders are organic and psychogenic or functional, the differential being the presence or absence of pathological change in the vocal folds or of neuropsychological control.

The laryngologist will refer patients to the voice specialist for assessment and remediation of symptoms, usually vocal fatigue, weakness, pitch change, or quality change with or without accompanying feelings such as a lump in the throat, tightness across the chest, pain over the sternum, or breathlessness being reported.

Assessment of the voice problem must embrace the way in which the voice has been used as well as the acoustic properties and the patient's attitudes to the voice and to therapy. It is the writer's experience that all too often assurance from the doctor that there is nothing wrong (cancer being the overriding fear) is not enough to allay fears, since the problem has not been given a label that the patient understands and accepts. Empathy and adequate explanations are usually effective, but the question remains, is this person justifiably anxious because of the problem, or did a propensity to anxiety provoke the problem? While recognizing the relationship between voice and personality, the therapist must not be judgemental. The voice specialist is unlikely to meet the patient until the problem is manifest, by which time its very existence will be influencing and affecting the patient, and will have already given rise to very real anxieties and fears. The therapist must listen and watch, put the patient at ease, and elicit information about the way in which the voice is used at work and at home, how much it is used, and in what circumstances and under what conditions. This will enable identification of any aggravating and contributory factors, which may at first sight seem innocuous, such as, almost-constant speaking at work and at home; being in a smoky, dusty, or dry atmosphere; speaking over noise (the sound level at the rear of an aircraft is 90 db, yet travellers are quite unaware of having raised their voices to overcome this); speaking to a hearing-impaired relative or noisy children; or frequent throat-clearing. Fluid intake and general dietary habits are also relevant; excess alcohol and/or insufficient fluid intake have a detrimental affect. Referral to a dietitian may be advisable.

10. Observation

Patients all too often report a hectic life-style at work and at home, feeling constantly pressured to achieve their goals, and always "on the go." These feelings of urgency may be reflected in behavior and in postural habits. These may include overt fidgeting or clock-watching, or less obvious behaviors, such as, crossing arms over the chest, clenching fists, tensing shoulder and neck muscles, rippling face muscles suggesting a clenched jaw, tightly pursing lips, or having a shallow, inadequate breathing pattern with residual air use or an ingressive gasp as a few more words are squeezed in.

Gould's definition (1971) previously referred to (see Section 8) provides a useful foundation for the evaluation of voice disorders and also explains to the patient the significance of a holistic approach, emphasizing the role of the way the voice is used, the framework within which it operates, the musculature instrumental in implementing it, and environmental influences. Any other problems have usually been confided by this stage and the therapist can discuss with the patient whether the help of other professionals should be enlisted. The therapist must not make any assumptions, especially regarding breathing disturbance, but must monitor responses to therapy and be alert to the changes the patient reports. If any other symptoms are identified, such as circulatory complaints (especially in older patients), referral to the appropriate specialist is essential. In the absence of pathology, vocal dysfunction produces predictable patterns of disturbance: shoulders tense and slightly elevated; neck muscles tight; jaw slightly elevated with tight lip posture and tense tongue root; and a disruption of the breathing pattern, which has moved up from intercostal diaphragmatic to clavicular.

11. Vocal Dysfunction

Patients' perceptions of the voice are intriguing. Many are unaware of the connection between voice and breathing. Abnormal breathing patterns are recog-

nized to be associated with psychogenic dysphonia. Gordon *et al.* (1978) reported that 53.4 percent of all dysphonic patterns presented a disturbance of quiet
breathing, and 47.9 percent of patients with mechanical (i.e., nonorganic) dysphonia showed disturbed breathing at rest.

Voice therapists must be conversant with the diverse symptoms produced by
hyperventilation and alert to the possibility that the patient is presenting them
(Chapter 6).

The proposition that some dysphonic patients may be hyperventilators has
been explored (Greene *et al.,* 1984). However, in this author's view, many
patients presenting with breathing disorders, regardless of etiology, also
have unrecognized disorders of phonation, which on examination by a speech
therapist will be evident as a limited ability to sustain phonation, the inability to
effect adequate volume changes, reduced range of pitch, and lowered habitual
pitch.

Hyperventilation symptoms may be reported by a patient with vocal fold
palsy. The paralyzed fold fails to make contact with the healthy fold, leaving a
gap or glottic chink. This causes air wastage, and the patient may overbreathe as
part of the effort to improve phonatory volume. The importance of breathing
applies equally to other disorders of speech, such as dysarthria—resulting from
cerebrovascular accidents, motor neuron disease, Parkinson's disease, or other
neurological disorders.

The final part of the assessment is the evaluation of the acoustic elements
(the ability to initiate and sustain phonation and to change loudness and pitch)
and the identification of exactly how the quality has changed. Certain parameters
of vocal function can be measured with instrumentation such as the electro-
laryngograph, which uses electrical impedance to monitor vibratory fold closure,
identify irregularity of vocal fold activity, and obtain information on pitch range
and distribution. Judgments of quality of voice are essentially subjective; it is
difficult to define "normal" voice, the range and diversity being so colorful. The
identifying characteristic of an individual's voice is the elusive quality that defies
definition because it is unique to that individual. However, there is usually
agreement on the use of terms such as hoarse, creaky, or breathy.

Most people are unable to describe their voices and, if a feature such as a
creaky quality is brought to their attention, will report that it is a lifelong characteristic. It should not be inferred that it is therefore appropriate, but it may
indicate long-standing strained voice production.

12. Therapy

Therapy begins as soon as the patient arrives at the clinic. Any contributory
factors having been identified, the therapist will discuss ways in which patients
can modify their behavior—often only a matter of changing habits, to avoid or

overcome aggravants—and will encourage them to talk through the problems, supporting and guiding them, often enabling them to find solutions themselves. Speech therapists are trained in counseling, and consequently are adept at recognizing when a person's problems need help beyond their own skills. The aim of therapy is to restore the balance and reestablish the posture as defined by Gould (1971).

12.1. Relaxation

The role of relaxation therapy is acknowledged and enjoying a revival after a decline, brought about not only by the advent of tranquilizers, but also by the yearning of voice specialists to be scientific; they would often abandon conventional therapy in favor of technology. The two approaches should ideally complement each other.

There are various schools of relaxation techniques. Therapists must apply that which is appropriate to the patient, and the technique with which they are completely conversant and confident. When excess muscle tone is eradicated, and appropriate tone restored, the mechanism can begin to function effectively.

12.2. Breathing

A pattern of breathing must be stabilized before being applied to speech. The patient is encouraged to focus on the lower chest and to experience the gentle expansion as the lungs fill. The concept of the rhythm of breathing is instilled so this can be modified for speech, by extension of the expiration phase to carry the utterance, with short inspiration, inconspicuous in the flow of speech. If necessary, the rate of speech is modified. If too rapid, the speaker has insufficient time to pause; breathing and delivery must be coordinated.

12.3. Voice Exercises

Finally, voice exercises are introduced, although few may be needed. Retrieving appropriate muscle tone and establishing good breath support may be sufficient to restore vocal function. Starting with a gentle hum eliminates a hard attack; controlled expiration produces steady phonation without quavering; and more forceful expiration with relaxed musculature effects volume increase and maximum resonance. However, if increased tension has resulted in a lowering of the habitual pitch, this may need specific attention. Patients are encouraged to *feel* the voice, to achieve the sensation that it just comes out on its own without deliberate effort on their part. Apprehensions about changing the note to which they have become accustomed are soon assuaged, since the variation is marginal to the ear. Those who have deliberately altered their pitch to create a desired image are advised accordingly. Therapy must equip the patient to use the voice to prevent any recurrence of symptoms. Changed awareness and perceptions contribute much to this end, and if the patients' needs go beyond normal daily voice use, then they would be advised to take an appropriate course of voice training.

13. Conclusion and Guidelines for Therapists

Breathing should be considered as the foundation of good voice production. If this foundation is unsteady, as in the patient with asthma or hyperventilation, it will be reflected in the vocal mechanism. A disturbance of the breathing mechanism will inevitably induce a disturbance of the laryngeal function. In the absence of obviously abnormal performance or quality, skilled assessment is a crucial part of the evaluation.

Therapists working with patients with a breathing disorder would find it helpful to liaise with a speech and voice therapist to agree on a methodology for identifying vocal dysfunction. A questionnaire such as the one shown in Table 1 is suggested.

Table 1
Voice Function Screening Questionnaire

1. Is there frequent throat clearing?	No	Yes
2. What is the rate of utterance?	Normal	Slow
		Fast
3. Does the patient pause when speaking?	Yes	No
(a) Are the pauses appropriate to place in utterance and frequency?	Yes	No
(b) Does the patient take quick "topping up" gasps?	No	Yes
4. Does the vocal pitch appear appropriate for the patient's age and sex?	Yes	No
5. Is there appropriate use of intonation?	Yes	No
6. Are there any conspicuous features of vocal quality?		Hoarse
		Creaky
		Breathy
		Other
7. Is the volume appropriate for the situation?	Yes	No
8. Does the patient report any changes in his/her voice?	No	Yes
9. Does the voice fade or appear to fatigue?	No	Yes
10. Is the jaw posture elevated or tight?		
(a) Observed	No	Yes
(b) Reported	No	Yes
11. Do you feel comfortable listening to the patient's voice?	Yes	No

If the responses to any of the questions fall in the right-hand column, it would be advisable to refer the patient for a full ENT examination and voice assessment.

14. References

Aronson, A.E. *Clinical voice disorders.* New York: Thieme Stratton, 1980.

Barlow, W. *The Alexander principle.* London: Arrow Books, 1973.

Boone, D.R. *The voice and voice therapy.* New Jersey: Prentice Hall, 1977.

Bunch, M. *Dynamics of the singing voice.* New York: Springer Verlag, 1982.

Gordon, M.T., Morton, F.M., and Simpson, I.C. Airflow measurements in diagnosis, assessment and treatment of mechanical dysphonia. *Folia-Phoniatrica,* 1978, *30,* 161–174.

Gould, W.J. Effect of respiratory and postural mechanisms upon action of the vocal cords. *Folia-Phoniatrica,* 1971, *23,* 211–224.

Greene, M.C.L., Timmons, B.H., and Glover, J.H.M. The significance of anxiety and breathing disorders in functional dysphonias. *Bulletin Européan Physiopathologie Respiratoire,* 1984, *20,* 94.

Moses, P.J. *The voice of neurosis.* New York: Grune and Stratton, 1954.

Sundberg, J., Leanderson, R., and von Euler, C. Voice source effects of diaphragmatic activity in singing. *Journal of Phonetics,* 1986, *14,* 351–357.

Taggart, P., Carruthers, M., and Sommerville, W. Some effects of emotion on the normal and abnormal heart. *Current Problems in Cardiology,* 1983, *7,* 9–29.

15. Further Reading

Baken, R.J. *Clinical measurement of speech and voice.* London: Taylor & Francis, 1987.

Dejonckere, P.H., Van-den Eeckhaut, J., and Sneppe, R. Lack of pneumorphonic co-ordination as a factor of functional dysphony. *International Journal of Rehabilitation and Research,* 1980, *3,* 81–82.

Fourcin, A. Electrolaryngographic assessment of vocal fold function. *Journal of Phonetics,* 1986, *14,* 435–442.

Husler, F., and Rodd-Marling, Y. *Singing, the physical nature of the vocal organ.* London: Hutchinson, 1976.

Okamura, H., Gould, W.J., and Tanabe, M. The role of respiratory muscles in phonation. In E. Loebell (Ed.), *XVIth International congress of logopedics and phoniatrics.* Basal: Karger, 1974.

Schutte, H.K., and Miller, R. Breath management in repeated vocal onset. *Folia-Phoniatrica,* 1984, *36,* 225–232.

Shipp, T., and McGlone, R. Laryngeal dynamics associated with voice frequency change. *Journal of Speech and Hearing Research.* 1971, *14,* 761–768.

Woo, P., Colton, R.H., and Shangold, L. Phonatory airflow analysis in patients with laryngeal disease. *Annals of Otology Rhinology and Laryngology,* 1987, *96,* 549–555.

Yanaginara, N., Koike, Y., and Von-Leden, H. Phonation and respiration function study in normal subjects. *Folia-Phoniatrica,* 1966, *18,* 323–340.

Respiratory System Involvement in Western Relaxation and Self-Regulation

PAUL M. LEHRER AND ROBERT L. WOOLFOLK

1. Introduction

Respiratory changes are consistently found during the practice of almost all relaxation techniques and specific manipulation of respiratory activity is employed in many of them. The purpose of this chapter is to review several Western relaxation techniques, and to describe the involvement of the respiratory system in each.

2. Progressive Relaxation

There are two major versions of progressive relaxation: the method used originally by Edmund Jacobson (1938), and the technique as taught by most modern behavior therapists (e.g., Bernstein and Borkovec, 1973; Paul, 1966; Wolpe and Lazarus, 1966). Descriptions of and contrasts between the two techniques have been detailed elsewhere (Lehrer *et al.*, 1986b; Lehrer and Woolfolk, 1993). The role of breathing in both approaches will be discussed here.

Jacobson's technique is oriented to teaching recognition and control of the most subtle levels of skeletal muscle tone. To do this the method of diminishing

PAUL M. LEHRER • Department of Psychiatry, Robert W. Johnson Medical School, University of Medicine and Dentistry of New Jersey, Piscataway, New Jersey 08854-5635.   *ROBERT L. WOOLFOLK* • Department of Psychology, Rutgers—the State University, Piscataway, New Jersey 08854.
Behavioral and Psychological Approaches to Breathing Disorders, edited by Beverly H. Timmons and Ronald Ley. Plenum Press, New York, 1994.

tensions is used (Jacobson, 1970). In this method, the subject is instructed to perform highly specific muscle flexions at intensities so low that an outside observer may not even recognize that anything is being done at all. To differentiate *actual* muscle tension from *perceived* tension, the trainee is not told where in the body the muscular sensations should be felt. In this method, control of respiration is not taught directly. Rather, just as the individual is trained to relax all the other muscles of the body, the individual is trained to relax the skeletal muscles involved in respiration. Jacobson does not advise giving specific suggestions to trainees about where in their bodies or when in the respiratory cycle they will experience tension, nor does he advise that any instruction be given about changing the rate or depth of respiration. Instead, he advises that, after the person has been trained to recognize muscle proprioceptions in other areas of the body (i.e., the arms, legs, and skeletal muscles in the trunk region), the individual assess the tension that occurs during normal respiration, in the generally relaxed state. The trainee is advised to "switch off" tension during each exhalation.

The revised progressive relaxation methods place greater emphasis on suggestion and the *perception* of relaxation, rather than relaxation per se. Larger muscular contractions are used, combining diverse *groups* of muscles, and subjects are given detailed descriptions of the sensations that should accompany relaxation. In training to relax the respiratory apparatus, the trainee is advised to breathe shallowly, regularly, and slowly, and to become aware of the tension in the chest and/or abdomen during each inspiration. Suggestions such as, "Ride the wave of relaxation each time you breathe out, and feel yourself become more and more relaxed," are often added. Sometimes hypnotic procedures are included, such as, "Now I shall count from ten back to one. At each count you will become more relaxed. When I reach one you will be completely relaxed" (cf. Bernstein and Given, 1984). At this point the therapist often gives one count with each exhalation.

There is some evidence that muscular relaxation can have specific effects on the respiratory system. These are seen most clearly in asthma, a reversible obstructive airway disease caused by reactive bronchoconstriction (Chapters 6 and 14). Although several literature reviews have shown relaxation to have very inconsistent effects on asthma as measured by the forced expiratory volume during the first second (FEV_1) of a maximal-effort forced expiration maneuver from full vital capacity (Alexander, 1981; Erskine and Schonell, 1981; King, 1980), two studies have found that relaxation produces decreases in airway reactivity to a methacholine challenge test (Lehrer *et al.*, 1986a; Philip *et al.*, 1972). In the study by Lehrer *et al.* (1986a), only subjects showing primarily large-airway constriction showed improvement in the methacholine challenge test, which is considered to be the "gold standard" measure of asthma, because it directly measures airway reactivity. The authors interpreted the results as suggesting that relaxation decreases parasympathetic reactivity, hence reactivity of the primarily parasympathetically controlled upper airway passages. In one controlled study of chronic obstructive pulmonary disease, progressive relaxation was found to produce significant reductions in sensations of dyspnea (Renfroe, 1988).

3. Hypnosis

Although methods of hypnosis are quite varied, many hypnotic inductions involve instructions in relaxation (Edmonston, 1981). An important element in hypnotic technique is to tell the subject to experience something that will be experienced naturally if the subject carries out the instructions of the hypnotist. Thus, hypnotic inductions often capitalize on the link experienced between slow deep respiration, and the waves of relaxation that sometimes are experienced during the deceleratory phase in respiratory sinus arrhythmia. As the subject breathes slowly and deeply, the hypnotist gives suggestions of relaxation. The relaxed feelings experienced by the subject then reinforce the credibility of the hypnotist's commands, and encourage compliance with the hypnotic process. An example of such hypnotic instructions during trance induction is given by Barber (1993):

> "Let's take a deep breath, and as we breath out slowly, we feel all the tensions leaving. . . Take another deep breath, and as we breathe out slowly we feel calm. . . at ease. . . at peace. . . waves of deep calmness. . . waves of deep peace and relaxation flowing throughout body and mind. . . lots of time. . . so much time . . . more and more time. . . feeling so good. . . floating. . . at peace. . . flowing calmly and gently through every muscle, organ, and cell. . . absolutely calm. . . waves of deep relaxation. . . lots of time. . . so much time. . . feeling so good. . . deep peace. . .deeper and deeper relaxation."

4. Autogenic Training

Autogenic training is a method of self-regulation derived from an amalgam of yoga and hypnosis. A detailed presentation of the autogenic technique, its rationale, and early research on it can be found in a six-volume work edited by Luthe (1969). Updated presentations have been made by Linden (1977, 1993). Although it is often used as a relaxation technique, its purpose is not simply (or necessarily) to produce relaxation. Rather, the putative rationale of the technique is to achieve a desirable state of homeostasis, in which the body's needs for relaxation and expression of tension are balanced (Schultz and Luthe, 1969). The method involves learning to concentrate passively on a series of autogenic formulae concerning various body sensations (e.g., heaviness, warmth, or coolness in various parts of the body). While doing this, the individual is told not to *try* to produce any specific changes, but just to lie or sit in a specifically prescribed relaxed position, to imagine what various body sensations might be like, to repeat the formulae (e.g., "My right hand is heavy and warm"), and to remain open to whatever experience might ensue. The initial standard autogenic formulae were derived from Schultz's research on hypnotic relaxation. When people are deeply calm, he found, they most often experienced heaviness and warmth in the limbs, coolness in the forehead, a calm and regular heartbeat, automatic breathing, and warmth in the solar plexus. From these, he developed the following standard formulae:

1. My arms and legs are heavy (said individually for each limb);
2. My arms and legs are warm (said individually for each limb);
3. My heartbeat is calm and regular;
4. It breathes me;
5. My solar plexus is warm;
6. My forehead is cool.

Training progresses slowly, with one instruction added in each session. Since each of these formulae describes a state of lower sympathetic activation and greater muscular relaxation, actually experiencing the sensations described in them should be accompanied by an experience of calmness and decreased physiological arousal. In order to train for this effect more explicitly, the technique is often combined with finger temperature biofeedback (Norris and Fahrion, 1993), although this is not part of the original regimen. Failure to attain these sensations is not necessary for treatment success; even experience of the *opposite* sensations or such negative occurrences as anxiety, tearfulness, or pain (the last two of which are considered to be part of the body's mechanism for releasing tension and restoring homeostasis) is not regarded as a treatment failure. Usually, tearfulness and pain are transient and yield to sensations of calmness and well-being, although, in some instances, their severity may interfere with treatment, in which case precautions must be taken (Chapter 17).

The fifth formula above is the one most relevant to respiration. Although it is rather awkward in English, it conveys the feeling of automatic breathing. Usually respiration becomes slower and deeper after sufficient experience with this formula (Linden, 1977; Luthe, 1969, Vols. I and IV).

5. The Alexander Method

F.M. Alexander was an Australian actor who, when faced with a functional aphonia that threatened to end his career, examined his body carefully in a mirror and retaught himself how to carry himself and how to "use" his body so as to minimize strain and tension. As a result of this self-training, his voice returned. He developed his method into a technique of body reeducation, which is widely used among actors, artists, and musicians, but which is known hardly at all in the scientific or medical community. Among its proponents were Tinbergen (1974), Huxley (1937), and Dewey (Jones, 1976). The few published scientific studies and clinical reports available on the technique are described by Jones (1976) and by Barlow (1977).

Although the technique has profound effects on the vocal apparatus (Jones, 1977), produces measurable improvement in pulmonary function (Austin and Ausubel, 1992), and possibly has a therapeutic effect on asthma (Barlow, 1977, 1978; Jones, 1977), the Alexander method does not work directly on the respiratory system. Rather, through gentle manipulation and positioning, the Alexander teacher instructs the trainee how to stand, walk, sit, etc., in such a way that minimum strain is placed on the body. Training includes verbal instructions to keep the head forward and up, and the spine straight and back. The goal of training is to teach the trainee to balance the head and torso such that minimum effort is required to keep the body erect. At the same time, the joints are stretched slightly, which probably relaxes isometric tension in the adjacent muscles. Although no electromyographic (EMG) studies have been reported, it is probable that the muscles of the speech region become particularly relaxed, and, with the head up, the upper air passages are less constricted. This method also has been applied in programs for prevention and rehabilitation of back pain (Hall, 1988; Jones, 1992; Prentice *et al.*, 1992). It has been applied in educational programs for improving motor performance in athletics, dance, etc., as well (Chazelton, 1985).

We have included a discussion of the Alexander technique because of its wide use in the artistic community and because of the power reported in demonstrations of the technique. Considerably more research is needed, however, in order for this technique to gain the scientific respectability of other methods described in this chapter.

6. Meditation

Meditation has been an integral feature of Oriental culture for many centuries. Only recently have Western scientists attempted to estimate the effects of the specific meditative techniques practiced by such traditions as Zen Buddhism and yoga, independent of the religious context in which they are normally practiced (Chapter 15). Three secular Western meditative techniques have been the subject of the most research: (1) Benson's Relaxation Response; (2) Carrington's Clinically Standardized Meditation; and (3) Woolfolk's breathing method. Each of these techniques has been found to contribute to the control and reduction of stress (Lehrer and Woolfolk, 1993).

Benson's Relaxation Response involves a focus on breathing, and the linking of a mantra with exhalation. Practitioners of this method sit quietly with eyes closed, skeletal musculature relaxed, and attention concentrated on their breathing. While exhaling they say the word "one" to themselves. In this method the "one" functions as a mantra, the utterance of which is regulated by the breath (Benson, 1975).

Carrington's Clinically Standardized Meditation is similar to Transcendental Meditation except that it is devoid of religious trappings and it is very explicit in all phases of instruction. It utilizes a focus upon a mantra, but attempts to impose no connection between the mantra and breathing. Trainees are told that the internal sounds may or may not naturally link themselves with the breath, and that either variation is permissible (Carrington, 1984, 1993).

Woolfolk's breathing method (Woolfolk and Richardson, 1978; Woolfolk *et al.*, 1976) requires individuals to direct all attention to their breathing, but without any attempt to alter its pace or depth. This is done while the trainee is seated, with eyes closed. During inhalation, the meditator silently utters the word "in," and during the exhalation, the word "out" is covertly spoken. Supplementary visualization exercises are utilized with trainees who respond to such exercises. One such visualization involves an image of a balloon that expands during the inhalation and contracts during the exhalation. In this method any verbal or imaginal focus is always paced by respiration.

7. Paced Slow Respiration

Although regulation of breathing figures more or less prominently in a variety of relaxation methods, notably yoga, it was only in the mid-1970s that systematic attempts were made to determine the effects of slow, regular breathing per se on psychophysiological variables. In the prototypical paced respiration study, nonclinical subjects are monitored initially by physiological recording equipment during a baseline period to allow for adaptation to instrumentation and to determine response levels at rest. Subjects are then given brief instructions followed by a period in which their breathing is paced at a slow rate by some external stimulus. There may be one or more intervals of paced respiration interspersed with control periods. Control groups may include the following: a group paced at normal rates; an attention control group that might monitor the pacing stimulus, or attend to an alternate stimulus, with no attempt to regulate breathing; and/or a group that receives no special instructions. A variety of laboratory stressors usually is administered to subjects at some time during the study. In this kind of design subjects serve as their own controls as well as being experimental treatment designees.

The effects of paced slow respiration have been examined to date in a number of investigations. Harris *et al.* (1976) measured electrodermal reactivity to a tone signaling the imminent onset of electric shock; they found that a group paced at eight respiratory cycles per minute (cpm) exhibited lower reactivity than did either an attention-control group or a no-pacing group. McCaul (1979) crossed three respiration conditions—(1) 8-cpm-paced respiration, (2) 16-cpm-paced respiration (a normal rate), and (3) a no-pacing-attention control—with either high or low experimentally manipulated expectations that subjects would experience lowered stress. Subjects were given the expectation of an electric shock as a stressor, but no actual shocks were delivered. Subjects in the 8-cpm condition showed a pattern that indicated greater stress reduction than that seen in the other two groups, as reflected in skin resistance, finger pulse volume, and self-reported anxiety. Clark (1979) found that subjects high in dental anxiety reported less discomfort while practicing 8-cpm-paced respiration during the viewing of a stressful film, depicting a dental procedure, than did subjects (also high in dental anxiety) from either of two other paced respiration groups (24-cpm and 16-cpm) or two control conditions. Clark and Hirschman (1990) found that, among a population of alcohol-dependent inpatients who scored high on trait anxiety, paced respiration at the rate of 10 cpm produced greater decreases in self-reported anxiety and tension than did simple uninstructed relaxation.

Lane (1980), however, found no intergroup differences among a paced slow respiration (7.5-cpm) condition, a 30-cpm condition, and a no-pacing control, in responses to a cold pressor test. Nelson (1980) failed to find evidence that 8-cpm-paced respiration lowered arousal during actual dental treatment, compared with arousal in a 16-cpm condition or an attention-control condition. Batey (1984) found that 3.75-cpm breathing tended to produce more variable responses than 7.5-cpm breathing on self-report measures of anxiety, but the 3.75 cpm group reliably produced elevated peak-to-trough heart rate variability, suggesting greater vagal tone in that condition.

Slow paced respiration (usually combined with abdominal breathing) has increasingly been used as one component of a multifaceted treatment program for panic attacks and has proven to be highly effective (Bonn et al., 1984; Clark et al., 1985; Fried, 1990; Salkoviskis et al., 1986). Other elements in this treatment sometimes include deliberate exposure to the physiological sensations thought to accompany panic, and cognitive therapy oriented to reattribution of these cues to normal and controllable processes. In some recent theoretical formulations, panic disorder has been viewed as synonymous with hyperventilation syndrome (Fried, 1987; Lum, 1975; and Chapter 5).

8. Abdominal Breathing

When the abdomen expands with each breath and there is little involvement from the muscles of the chest and shoulders, respiration requires minimum effort (Chapter 11). The fight-flight reflex naturally tends to be accompanied by increased skeletal muscle tension in the abdomen, lower back, and perineum. Tension in these areas necessitates involvement of the thoracic muscles in the respiratory process to allow inspiration, since free movement of the diaphragm is met by resistance in the lower abdomen. With thoracic breathing, the muscles in the lower trunk of the body work against each other, while additional effort must be expended by muscles of the thorax (Chapter 11). Abdominal breathing has been found to improve ventilation in the lower lobes of the lung (Hughes, 1975). For conditions in which respiratory effort and/or elevated muscle tension in the lower portion of the trunk are problematic, abdominal breathing may be therapeutic. Such conditions may include muscular spasms, back or abdominal pain, and various chronic respiratory disorders. Abdominal breathing has also been recommended for manifestations of irritable bowel syndrome. Clinical observations have suggested that slow abdominal breathing approaching the rate of 3 cpm has been found to aid in reestablishing electrogastrogram (EGG) rhythms at this frequency. The presence of 3 cpm EEG rhythms has been found to be associated with the normally functioning gut (Grove, 1988). Bacon and Poppen (1985) found that abdominal breathing appeared to decrease the peripheral vasoconstrictive response to sitting in a chilly room, compared with thoracic and uninstructed breathing. Thus abdominal breathing appeared to dampen sympathetic reactivity.

9. Biofeedback

EMG biofeedback training to reduce tension in the skeletal muscles of the face may affect the respiratory system. After receiving this training, subjects tend to show associated increases in air flow (Glaus and Kotses, 1983). Such respiratory effects do not occur in conjunction with EMG biofeedback to the limbs. It has been hypothesized (Glaus and Kotses, 1983) that the respiratory changes are mediated by a vagal-trigeminal reflex, through which facial muscle relaxation may produce bronchodilation.

Direct biofeedback of respiratory activity also appears to affect bronchial tone. Several investigators have provided subjects with continuous feedback of respiratory resistance, via the forced oscillatory pneumograph, and found substantial improvements in some subjects (Janson-Bjerklie and Clark, 1982; Steptoe et al., 1985; Vachon and Rich, 1976). Earlier investigators had found reliable increases in the more effort-dependent measure of FEV_1, despite the fact that this measure cannot be taken continuously (Kahn, 1977). Although biofeedback produces bronchial changes in many asthmatics, no reliable biofeedback results have been obtained among normal subjects.

Peper (1988) combines several biofeedback techniques to teach relaxation and increased respiratory flow simultaneously. He teaches muscle relaxation and abdominal breathing, using instructions influenced by the Alexander technique, designed to position the body in an erect, symmetrical, and relaxed position. Simultaneously, he applies EMG biofeedback to the trapezius area in order to alert subjects to undesirable thoracic involvement in respiration. These procedures are carried out while subjects are given respiratory feedback through an incentive inspirometer. Through this technique, he teaches asthmatic subjects to breathe with greater sustained inspiratory force, without thoracic involvement in breathing.

Tiep et al. (1986) use biofeedback of blood oxygen via an ear oximeter to teach patients with severe chronic obstructive pulmonary disease to increase oxygenation. Patients are simultaneously taught to breathe through pursed lips. A similar technique combining resistive ventilatory muscle training with biofeedback has also been found to improve ventilatory function (Belman and Shadmehr, 1988). Zeier (1984) combined respiratory biofeedback with other relaxation and self-control methods, and found greater decreases in heart rate and relaxation rate than he found with relaxation instructions alone. In another study, the same investigator found no within-session incremental physiological effects of respiratory biofeedback over autogenic training alone, but found that subjects spent more time practicing their technique at home when biofeedback was included (Zeier, 1985).

10. Relaxation and Hyperventilation

Among the many facets of the fight–flight reflex are various bodily changes having the effect of increasing blood oxygenation. These include increased bronchodilation, increased ventilation, and increased tendency of red blood cells to absorb oxygen from the lung. These changes tend to be accompanied by a decreased blood level of carbon dioxide, which, in turn, triggers the symptoms of hyperventilation in the absence of appropriate metabolic demand. It has been widely commented upon that these symptoms are almost identical with those of panic disorder (Fried, 1986; Hardonk and Beumer, 1979; Ley, 1985; Lum, 1975; also, see Chapter 5). Some individuals have been observed to experience anxiety attacks more frequently during relaxation training. While this has been observed in most relaxation techniques, it occurs less frequently in progressive muscle relaxation than in meditation (Heide and Borkovec, 1983; Lehrer et al., 1983). Ley (1988) has hypothesized that this relaxation-produced anxiety results from an inability to adapt blood oxygen levels properly to changing metabolic needs, through appropriate changes in respiration. This observation is consistent with findings of Fried (1987) that, during deep relaxation induced by imagery and diaphragmatic breathing in 15 patients with various psychosomatic disorders, $PETCO_2$ decreased while various other data indicated decreased levels of arousal. Similar effects have been found in mantra meditation (Beary and Benson, 1974; Fenwick et al., 1977). Other studies, however, reported evidence of increased blood and expiratory levels of CO_2 during autogenic training (Linden, 1977) and slow paced respiration (Salkoviskis et al., 1986).

11. Conclusion

Relaxation has long been known to affect respiratory patterns and vice versa. Western relaxation techniques have been designed to be particularly amenable to empirical study, and research has been proceeding on the mechanisms for this interaction. Although it is possible that changes in respiratory strategies are *critical* elements in the effectiveness of all relaxation techniques, this is yet to be established. Other possible mechanisms include cognitive changes produced by engaging in various methods, and direct effects of muscular or other peripheral physiological changes on central processes. Future research may also show that, because of the interaction between relaxation and breathing, these techniques may find important applications in the treatment of various pulmonary disorders.

ACKNOWLEDGMENTS. This work was supported in part by Grant number RO1-HL34336 from the National Institutes of Health.

12. References

Alexander, A.B. Behavioral approaches in the treatment of bronchial asthma. In C.K. Prokop, and L.A. Bradley (Eds.), *Medical psychology: Contributions to medical psychology.* New York: Academic Press, 1981, pp. 373–394.

Austin, J. H., and Ausubel, P. Enhanced respiratory muscular function in normal adults after lessons in proprioceptive musculoskeletal education without exercises. *Chest,* 1992, *9,* 6–16.

Bacon, M., and Poppen, R. A behavioral analysis of diaphragmatic breathing and its effects on peripheral temperature. *Journal of Behavior Therapy and Experimental Psychiatry,* 1985, *16,* 15–21.

Barber, T.X. Hypnosis, deep relaxation, and active relaxation: Data, theory, and clinical applications. In R.L. Woolfolk and P.M. Lehrer (Ed.), *Principles and practice of stress management.* New York: Guilford, 1984.

Barlow, W. *The Alexander technique.* New York: Alfred A. Knopf, 1977.

Barlow, W. Medical aspects of the Alexander Technique. In W. Barlow (Ed.), *More talk of Alexander: aspects of the Alexander Principle.* London: Victor Gollancz Ltd., 1978.

Batey, D.M. *The physiological effects of 3.75 and 7.5 cycle per minute paced respiration in stressful and nonstressful contexts.* Doctoral Dissertation, 1984, Rutgers University. *Dissertation Abstracts International,* 1985, *46,* (633-B). Order # DA8507092.

Beary, J.F., and Benson, H. A simple psychophysiologic technique which elicits the hypometabolic changes of the relaxation response. *Psychosomatic Medicine,* 1974, *36,* 115–120.

Belman, M.J. and Shadmehr, R. Targeted resistive ventilatory muscle training in chronic obstructive pulmonary disease. *Journal of Applied Physiology,* 1988, *65,* 2726–2735.

Benson, H. *The relaxation response.* New York: Morrow, 1975.

Bernstein, D.A. and Borkovec, T.D. *Progressive relaxation training: A manual for the helping professions.* Champaign, IL: Research Press, 1973.

Bernstein, D.A. and Given, B.A. Progressive relaxation: Abbreviated methods. In R.L. Woolfolk and P.M. Lehrer (Eds.), *Principles and practice of stress management.* New York: Guilford Press, 1984.

Bonn, J.A., Readhead, C.P.A., and Timmons, B.H. Enhanced adaptive behavioural response in agoraphobic patients pretreated with breathing retraining. *The Lancet,* 1984, *2,* 665–669.

Carrington, P. *Freedom in meditation.* Kendall Park, N.J.: Pace Educational Systems, 1984.

Carrington, P. Modern forms of meditation. In P.M. Lehrer and R.L. Woolfolk (Eds.) *Principles and Practices of Stress Management,* 2nd ed. New York: Guilford Press, 1993.

Clark, M.E. Therapeutic applications of physiological control: The effectiveness of respiratory pacing in reducing autonomic and subjective distress. *Dissertation Abstracts International,* 1979, *39,* (9-B), 4571.

Clark, D.M., Salkovskis, P.M., and Chalkley, A.J. Respiratory control as a treatment for panic attacks. *Journal of Behavior Therapy and Experimental Psychiatry,* 1985, *16,* 23–30.

Clark, M.E., and Hirschman, R. Effects of paced respiration on anxiety reduction in a clinical population. *Biofeedback and Self-Regulation,* 1990, *15,* 273–284.

Edmonston, W.E. *Hypnosis and relaxation.* New York: Wiley, 1981.

Erskine, J.M. and Schonell, M. Relaxation therapy in asthma: A critical review. *Psychosomatic Medicine,* 1981, *43,* 365–372.

Fenwick, P., Donaldson, S., Gilles, L., Bushman, J., Fenten, G., Perry, I., Tilsley, C., and Serafinowicz, H. Metabolic and EEG changes during transcendental meditation. *Biological Psychology,* 1977, *5,* 101–118.

Fried, R. *The hyperventilation syndrome.* Baltimore: Johns Hopkins University Press, 1986.

Fried, R. Relaxation with biofeedback-assisted guided imagery: The importance of breathing rate as an index of hypoarousal. *Biofeedback and Self-regulation,* 1987, *12,* 273–279.

Fried, R. *The breath connection.* New York: Plenum, 1990.

Glaus, K.D., and Kotses, H. Facial muscle tension influences lung airway resistance—Limb muscle tension does not. *Biological Psychology,* 1983, *17,* 105–120.

Grove, R. *Digestive physiology and the clinical electrogastrogram.* Paper presented at the annual meeting of the Biofeedback Society of America, Colorado Springs, March 25-30, 1988.

Hall, D. Bad backs—uncovering the real problem: the Alexander technique sheds new light on a sore situation. *Lamp,* 1988, *45,* 24–28.

Hardonk, J., and Beumer, H. Hyperventilation syndrome. In P. Vinken and G. Bruyn (Eds.), *Handbook of clinical neurology.* Amsterdam: North Holland, 1979, pp. 309–360.

Harris, V.A., Katkin, K.D., Lick, J.R., and Habberfield, T. Paced respiration as a technique for the modification of autonomic response to threat. *Psychophysiology,* 1976, *13,* 386–391.

Hazelton, J.E. The purpose and relevance of nonclinical biofeedback relaxation and the Alexander Principle. *Clinical Biofeedback and Health: An International Journal,* 1985, *8,* 52–67.

Heide, F.J., and Borkovec, T.D. Relaxation-induced anxiety: Paradoxical anxiety enhancement due to relaxation training. *Journal of Consulting and Clinical Psychology,* 1983, *51,* 1–12.

Hughes, R.L. Does abdominal breathing affect regional gas exchange? *Chest,* 1979, *76,* 288–293.

Huxley, A. *Ends and means.* New York: Harper Brothers, 1937.

Jacobson, E. *Progressive relaxation.* Chicago: University of Chicago Press, 1938.

Jacobson, E. *Modern treatment of tense patients.* Springfield, IL: Charles C. Thomas, 1970.

Janson-Bjerklie, S., and Clark, E. The effects of biofeedback training on bronchial diameter in asthma. *Heart and Lung,* 1982, *11,* 200–207.

Jones, F.P. Voice production as a function of head balance in singers, *Journal of Psychology,* 1972, *82,* 209–215.

Jones, F.P. *Body awareness in action.* New York: Schocken Books, 1976.

Jones, P.R. Psychology for physically disabled people. *Educational and Child Psychology,* 1992, *9,* 6–16.

Kahn, A.V. Effectiveness of biofeedback and counter-conditioning in the treatment of bronchial asthma. *Journal of Psychosomatic Research,* 1977, *21,* 97–104.

King, N.J. The behavioral management of asthma and asthma-related problems in children: A critical review of the literature. *Journal of Behavioral Medicine,* 1980, *3,* 169–189.

Lane, J.D. The effects of self-control of respiration upon experimental pain. *Dissertation Abstracts International,* 1980, *40,* (10-B), 5066.

Lehrer, P.M., Hochron, S., McCann, B., Swartzman, L., and Reba, P. Relaxation decreases large-airway but not small-airway asthma. *Journal of Psychosomatic Research,* 1986a, *30,* 13–25.

Lehrer, P.M., and Woolfolk, R.L. *Principles and practice of stress management.* (2nd ed.). New York: Guilford Press, 1993.

Lehrer, P.M., Woolfolk, R.L., and Goldman, N. Progressive relaxation then and now: Does change always mean progress? In R. Davidson, G.E. Schwartz and D. Shapiro (Eds.), *Consciousness and self-regulation.* Vol. IV. New York: Plenum, 1986b.

Lehrer, P.M., Woolfolk, R.L., and Rooney, A. Progressive relaxation and meditation: A study of psychophysiological and therapeutic differences between two techniques. *Behaviour Research and Therapy,* 1983, *21,* 651–662.

Ley, R. Blood, breath and fears: A hyperventilation theory of panic attacks and agoraphobia. *Clinical Psychology Review,* 1985, *5,* 271–285.

Ley, R. Panic attacks during relaxation and relaxation-induced anxiety: A hyperventilation interpretation. *Journal of Behavior Therapy and Experimental Psychiatry,* 1988, *19,* 253–259.

Linden, M. Longitudinal study of changes in respiratory frequency and amount of CO_2 exhaled during the learning stage of autogenic training. *Psychotherapie und Medizinische Psychologie.* 1977, *27,* 229–234.

Linden, W. The autogenic training method of J.H. Schultz. In P.M. Lehrer and R.L. Woolfolk (Eds.) *Principles and practice of stress management,* 2nd ed., New York: Guilford Press, 1993.

Lum, L.C. Hyperventilation: The tip of the iceberg. *Journal of Psychosomatic Research,* 1975, *19,* 375–383.

Luthe, W. (Ed.), *Autogenic therapy.* Volumes I, II, and IV. New York: Grune & Stratton, 1969.

McCaul, K.D., Solomon, S., and Holmes, D.S. Effects of paced respiration and expectations on physiological and psychological responses to threat. *Journal of Personality and Social Psychology,* 1979, *27,* 229–234.

Morrow, F. William James and John Dewey on consciousness: Suppressed writings. *Journal of Humanistic Psychology,* 1984, *24,* 69–79.

Nelson, C.S. The effects of respiration pacing on distress and anxiety in dental treatment. *Dissertation Abstracts International,* 1980, *41,* (4B), 1518.

Norris, P., and Fahrion, S. Autogenic biofeedback in psychophysiological therapy and stress management. In P.M. Lehrer and R.L. Woolfolk, (Eds.), *Principles and practice of stress management.* (2nd ed.), New York: Guilford, 1993.

Paul, G.L. *Insight versus desensitization in psychotherapy.* Stanford, CA: Stanford University Press, 1966.

Peper, E. Strategies to reduce the effort of breathing: Electromyographic and incentive inspirometry feedback. In C. Von Euler and M. Katz-Salamon (Eds.), *Respiratory psychophysiology.* London: McMillan Press, Ltd., 1988.

Philip, R.L., Wilde, G.J.S., and Day, J.H. Suggestion and relaxation in asthmatics. *Journal of Psychosomatic Research,* 1972, *16,* 193–204.

Prentice, C., Canty, A.M., and Janowitz, I. Back school programs. The pregnant patient and her partner. *Occupational Medicine,* 1992, *7,* 77–85.

Renfroe, K.L. Effect of progressive relaxation on dyspnea and state anxiety in patients with chronic obstructive pulmonary disease. *Heart-Lung,* 1988, *17,* 408–413.

Salkoviskis, P.M., Jones, D.R., and Clark, D.M. Respiratory control in the treatment of panic attacks: Replication and extension with concurrent measurement of behaviour and pCO_2. *British Journal of Psychiatry,* 1986, *148,* 526–532.

Schultz, H., and Luthe, W. (Eds.) *Autogenic methods.* In W. Luthe, (Ed.), *Autogenic therapy.* Vol. I. New York: Grune and Stratton, 1969.

Steptoe, A., Phillips, J., and Harling, J. Biofeedback and instructions in the modification of total respiratory resistance: An experimental study of asthmatic and non-asthmatic volunteers. *Journal of Psychosomatic Research,* 1981, *25,* 541–551.

Tiep, B., Burns, M., Kao, D., Madison, R., and Herrera, J. Pursed lips breathing training using ear oximetry. *Chest,* 1986, *90,* 218–221.

Tinbergen, N. Ethology and stress diseases. *Science,* 1974, *185,* 20–27.

Vachon, L., and Rich, E.S. Visceral learning in asthma. *Psychosomatic Medicine,* 1976, *38,* 122–130.

Wolpe, J., and Lazarus, A.A. *Behavior therapy techniques.* New York: Pergamon, 1966.

Woolfolk, R.L., Carr-Kaffashan, L., McNulty, T.F., and Lehrer, P.M. Meditation training as a treatment for insomnia. *Behavior Therapy,* 1976, *7,* 359–365.

Woolfolk, R.L., and Richardson, F.C. *Stress, sanity, and survival.* New York: Sovereign Books, 1978.

Zeier, H. Arousal reduction with biofeedback-supported respiratory meditation. *Biofeedback and Self-Regulation,* 1984, *9,* 497–508.

Zeier, H. Entspannung durch biofeedbackunterstutze Atemmeditation und autogenes Training [Relaxation through feedback-supported respiratory meditation and autogenic training.] *Zeitschrift für Experimentelle und Angewandte Psychologie,* 1985, *32,* 682–695.

14

Behavioral Management of Asthma

JONATHAN H. WEISS

1. Introduction

Asthma is a physical, not an emotional, illness. Its primary treatment must be medical. However, psychological factors influence the frequency, severity, and impact of asthma, and must be attended to if the result of medical care is to be optimal. Physicians often neglect this fact, perhaps because they have been disappointed by "psychosomatic" theories and therapies that are based upon the misconception that asthma is caused, rather than influenced, by psychological factors (see Weiss, 1974, for a critical evaluation of such theories). However, the opportunity exists to put that neglect behind us. Behaviorally based approaches (e.g., Creer, 1979; Weiss, 1983; and see Chapter 13)—that recognize the physical basis of asthma and work to reduce the negative effect of psychological variables—have been successful in reducing the severity of asthma and its impact in many patients. The purpose of this chapter is to introduce clinicians to the behavioral approach. I will introduce the reader to basic facts about asthma and its symptoms; discuss how psychological variables can affect its course; describe how to probe for such variables; suggest how to target them for treatment; and outline what I consider to be the basic goals for behavioral intervention in asthma.

2. Description of Asthma

Asthma is a chronic respiratory disease of unknown origin. It is characterized by aperiodic "attacks" of symptoms during which breathing is impeded

JONATHAN H. WEISS • Department of Psychiatry, New York Hospital, Cornell University Medical Center, New York, New York 10021.
Behavioral and Psychological Approaches to Breathing Disorders, edited by Beverly H. Timmons and Ronald Ley. Plenum Press, New York, 1994.

by the constriction of airway muscles and swelling of mucus membranes and other tissues that line the airways, and by the accumulation of mucus and other matter in the airways. An asthma attack can be mild, moderate, or life threateningly severe (status asthmaticus), depending upon how impeded the airways are and how responsive they are to medication.

Epidemological data suggest that in the United States about 5 percent of the population has asthma and that the prevalence is rising. They also reveal a small, but—for some unknown reason—growing, mortality rate associated with asthma, especially in older patients.

In the United States, asthma is the leading cause of school days lost because of chronic illness. It also accounts for 38 million days spent in bed each year, 111 million days of restricted activity and 9 million lost work days. In money, asthma cost about 4 billion dollars in 1986.

In addition to the physical and financial toll exacted by asthma, there are also emotional difficulties and disruptions of daily life engendered by the illness, although not, to be sure, in all patients.

The onset of asthma is usually in childhood, but it can begin at any age. About one third of all asthmatics are below the age of 17, and in that age range there are about twice as many boys with asthma as girls. There is evidence that asthma can remit, or at least diminish in severity, during adolescence. The chance of relapsing, however, increases with age.

The typical symptoms of asthma include sensations of tightness in the chest, air hunger, and an inability to breathe without deliberate, even great, effort. The patient's struggle to inhale is marked by a hunched-over posture, hands pressed against a table top, chair back or other surface (as if to get leverage in the effort to breathe), shoulders drawn up and back and chest heaving. Associated with the problem in breathing *in* is the patient's inability to *exhale* normally, which results in air being trapped in the lungs, thus reducing *vital capacity* (see Chapter 1) to breathe in and out. Paradoxically, the harder patients try to breathe, the more resistance they may feel, the more frightened they may become, and the harder they may try. An important goal of the behavioral treatment of asthma is to reverse this cycle.

Breathing during an asthma attack is characteristically "wheezy," the result of air being forced through narrowed passages that resonate like whistles. In the most severe attacks, however, the lungs may become so hyperinflated that too little air is moved to generate any wheezing.

An asthma attack begins with the occurrence of one or more precipitating events (see Table 1). Usually within minutes, but sometimes more slowly, a chemical response within the patient releases a variety of mediators into the airways. Some of these mediators cause the changes described above that impede breathing. These changes and their accompanying symptoms constitute the early phase of an attack. The medications most often prescribed during this phase are

Table 1

Asthma Precipitants

Overexertion, exercise
Weather (including change in season, heat, cold, damp)
Nocturnal asthma (patient goes to sleep clear and wakes up with symptoms)
Excitement (positive affect)
Emotions (worry, upset, anger, anxiety, sadness)
Laughing
Crying
Coughing
Foods
Pollens
Colds, viral infections
Dust
Molds
Smoke
Strong smells
Seeing somebody else having trouble breathing
"Just get it"
Animals
Other allergies

---

bronchodilators (e.g., Alupent, Proventil, Slo-bid, Theo-Dur) designed to relax the constricted smooth muscles and thereby help to restore breathing. However, even as the early phase is subsiding, other mediators are causing changes that can prolong the attack or cause a second set of late phase reactions. Those mediators call white blood cells to the airways, cells that stimulate responses that can inflame and damage the lining of the airways. This, in turn, can cause further narrowing and blocking and, as a result, more severe symptoms.

Late phase asthma can last for a day or more and require anti-inflammatory steroid medication (e.g., Azmacort, Vanceril) in order to be controlled. Late phase asthma is the cause of most hospitalizations. Neglecting to anticipate it, because the early phase was mild or quickly responsive to bronchodilators, can be a serious error that patients must be taught to avoid.

Recent evidence suggests that chronic airway inflammation is an important underlying condition in asthma, and is at least as important to treat as is the acute exacerbation of symptoms.

3. The Role of Psychological Factors in Asthma

What patients (and their families) know, feel, and do about their asthma can have either beneficial or deleterious effects. In what follows, I will suggest how cognitive, affective and behavioral variables operate in asthma. My purpose is to alert the clinician to what to look for, using the assessment procedures that will be described next.

3.1. Cognitive Variables

Accurate information, appropriate alertness and self-efficacy are important ingredients in patients' efforts to control asthma and to keep its impact on their life style to a minimum. Patients who know their symptom precipitants and aggravants can try to minimize their exposure to them. Patients who are alert to symptoms but avoid excessive worry about them are less likely to restrict themselves unnecessarily or to panic during an attack. Patients who know the early warning signs (see Section 5.3) of symptom onset, and what to do about them, are better positioned to abort or control an attack. And patients who value their health, who believe they can participate in their treatment effectively, and who understand their treatment accurately are less likely to feel helpless, deny their illness, avoid treatment, be erratic in their compliance, or seek out unproved miracle cures.

Unfortunately, patients who demonstrate these desirable characteristics are in the minority. Many doctors have neither the time nor the training to teach effective health management skills to patients. And too many patients are afraid to express confusion, frustration, or anxiety. Instead of working out an effective partnership with their physicians, they accept the well-meant, but too often inappropriate, advice of friends, neighbors, or relatives, all of whom know a remedy that "works."

The behavior therapist who undertakes to treat patients with asthma should be prepared to teach the facts about the illness in collaboration with the doctor and the other members of the treatment team. The therapist should also be prepared to act as liaison between patients and the team until the patients (or their families) have learned to fend for themselves.

3.2. Emotional Variables

Emotions, both positive and negative, are reported by patients to precipitate and aggravate their asthma attacks. How emotions do that, however, varies, often involving nonemotional mediators, without which the emotions per se would have no effect. For example, excitement is reported by some patients to trigger asthma directly. It is reported by others to trigger asthma only if it is accompanied by laughing, shouting, jumping, or some other vigorous activity.

The distinction between the direct elicitation of symptoms and that which is mediated by other events is important because it suggests different treatments. It is one, however, that is often missed by patients, their families, and even doctors. Patients are told to "calm down" when advice on how to *express* their feelings would be more helpful (Chapter 17).

I have observed four distinct patterns of emotion-triggered asthma that I believe the clinician should look for.

1. Emotions → Asthma. In this pattern there is a (nearly) simultaneous occurrence of the emotion and the symptoms of asthma. For example, one patient described her chest "tightening up" on a trip at the moment she noticed that she had left her medicine at home. Another described getting symptoms as soon as she learned that she had been elected to be a class officer.

In instances of this kind, close questioning fails to elicit any intervening events (e.g., exertion or hyperventilation) that could explain the onset of symptoms, and it appears that the emotion and the breathing changes are two sides of one coin. In my experience such instances are relatively rare.

2. Emotions → Behavior → Asthma. In this pattern, excitement leads to exertion, anger leads to shouting, anxiety leads to hyperventilation, and so on. It is the behavior, i.e., the exertion, the shouting, or the hyperventilation, that triggers the symptoms. Patients who report this pattern need help in learning how to show their feelings in nonprecipitating ways, rather than how to avoid having the feelings.

Clinicians should bear in mind that the behavior in this pattern can be a negative behavior, i.e., a behavioral deficit. For example, patients who are embarrassed may avoid taking their medicine at the prescribed time if there are people around. Patients who are frightened of asthma may deny their symptoms and do nothing until the symptoms are too severe to overlook. And patients who have experienced unpleasant side effects of asthma medication may avoid taking it when they shouldn't do so. I knew one man whose death during a severe asthma attack might have been avoided had he not refused to take steroids because of his exaggerated fear of their side effects.

3. Emotions → Behavior → Physiological Stimuli → Asthma. Neither the emotion nor the behavior in this pattern would affect patients' asthma if the behavior did not expose them to noxious stimuli. For example, jumping up and down excitedly might have no ill effect if it did not take place on a dusty couch. And feeling or acting shy might have no ill effect if it didn't make it hard for the patient to refuse a cigarette or some allergenic food.

4. Asthma → Reaction (→ Secondary Symptoms). This final variation on the theme of emotions and asthma starts with the patient have symptoms for whatever reason and reacting to them in a way that aggravates their severity and sometimes leads to secondary complications. For example, patients who are frightened by the onset of asthma can react to it by hyperventilating or resisting treatment. They may also inhibit themselves unnecessarily in an exaggerated attempt to prevent symptoms. Adult onset asthmatics, who have not had a

lifetime in which to adapt to the illness, are particularly prone to show this pattern.

The reactions of others to patients' asthma should also be considered when assessing this pattern. Frightened family members can complicate the handling of an attack quite as much as can panicky patients. And parents who exempt their asthmatic children from chores that are well within their capability on grounds that they are "too sick," are rewarding illness behavior and are shaping manipulation, hypochondriasis, or both.

3.3. Behavioral Variables

Behaviors that can lead to asthma include strenuous sports, hobbies—such as painting or woodworking—that expose patients to noxious stimuli or irritants, and habits such as smoking. Skill deficits, such as an inability to use diagnostic or therapeutic devices or to keep track of medicines, are also included in this category.

A very important behavior that should be looked for in all asthmatic patients is hyperventilation (Chapter 6). I have discussed this breathing pattern and its management in detail elsewhere (Weiss, 1989) and the reader is urged to acquaint himself with that discussion or with others in the burgeoning literature on the topic (e.g., Fried, 1987; Lum, 1976; and Chapters 7–12).

In brief, hyperventilation is defined as primarily thoracic breathing that results in excessive loss of carbon dioxide as well as cooling and drying of the airways, and sets in motion a chain of events that can trigger a bewildering array of symptoms, including asthma. It can be an acute response to stress or a chronic habit, acquired for any of a variety of reasons, that has become the patient's preferred way of breathing.

3.4. Background Variables

Background variables that can influence the severity of symptoms as well as their impact and management include the following: the overall level of tension in patients' lives; the degree of value placed upon matters of health and hygiene; the level of nutrition; the presence of smokers in the patient's family; the availability and adequacy of medical care; the inclination of patient and family to be cooperative; the availability of social support; and environmental pollution. Age may be considered to be a background variable, teenagers often being harder to treat and adult onset asthmatics often being more frightened and depressed.

4. Assessing Psychological Variables in Asthma

There are several assessment techniques that I have found to be useful supplements to the standard diagnostic interview. I will describe them briefly and refer the reader to more detailed accounts.

4.1. Asthma Interview

The purpose of this interview is to obtain detailed information about the precipitants and aggravants of patients' asthma, their preferred methods of coping with symptoms, the reactions of others to their symptoms, and the impact of asthma on their lifestyle.

The interview is started by asking patients (and/or other informants) to tell what they can remember brings on or aggravates their asthma. They are asked to report only those things that they can remember experiencing, *not* what others, including doctors, may have told them could affect their asthma. Patients are encouraged to list as many things as they can remember, not only major precipitants and aggravants. When this has been done, the clinician can jog their memories by reading to them from the list of precipitants (Table 1) and asking if any of the items not already mentioned apply.

When a complete list has been obtained, patients are asked to describe at least one experience with each precipitant. The purpose is to find out as much as possible about what happened between the occurrence of the precipitant and the onset or worsening of symptoms. This will help the clinician to determine if the "active ingredient" was the precipitant named or something else in the chain of events that led up to the asthma. For example, patients may report that cold weather makes their asthma worse. On inquiry, it may turn out that during cold weather some patients get more upper respiratory infections, and these trigger their symptoms. When it is cold and those same patients have no upper respiratory infections, their asthma is fine.

The inquiry is especially useful in finding out which pattern(s) of emotionally precipitated asthma is (are) at work. For example, one young man reported that getting scared triggered his asthma. On inquiry, he described being alone at home, being frightened by a strange noise, and getting asthma within a few minutes. What happened during those few minutes? The patient investigated the source of the noise by climbing three flights of steps and looking around in a dusty attic. Since he also listed exertion and dust as precipitants, the role of the fright was unclear. Had he ever been frightened, done nothing and gotten asthma? He could remember no such experience.

Clinicians should pursue the inquiry until they believe they have enough information from which to draw conclusions about what precipitated or aggravated their patients' asthma. This is not complicated or very time-consuming, rarely taking more than 40 minutes.

Following the precipitant inquiry, patients are asked to describe what, if any, measures they (or their families) have taken to minimize exposure to each precipitant. At this point the clinician can inquire into background variables as well. Attention is then turned to how patients cope with attacks of asthma. The clinician can start by asking patients how they know when they are getting asthma, i.e., what early warning signs (EWSs) do they recognize (see Section

5.3 for a description of common EWSs), and what they do when they become aware of one. They should be asked what suggestions their doctors have made, and if they have tried them? With what success? Finally, patients should be asked to describe what they and their families do when full-blown symptoms occur. Do they ever call the doctor or go to the emergency room? Why? What do they do if they are away from home (e.g., at school, on a trip, at somebody else's home)? Have they experienced any interferences with their attempts to cope with symptoms (e.g., other family members getting upset, friends poking fun, etc.)?

The asthma interview is brought to a close with questions about the effects of asthma on lifestyle. For example, has it affected school or work attendance, socializing, participation in sports, going on vacation, finances, etc.? What strains has it imposed on the family, e.g., do siblings feel resentful that patients get preferred treatment?

More detailed descriptions of asthma interviews can be found in Purcell and Weiss (1970) and Creer (1979).

4.2. Asthma Problems Checklist (APCL)

This pencil and paper questionnaire (Creer, 1979) inquires into eight problem areas: use of asthma medications; early signs of asthma; triggers of asthma; child's behavior during an attack; behavior of others during an attack; effects of asthma on social development; effects on school; and effects on the family. The 62 questions that comprise the checklist are each rated on a five-point scale (0 = never a problem; 4 = always a problem). Subscale scores can be calculated as well as a full scale score. The APCL has a reported test-retest reliability of about .90 (Creer *et al.*, 1983). It can be administered prior to the Asthma Interview and serve as a guide to areas that merit detailed inquiry, or serve as an additional source of information that the clinician may not have fully covered in the interview. It can also be mailed to informants who are not able to come in for an interview.

4.3. Asthma Attitude Survey (AAS)

This instrument (see Creer, 1979) contains a parents' scale and a child's scale. The parents' scale has 24 questions that break down into two subscales: (1) what the child and parents can do to manage the child's asthma; and (2) the asthmatic child's relationship to the outside world. The child's scale contains 28 questions and two subscales, one covering the child's attitude toward self-management of asthma, and the other covering the child's sense of how asthma has influenced self-perception and their perception of relations with others. AAS items are rated on a five-point scale (0 = most negative; 4 = most positive). The

AAS, like the APCL, can be used as a guide or a supplement to the Asthma Interview.

4.4. Asthma Diary

If one can get patients' cooperation, it is very useful to have them keep a daily diary in which they record if and when symptoms occurred, their best guess about what brought the symptoms on, how severe the symptoms were and how long they lasted, and what medications and/or other interventions were used. Patients who use a peak flow meter (a device that measures how fast air can be exhaled with maximum effort) at home, can record the readings also. Information from the diary can be used to check patients' impressions about the pattern of their asthma.

Having patients keep a diary is a good way to train them to attend to relevant asthma variables. It also generates a record of progress (or lack thereof) that will be useful to both the therapist and patients' physician.

Many patients balk or are erratic at keeping an asthma diary. I have found it helpful in such cases to phone my patients one or more times a week to collect data and to reinforce cooperation. A call can last anywhere from 30 seconds to 4 or 5 minutes.

5. Treating the Psychological Contributors to Asthma

The physiology of emotion, thought, or action interacts with the physiology of asthma. The two are not, however, identical. Treating the psychological contributors to asthma, then, is not the same as treating asthma. The latter must be handled by a skilled allergist, pulmonologist, or both. The behavioral clinician should be sure that such treatment is ongoing before undertaking to work with an asthmatic patient. I have refused treatment to patients who, for whatever reason, were not under medical care and wanted their asthma treated only behaviorally. I have also refused referrals from frustrated physicians who proposed to discharge their difficult patients from medical care into mine.

Treatment planning begins with a diagnostic formulation, that is essentially a hypothesis about what is maintaining the observed pattern of symptoms and what would be the most effective point of intervention, i.e., the core problem. A device that may be helpful in arriving at a formulation is a flow chart that shows the give and take of asthma and its functionally related antecedents, concomitants and consequences. An example of such a flow chart is given in Figure 1. The case from which it is drawn has been described in detail elsewhere (Weiss, 1983); it involved a teen-age boy whose asthma and medication usage were considered to be out of control. The results of the assessment suggested that the

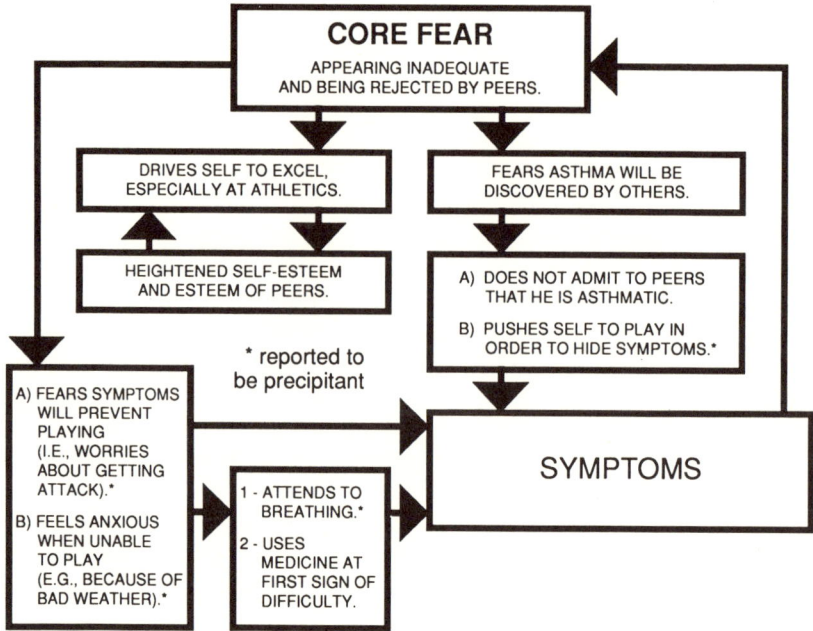

Figure 1. Behavioral formulation, showing hypothesized relationships of cognitive, emotional and behavioral variables to symptoms in a case of asthma. From Weiss (1983), with permission.

core problem was the patient's fear of being rejected by his peers. That fear gave rise to thoughts, feelings, and actions that affected the patient's asthma adversely but that were, paradoxically, maintained by the esteem he felt he derived from them. The intervention suggested by the formulation was a program of assertiveness training and support that helped the patient to say "no" to strenuous sports on days when he didn't feel well. The patient discovered that he did not become the outcast he feared he would be, and his asthma improved dramatically.

Core problems can be simple or complex, reside within the patient or stem from somebody or something in his environment. A relatively simple problem that resides within the patient is often seen in people with adult onset asthma, viz., anticipatory anxiety about symptoms and feelings of fear and helplessness when symptoms occur. Problems that impinge upon the patient's asthma from the environment are exemplified in the case of a girl whose mother was convinced that her poor child-rearing skills were responsible for her child's asthma. In an attempt to compensate for having caused her to suffer, the mother permitted the child anything she wanted, including the chocolate, nuts, and pets that precipitated her symptoms!

There can be more than one core problem. For example, a patient's (symptom-induced) anxiety may need to be controlled and, at the same time, the patient may need to be taught to be assertive toward people who smoke in his presence.

No two cases of asthma will be exactly alike. However, there are certain skills that all patients should have and for which training should, if necessary, be incorporated into the treatment plan. They are:

1. Knowing the facts and fallacies about asthma and its management.
2. Knowing one's symptom precipitants and aggravants.
3. Knowing and attending to one's early warning signs, and knowing what to do about them.
4. Knowing how to relax and breathe abdominally (at all times, but especially during an attack).
5. Knowing how to gather useful information about one's asthma, and being able to conduct a productive dialogue with members of the treatment team.

Patients who use these skills, alone or with family cooperation, have been shown to: use medication more appropriately; miss less school; require fewer hospitalization or emergency room visits; incur lower asthma-related costs; handle their illness with fewer problems; feel better about themselves; and relate better to others.

5.1. Knowing the Facts and Fallacies about Asthma and Its Management

It is likely, as suggested above, that the failure to take appropriate preventive action, to handle attacks calmly and effectively, and to avoid unnecessary secondary problems, are, at least in part, due to limited information about the illness and how to care for it. Such failures may also be due to inaccurate "information" supplied by misinformed friends, family, or neighbors. Among the more common fallacies about asthma are: it is an emotional illness; it is somebody's "fault"; asthma can be turned on and off voluntarily; all children outgrow asthma so there is nothing to worry about; asthma is contagious; asthmatics must always "take it easy" and avoid athletics or exercise; asthmatics must never allow themselves to become upset; asthmatics must avoid nuts, chocolate, wheat, etc., even if they have never been shown to be allergic to them; chihuahua dogs cure asthma.

Publications available from the American Lung Association,* can help patients get accurate information about asthma. Conferences with the doctors will also help to accomplish that purpose. Clinicians should help their patients to

*1740 Broadway, New York, New York 10019.

formulate specific questions or issues to be raised with their doctors. They should also prepare their patients for the sorts of questions the doctors are likely to ask (these will be described in Section 5.5).

Clinicians should enlist the doctors' cooperation in their efforts to help patients become more competent asthma managers. Some doctors will be skeptical of such efforts. Others will worry that their patients will become overly self-reliant and put off getting professional help when they need it. I have found that when I have taken time to talk with doctors and to understand their concerns, it has been possible to educate them about the role of behavior in asthma, and to persuade them that adjunct behavioral care will enhance, not undermine, their efforts. I have seen the patient at hand benefit, and I have also seen doctors go on to make useful behavioral observations in other patients as well. Not infrequently they have also gone on to make appropriate referrals for behavioral treatment.

5.2. Knowing One's Symptom Precipitants and Aggravants

Effective and reasonable preventive actions can only follow from accurate knowledge about what precipitates the patient's symptoms. Patients who see precipitants virtually everywhere are likely to restrict themselves unnecessarily. And patients who, on the other hand, know too little about what brings on or aggravates their symptoms are likely to suffer entirely avoidable attacks. Medications such as sodium cromolyn now exist that can prevent certain attacks if used appropriately.

Participating in the asthma assessment can start the uninformed patient on the road to a more accurate awareness of symptom precipitants. Keeping an asthma diary can sharpen that awareness. Knowing the results of medical diagnostic tests is another way to broaden the patient's knowledge of this important matter.

5.3. Knowing and Attending to Early Warning Signs, and Knowing What to Do in Response to Them

Patients and families can err in two ways regarding EWSs. They can be hypervigilant—see asthma in every slight change in breathing, sign of fatigue, sniffle, etc., and then overmedicate, run to the emergency room, take to bed, or panic themselves into a full-blown attack. Alternatively, they can ignore the signs and symptoms of an impending attack, and fail to take actions that might have headed it off or controlled its severity. An important goal of treatment is to help patients and their families learn what to look for and how to be alert but calm. (A list of common EWSs is given in Table 2.) Family members can learn how to listen to the patient's chest for wheezing sounds and how to use a peak flow meter at home. With the doctor's help, they can learn how to respond to

Table 2
Early Warning Signs of Asthma

Paleness, sweating
Fatigue not caused by working or playing hard
Restless sleep
Anxiety
Fast breathing
Vomiting
Hunched over posture
Flared nostrils while breathing in[a]
Pursed lips breathing (breathing out by blowing air through tightened lips)
Space at the base of the throat and the spaces between the ribs sink in during
    inhalation
Coughing
Throat clearing (a lot)
Irregular breathing
Wheezing
Noisy, labored breathing[a]

---

[a]These are not, strictly speaking, *early* warning signs of asthma as much as indices of the severity of airway obstruction. They are included because they may be the first thing another person may notice in the patient.

different warning signs by relaxing, drinking liquids, doing abdominal breathing exercises, taking appropriate extra medication, doing postural drainage (a technique for helping the patient to clear mucus from the airways) and calling the doctor for advice.

5.4. Relaxing and Doing Abdominal Breathing

Relaxing and breathing abdominally can control anxiety and facilitate slower, easier, and deeper breathing. They are important skills for the patient to use between as well as during asthma attacks.

There are many relaxation exercises readily available for use with children and adults. Abdominal breathing training has also been described in detail elsewhere (Weiss, 1989, and Chapter 11), and I will only mention two interim techniques that can be used while the patients learn the more comprehensive skill. First, patients place their fists on the back of their hips and try to bring their elbows together behind them. A family member can help by grasping the patient's elbows and gently pushing them towards each other. Second, the patient gets down on all fours with the abdomen relaxed. In this position, it is almost impossible not to breathe abdominally and I have had patients report that it was easier for them to get air in that position.

5.5 Talking to the Doctor and Other Members of the Treatment Team

It can take anything from a simple suggestion to do so, all the way to assertiveness training and role playing to get the patients to talk openly with their doctors. Patients should be made aware that, as (paying) consumers, they are entitled to receive specific, clear instructions, and to question the doctor if treatment appears not to be helping. The tension that builds when patients are afraid to assert themselves can undermine their relationship with the doctor and compromise the treatment. However, patients must understand that a dialogue is a two-way matter and the more information they bring to that dialogue, the more likely it is to be productive.

Patients should be encouraged to call their doctors before going to the office or the emergency room for an apparent emergency. At such times they should be prepared to tell the doctor about the signs and symptoms of their condition, to state when, how much, and what medication they last took, what others measures were tried, and when they last saw the doctor. With that information, the doctor can better determine if the patient should come in immediately or if there are procedures that could be safely tried at home first. I have seen cases in which emergency visits were drastically reduced by this simple measure.

6. Conclusion

Asthma cannot be cured. Its physical, emotional, and financial costs can, however, be reduced. Behavioral intervention contributes to that end by helping patients and their families to become more effective self-managers and more competent participants in their medical care. The rewards of successful interventions are enjoyed not only by patients and their families; therapists partake of them as well. I remember how I felt one morning some years ago when I appeared on network television with a young lady who had been chosen to represent *Superstuff*, an asthma self-management program that I had developed in cooperation with the staff of the American Lung Association. Using *Superstuff*, this young lady had learned to work her way around the obstacles of her asthma. That morning she smiled into the camera and offered encouragement to millions of her peers and elders. She simply said, "I'm not afraid any more."

ACKNOWLEDGMENT. Robert B. Mellins, M.D., read and commented on the first draft of this chapter. His insights and suggestions are gratefully acknowledged.

7. References

Creer, T. *Asthma Therapy: A behavioral health care system for respiratory disorders.* New York: Springer, 1979.

Creer, T., Marion, R.S., and Creer, P.P. Asthma problems behavior check list: Parental perceptions of the behavior of asthmatic children. *J. Asthma,* 1983, *20,* 97–104.

Fried, R. *The hyperventilation syndrome.* Baltimore: Johns Hopkins University Press, 1987.

Lum, C. The syndrome of habitual chronic hyperventilation. In O. Hill (Ed.), *Modern trends in psychosomatic medicine.* Boston: Butterworth, 1976, pp. 196–230.

Purcell, K., and Weiss, J.H. Asthma. In C.G. Costello (Ed.), *Symptoms of psychopathology.* New York: Wiley, 1970, pp. 597–623.

Weiss, J.H. The current status of the concept of a psychosomatic disorder. *International Journal Psychiatry in Medicine,* 1974, *5,* 473–482.

Weiss, J.H. Managing psychosomatic symptoms: The case of George. In H. Fensterheim and H. Glazer (Eds.), *Behavioral psychotherapy.* New York: Brunner Mazel, 1983, pp. 207–227.

Weiss, J.H. Breathing control. In C. Lindemann (Ed.), *Handbook of phobia therapy.* New York: J. Aronson, 1989, pp. 299–326.

15

Respiratory Practices in Yoga

FRANK A. CHANDRA

1. Introduction

In the West changes in respiration have been regarded primarily as signs and symptoms of disease. Mechanisms for abnormal ventilation—malfunction of the respiratory control centers, neuromuscular disease, or excess work of breathing—have been elucidated and therapeutically modified (Guenter, 1984). In the East, however, voluntary modifications of breathing have long been used for treatment of disease and for influencing physiological function of the nervous and other systems of the body. The methods were drawn from disciplines practiced by esoteric communities for spiritual purposes, especially in India. A statuette found in an Indus valley excavation suggested that yogic breath control was well developed in the third millennium BC and was associated with physical and spiritual well-being (Rowland, 1953).

2. Pranayama

As a stage toward meditation, yogis practice a special breathing technique known in Sanskrit as *pranayama*. The essentials of this technique include (1) slowing and regularizing the breath by prolonging the expiratory phase, (2) enhancing abdominal/diaphragmatic breathing, and (3) imposing resistance to both inspiration and exhalation.

FRANK A. CHANDRA (1925–1993) • Formerly, Department of Health, London, England.
Behavioral and Psychological Approaches to Breathing Disorders, edited by Beverly H. Timmons and Ronald Ley. Plenum Press, New York, 1994.

3. Prolonged Expiration

In ordinary life, prolonged expiration is associated with diminished cerebral and physical activity and tone (e.g., in yawning, sighing, smoking, or counting to ten in crises). Yogi masters assumed, without investigating causal relationships, that prolonged expiration in breathing exercises would induce mental and physical relaxation. Expiration is therefore usually prolonged to twice the duration of inspiration.

4. Abdominal/Diaphragmatic Breathing

In yogic practice, both the diaphragm and the lower ribs are used, in contrast to the use by some singers of the diaphragm alone with chest fully expanded. Abdominal breathing is practiced by concentration on restricting the movement of the upper ribs and on bulging of the upper part of the abdominal wall. Breath-holding in submaximal inspiration is introduced as expertise in the method is developed and it can be done safely.

5. Increased Resistance

Resistance to breathing may be imposed at the nose (by closing one nostril with the fingers), or at the mouth (by mouth-breathing through different configurations of lips and tongue) or at the larynx (by voluntarily narrowing the glottic aperture). Pressure on the nostril due to inward compression by the fingers stimulates the mucous membrane and results in increased patency of the nostrils by constriction of resistive and capacitative blood vessels, as also occurs in exercise (Girgis et al., 1974). In addition, it may assist voluntary partial closure of the glottis and may slow the pulse. These effects are mediated through a reflex having the fifth cranial nerve as afferent, and the vagus nerve as efferent (Gooden et al., 1978).

6. Alternate Nostril Breathing

Various combinations of alternate nostril occlusion during inhalation or exhalation are used, resulting in stimulation of both nasal cavities and producing changes in temperature, pressure, and airflow characteristics. From experiments in animals, Whicker et al. (1978) showed that nasal stimulation caused changes in breathing patterns, which altered resistance without actual change in the intrinsic behavior of the lung airways. It was thought that subtle relations between the upper and lower respiratory tract were probably important to respiratory health (Chapter 2). An increase in pulmonary airflow resistance allows efficient gas exchange in the alveoli and, to maintain this, nasal respiration and stimulation are important (Strong, 1979). Negus *et al.* (1970) showed that if one nostril is closed there is decreased air intake and output and increased intratracheal and intrathoracic negative and positive pressures. The alteration of pressure on the great veins and right atrium helps onward flow of the blood during inspiration. With the right nostril closed, swings of pressure from -10 to $+10$ mm Hg were measured in the right atrium during inspiration and expiration, respectively. In strong inspiration against resistance, intrapleural pressure can reach -30 mm Hg (Feely *et al.*, 1975).

7. Nasal Passages and Nasal Cycles

Yogic theory consistently states that there are important connections between the nasal passages and the psyche. During spontaneous breathing, inhaling through the left nostril is said by most people to have a calming, beneficial, stabilizing effect, while breathing through the right nostril is destabilizing, excitatory, and ultimately enervating. A balance between the two modes is thought to be most suitable for the challenges of daily life, and is put forth as a teleological explanation for the ultradian rhythm of congestion/decongestion that occurs in the nose throughout the day. This cycle of naturally occurring congestion in one nostril with relative decongestion in the other nostril, followed by the reverse, occurs every $1^{1}/_{2}$–4 hours and has been described by yogic practitioners for hundreds of years. Confirmation of this finding has been made in the West (Stoksted, 1952), and central nervous system correlates of nostril laterality documented by Werntz *et al.* (1983). Such cycling might be regulated from a nasal center in the hypothalamus or the medulla, and Eccles (1978) suggests that persons trained in yogic breathing exercises could alter dominance of nasal airflow from one nostril to the other, presumably by developing voluntary control of this autonomic nasal center. Persistence of airflow through one nostril instead of alternation has been shown in allergic rhinitis, septal deviation, and upper respiratory infection (Gray, 1977). A summary of proposed physiological and clinical effects (including hemispheric lateralization) produced by changes from normal nasal breathing are described by Backon (1989).

8. Asthma

In asthma, strong, active expiratory effort does not necessarily reduce the hyperinflation of the lungs since dynamic compression of the airways may further increase resistance (des Jardins, 1984). A low level of positive pressure applied to the expiratory phase of tidal breathing should decrease or prevent premature closure, by increasing the transmural pressure across the intrathoracic airways (Mead, 1960). Thus, slow expiratory effort against resistance, as in the pranayamic expiration, should increase pressure in the airways and delay dynamic compression, allowing a stronger contraction of the expiratory muscles to reduce hyperinflation to some extent.

Nagarathna and Nagendra (1985) found significant improvements in number of attacks, drug use, and peak flow rate in a group of 53 asthmatic patients on yoga therapy, compared with matched control patients. The yoga subjects practiced daily—after training—in a series of breathing, postural, mental, and spiritual exercises. The authors speculated that the physical and mental relaxation produced by yoga had a stabilizing effect on bronchial reactivity, through reduction of vagal efferent activity.

9. Effects of Pranayama on Carbon Dioxide Levels

Using inspiration against resistance for 5 seconds, followed by breath-holding for 20 seconds, then expiration against resistance for 10 seconds, Kuvalayananda (1933) found that alveolar CO_2 rose from about 5.5 percent to approx 6.5 percent (i.e., mild respiratory acidosis; see Chapter 7) by about the sixth breath and remained at this level during the final four breaths of the ten-breath cycle. Many of the effects claimed for this type of breathing may be attributable to the rise in alveolar CO_2 and arterial Pa_{CO_2}. Among these effects are:

- Tranquilizing of the cerebral cortex with stimulation of the reticular activating system, resulting in a calm but alert mind.
- Increase in cerebral blood flow without causing headache.
- Vasodilation of the skin blood vessels, producing a sensation of warmth moving over the body.
- In some persons, vasoconstriction of digital blood vessels, resulting in cold fingers.
- Stimulation of certain exocrine glands, producing, for example, increased flow of saliva and sweat.
- Elevation of the threshold of the high pressure baroreceptor in the carotid sinus.
- Shunting of blood from the internal abdominal areas to skin and skeletal muscles.
- Decreased contractility of the inspiratory muscles (Cohen et al., 1982), the laryngeal muscles (Dixon et al., 1974), and the cardiac and skeletal

muscles in general (Cingolani *et al.*, 1969). This does not appear to be due merely to the sense of relaxation produced by the effect of CO_2 on the brain, but may be a direct effect on muscle due to alteration of pH (Juan *et al.*, 1984).

Raised levels of alveolar CO_2 do not result in increased rate and depth of respiration in the trained yoga practitioner because volume is voluntarily controlled to about 50–75 percent of the inspiratory capacity, and rate is fixed at about two breaths per minute in adepts practicing the recommended cycle (5, 20, and 10 seconds, respectively, for inspiration, breath-holding, and expiration).

Yogis attribute their ability to resist the normal stimulus for increased ventilation—a rise in alveolar CO_2—to voluntary control over automatic and reflex actions and thus a desirable dominance of mind and will over bodily urges. Stanescu *et al.* (1981), however, attribute these striking changes in fundamental ventilatory responses (to increased alveolar CO_2) to chronic overstimulation of the stretch receptors of the lung. This overstimulation results, through habituation, in decreased vagal information from the receptors.

Pietroni and Pietroni (1989) reviewed the evidence and concluded that respiratory modulation of the autonomic nervous system had a central, and a peripheral, component. Shallow inspiration increased arousal (as shown, for example, by reaction time or the knee jerk reflect), but deep inspiration decreased arousal. Arousal was associated with increased sympathetic, and decreased parasympathetic, discharge. The pranayamic deep inspiration, followed by some seconds of breath holding and then slow expiration, might therefore prolong the inhibition of arousal and contribute to the long-lasting modulation of autonomic activity noted in such an exercise.

An alternative explanation is that the yogi's entire sympathetic nervous system may become less active, as shown by the low blood pressure and metabolic rate seen in many practicing yogis. Medical investigators of yogic physiology have repeatedly observed that these practices produce a decrease in sympathetic tone (Patel, 1975).

10. Underbreathing, Normal, and Overbreathing

Panting is used by dogs and other hairy mammals to cool the body. Stable levels of Pco_2 (*eucapnia*) are maintained because it is primarily dead space that is ventilated (see Chapter 2). An analogue in yoga is an advanced practice, bellows breathing (*Bhastrika*), in which adepts breathe at a rate of about 60 (or 120) breaths per minute, using abdominal and expiratory muscles, the latter working from rest point to greater expiration, with the subsequent inspiration being due to reflexive recoil. It has been documented that stable levels of Pco_2

are maintained during Bhastrika (Kuvalayananda and Karambelkar, 1957). If rapid respiration is too shallow, there is primarily dead space ventilation and inadequate alveolar ventilation; therefore, CO_2 is retained (Bradley et al., 1984). On the other hand, deep rapid respiration will produce hypocapnia and the familiar unpleasant sequelae of hyperventilation. It must be borne in mind, however, that some persons find hypocapnia attractive because of the alteration of consciousness or "high" it can cause. In some communities it is actively practiced in rituals, for inducing trances and psychic states that give the performer an enhanced status among his people. A relative insensitivity to pain can occur during these trances, enabling the performer to execute impressive feats, such as, skewering his flesh or suffering beating with whips, without any apparent discomfort (Lum, 1981). In many parts of the world certain nonyogic groups, e.g., some of the cult groups of African origins in Jamaica, use overbreathing and the resulting hypocapnia to procure or enhance trancelike states. West Indians are sometimes admitted to accident and emergency departments in the United Kingdom for "epilepsy," but have no detectable organic lesions. Their histories strongly suggest ritual overbreathing as a causative factor.

The potential value of pranayama in the treatment of hyperventilation is evident, not only because of the slight degree of hypercapnia induced, but also because of the tranquilizing effect and the retraining of respiratory patterns that results. Hyperventilating agoraphobics had an improved response to conventional behavior therapy when the latter was supplemented with breathing retraining (Bonn et al., 1984). Patients were instructed in abdominal/diaphragmatic breathing, slowed to 8–10 breaths per minute.

11. Respiratory Muscles

Various phases of pranayamic breathing have potential for increasing endurance of respiratory muscles in certain circumstances. Inspiratory resistance was used to improve exercise performance in cystic fibrosis (Pardy et al., 1981a,b) and to increase the strength of inspiratory muscles in quadriplegia (Gross et al., 1980). Breath holding after inspiration is advocated by swimming coaches—one deep breath per four arm cycles. The resulting improved performance is said to be due to physiological adaptations facilitated by increased blood CO_2 (Counsilman, 1981).

12. Valsalva Maneuver

This procedure, which involves an expiratory effort with the glottis closed after a full inspiration, is avoided in Eastern breathing practices because of its possible harmful effects. The Valsalva maneuver can produce intrathoracic pressures of up to 100–150 mm Hg (Charlier *et al.*, 1974). To prevent syncope from an unintentional Valsalva effect, pranayama practitioners are advised to breathe in submaximally (i.e., less than the inspiratory capacity), especially when breath holding follows the end of inspiration.

13. Comparison of Pranayama and Mechanically Assisted Ventilation

Although resembling, in the *expiratory* phase, various forms of mechanical respiratory assistance now in clinical use, the yogic *inspiratory* phase is quite different from that in any form of assisted ventilation, even intermittent positive pressure ventilation (IPPV), in which positive pressure is given during inspiration only. Unlike mechanical ventilation, pranayamic breathing does not embarrass the venous return and cardiac output during each cycle of respiration. Its full use in clinical medicine awaits exploration.

14. Abdominal Pressures

During performance of yogic postures (*asanas*), breathing is controlled primarily to adjust pressures in the abdomen. Forward bending of the spine tends to increase intraabdominal pressure. The performer is therefore advised to let the breath out slowly and gradually during a full forward bending posture (head on fully extended knees while standing (Fig. 1A) or sitting (Fig. 1B); to hold the breath in expiration during maintenance of this full spinal flexion; and then to breathe slowly in as the spine is straightened again into the erect standing or sitting position. Adepts who can hold the full position for several minutes are advised to breath normally during this time. Conversely, when doing exercises causing extension of the spine beyond the upright position, the performer gradually breathes in; holds the position while breathing naturally; and then breathes out while straightening up. Thus, in the extreme flexion of the spine known as the *plough* (Fig. 1C), intraabdominal pressure remains at approx 10 mm Hg, as it does in a spinal extension posture, the *fish* (1D).

Riemenschneider and Shields (1981) described the movement of lymph through the valves of the thoracic duct during the negative intrathoracic pressure of inspiration. This effect is likely to be enhanced by the ancient yogic exercise of maximal inspiratory effort against the closed glottis after full expiration, recently termed the *Mueller maneuver* (Mines, 1986). Subsequent diminution of the negative pressure, as normal breathing is resumed, will move the lymph upwards out of the chest into the subclavian veins, as the valves of the thoracic duct prevents reflux. This upward movement of lymph increases as intrathoracic

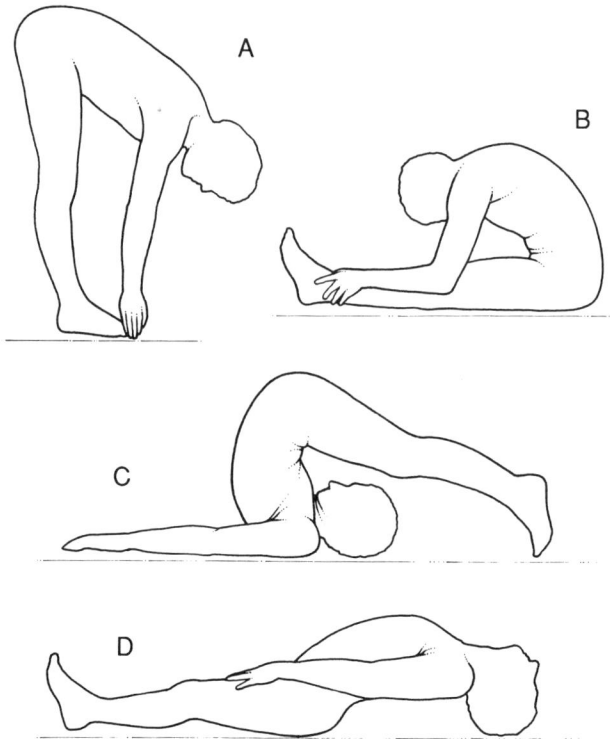

Figure 1. Yoga postures (asanas).

pressure becomes positive with the next expiration, and more so if this expiration is against resistance. This enhanced movement of lymph has nutritive and immunological significance (Damshek, 1963).

Negative intrathoracic pressures are transmitted to the abdomen via the diaphragm, and to the soft walls and interiors of the viscera of the abdomen and the chest. An increase in transmural pressures would be expected in blood vessels, gut, gall bladder, pelvis of the kidneys, urethra, and urinary bladder. Hypotheses have been generated that such effects would dilate extensible tubular structures, causing increased blood flow in organs of the chest and abdomen, and clearance of obstructing debris from ducts and hollow viscera, etc.

15. Hormonal Effects

Yogic physicians claim that breathing practices can affect many physiologic parameters, including output of several hormones. Udupa and colleagues' subjects practiced pranayamic breathing for seven minutes, rest for five minutes and then Bhastrika for ten minutes. After six months of daily practice, decreased total serum lipids and increased plasma cortisol, urinary 17-hydroxy- and 17-keto-steroids were observed (Udupa *et al.*, 1975).

16. Meditation

Most types of meditation can be assigned to either one or two major classes: the excitatory (ergotropic), hyperarousal class and the calming (trophotropic), hypoarousal class (Fischer, 1971), each associated with appropriate changes in blood pressure, pulse, respiratory and metabolic rates, and EEG. The excitatory (Kundalini) types (Eliade, 1958) of meditation may use the Bhastrika breathing or else a mild overbreathing, while the calming types of meditation [expounded by the sage Patanjali (late BC to early AD)] involve special types of slow, controlled breathing, often with breath retention. The latter are practiced in the early stages of diaphragmatic breathing (pranayama) and later during the induction of meditation.

In a Western study documenting central nervous system correlates of breathing patterns, Timmons *et al.* (1972) found that the relaxed presleep state (characterized by EEG alpha activity) was usually associated with abdominal-dominant breathing. In stage I or stage II sleep, thoracic breathing tended to increase in amplitude while abdominal breathing decreased. In the transition from wakefulness to sleep, changes in EEG patterns (waxing and waning of alpha activity, appearance of theta waves, etc.) were tightly linked to changes in abdominal/thoracic amplitudes. The authors concluded that their findings were compatible with claims of yogis, Zen Buddhists, and others who use breathing techniques to facilitate attainment of special states of consciousness. The findings are also relevant to anecdotal accounts of yogis who claim that pranayama induces calmness and relaxation but increases mental alertness: neurophysiologists recognize the EEG alpha state as compatible with relaxed wakefulness.

17. Conclusion

This brief account of the effects of a few pranayamic breathing techniques suggests that the traditional teachings of yogic masters can prove to be an interesting and rewarding field for scientific investigation. Such studies would not only increase our knowledge of basic physiological mechanisms, but would also point the way to new, simpler, and less costly methods for treatment of respiratory and other disorders.

18. Guidelines for Therapists

Pranayamic type breathing is likely to be of some benefit to people suffering from anxiety disorders, hyperventilation, cystic fibrosis, emphysema, cardiac failure, asthma, and some forms of epilepsy. Bhastrika type breathing may help mild depressives and asthmatics, and perhaps assist in evacuation of excess liquid and semiliquid material from the lungs in chronic obstructive pulmonary disease and bronchiectasis. However, patients should not be referred to yoga teachers unless a firm medical diagnosis has been made, and the teacher is known to understand the condition. Great care should be taken not to use inappropriate treatment; e.g., Bhastrika should not be taught to hyperventilators, epileptics, or cases of angina pectoris, nor should pranayama be used by depressives.

19. References

Backon, J. Nasal breathing as a treatment for hyperventilation: Relevance of hemispheric activation. *British Journal of Clinical Practice,* 1989, *43,* 161–162.

Bonn, J.A., Readhead, C.P.A., and Timmons, B.H. Enhanced adaptive behavioural response in agoraphobic patients pretreated with breathing retraining. *Lancet,* 1984, *2,* 665–669.

Bradley, T.D., Day, A., Hyland, R.H., Webster, P., Rutherford, R., McNicholas, W., and Phillipson, E.A. Chronic ventilatory failure caused by abnormal respiratory pattern generation during sleep. *American Review of Respiratory Diseases,* 1984, *130,* 678–680.

Charlier, A.A., Javmin, P.M., and Pouleur, H. Circulatory effects of deep inspirations, blocked expirations and positive pressure inflations at equal transpulmonary pressures in conscious dogs. *Journal of Physiology,* 1974, *241,* 589–605.

Cingolani, H.E., Blesa, E.S., Gonzalez, N.C., and Mattiazzi, A. Extracellular vs. intracellular pH as a determinant of myocardial contractility. *Life Sciences,* 1969, *8,* 775–781.

Cohen, C.A., Zagelbaum, G., Gross, D., Roussos, C.H., and Macklem, P.T. Clinical manifestations of inspiratory muscle fatigue. *American Journal of Medicine,* 1982, *73,* 308–316.

Counsilman, J.E. Competitive swimming and controlled breathing. *Journal of the American Medical Association,* 1981, *246,* 1967.

Damshek, W. William Hewson: Thymicologist: Father of hematology? *Blood,* 1963, *21,* 513–516 (Editorial).

des Jardins, T.R. *Clinical manifestations of respiratory disease.* Chicago: Year Book Medical Publishers, Inc, 1984.

Dixon, M., Szereda-Przestaszewska, M., Widdicumbe, J.G., and Wise, J.C.M., Studies on laryngeal calibre during stimulation of peripheral and central chemoreceptors, pneumothorax and increased respiratory loads. *Journal of Physiology,* 1974, *239,* 347–363.

Eccles, R. The central rhythm of the nasal cycle. *Acta Otolaryngologica,* 1978, *86,* 464–468.

Eliade, M. *Yoga: Immortality and freedom.* Princeton, New Jersey: Princeton University Press, 1958.

Feely, T.W., Saumarez, R., Klick, J.M., McNabb, T.G., and Skillman, J.J. Positive and expiratory pressure in weaning patients from controlled ventilation: A prospective randomised trial. *Lancet,* 1975, *2,* 725–729.

Fischer, R. A cartography of the ecstatic and meditative states. *Science,* 1971, *174,* 897–904.

Girgis, I.H., Yassin, A., Hamdy, H., and Moris, M. A method for assessment of the nasal circulation. *Journal of Laryngology and Otology*, 1974, *88*, 1149–1158.

Gooden, B.A., Holdstock, G., and Hampton, J.R. The magnitude of the bradycardia induced by face immersion in patients convalescing from myocardial infarction. *Cardiovascular Research*, 1978, *12*, 239–242.

Gross, D., Ladd, H.W., Riley, E.J., Macklem, P.T., and Grassino, Λ. The effect of training on strength and endurance of the diaphragm in quadriplegia. *American Journal of Medicine*, 1980, *68*, 27–35.

Gray, L.P. The T's and A's problem—assessment and re-assessment. *Journal of Laryngology and Otology*, 1977, *91*, 11–32.

Guenter, C.A. Altered regulatory mechanisms in disease. In E.D. Frohlich (Ed.), *Pathophysiology*. Philadelphia: J B Lippincott, 1984.

Juan, G., Calverly, P., Talamo, E., Schnader, J., and Roussos, C. Effect of carbon dioxide on diaphragmatic function in human beings. *New England Journal of Medicine*, 1984, *310*, 874–879.

Kuvalayananda, Swami. Oxygen absorption and carbon dioxide elimination in Pranayama. *Yoga Mimamsa*, 1933, *4*, 267–289.

Kuvalayananda, Swami, and Karambelkar, P.V. Studies in alveolar air during Kapalabhati. *Yoga Mimamsa*, 1957, *7*, 87–97.

Lum, L.C. Hyperventilation and anxiety state. *Journal of the Royal Society of Medicine*, 1981, *74*, 1–4.

Mines, A.H. *Respiratory physiology*. New York: Raven Press, 2nd ed., 1986.

Mead, J. Volume displacement body plethysmograph for respiratory measurements in human subjects. *Journal of Applied Physiology*, 1960, *15*, 736–740.

Nagarathna, R., and Nagendra, H.R. Yoga for bronchial asthma: A controlled study. *British Medical Journal*, 1985, *291*, 1077–1079.

Negus, V.E., Oram, S., and Bank, D.C. Effect of respiratory obstruction on the arterial and venous circulation in animals and man. *Thorax*, 1970, *25*, 1–10.

Pardy, R.L., Rivington, R.N., Despas, P.J., and Macklem, P.T. Inspiratory muscle training compared with physiotherapy in patients with chronic airflow limitation. *American Review of Respiratory Diseases*, 1981a, *123*, 421–425.

Pardy, R.L., Rivington, R.N., Despas, P.J., and Macklem, P.T. Inspiratory muscle training on exercise performance in chronic airflow limitation. *American Review of Respiratory Diseases*, 1981b, *123*, 426–433.

Patel, C. Twelve-month follow-up of yoga and biofeedback in the management of hypertension. *Lancet*, 1975, *2*, 62–64.

Pietroni, P.C., and Pietroni, M. Respiratory mechanisms and clinical syndromes. *Holistic Medicine*, 1989, *4*, 67–79.

Reimenschneider, P.A., and Shields, J.W. Human central lymph propulsion. *Journal of the American Medical Association*, 1981, *246*, 2066–2067.

Rowland, B. The art and architecture of India: Buddhist, Hindu, Jain. In N. Pevsner (Ed.), *Pelican history of art*. Melbourne: Penguin Books, 1953.

Stanescu, D.C., Nemery, B., Veriter, C., and Marechal, C. Pattern of breathing and ventilatory response to CO_2 in subjects practising Hatha-Yoga. *Journal of Applied Physiology*, 1981, *51*, 1625–1629.

Stoksted, P. The physiologic cycle of the nose under normal and pathologic conditions. *Acta Otolaryngologica*, 1952, *42*, 175–179.

Strong, M.S. Nasopulmonary reflex: Evaluation in the non-paralyzed and paralyzed anaesthetized dog (Editorial comment). In M.M. Paparella and M.S. Strong (Eds.), *Year book of otolaryngology*. Chicago and London: Year Book Medical Publications, Inc., 1979.

Timmons, B., Salamy, J., Kamiya, J., and Girton, D. Abdominal-thoracic respiratory movements and levels of arousal. *Psychonomic Science,* 1972, *27,* 173–175.
Udupa, K.N., Singh, R.H., and Settiwar, R.M. Studies on the effect of some yogic breathing exercises (Pranayama) in normal persons. *Indian Journal of Medical Research,* 1975, *63,* 1062–1065.
Werntz, D.A., Bickford, R.G., Bloom, F.E., and Shannahoff-Khalsa, D.S. Alternating cerebral hemispheric activity and the lateralization of autonomic nervous function. *Human Neurobiology,* 1983, *2,* 39–43.
Whicker, J.H., Kern, E.B., and Hyatt, R.E. Nasopulmonary reflex: Evaluation in the non-paralyzed and paralyzed anaesthetized dog. *Annals of Otology, Rhinology and Laryngology,* 1978, *87,* 91–98.

20. Further Reading

The Gheranda Samhita. London: Theosophical Publishing House Ltd, 1976.
The Hatha Yoga Pradipika. New Delhi: Oriental Books Reprint Corporation, 1975.
Iyengar, B.K.S. *Light on yoga.* London: George Allen and Unwin Ltd, 1968.
Iyengar, B.K.S. *Light on pranayama.* London: George Allen and Unwin Ltd, 1981.
Kuvalayananda, Swami. *Pranayama.* Bombay: Popular Prakashan, 1966.
Rama, Swami, Ballentine, R., and Hymes, A. *Science of breath.* Honesdale, Pennsylvania: Himalayan International Institute of Yoga Science and Philosophy, 1979.
Satyananda Saraswati, Swami. *Asana, Pranayama, Mudra, Bandha.* Monghyr, Bihar, India: Sivanand Ashram, 1973.
Vivekananda, Swami. *Raja yoga.* Calcutta: Advaita Ashrama, 1973.

For further information about yoga and its practices, please refer to:

Yoga Journal (published by the California Yoga Teachers Association, 2054 University Avenue, Berkeley, California 94704).

Yoga and Health (published by Yoga Today Ltd, 21 Caburn Crescent, Lewes, East Sussex BN7 INR England).

Yoga Biomedical Trust
P.O. Box 140
Cambridge CB4 3SY
England

Styles of Breathing in Reichian Therapy

DAVID BOADELLA

1. Introduction

The Austrian psychoanalyst Wilhelm Reich was a colleague of Freud's in the 1920s. Whereas his fellow psychoanalysts worked with patients essentially by the analysis of the *contents* of their communications, Reich analyzed in addition the *form* of the communication. This led him to a detailed study of muscle tone, posture, and patterns of breathing. He found chronic patterns of muscle tension (which he called *armoring*), consistently associated with breathing disturbances, in all the patients he treated. He came to the conclusion that deficient expansion on inspiration or deficient relaxation on expiration, or both, was a central mechanism of neurotic repression. By 1934, he had begun to counteract the dysfunctional breathing with a special style of massage and manipulation. Typically, his clients released a range of repressed emotions. Emotional release was followed by more rhythmic breathing. From 1933 onwards, Reich developed *character* (ego structure) *analysis* as a way of focusing on the "gestalt" of a person's neurotic defence patterns, and interpreting these in the same way that Freud had interpreted the neurotic symptoms.

The autonomic nervous system (known in Germany as the "vegetative" system) has a strong influence both on respiratory rhythms and on an individual's emotional balance (Chapter 1). When Reich first discovered the basic role of

DAVID BOADELLA • Psychotherapy Training, Biosynthesis Center, CH 8049 Zurich Switzerland.

Behavioral and Psychological Approaches to Breathing Disorders, edited by Beverly H. Timmons and Ronald Ley. Plenum Press, New York, 1994.

inhibited breathing in every neurotic character, he described his insight as a "breakthrough into the vegetative realm." He went on to develop what he called *vegetotherapy,* a method of working directly with the somatic expression of neurosis. It led him to investigate the hidden, inner rhythms of the body, the pulse of life through the arteries, the beating of the heart, the flow of secretions from glands, and the peristaltic pulsation in the gut. Wherever there were chronic patterns of disturbed breathing he found disturbances in these internal rhythms, blocks to the smooth, harmonious pulsation of the internal organ systems.

In a temporary emergency, an animal experiences acute states of stress during which these basic metabolic rhythms are altered or interrupted; the smooth rhythms that characterize the body when it is in a state of relaxation and well-being return as soon as the challenge or threat has passed. But human beings, from the earliest stages of childhood onwards, are often exposed to long term stressors; for example, the difficult conditions of a deprived, overprotective, or frustrating upbringing. A baby who is left to cry unnecessarily for long hours, an infant who learns tension and guilt over toilet functions, a child who is smacked or shamed for being sexually alive—such children experience decades of conditioning in how to suppress or distort natural feelings. Such conditions constitute chronic stress.

Awareness of the relation between muscular tension and stress is not new, and many forms of relaxation therapy have been developed. But all of these differ in important ways from the therapy that Reich developed as a means of releasing pent up vegetative energy and restoring the natural rhythms of the body. As blocked emotions are released and tense muscles give up their defensive function in the course of a vegetotherapeutic treatment, spontaneous movements in both the skeletal and smooth muscles take place. The relationship between the tension of the main muscle sheets of the body and the internal organ systems is a very complex one and has been addressed directly by some neo-Reichian therapists (e.g., Boyesen, 1985).

Many other contemporary forms of somatically oriented psychotherapy have been profoundly influenced by Reich. Fritz Perls, who trained with Reich, subsequently developed the method of *gestalt therapy* (Perls *et al.,* 1951). Lowen, an American psychiatrist, developed *bioenergetics* in the 1950s, after his studies with Reich (Lowen, 1958). Lowen also focused on the role of dysfunctional breathing in the maintenance of neurotic repression. He used stress positions and expressive movements as a way of mobilizing his patients to give up their muscular holding patterns and to liberate more spontaneous rhythms of breathing. Many therapists, however, have not acknowledged their debt to Reich, and his influence is far more pervasive than is generally known.

2. Breathing Patterns

Observing the breathing of a healthy baby or well-functioning adult, one will see the whole trunk expand on the in-breath and deflate on the out-breath. Healthy breathing follows a wavelike rhythm, is pleasurable, and is in good balance to the needs of the organism (Glaser, 1980). There are four principal ways in which this healthy rhythm may be disturbed:

1. Overinflation of the chest on inspiration with underinflation of the abdomen, coupled with underdeflation of the chest on expiration. The chest is hard, firm and cagelike. This pattern has been found to correlate closely with Type A behavior in persons prone to coronary artery disease (Friedman and Rosenmann, 1960).

2. Overinflation of the abdomen on inspiration with undcrinflation of the chest. There may be underdeflation of the abdomen on expiration. The abdomen feels congested, tense or spongy. This is associated with the *masochistic* temperament in Reichian characterology: the person who typically "swallows down" feelings and holds them in. Occasionally this pattern is linked to *aerophagia*—swallowing air as well as feelings.

3. Underinflation of chest or abdomen or both on inspiration. The breathing is scarcely visible (see Section 6).

4. Forced expiration with a tendency to some form of hyperventilation, the mechanism for which is as follows: If a person is shocked, a startled reflex follows, with increased muscle tone and a tendency for the respiration to become shallow and inhibited. In relaxation, muscle tone returns quickly to its normal state, and breathing, to a harmonious rhythm. People with an anxious attitude toward life retain their startle-reflex patterns and may consequently develop a chronic hyperventilatory tendency.

These are the basic physiological choices that patients may show as deviations from an emotionally balanced and muscularly relaxed breathing rhythm. Some breathing patterns will now be described in their clinical setting, with more attention to the emotional context of the disturbed rhythm.

3. Muscle-Bound Breathing

The type of breathing that Reich first described was characterized by stiffening of the chest muscles and tightening of the rib cage, with a corresponding reduction of the free mobility of the diaphragm:

> The muscles that take part in the armouring of the chest are the intercostals, the large
> chest muscles (pectorals), the shoulder muscles (deltoids), and the muscles on and

between the shoulder blades. The expression of the chest armouring is essentially that of "self-control and restraint." The pulled-back shoulders literally express "holding back." Together with neck armouring, the chest armouring expresses suppressed "spite" and "stiff-neckedness," again to be taken literally. In the presence of armour, the expression is that of "immobility" or "being unmoved." (Reich, 1949)

The kind of defense pattern described above is fairly specific to rigid patterns of armoring, where marked stiffening and tenseness of the large muscle sheets of the body is a pronounced characteristic. The breathing of such people is *unfeeling* breathing. The breathing is reduced by tensions. It neither expresses strong emotion nor responds easily to it. The breathing has a mechanical regularity—inspiration and expiration occur to predictable degrees, the breathe expanding and contracting within the fixed limits imposed by the pressure of the rib cage and the abdominal wall.

Chronic expansion of the thorax creates a range of problems to which people with a tendency to rigid, muscularly armored bodies are particularly prone. Reich includes among them "a tendency to increased blood pressure, palpitations and anxiety, and in severe cases of long standing, also to enlargement of the heart. Various kinds of heart disease result either directly from chronic expansion or indirectly as a result of the anxiety syndrome. Pulmonary emphysema is an immediate result of chronic expansion of the thorax" (Reich, 1942).

Reich also points out how militarism makes use of the expression embodied in this kind of armoring. Alexander (1932; and see Chapter 13) described how methods of physical education stressing "stomach in, shoulders back, chest out" reinforced the body attitude of the stiff automaton responding to mechanical drill. Barlow, a medical practitioner of the Alexander method, wrote that in all his cases of coronary thrombosis, "I have never yet seen a case in which the upper chest was not markedly raised and overcontrolled. The 'powerful' tycoon impression is often accompanied by the blown-up, overfilled chest" (Barlow, 1973).

4. Intestinal Breathing

Reich also describes a form of armoring centered in abdominal pressure:

Patients complain of an intolerable "pressure" in the stomach or of a girdle which "restricts." Others have a certain spot in the abdomen which is very sensitive. Everyone is afraid of getting punched in the belly. This fear becomes the centre of very rich phantasies. Others have the feeling that "there is something in the belly that can't get out"; "it feels like a dinner plate in my belly"; "my belly is dead"; "I have to hold on to my belly," etc. Most of the phantasies of small children about pregnancy and childbirth centre around the vegatative sensations in their abdomen. (Reich, 1942)

There are specific ways of using the gut as a way of suppressing feeling. The gut can be constricted by abdominal pressure, by contraction of the anal sphincter, by "swallowing down" of feelings, and by tension in the diaphragm, which the upper part of the alimentary canal must pass through to get from chest to abdomen. Reich discusses this in relation to the energetics of vomiting:

> In many cases of diaphragmatic block there is, together with the inability to vomit, more or less constant nausea. There can be no doubt that so-called "nervous stomach" disorders are the direct result of armouring in this region. Vomiting is a biological expressive movement, the function of which achieves exactly what it "expresses": convulsive expulsion of body contents. It is based on a peristaltic movement of stomach and oesophagus in the opposite direction of its normal function, that is, towards the mouth (anti-peristalsis). The *gag reflex* dissolves the armouring of the diaphragmatic segment quickly and radically. Vomiting is accompanied by a convulsion of the body, a rapid folding in of the epigastrium, with a forward jerk of the head as well as pelvis. In the colic of infants, vomiting is accompanied by diarrhoea. Energetically speaking, strong waves of excitation run from the middle of the body upwards and downwards toward mouth and anus . . . These convulsions go with deep expiration. (Reich, 1942)

A child who is made to feel ashamed or guilty about expulsion of body contents learns to swallow down bad tastes as well as bad feelings, rather than spit them out, and to inhibit the peristaltic movements of the colon. He often develops a specific pattern of breathing that accompanies and supports the anti-peristaltic pattern. We could speak of *intestinal breathing*. I noticed it in a patient who, when she breathed out, filled up and pressurized the abdomen, even while her chest relaxed and moved downwards. This is an example of *paradoxical* breathing mentioned by Waal *et al.* (1976):

> The direction of movement in the thorax and the abdomen are in this case in opposition to each other. When the chest goes out the abdomen goes in and vice versa. The abdomen is pulled in during inspiration and presses out under expiration; diaphragmatic movements are quite out of touch with movements of the chest.

Such breathing was independently described by Lowen:

> In paradoxical breathing inspiration is produced by an upward movement rather than an outward one . . . Thus the expansion of the chest is accompanied by a narrowing of the abdominal cavity. Sometimes one observes that the belly is sucked in during inspiration and let out in expiration. (Lowen, 1967)

Lowen reported a related pattern in a masochistic patient:

> When he attempted to make a deep expiration, as in a deep sigh, the chest relaxed but the descending wave piled up into a hard knot in the middle of the abdomen . . . It made me think of someone straining at stool. He looked as if he were trying to push something out against a resistance. (1958)

We have here a pattern transferred to the respiratory system from the intestinal system, a breathing pattern that would be particularly expected in association with people exposed to nauseating situations that make them want to throw up *the poison of paranoia,* or with people exposed to situations of anal humiliation and disgust over abdominal contents (*the morass of masochism*).

5. Breathing as Sucking

In the oral character, Lowen describes the opposite of the inflated chest of the rigid character. "Marked muscular tension seems absent from the front of the body but this is only because of the *deflated condition of the chest and abdomen.*" In contrast to the pattern just described, "the gag reflex is fairly easy to elicit. This may be due to early feeding disturbances with persistent tendencies to vomit." It is as though the oral defence is an acclimatization to emptiness. "The chest is generally deflated, the belly is without turgor and *feels soft and empty to palpation.*" (Lowen, 1958.)

The deflation of the oral body structure and personality characteristics, which Lowen has described so clearly, is found in the breathing pattern. We can recognize a specific type of oral breathing distinguished by fear and reluctance to express greed. It seems to be a learned attitude transferred from suckling behaviours. "Any disturbance in the function of sucking," Lowen wrote (1967), "will have an immediate repercussion upon the function of breathing." The child learns to be disappointed and left feeling hungry, not only in relation to food, but in relation to air. His experience that reaching out for what you want does not get you what you want, that you are left unfilled and uncharged, is learned in relation to the flow of milk from the mother, which is a flow he cannot regulate. When this is transferred to breathing, it means that such a person starves himself of air; he is afraid to gulp it in and suck it down. The oral attitudes of sucking nourishment from other people or from the substitutes provided by various addictions stem from the refusal to let nourishment rush in from the air.

6. Schizoid and Hysterical Breathing

Reich has described another breathing pattern in a case of schizophrenia that he treated. Although this pattern also seems to be based on a reluctance to breathe in, its origins and dynamics are very different.

> I tried to approach her dysfunction of respiration. The problem was not as in the armoured neurotic, to break down the armouring of the chest. *There seemed to be no armour.* The problem was how to make her draw in and expel air through the larynx. She began to.struggle severely whenever I tried to bring about full respiration. I had the impression that the function of respiration was not stopped by any immobility due to armouring, but was inhibited as if by a *strong conscious effort.* (Reich, 1949)

Reich describes how one of the functions of this breathing inhibition is to cut off the pleasure sensations and anxiety feelings moving in the body, and that his patient fought these "by not permitting the passage of air to and from the lungs." But since schizophrenics cannot refuse to take in air, the specific dynamic of this breathing seems to involve minimizing the movements of breathing. In other words, the intake of air and its explusion does take place but is made as imperceptible as possible. It is interior, invisible breathing, as compared with the breathing of someone who confidently breathes out into the world. It is not that a person living in this way does not feel entitled to be nourished orally and therefore reduces his demand on the air, as in the situation described above. Imperceptible breathing is a denial not of the air, but of the breathing process itself, which is the prerequisite of life outside the womb. The schizophrenic breathing movements are a duplication, as closely as it is possible to do so, of the inactivity of the breathing apparatus inside the womb. The soft, imperceptible breathing that Reich described is "uterine respiration." It is the breathing of someone reluctant or unable to be born.

Breathing vigorously for a schizoid person may arouse sensations of dying through drowning. Lowen explains this as follows:

> Opening the throat wide to breathe evoked feelings of drowning in several patients. One patient reported this sensation on a number of occasions. Yet the patient could not find any incident in his memory which could give rise to such an experience. The logical interpretation was that the feeling of drowning represented his reaction to a flood of tears and sadness which welled up in his throat when its tensions were relaxed. In the same way, the choking sensations commonly reported by patients could be interpreted as the "choking off" of these overwhelming feelings of sadness. (Lowen, 1967)

Another form of schizoid breathing pattern described by Lowen appears to be the opposite of that shown by Reich's patient and by the patient above. It is when a person immobilizes breathing around the inbreath.

> This kind of schizophrenic respiration has an emotional sign. If you duplicate it in yourself (inflate your chest and pull in your belly), you will hear a gasp as air enters your lungs. It is not difficult to recognize this as an expression of fright. The schizophrenic breathes as if he were in a state of terror. (Lowen, 1958)

If this gasp, once taken in, is let out imperceptibly, then the expression of fear is frozen and inturned. The schizophrenic breathes like a man who plays dead on a battle field and who will be shot if he betrays he is alive through his breathing movements. He can breathe but he must not be seen to breathe.

The hysterical breathing attitude shows the opposite tendency: at all costs one must be seen to breathe. Breathing at least proves one is alive and out of the womb, but it is anxious, panicky breathing, the breathing of someone who only just made it. Anxiety means constriction, and hysterical breathing is constricted breathing in which the breathing struggles to assert itself.

> Let us imagine that one is frightened or in anticipation of great danger. Instinctively one will draw in one's breath and remain in this attitude. As one cannot continue to do this one will soon breathe out again. However, expiration will be incomplete and shallow; one does not breathe out completely in one breath, but in fractions, in steps, as it were . . . What is the function of this attitude of "shallow respiration?" If we

look at the position of the inner organs and their relation to the solar plexus, we see immediately what we are dealing with. In fright one involuntarily breathes in, as for instance in drowning, where this very inspiration leads to death. (Reich, 1942)

Reich goes on to describe how children learn to fight anxiety states by restricting their breathing and suppressing the anxious feelings. If they succeed, the resulting pattern of affect block and rigid holding leads to the muscle-bound thoracic block already described. The hysterical body pattern copes with stress by expressing some of the anxiety symptoms and learning to manipulate the environment through them. The breathing pattern is close to what Waal *et al.* (1976) described as *flutter breathing:* the movements are irregular and uneven and there is total lack of rhythm. It leads to hyperventilation and a sensation of being short of breath. When Freud asked his patient Katherina, "What is it you suffer from?" she answered, "I get so out of breath. Not always. But sometimes it catches me so that I think I shall suffocate."

Freud comments:

This did not, at first sight, sound like a nervous symptom. But soon it occurred to me that probably it was only a description that stood for an anxiety attack: she was choosing shortness of breath out of the complex of sensations arising from anxiety and laying undue stress on that single factor. (Freud, 1975)

The conversation between Freud and Katherina goes on as follows:

"Sit down here. What is it like when you get 'out of breath'?"

"It comes over me all at once. First of all it's like something pressing on my eyes. My head gets so heavy, there's a dreadful buzzing, and I feel so giddy that I almost fall over. Then there's something crushing my chest so that I can't get my breath."

"And you didn't notice anything in your throat?"

"My throat's squeezed together as though I were going to choke."

"Does anything else happen in your head?"

"Yes, there's a hammering, enough to burst it."

"And don't you feel at all frightened while this is going on?"

"I always think I'm going to die. I'm brave as a rule and go about everywhere by myself, into the cellar and all over the mountain. But on a day when that happens I don't dare to go anywhere. I think all the time someone's standing behind me and going to catch hold of me all at once." (Freud, 1975)

This gives a lot of insight into the transition between hysterical and schizoid breathing patterns. When she chokes and cannot get her breath the head pressure builds. Reich describes how:

if the attitude of anxious anticipation is maintained for some time, a pressure in the forehead appears. I have had several patients in whom it was not possible to eliminate the pressure in the forehead until I discovered their attitude of anxious anticipation in the chest musculature. (Reich, 1942)

The hysterical tendency, however, is to abreact some of the panic, to come out of the sense of choking into the flutter breathing, flirting with dying but always demonstrating a racy aliveness. The hysteric breathes with the hesitant, panicky breath of a baby that had a difficult birth struggle.

I am not suggesting that we can rigidly classify styles of breathing and allocate them mechanically to specific character patterns. People have unique experiences that lead to all gradations of coloration by differing character tendencies and bodily attitudes. Styles of breathing shade into each other and even polar extremes can exist in the same person as that person crosses the margin of stress, under fluctuating conditions of anxiety or tension. But looking on patterns of breathing in terms of uterine and birth experiences, intestinal conflicts, and muscular boxing-in, seems to me to increase the understanding of some of the dynamics we see when we work with people who struggle with the tensions and guilts and existential crises of letting out or taking in air.

7. Words of Caution for Therapists

Nearly all strong emotions, crying, anger, fear, and pleasure, involve increased breathing. So it is not surprising that if a person seeks to repress emotion, breathing reduction is a central dynamic. In Reich's work the therapist seeks to deepen breathing beyond the level of the repression. In doing so he has to be sensitive to the natural rhythms of the breath cycle and to the thresholds of anxiety in the client. Inexperienced therapists trying to provoke a patient to deeper breathing can easily induce a hyperventilation crisis and not recognize it as such. Skill is required in this work since a patient with chronically reduced breathing may easily go into hyperventilation as a response to the therapeutic situation. The crisis is avoided either by careful pacing of the rate of respiratory changes or by the patient becoming more expressive, either muscularly, emotionally, or both.

Tension of the respiratory muscles is found in the pectorals, intercostals, and other muscles of the upper chest and back. Diaphragmatic tension is extremely frequent in many neurotic states. Since the diaphragm is attached to the spine, methods of mobilizing the spine and the *psoas* muscle are used as a principle means of opening the diaphragm. These methods are not "exercises" and cannot be done mechanically. There is always an emotional context to the repression, which needs to be sensed, elicited, and resolved *before* the dysfunctional patterns of breathing can be altered.

Reich warned that changing the patterns of a person's breathing was tantamount to emotional surgery and should only be attempted by those experienced in his methods. His teachings, as mentioned above, may already have influenced the therapies practiced by many readers. Any clinician responsible for retraining the breathing patterns of patients will find a wealth of information, based on decades of experience, in the Reichian and neo-Reichian literature.

8. References

Alexander, F.M. *The use of the self.* London: Metheun, 1932.

Barlow, W. *The Alexander principle.* London: Victor Gollancz, 1973.

Boyesen, G. *Entre psyche et soma.* Paris: Payot, 1985.

Friedman, M. and Rosenmann, R.H. Overt behavior pattern in coronary disease. *Journal of the American Medical Association,* 1960, *173,* 1320–1325.

Freud, S. *Studies in hysteria.* London: Penguin Books, 1975.

Glaser, V. *Eutonie.* Heidelberg: Haug Verlag, 1980.

Lowen, A. *Physical dynamics of character structure.* New York: Grune and Stratton, 1958.

Lowen, A. *Betrayal of the body.* New York: Collier MacMillan, 1967.

Perls, F., Hefferline, R., and Goodman, P. *Gestalt therapy,* New York: Julian Press, 1951.

Reich, W. *The function of the orgasm.* New York: Orgone Institute Press, 1942.

Reich, W. The expressive language of the living. In *Character analysis.* London: Vision Press, 1949.

Waal, N., Grieg, A., and Rasmussen, M. Psychodiagnosis of the body. In D. Boadella (Ed.), *In the wake of Reich,* London: Coventure, 1976.

9. Further Reading

Boadella, D. *Lifestreams.* London: Routledge & Kegan Paul, 1987.

17

Breathing and Feeling

ASHLEY V. CONWAY

1. Introduction

Models attempting to explain the relationship between hyperventilation and acute anxiety or panic frequently involve a trigger precipitating a vicious circle, such as: *trigger → hyperventilation → symptoms → misattribution → anxiety → further hyperventilation, and so on* (e.g., see Clark *et al.*, 1985; Lum, 1976). However, it seems unlikely that either panic (Lelliott and Bass, 1990; Ley, 1990, 1992) or hyperventilation (Conway *et al.*, 1988) are unitary disorders. Pollard *et al.* (1989) found that major life events were reported by agoraphobics in greater numbers and at a higher percentage during a time period around panic onset than they were reported during either a within-subjects or a between-subjects control period; these results provided evidence of a contiguous relationship between life events and onset of panic attacks associated with agoraphobia. This paper intends to explore the significance of an initiating event for some patients and the emotional response to it, the relevance of the trigger to episodes of acute hyperventilation, and the consequent implications for therapy.

Studies using hypnosis have demonstrated that breathing can be influenced by suggestion. Sato *et al.* (1986) found that verbal suggestion can be used to decrease the response to CO_2 inhalation and that hypnotic suggestion augments this effect. Dudley *et al.* (1964) found changes in respiration associated with hypnotically suggested exercise and suggested emotion. Suess *et al.* (1980) demonstrated the occurrence of hyperventilation in response to experimentally induced psychological stress in normal subjects, with the degree of response

ASHLEY V. CONWAY • Department of Psychiatry, Charing Cross and Westminster Medical School, London W6 8RP, England.
Behavioral and Psychological Approaches to Breathing Disorders, edited by Beverly H. Timmons and Ronald Ley. Plenum Press, New York, 1994.

varying widely. Freeman *et al.* (1986a) also found some degree of hyperventilation as a normal response to stress. Stevenson and Ripley (1952) asked patients with asthma or anxiety states to think about topics relevant to individual patients. They found that there were alterations in the breathing pattern accompanying changes in emotion in all subjects: "Symptoms which arose during the interviews were always related to variations both in emotional state and in respiration" (p. 478). Bass and Gardner (1985) have reviewed the literature on emotional influences on breathing, specifying some of the pathways of the feedback control system, and report that there is general agreement that under conditions of psychological stress there are decreases in blood CO_2 levels compared with baseline conditions. They review evidence suggesting that there is a continuum of susceptibility to overbreathe in stressful situations, rather than a specific over-responsiveness of the respiratory system in certain individuals.

There seems little doubt then, that breathing changes in response to emotional arousal (see also Nixon and Freeman, 1988). It seems likely that the degree of change in respiration on this continuum will be related to the degree of emotion generated. Events of major emotional impact would be expected to produce greater change in respiration than would events of negligible emotional impact. An explanation of the influence of a discrete, identifiable, emotionally significant life event on respiration would therefore be appropriate. Bereavement provides such an example.

The model proposed below employs the illustration of emotional response to bereavement and its relationship to hyperventilation and anxiety. Although for the sake of brevity the example will be concerned primarily with sadness, the effect may also apply to other emotions and other stressful life events.

2. Life Events, Hyperventilation, and Anxiety:
An Integrative Model

There is evidence that the experience of bereavement has an adverse effect on both health (Parkes, 1987–8) and mortality. Rees and Lutkins (1967) found a sevenfold increase in risk for mortality for the first year following a bereavement, compared to a control group. Burns and Nichols (1972) compared groups of depressed patients with chest symptoms to those without. They found that recent bereavement was much more common to the chest symptom group, as was witnessing the death with gross emotional impact. Pollard *et al.* (1989) provide data that include a simple analysis across four categories of life events; they found that in their sample a majority of agoraphobics had experienced panic-related life events involving separation or interpersonal conflict. More specifically, Conway *et al.* (1988) used hypnosis to explore triggers in patients showing acute episodes of hyperventilation, and found that recall of a bereavement was a trigger to hyperventilation in one-third of their cases. Reporting detailed clinical observations, Lazarus and Kostan (1969) have stated that ". . . in no instance is the relationship between loss and illness more clear-cut than in the case of psychogenic hyperventilation."

Why do some people react to bereavement with hyperventilation and suffer its physiological and psychological consequences, while others do not? Conway (1989) has suggested that it is not just the occurrence of the event itself, but rather the *failure to express emotion* that is the important factor. These patients show characteristics of emotional suppression similar to the characteristics of a group identified by Parkes (1982) as those predisposed to avoidant or delayed responses to bereavement. Empathetic probing usually reveals a failure to grieve for the lost person. Reasons for such failure to acknowledge and/or express feelings may be many: "Men don't cry," "I didn't have time for my own feelings," "I had the children to look after," "I had to keep in control to take my exams / start my new job / prepare for the baby," etc. Parkes also pointed out that there may be a social attribution of "breakdown" to any loss of emotional control. The fear of madness associated with loss of control over emotional expression may cause some people to inhibit the expression of grief and avoid situations that evoke it. Social influences, whether from family or wider cultural pressures, may play an important role in the perceived acceptability of emotional expression. A failure to express emotion has been found to be associated with increased reports of physical symptoms in general (Malatesta *et al.*, 1987), and, in asthmatic children, with adverse effects on ventilation in particular (Florin *et al.*, 1985; Hollaender and Florin, 1983).

A traumatic event such as a bereavement may stimulate emotional arousal and consequent hyperventilation. In a healthy response, the emotion is expressed, the breathing slows again, equilibrium is restored. If, however, there is emotional suppression rather than expression, the proposition here is that the hyperventilation, or at least the tendency to hyperventilate, is maintained. Acute episodes of hyperventilation may be triggered by any reminder of the loss *whether or not this is consciously processed* (see below). Whatever the reason for the suppression, it is likely to be accompanied by denial of the emotion (Lazarus and Kostan, 1969). Symptoms will inevitably be misattributed as a result of suppression and denial, anxiety will increase, stimulating further hyperventilation, and so on (see Fig. 1).

Pennebaker and Susman (1988) propose a general theory of inhibition and psychosomatics:

> . . . if individuals are unable to disclose the traumas. . . . they must constantly hold
> back or inhibit their thoughts, feelings, and behaviours from others and, on occasion,
> themselves. Not discussing traumatic events with others, then, represents a significant
> long-term physical stressor. (p. 327)

MAJOR EMOTIONAL LOSS

↓

Emotional Arousal

+

Hyperventilation

(a) ————————————————————————— (b)

Emotional Expression   Emotional Suppression

                                                                              +

                                                                           Denial

↓   ↓

Psychophysiological   Continued Psycho-
equilibrium   physiological
and well-being   instability

                                                                              ↓

                                                                   Vulnerability to
                                                                        "trigger"

                                                                              ↓

                                                      ┌→ Hyperventilation ┐

                                                anxiety   symptoms

                                                      └─ misattribution ←┘

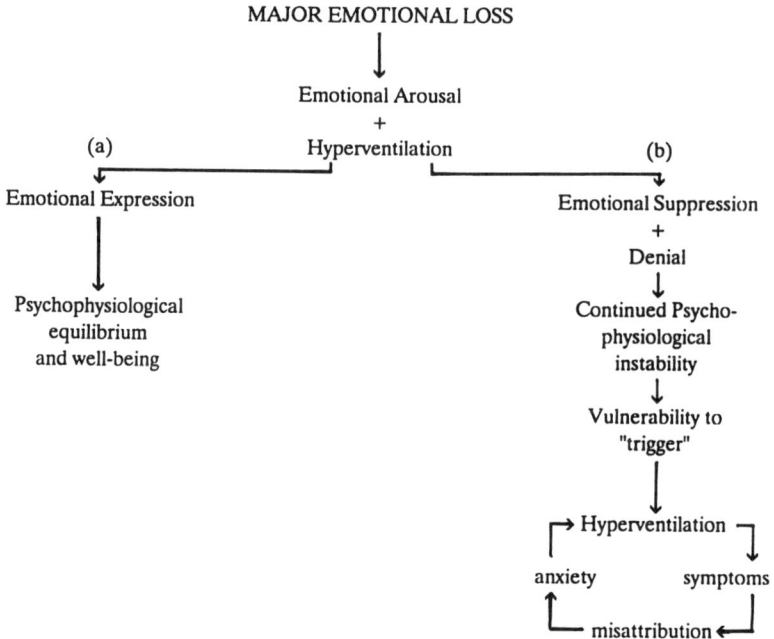

Figure 1. Two possible outcomes of major emotional loss: pathway (a) restores health through emotional expression, whereas (b), involving suppression of emotion, results in a cycle of hyperventilation and anxiety.

    The proposal here is that hyperventilation is an example of such a physical stressor—a direct consequence of prolonged emotional suppression. Examining the effects of bereavement on surviving spouses, Pennebaker and Susman (1988) report that subjects who talked more about their spouses' deaths had fewer health problems in the following year. They found that confiding about traumatic events may be immediately anxiety-provoking or depressing, but has positive physical and psychological effects in the long run; the investigators suggest that, on the other hand, inhibition can be viewed as a source of stress that, over time, is cumulative and increases the probability of disease.

    The patient may become acutely vulnerable to stimuli that evoke the suppressed emotion. Burns and Nichols (1972) report of patients who ". . . would continue to hyperventilate when they were reminded of the loss" (p. 408). Braeshear (1983) proposes a mechanism: the hyperventilation first occurs in the context of a real or threatened loss and this initial event establishes a set of various internal sensations (feelings, images, sounds, etc.) associated with the hyperventilation. Subsequently, the patient may deny, repress, rationalize, or cover up the actual event. However, since the hyperventilation is anchored to a particular set of internal sensations, any time the internal sensations are accessed, for whatever reason, the hyperventilation is also accessed.

Mathews and MacLeod (1986) compared anxious subjects to nonanxious controls in a dichotic listening situation, where threat or nonthreat words were presented in the unattended channel. Anxious, but not control, subjects experienced interference in a simultaneous reaction-time task, when the unattended words were threatening in content, although neither group could report or recognize the words to which they had been exposed. The proposal here is that a threat cue (trigger) will be any stimulus that threatens access to the suppressed emotion, and that this cue may be processed outside of conscious awareness. The physiological response of hyperventilation, however, remains undiminished.

If the emotion is being suppressed, then there is likely to be conscious denial of its relevance or importance. Therefore the patient's own interpretation of the reasons for symptoms *must* be incorrect. The patient's interpretation cannot be "I'm feeling bad because I'm upset," but is more likely to be "I am having a lot of strange feelings, there must be something wrong with me, I am ill or going mad." Conway *et al.* (1988) found that the use of hypnosis helped to identify triggers to acute episodes of hyperventilation, and patients frequently reported being previously unaware of the nature of such stimuli. This ignorance of the trigger is not a chance event, nor is the patient being deliberately misleading. The ignorance of the trigger is what makes the acute hyperventilation appear to arise spontaneously. The emotion is accessed outside of conscious awareness but the physiological response is still triggered.

Two other factors may each be playing a role in maintaining the process of emotional suppression, hyperventilation, and anxiety:

1. Anxiety may be worsened if there is a similarity of symptoms to those suffered by the deceased, particularly where there is a familial relationship. A patient's belief in genetic transmission of vulnerability may escalate and perpetuate the vicious cycle of anxiety and symptoms. Palpitations, breathlessness, or dizziness actually produced by the hyperventilation may be interpreted catastrophically by the patient as heart disease, respiratory failure, or a serious neurological problem comparable to that which brought about the bereavement.
2. Pain is known to stimulate hyperventilation, which seems to produce some analgesic effect (Clutton-Brock, 1957; Glynn *et al.,* 1981). Whatever the physiological explanation for this phenomenon, the same process may also apply to emotional suffering where hyperventilation might prove beneficial by helping to numb emotional "pain." Thus, the physiological consequence of the process of inhibition might then become an adaptive response.

3. Implications for Therapy

Therapy necessarily begins with a sensitive history taking. Open-ended questioning about the client's symptoms ("When did things seem to start going wrong?" rather than, "When did you first experience the parasthesia?") will often elicit spontaneous replies such as, "Ever since Mum died. . . ." Often this kind of remark will be qualified by, "*I don't know why,* but ever since Mum died. . . ." Finding ways to deal with bottled up thoughts and feelings is often very helpful. Pennebaker and Susman (1988) report that ". . . talking or writing about traumas can promote adaptive psychological responses to these memories by facilitating habituation or extinction." It is interesting to note that the irregular, jerky thoracic breathing patterns seen when suppressing the expression of sadness is very similar to the breathing pattern of someone who is actually crying.

The initial target of therapy will often be to enable the patient to express grief and cry. Later, or at subsequent meetings, connections can be made between the recall of the bereavement and its effect on breathing and consequent symptom production. This is particularly powerful if the session evoking sadness has included ongoing capnographic monitoring, so that the patient can be shown on a printout how the emotion affects breathing and CO_2 levels. If the emotional pain is expressed/released/relieved, there will no longer be any hyperventilation as a physical consequence of the "work" of maintaining the suppression. Additionally, if there had been a secondary gain of hyperventilation as an analgesic to the emotional pain, then when the pain is gone, the hyperventilation would no longer be psychophysiologically adaptive, and could therefore be relinquished.

Anxiety about losing control in one way or another may also be a factor that is helped by this process. If emotional expression has been associated with loss of control, and/or threat to sanity, then any trigger that evokes feelings therefore becomes threatening. The ability to experience the feeling, express it, and then come away from it and talk about feelings, increases the sense of control and defuses the escalation, relieving the anxiety and its attendant hyperventilation. The patient's understanding of the link between emotion and breathing helps to end the deadlock of, "Is it something wrong with my body or is it all in my mind?" Misattributions of symptoms can then be corrected. Allowing and encouraging the patient to cry has been reported to stabilize and slow the rate of respiration; clinical observation suggests that this effect is evident within minutes after crying has stopped, and over a longer term, too (Conway, 1989). Breathing retraining may be easier after feeling has been acknowledged and expressed.

This kind of intervention clearly makes demands on the therapist, particularly on his or her own capacity to tolerate the patient's expression of emotion. It is also important that individual differences between patients be acknowledged. Dudley *et al.* (1964) report that hyperventilation occurred only on suggestion of a stimulus that was meaningful to the subject. Mathews and MacLeod (1985) report that disruption of cognitive performance is greatest when threat cues are of greatest concern *to that individual*. As well as being sensitive to the needs of the individual, the therapist should have other qualities. Lazarus and Kostan (1969) say that the physician must be patient, tolerant and understanding, and Pennebaker and Susman (1988) recommend that ". . . the positive effects of disclosure are most likely to accrue if the target is viewed as both accepting and trustworthy."

The types of therapy currently fashionable are cognitive, behavioral, pharmacological, and physiological (such as breathing retraining), all of which may have their benefits. However, treating a life event and its consequence of emotional arousal as if they were an illness or a simple problem of behavior or cognitive function may be making an important omission. Breathing retraining alone, without concomitant psychological counseling, may be ineffective in some hyperventilation patients (Freeman *et al.*, 1986b). The preconscious processing of emotionally significant cues may be an important determinant of the unexplained variability in frequency of "spontaneous" panic. Therapy might be appropriately directed to the cause of the problem as well as the symptoms arising as a result of it. Mathews and MacLeod's data (1986) suggest that anxiety can arise from threat cues of which patients may remain unaware. This presents a difficulty for the theory and practice of both cognitive and behaviour therapy. If anxious patients in therapy are unable to report on cues of emotional significance that occurred prior to periods of acute anxiety or panic, this should not necessarily be taken as evidence that no such cues existed.

Therapy attending to feelings is not being presented here as an alternative to breathing retraining, cognitive, or behavioral techniques. However, in the same patient there may be a number of different levels at which it is appropriate to intervene.

What happens if an emotional aspect of the process is ignored? What are the consequences of colluding with a bereaved patient and giving the implicit message that feelings should be suppressed or ignored, or are not important? What would be the consequences of patients having their symptoms or cognitive attributions treated as if they were the problem itself? Even if a therapeutic intervention ignoring feeling is successful in reducing the incidence or reported severity of panic, what would be the consequences overall? If the model of psychosomatics proposed by Pennebaker and Susman (see Section 2) is correct, then the suppression of emotion is maintained, and there is a danger that there would be breakdown of another psychological or physiological system, whereas therapy encouraging disclosure of emotionally significant material would be expected to promote health in the long run.

A relevant example is the experience of Charles Darwin. With regard to his reaction to the death of his father, he wrote, "All this winter I have been bad enough and my nervous system began to be affected, so that my hands trembled, and my head was often swimming" (see Hubble, 1943). There are good reasons to believe that many of Darwin's symptoms were a result of hyperventilation (Bowlby, 1990). There have been criticisms that psychological factors do not explain Darwin's repeated illnesses when his life was apparently going smoothly, while he stayed healthy during the profound crisis of the death of his ten-year-old daughter Annie (Cowley, 1991). Colp (1991) replies that following the death of his mother in 1817, when he was eight years old, Darwin was taught by his sisters not to verbalize his feelings of grief and anxiety; for the most part, he expressed his disturbed feelings in physical symptoms. Colp goes on to state that when Annie died in 1851, Darwin openly and intensely wept for her.

> This marked the first occasion when he openly mourned for another person. When his father had died, three years previously, he had not done so, and had expressed his grief in an exacerbation of symptoms of physical illness. And because he was able to express his feelings for Annie by weeping, he did not suffer an exacerbation of his physical symptoms when she died. (Colp, 1991)

Emotional response to a major life event is hard to measure and assess, and even more so if it is not acknowledged by the subject. However, for reasons both scientific and ethical it is no longer appropriate for researchers or clinicians to ignore the significance of emotional responses to distressing life events, and of patients' consequent vulnerability to psychological triggers. Further research is needed to address these issues.

4. References

Bass, C., and Gardner, W. Emotional influences on breathing and breathlessness. *Journal of Psychosomatic Research*, 1985, *29*, 599–609.

Bowlby, J. *Charles Darwin: A New Biography.* London: Hutchinson, 1990.

Braeshear, R. Hyperventilation syndrome. *Lung*, 1983, *161*, 257–273.

Burns, B.H., and Nichols, M.A. Factors related to the localisation of symptoms to the chest in depression. *British Journal of Psychiatry*, 1972, *121*, 405–409.

Clark, D.M., Salkovskis, P.M., and Chalkley, A.J. Respiratory control as a treatment for panic attacks. *Journal of Behaviour Therapy and Experimental Psychiatry*, 1985, *16*, 23–30.

Clutton-Brock, J. The cerebral effects of overventilation. *British Journal of Anaesthesia*, 1957, *29*, 111–113.

Colp, R. Darwin's anxieties. Letter to *New York Times*, August 4, 1991.

Conway, A.V. Blood, breath and tears. Poster presentation at the *9th Annual Symposium on Respiratory Psychophysiology.* London, England, 1989.

Conway, A.V., Freeman, L.J., and Nixon, P.G.F. Hypnotic examination of trigger factors in the hyperventilation syndrome. *American Journal of Clinical Hypnosis*, 1988, *30*, 296–304.

Cowley, D.S. Review of *Charles Darwin-A New Biography, New York Times*, July 14, 1991.

Dudley, D.L., Holmes, T.H., Martin, C.J., and Ripley, H.S. Changes in respiration associated with hypnotically induced emotion, pain and exercise. *Psychosomatic Medicine*, 1964, *26*, 46–57.

Florin, I., Freudenberg, G., and Hollaender, J. Facial expressions of emotion and physiologic reactions in children with bronchial asthma. *Psychosomatic Medicine*, 1985, *47*, 382–393.

Freeman, L.J., Conway, A.V., and Nixon, P.G.F. Physiological responses to psychological challenge under hypnosis in patients considered to have the hyperventilation syndrome: Implications for diagnosis and therapy. *Journal of the Royal Society of Medicine*, 1986a, *79*, 76–83.

Freeman, L.J., Conway, A.V., and Nixon, P.G.F. Heart rate response, emotional disturbance and hyperventilation. *Journal of Psychosomatic Research*, 1986b, *30*, 429–436.

Glynn, C.J., Lloyd, J.W., and Folkhard, S. Ventilatory response to intractable pain. *Pain*, 1981, *11*, 201–211.

Hollaender, J., and Florin, I. Expressed emotion and airway conductance in children with bronchial asthma. *Journal of Psychosomatic Research*, 1983, *27*, 307–311.

Hubble, D. Charles Darwin and psychotherapy. *The Lancet*, 1943, *244*, 129–133.

Lazarus, H.R., and Kostan, J.J. Psychogenic hyperventilation and death anxiety. *Psychosomatics*, 1969, *10*, 14–22.

Lelliott, P., & Bass, C. Symptom specificity in patients with panic. *British Journal of Psychiatry*, 1990, *157*, 593–597.

Ley, R. The anatomy of a hyperventilatory panic attack. Paper presented at the *13th Annual Meeting of the Society for Psychophysiological Research*. Boston, Massachusetts, 1990.

Ley, R. The many faces of Pan: Psychological and physiological differences among three types of panic attacks. *Behaviour Research and Therapy*, 1992, *30*, 347–357.

Lum, L.C. The syndrome of habitual chronic hyperventilation. In O.W. Hill (Ed.), *Modern trends in psychosomatic medicine*. London: Butterworth, 1976.

Malatesta, C.Z., Jonas, R., and Izard, C.E. The relation between low facial expressivity during emotional arousal and somatic symptoms. *British Journal of Medical Psychology*, 1987, *60*, 169–180.

Mathews, A., and MacLeod, C. Selective processing of threat cues in anxiety states. *Behaviour Research and Therapy*, 1985, *23*, 563–569.

Mathews, A., and MacLeod, C. Discrimination of threat cues without awareness in anxiety states. *Journal of Abnormal Psychology*, 1986, *95*, 131–138.

Nixon, P.G.F., and Freeman, L.J. The 'Think test': A further technique to elicit hyperventilation. *Journal of the Royal Society of Medicine*, 1988, *81*, 277–279.

Parkes, C.M. Attachment and the prevention of mental disorders. In C.M. Parkes, and Stevenson-Hinde (Eds.), *The place of attachment in human behaviour*, New York: Basic Books, 1982.

Parkes, C.M. Research: Bereavement. *Omega*, 1987-8, *18*, 365–377.

Pennebaker, J.W., and Susman, J.R. Disclosure of traumas and psychosomatic processes. *Social Science in Medicine*, 1988, *26*, 327–332.

Pollard, C.A., Pollard, H.J., and Corn, K.J. Panic onset and major events in the lives of agoraphobics: A test of contiguity. *Journal of Abnormal Psychology*, 1989, *98*, 318–321.

Rees, D., and Lutkins, S.G. Mortality of bereavement. *British Medical Journal*, 1967, *4*, 13–16.

Sato, P., Sargur, M., and Schoene, R.B. Hypnosis effect on carbon dioxide chemosensitivity. *Chest*, 1986, *89*, 828–831.

Stevenson, I., and Ripley, H.S. Variations in respiration and in respiratory symptoms during changes in emotion. *Psychosomatic Medicine*, 1952, *14*, 476–490.

Suess, W.M., Alexander, A.B., Smith, D.D., Sweeney, H.W., and Marion, R.J. The effects of psychological stress on respiration: A preliminary study of anxiety and hyperventilation. *Psychophysiology*, 1980, *17*, 535–540.

18

Breathing Therapy

MAGDA PROSKAUER

My present approach to human growth is the outcome of early childhood experiences. When I was young, I loved to skate. Once the river in my home town was solidly frozen, I spent every free minute on the ice. As my body glided effortlessly, it seemed I was carving handwriting on the mirrorlike surface. After I had practiced ardently for hours, all restraint fell away, and the smooth shift of balance brought with it a sense of weightlessness. The joy of life that flowed through me in those days has never been forgotten. Thinking of it years later evoked the question: what is it that releases life?

In those early experiences was a first realization of discipline leading to spontaneity, of effort leading to effortlessness. In those frosty hours, tireless concentration led to the kind of delicate balance that is a prerequisite for figure skating. Once the willpower had been summoned to provide the skill, the same willpower could be shed; nature took over once more, so that the genuine movement came through, bringing the sort of release I was looking for unconsciously. The spontaneous motion brought with it the "e-motion" of joy, of being fully alive.

It is a long way from one's own experience to teaching a new sense of awareness to others. The way led me to a degree in physiotherapy from Munich University, through hospital work in Germany, Yugoslavia, New York Medical Center, and private practice. In these years I had ample opportunity to explore traditional ways of treatment with the application of breathing therapy to asthma, polio, cerebral palsy, and related diseases. Often we witnessed strange and

---

This chapter is reproduced with permission from Otto H., and Mann, J. (Eds.), *Ways of growth*. New York: Grossman, 1968.

MAGDA PROSKAUER (1910–1990) • Formerly in Private Practice, San Francisco, California.
Behavioral and Psychological Approaches to Breathing Disorders, edited by Beverly H. Timmons and Ronald Ley. Plenum Press, New York, 1994.

unpredictable results from the breathing exercises that were prescribed for our patients. With one patient the cure seemed miraculous and lasting; with another, a quick recovery would reverse itself all too soon into the former misery. One patient would flatly refuse to collaborate, while another one would form an attachment to his therapist that developed into an unhealthy dependence or into a hopeless power struggle. We encountered these irrational responses only during breathing therapy and not in other kinds of treatment, because breathing reaches the unconscious.

Gradually it became clear that cure of symptoms could no longer be expected by predetermined means—fixed sets of exercises and arbitrary manipulations. The whole of the personality had to be taken into account. The question of the *meaning* of the disturbance entered the picture. What unfulfilled needs or underlying conflicts were being expressed by the symptom? The unfolding of the new therapeutic methods came as the development of psychoanalysis shed new light on the psychosomatic character of many disturbances. Orthodox therapy was confronted with challenging questions, and new schools of thought arose. Practical work with some of these schools shaped my techniques to a considerable degree. The strongest influence was the analytical psychology of C.G. Jung.

Experiments had to be created by which the patient became conscious of hindering influences, so that awareness of these obstacles could introduce the desired change. The same principle had to be applied as in psychotherapy, where patient and doctor work together in a common search for the unknown need of the patient. All expectations and former attitudes had to be set aside; each patient had to be met as a new challenge. *Only when subliminal feelings and sense perceptions were allowed to come to the surface could there be a change.*

To achieve this, new methods slowly evolved. Certain breathing techniques were combined with subtle motions to cultivate perception. The breathing function proved valuable because of its intimate connection with the emotions as well as with the two nervous systems: the voluntary, consciously directed one, and the autonomous or vegetative one, which works without the mind. Normally, we breathe automatically, but we can also take a breath or hold it for a time. In this respect, respiration is different from other autonomous functions, such as digestion. The stomach and intestines cannot be contracted at will. *The breath thus forms a bridge between the conscious and the unconscious systems.* By watching it, one can observe an unconscious function at work, learn to exclude interferences, and help self-regulating processes set it. One may be able to yawn before becoming overtired, to sigh before feeling overly restricted.

Because of its close relationship to the circulation, breath equals life. At the moment of birth, the first breath is the signal for amazing change to take place. The blood, until then supplied from the maternal source, becomes within seconds the independent, nourishing agent. With the environmental change, inhalation and exhalation begin to compress and dilate inner spaces as blood and lymph rush in and out of ever-changing vessels. The rhythmic filling and emptying acts like a compression wave, regulating the blood pressure and massaging the inner organs with gentle vibrations. At times of heightened sensitivity, some of these sensations can be experienced.

One wonders if this intricate process of birth might not better be named rebirth, since life exists already in the womb. Could it not be compared to the metamorphosis of certain animals and be a first transformation into a different kind of existence? From here on growth means constant change, continuing through a lifetime. It always implies abdication of nourishment by means of past methods in favor of the opening up of new resources. Being ready for the impending changes, like the infant's preparedness for meeting the atmosphere, leads in the direction of life. Resisting or evading the new situation leads to stagnation. Sensitivity and alertness are therefore valuable tools for dealing with the ever-changing demands of life.

Just as we behave, move, act, according to our specific makeup and express ourselves uniquely through gestures *so does our breathing pattern express our inner situation,* varying in accordance with inner and outer circumstances. The usual arrhythmic respiration goes with our normal diffusion of attention, and changes with emotional states: agitated in anger, stopped momentarily in fear, gasping with amazement, choking with sadness, sighing with relief, etc.

With neurotics, we frequently find the so-called reversed breathing pattern, which reduces the breath to a minimum. The abdomen is pulled in; no breath can enter, since there is no exhalation. The bottle is filled with consumed air.

Normally, when at rest one breathes more with the diaphragm, like the abdominal breathing of the infant. Complete chest breathing, where the ribs expand and lift, occurs only at times of maximum effort. It usually starts the moment we pull ourselves together for action, or if we focus our attention toward outer events. To put it in oversimplified terms: abdominal breathing goes with sleep, rest, inertia, letting things happen. Where it is disturbed, the inner life is disturbed: one is driven, unreceptive, and lives too intentionally.

On the other hand, those who cannot open their chest cage are often anxious, inhibited, self-conscious, and tend toward feelings of inferiority. In between, there are endless variations and combinations, slightly different in rhythm in each individual. Where the pattern is reversed, the chest is lifted abnormally high, which means that only the auxiliary breathing muscles are used, those we need for maximum adaptation, as in the effort of mountain climbing. The diaphragm is excluded and becomes flabby, so the circulation is disturbed and the inner organs suffer. By relearning the use of the diaphragm, the warmth of returning circulation can be sensed in different ares of the body when one concentrates on them.

Instead of correcting faulty habits one takes as the point of departure the individual breathing pattern, disturbed as it may be. One concentrates on the act of breathing, observing its inner movement until the breath, left to itself, can find the way back to its own rhythm. This kind of playful attitude counteracts purposive, directed movement, so that one learns to experiment with one's nature, and harmoniously trains the body for its own purpose. This is very different from training for any kind of performance or outward goal such as sports or other competitive exercises.

The technique lends itself to self-exploration by concentrating in an introverted attitude upon oneself. The mind is set aside, so that quiet contemplation can allow for awareness of one's inner state. One may, for instance, suffer from too spastic or too atonic (flabby) conditions in his system, or from both. Since these are often below the level of consciousness, we tend to feel these disorders only when they have already done some damage. Experiments are therefore set up by which we learn to feel and sense ourselves before a symptom is forced upon us. Gradually we recognize that every physical rigidity is simultaneously a psychic one, *that relaxation is not collapse, but the appropriate degree of contraction, the life-giving tension called tonus.* Through subtle movements, we discover for ourselves that in the simplest motion there are always two opposite muscle groups involved, which balance each other in their opposition. If an arm is stretched, one group contracts, the other extends and holds; both work, so there is a "yes" and a "no" in each action. Instead of making arbitrary corrections, we look together ingeniously for the simplest, most natural ways of making small movements.

Many intelligent people have developed in a one-sided manner, to the extent that they live without using their senses. Some do not taste the food they eat or see what is before their eyes. Some are unaware of the state of their own body.

Everyone knows that he can sharpen his perception, simply by having observed that he may not hear the ticking of a clock in a room or the singing of a bird under the window unless he concentrates on the sound. The sound is there all the time, but one becomes conscious of it only if he focuses his attention on it. Otherwise, the sound does not really exist; it is unconscious. The same is true of our physical sensations, pulse or heartbeat for example; normally they are not felt.

The sensory cortex of the brain is the storeroom of past impressions, which may rise to consciousness as images but which more often remain unconscious. A present sense perception may get linked to the store of earlier perceptions and evoke a response that belongs to the past. Memory can be held in the body and awakened by certain disciplines. A muscular contraction once caused by the emotion of fear or joy may exist long after the accompanying experience has subsided. With the physical release of that specific tension, the psychic experience may return, to become a steppingstone for further development. How far the message can be used in the direction of growth depends on the individual's psychological capacity. Here we enter the realm of psychotherapy.

All physical changes in this work occur spontaneously and may or may not lead to insights. The experience of a young musician illustrates that such recollections need not be highly charged events: This man recently returned to his vocation after having had to abandon it for a while because of external pressures. During his sessions, he visualized lovely sketches from his past life; these he looked at in a meditative mood, and felt greatly enriched by them.

It all depends on the attitude of consciousness how the unconscious reacts. If one is in tune with the unconscious, as it seems that this young man was at the time, the psyche reacts in a favorable manner and compensates the outer life in a pleasant, rather than a menacing, way. The process often comes close to the work of psychotherapy, where this kind of listening is encouraged, leading to the needed associations and images from which healing occurs. While psychotherapy starts on an intellectual level by using words, *the approach through the physical sensations is predominantly nonverbal.*

Practical work with artists has taught me over the years that the need can be of another kind. Creativity is easily buried under ambition and the strain of being trained for a specific skill. Certain schools of dance and drama, in striving for top performance, are often unable to consider individual inclinations. The very different discipline of concentrating on one's genuine responses helpfully balances this shortcoming and may prepare for more genuine modes of expression.

It becomes evident that body and psyche act as a unit, so awareness can come by approaching one or the other. This is so because body and psyche are two aspects of the same reality, two poles of life, two manifestations of the whole of the personality that are in steady interaction. To bridge the gap between these two extremes, we may start from the point of view that *our physical behavior corresponds to a psychic pattern, according to the law of synchronicity, not of causality.* With this in mind we need no longer explain a symptom reductively, but can try to grasp what it wants to convey and can thus discard any kind of criticism or attempt at arbitrary correction.

A sunken chest cage, when expanded, brings a natural sense of self-assertion; legs tightly held together in the manner of a Prussian soldier speak their own language. No explanations are needed once a person becomes aware of such habits. *The distortion will correct itself when it has been experienced, since consciousness has been brought to it.* The different techniques applied in this work permit the mind to be a quiet observer while feelings and sensations are questioned and imagination is used.

In attempting to describe a method designed to lead one toward genuine experience, much is omitted, since the living experience defies precise formulation. Therefore, it may be helpful to indicate a few of the subtle, simple directions that are given in our sessions.

For example, one experiments with the weight of one's body (or its parts) by trying to give it over to gravity. This leads to the experiencing of one's heaviness, and releases tensions.

One is asked to bend one's knees, to find the place where they are in balance, so that they have to be neither held in support of each other nor manipulated in any other way.

One learns to visualize an inner body space, while simultaneously concentrating on one's exhalation, as if the breath were sent into that particular space. This may change the blood pressure and lead to a sense of lightness.

One examines the distances between certain joints, or the relationship between one's limbs, which touches on the body image.

Experiments are introduced that involve contact with another person, by hand or by sitting back to back. By way of sensing the other person one learns to get in touch with one's own sensations.

One is asked to concentrate on scanning* a certain area of one's body and to combine this with one's inhalation. Gradually the two tasks will connect, as if one were breathing with that particular area, or being breathed by it.

The ways people describe their feelings are of endless variety, since no two experiences are ever quite the same. Often the pleasurable sensation evolves, that the breath carries one upright so that no effort is needed for sitting or standing in good posture.

In the use of motion and breathing as therapeutic agents, one can roughly distinguish two basic tendencies. One is the rigid, tensely controlled attitude, "running on rails," incapable of spontaneous reactions, and therefore out of touch with the deeper layers of the personality. This picture reflects a life lived as a product of one's environment and upbringing, performed according to what is expected by tradition and convention.

Such an attitude was apparent in a young dancer who came with the intention of learning my methods in order to use them in her field of teaching. She suffered from severe anxiety attacks from which long years of psychiatric care had brought no relief. She was an overly intellectual woman who relied exclusively on her reasoning capacity. When I asked her to exhale gently, then wait and observe how the next breath came in, she became extremely anxious. She realized through this experience that she could not trust anything to happen on its own accord, not even respiration. Only what she controlled could occur. After an initial sense of confusion, this insight brought her great relief. It led her to the roots of her fears, which she felt went back to her childhood, in which no father was present to counteract an overburdened, domineering mother who knew no natural tenderness. She saw how far she had parted from Mother Nature and was glad to find this new channel through which she hoped to regain the lost contact with herself.

The opposite tendency is shown by the flabby, overflexible, unstructured dreamer with too little life-giving tension in his system, the person who is too

---

*Scanning is defined as focusing one's energy on a particular part of the body—chosen at will. One mentally breaks up this area into small units or points and directs one's concentration progressively toward each successive point. This allows for a fresh sensory perception of the chosen area.

close to unconsciousness and easily collapses into it. With this type, one may expect quietude without repose, phlegmatic disinterest, apathy, inertia, and depression. Whereas the rigid type has deviated too far from his nature, this type has not yet evolved. His ego got stuck somewhere between the womb, nursery school, and adolescence; the world is taken either as the benign parent who is supposed to provide for its child, or as the evil one against whom one must rebel at any cost.

One finds many less extreme combinations of both tendencies in most people, probably because the growth process itself contains the two alternating phases. Parting from the natural, unconscious state so that a differentiated ego can emerge, and periodically returning to it, constitute the cycle of human development.

The one-sidedness, with its loss of balance, which is so typical of modern man's development, may arise from two opposite tendencies: On the one hand, it can come about by overconsolidation of the ego, which blocks the reception of impulses and messages. On the other hand, it can come about by a state of unconsciousness that threatens concentration and the continuity of the ego by unchecked emotionality, daydreaming, or instinctive drives. In nature itself, the balance is not firmly established. A sexually excited animal may endanger itself, forgetting security and hunger while following a single drive.

The acting out of every impulse is often mistakenly taken for freedom. In practical work, it is important to know the difference between acting out and befriending the suppressed instincts. It is only after having made our first adaptations that, in order to become individuals, we find it necessary to rediscover what has been left behind. By definition, *individual* means indivisible, a separate unit, a whole; not split; in psychological terms, comprising both the conscious and the unconscious elements of the personality.

Education toward the goal of individuality must cope with the difficulty of trying to prepare people for life's tasks *with the least interference with their inherent nature, so that the desire for further growth can remain the motivating force throughout life*. Repeatedly, in the different stages of life, patterns that once provided security have to be renounced so that new potentials can take their place. Since this cannot be brought about arbitrarily, it requires that time and again we return to our roots. In the past, religions took care of this need by enacting the periodic return and reemergence in the mystery rites of death and rebirth. Today there is confusion about this process.

We have to learn again that to contact one's depths is not to sink back into trancelike oblivion, but rather to submit to the difficult discipline of quiet attentiveness. This is a forgotten product of our culture that requires conscious effort. Culture means to tend to. Much as a gardener tends to the soil in order that his plants may grow in their own way and season, so attending to the depths of our own nature tills the soil in which, firmly rooted, we can develop into healthy individuals. The somatic approach of breathing therapy is aimed at providing the climate for this kind of growth.

19

Breathing-Related Issues in Therapy

BEVERLY H. TIMMONS

Therapy for breathing-related disorders is still a developing field; professional opinions on treatment strategies are divided, and there is even a lack of consensus among experts on diagnostic procedure for some of these disorders. Consequently much of this chapter, reflecting the state of an emergent field, reviews in detail the competing approaches, problem areas, and topics that are still being argued over and that need further research.

Breathing is first discussed in this chapter in the context of several issues of central importance to all therapists, including emotional and learning factors and ethical concerns. Other subjects that may not be so familiar are then introduced, in particular, the validity of breathing retraining (which is discussed at some length) and suggestions for the use of respiratory measurements in office practice.

1. Stress and Breathing

Some years ago a stress management therapist was perplexed to observe that almost all of his clients were "breathing at collarbone level." In Chapter 1 of this volume, Naifeh proposes an interesting hypothesis to explain this phenomenon; she describes a shift from the relative dominance of abdominal to thoracic breathing as one component of the physical response to stress. Naifeh's explanation of this shift is that under conditions of threat, the contraction of abdominal muscles for protection of organs in that part of the body serves as a survival mechanism.

BEVERLY H. TIMMONS • Department of Respiratory Medicine and Allergy, St. Bartholomew's Hospital, London EC1A 7BE, England.
Behavioral and Psychological Approaches to Breathing Disorders, edited by Beverly H. Timmons and Ronald Ley. Plenum Press, New York, 1994.

With the abdomen thus "splinted," however, the diaphragm cannot descend with inhalation and breathing is therefore restricted to the upper thoracic, rib cage area (K.H. Naifeh, 1991, personal communication). This response can be observed in infants and children (and in dogs and cats) whose rib cage movements become more prominent than abdominal movements when they are excited or upset. Some therapists now teach their clients that "chest breathing *is* stress breathing" (MacGregor, 1990).

In a recent book on stress management addressed to clients, Patel (1989, 1991) explains that both chest breathing and sensations of heightened arousal are part of the fight-or-flight response. If this mode of breathing occurs at rest, it can trigger unpleasant feelings of tension and anxiety. Lum (1975) has described the hyperventilator's typical pattern as the "breathing of stress or emotion." Lum reinforces his explanations of the fight-or-flight response to patients with a demonstration. He first brings on hyperventilation symptoms by having patients overbreathe at rest. He then asks them to walk up and down stairs to demonstrate that the symptoms of hyperventilation can be dissipated as a result of increased exertion, as in fight-or-flight (L.C. Lum, 1991, personal communication). Additional evidence regarding the relationship of breathing parameters to physiological arousal and stress may be found in laboratory studies (e.g., Suess *et al.,* 1980), which are reviewed by Ley in Chapter 5 of this volume.

There are other suggested links between stressful life situations and hyperventilation. Bereavement is one of the most severe stresses most individuals will ever experience. Conway discusses the role of hyperventilation in the expression of grief in Chapter 17 of this volume. While there are no studies of the prevalence of hyperventilation in bereaved persons, their complaints are often similar to the symptoms of hyperventilation, and those who work with bereaved clients have noted that many of them are overbreathing.

Combat has had a prominent role in the clinical history of hyperventilation. What Lum (1987) has called a "prototype" of hyperventilation syndromes was identified by Da Costa during the American Civil War, and was later studied by senior cardiologists to the British Army in World War I (Lewis, 1918) and in World War II (Wood, 1941) as well as by Sargent (1940). Lowry (1967), an American Airforce psychiatrist, has published studies of military recruits in a book entitled *Hyperventilation and Hysteria.*

The systematic use of torture by an increasing number of contemporary political regimes is another source of stress for people in many countries. Hough (1992) has described her therapy for torture survivors in whom hyperventilation is often observed.

Traditionally a mechanism for anesthesia or dissociation from pain during ritual ceremonies (Lum, 1981), hyperventilation can also serve similar purposes during torture. If overbreathing is continued after torture has ceased, however, survivors may experience the classic symptoms of hyperventilation interacting with the anxiety induced by their past experience.

Could hyperventilation be involved in the now well-documented effects of grief (or other emotions) on the immune system? Mooney *et al.* (1986) addressed this question by asking chronic hyperventilators and normal subjects to overbreathe for 3 min, following the Bonn *et al.* (1984) protocol (see Section 7.4.3). Patients showed a greater decrease in the ratio of T-helper to T-suppressor cells than did the subjects in the control group. Since a decrease in this ratio of lymphocyte subpopulations is indicative of immunological incompetence, the findings suggest that chronic overbreathing could compromise the immune system. While this was apparently the first study to look at the effects of a brief period of overbreathing on suppressor cells, hematological changes as a result of prolonged hyperventilation have been described in a series of papers by Stauebli and colleagues (1988).

2. Emotion and Breathing

In her early experiences as a physical therapist utilizing traditional methods, Proskauer describes how she encountered irrational responses and behavior as well as transference phenomena only when working with the breathing of patients and not in the course of other forms of physical therapy (see Chapter 18). Some readers may reject as fanciful her explanation that "breathing reaches the unconscious," but other physical therapists have confirmed her observation that breathing exercises can result in unpredictable emotional responses. Few practitioners other than Reich and the therapists influenced by him have explored the clinical implications of this phenomenon (Christiansen, 1972). The reverse of this effect, namely, the influence of emotional influences on breathing, has often been studied (see the review by Bass and Gardner, 1985). Clausen (1951) and Grossman (1983) have provided references to early clinical and laboratory studies of the relationship between breathing and affective states. One of the most dramatic of these studies was carried out by a cardiothoracic surgeon who used fluoroscopy to observe the effects of suggested states on diaphragmatic function in several of his patients (Faulkner, 1941). With positive suggestion, the diaphragm moved up and down by more than 3 inches; with negative thoughts, diaphragmatic movement decreased to less than 1 inch. These findings are compatible with a shift from abdominal to rib cage breathing. The results of Faulkner's work have been supported by Ancoli and Kamiya (1979), and Ancoli *et al.* (1980). Bloch *et al.* (1991) have described other respiratory parameters that are associated with basic emotions.

A recent interesting development that relates breathing to emotional arousal has emerged from a cardiology clinic where Dr. Peter Nixon headed an inter-disciplinary team. Conway, a team member and psychologist (and author of Chapter 17 of this volume), interviewed patients suspected of hyperventilating. He then asked them under hypnosis to recall episodes of individually significant emotional or psychological distress, while at the same time monitoring their exhaled P_{CO_2} and ECG (Freeman *et al.*, 1986a,b; Conway *et al.*, 1988). Personally relevant triggers were found to cause P_{CO_2} levels to drop below a criterion level.

Cardiologists Nixon and Freeman modified Conway's method in developing their *Think Test* (Nixon and Freeman, 1988; King *et al.*, 1990). By not using hypnosis, they enabled psychological stressing to be carried out in a more clinically realistic setting. This was accomplished by first looking for any changes in breathing patterns as the patient's history was taken. Then, while CO_2 levels were being monitored, patients were asked to mentally rehearse those topics that had previously disturbed their breathing (see Chapter 5).

While Nixon and colleagues were the first contemporary clinicians to label and suggest the diagnostic potential of the Think Test, the American physicians Stevenson and Ripley, and Dudley should be credited for using analogous procedures as early as 1952 and 1969, respectively. Other clinicians have applied similar methods in controlled studies of different patient populations. Bass, Lelliott, and Marks (1989) used a procedure called *Fear Talk* with agoraphobic patients. In cognitive therapy for panic attacks, Salkovskis and Clark (1991) asked patients to read lists of pairs of words and to dwell upon them in order to "activate negative interpretations."

These procedures could add yet another string to the diagnostic bow. As Gardner points out, multiple provocation tests may be needed to identify patients who hyperventilate episodically but whose P_{CO_2} levels are normal when measured at rest (see Chapter 6). The potential therapeutic value of patient-specific psychological probing seems self-evident but does not appear as yet to have been systematically investigated.

In Chapter 8 of this volume, Bass reminds us that Freud was among the first to recognize that anxious patients may present with somatic symptoms in the absence of demonstrable pathology ("anxiety equivalents") while they deny or minimize psychological distress. The term *somatization* is currently used to describe this process. Bass, in his recent book on this topic (1990), states that hyperventilation is an important mechanism in "somatization disorders."

The term *hyperventilation syndrome* was first used by the American psychiatrist Kerr and his colleagues (1937, 1938), who also suggested that suppression of emotions was an important factor in the development of this syndrome. In Chapter 17 of this volume, Conway takes up this subject that has received little attention since Kerr's suggestion more than a half century ago. The failure of some hyperventilators to express emotion was also observed by Pinney *et al.* (1987). Their study is also important for therapists to be familiar with because it is one of the few studies in which these patients have been offered a holistic treatment program. Suspected hyperventilators were referred from an accident and emergency department. In addition to instruction in abdominal breathing and relaxation, attention was given to all aspects of their life-style, including sleep, emotional arousal, and daily activities. Pinney, a nurse counselor, found that she often had to instruct her patients in "normal expression of feelings." After treatment (2 to 3 sessions for most patients), all but 6 percent of patients had improved. At followup, accident and emergency attendance was markedly reduced and valuable savings in both outpatient and casualty physician time were demonstrated. The authors also claimed that their therapy program was effective in a considerably shorter time than somatically based treatment without the counseling element.

The expression or repression of emotion is clearly an important factor in breathing disorders. In Chapter 16 of this volume, Boadella suggests mechanisms that may be involved, and he, Fensterheim, Conway, and Proskauer describe in their chapters (9, 17, and 18, respectively) the complexities and subtleties of dealing with breathing and emotions in the psychotherapeutic setting (see also Horowitz, 1967).

3. Placebo Responses and Breathing

There seems to be little doubt that arousal levels can be lowered in many ways: drugs, relaxation, explanations, reassurance, cognitive restructuring, insight, religious practices, meditation, hypnosis, and, in some subjects in some circumstances, placebo treatments. Since we know that emotional arousal causes changes in breathing, it is likely that these very same means can bring about relative normalization of breathing. Readers will note that many of the symptoms of hyperventilation listed in Table 1 of the Introduction to this volume are those known to respond to placebo treatments. It is suggested therefore that in persons who tend to hyperventilate, the reduction in arousal level effected by placebos may result in amelioration of symptoms because excessive ventilation is reduced. Thus the *cessation* or reduction of hyperventilation may be an undetected causal factor in placebo effects. The mechanisms by which placebo effects occur are as yet largely unexplained. While there is apparently no suggestion of reduced hyperventilation as a possible mechanism either in the literature on hyperventilation or on placebos (Richardson, 1989), the hypothesis seems well worth testing and, according to Richardson, could shed light on the inconsistency of findings with regard to the role of anxiety in placebo effects (P.H. Richardson, personal communication, 1992).

4. Panic Attacks and Breathing

Panic tends to be an enduring complaint which can progressively affect quality of life and at worst result in the sufferer becoming agoraphobic and even housebound. Panic also presents problems for health care providers, as panic patients may become habitual attenders at emergency and outpatient clinics. Many of these patients are now maintained on costly medications.

Despite early descriptions by da Costa and Freud of what we would now call panic attacks, the etiology, treatment, and even the issue of whether panic attacks should be considered a discrete phenomenon are currently subjects of debate. While there seems to be common agreement that hyperventilation plays a part in panic, there are several competing views on the precise role of hyperventilation and consequently how, and if, it should be treated. These models and their implications for therapy are outlined below.

4.1. Models of Panic

A biological model involving pharmacological treatment of panic emerged from the studies of Klein and associates that began in the 1960s. They made a distinction between panic and nonpanic anxiety and established that only patients of the former type responded to antidepressant medication. Out of this work also came the DSM-III classification *panic disorder,* a label that is unacceptable to some British psychiatrists and psychologists (see Chapter 10). It should be added that the role of hyperventilation receives little attention in this model.

Clark (1986), a cognitive psychologist, challenged the views of Klein and colleagues, claiming that their results could be reinterpreted within a cognitive model. In this model, the primacy of hyperventilation as a cause of panic attacks has also been called into question (see Chapter 10), with the implication that cognitive restructuring of catastrophic thoughts is more important than breathing retraining for these clients. Ley and others have, in turn, challenged the cognitive model, pointing out the accruing evidence that catastrophic thoughts do *not* necessarily precede panic attacks (see Chapter 5).

Ley began his theoretical studies of hyperventilation twenty years ago (Ley and Walker, 1973), and in a recent series of publications has increasingly turned his attention to panic attacks (see Chapter 5). While sharing others' concerns regarding the overinclusiveness of the diagnostic category *Panic Disorder,* Ley (1992) recommends the differentiation of several types of panic. Ley advocates a somatically based model of panic, but one which differs from that of Klein and colleagues; he argues that uncontrolled dyspnea plays a central role in the production of panic fear. In the context of Ley's model, therefore, an essential component of treatment for panic attacks is breathing retraining, in conjunction with cognitive corrections and deconditioning of fear.

British specialist physical therapists have described success in reducing or abolishing panic attacks as a result of their treatment of hyperventilation (see Chapter 11). Although only uncontrolled studies of their work are available (e.g., Evans and Lum, 1977), clinical impressions based on more than 25 years of application in the United Kingdom would support these claims, as do the results of Bonn *et al.* (1984). In the latter, at six months' follow up, a group of agoraphobics treated with breathing retraining and exposure were free of panic attacks, whereas a group treated with exposure alone were still having an average of one to two panic attacks per week.

The treatment protocols developed in Britain are now being recognized in the United States. At a center for management of anxiety and depression, Cowley and Roy-Byrne (1987) found that "breathing . . . treatments offer an exciting alternative or adjunct to medication in these patients since they involve imparting a sense of mastery to the patient and since many patients with panic disorder seem particularly sensitive to medication side effects."

In clinical practice, of course, the above described approaches are often combined. The importance of cognitive elements in multifactorial treatment was emphasized by Patel in the Foreword to this book. And, as Bass points out in Chapter 10, drugs can, of course, be used with any of the psychological therapies. In some treatment studies, various components have been systematically combined. For example, Clark (1986) reviewed those using behavioral–cognitive and behavioral approaches. In Bonn *et al.* (1984) and de Buers *et al.* (1990) treatment of agoraphobic patients included both breathing retraining and exposure therapy. In a study that has as yet been only partially reported, Timmons, Somerville, and Bonn (1990) gave panic attack patients multimodal treatment comprised of physical therapy, a behavioral/cognitive program, and group counseling.

The recognition that there are different types of panic attacks, as argued by Ley, and that those suffering such attacks may be treated successfully by various clinicians (physical therapists and clinical psychologists, among others) may prevent many clients from being unnecessarily labeled as "psychiatric cases" requiring treatment with drugs.

4.2. Assessing Treatment Outcome Studies

Further clinical trials testing the models described above are obviously necessary in order to guide therapists' approaches to panic and to determine the role of breathing in this disorder. When treatment modalities are combined, it is difficult to compare the results of trials, as emphasized by Bass: "One of the problems in assessing the efficacy of cognitive–behavioral therapy in patients with hyperventilation-related disorders, is that the treatments are often given with some kind of breathing retraining" (see Chapter 10 of this volume). The reverse situation, however, is even more confounded. Breathing-retraining-centered treatment of hyperventilators (see Chapter 11) contains, as essential and inextricable components, the very elements described by Bass as comprising cognitive–behavioral therapy: replication experiments, reattribution of symptoms, and coping strategies. In fact, psychiatrists and other physicians caring for hyperventilators have, from the 1930s onward, relied upon these methods, albeit with less specific labels and structured protocols than those provided recently by cognitive psychologists. It was not until the 1960s that Lum and his colleagues added their breathing retraining protocols to earlier treatments. As currently administered by experienced, specialist physical therapists, breathing retraining is inseparable from relaxation training and behavioral–cognitive elements (see Chapter 11). In the words of the physical therapist Bradley (1991), "50% of the cure is knowing about and understanding the nature of the hyperventilation syndrome" (see also DeGuire *et al.*, 1992).

A scientific demonstration of the effectiveness of any multifactorial treatment, including physical therapy, will be difficult. To devise a credible control group activity for double blind, randomized trials of these treatments seems as improbable as it would be for testing the effectiveness of surgical procedures. Given the typically chronic nature of panic attacks and hyperventilation, waiting-list control groups seem a valid (and perhaps the only) alternative, but as yet few studies of this design have been published in this field (e.g., Jongmans *et al.*, 1990).

Unfortunately, it has to be said that the problems inherent in the research process, as described by Ley in Chapter 5 of this volume, make it unlikely that there will be any quick and simple answers. While trials of different interventions or combinations thereof may not be directly comparable, and control methods inadequate, scrutiny of certain factors common to research in this field as described below may be helpful in assessing new studies.

4.2.1. Symptom, Panic Attack, and Anxiety Ratings

There are apparent differences in emphasis between the breathing-retraining and cognitive schools regarding outcome measurements. The objective of physical therapists using the Lum/Papworth methods (as described in the Introduction as well as in Chapter 11) is to abolish symptoms including panic attacks and to teach patients to control any symptoms which might recur under conditions of unusual stress. In Lum's view, any therapy which does not at least aim at such results is merely palliative (L.C. Lum, 1991, personal communication).

Cognitive therapists have usually reported the frequency of panic attacks as their principle dependent variable (e.g., Salkovskis *et al.*, 1991). Consequently, one may question whether clients who have been convinced that there is a "suitable alternative explanation" for their distressing symptoms (see Bass, Chapter 10) therefore tolerate the persistence of some of these symptoms because the cause has been relabeled and anxiety thus reduced? Only a few studies have provided baseline and posttherapy ratings of the frequency and/or severity of symptoms (e.g., Bonn *et al.*, 1984; Pinney *et al.*, 1987; Jongmans *et al.*, 1990) in addition to panic attack frequency and anxiety ratings. Persistence of complaints is thus an issue which remains to be clarified.

4.2.2. Qualifications of Therapists

Salkovskis and Clark (1991) recommend the use of their "therapist competency check list," pointing out that studies of cognitive and behavioral treatments have too often placed little emphasis on the qualifications and training of therapists. The same problem prevails in research involving a "breathing therapy" element, where the need for specialist skills has not generally been recognized. The training and experience of therapists are either not described òr are, one must say, apparently inadequate. In one recent study, for example, breathing retraining was done by "junior clinical psychologists." While it is obvious that we cannot teach someone to play the piano unless we know how to play ourselves, we may wrongly assume that because we all breathe, we are therefore qualified to help our clients improve their breathing. Many physical therapists believe, in fact, that breathing retraining of patient populations should be done only by those with a knowledge of anatomy, the mechanics of breathing, and respiratory diseases. Moreover, therapists should ideally be in themselves models of relaxed abdominal breathing (see Chapter 11 and Hough, 1991). Finally, as Lum has often emphasized in his teachings, the single most important characteristic of therapists in this field is *empathy*.

4.2.3. Methods of Assessing Hyperventilation

In a recent series of papers, Gardner and Bass have suggested diagnostic protocols for hyperventilation that are appropriate for clinical trials (see Chapters 6, 8, and 10). In Chapter 6, Gardner puts these procedures into a clinical context and describes the path therapists must follow to achieve diagnosis without over-investigation. He recommends using multiple provocation tests when necessary. Unfortunately, current treatment studies, including some that have been cited in criticism of the "hyperventilation school" by cognitive therapists, do not as yet reflect recent advances. Investigations of hyperventilation that rely on inadequate assessment should therefore be viewed reservedly. For example, in several recent publications, hyperventilation has been "diagnosed" either solely on the basis of voluntary overbreathing, on a single resting measurement of P_{CO_2}, or on a hyperventilation symptom list. Finally, and perhaps most important, the evidence from Dudley's early studies (1969), recently confirmed by Nixon and Freeman (1988), is often overlooked. Trials are still being designed without taking into account that hyperventilation is triggered by *personally relevant* stimuli.

4.2.4. Follow-up Studies

Panic tends to be a chronic condition, and it is therefore important to note that there are not yet any long-term follow-ups of controlled studies of patients treated with physical therapy for hyperventilation, or long-term controlled studies of cognitive treatments for either panic attacks or even for generalized anxiety. Such follow ups, preferably of five years' duration, will be necessary to establish treatment efficacy, given the possibility of relapse or symptom substitution with either approach, as suggested below.

5. Breathing Patterns: Their Significance for Therapists

A skilled observer can estimate not only the rate of breathing but also its regularity; the relative amplitudes of rib cage versus abdominal movements; and the duration of inspiration, expiration, and pauses. Variations in these parameters of breathing in persons free of lung disease have been of interest to somatotherapists and yogis as described in previous chapters of this volume, but to only a few in Western medicine (e.g., Dudley *et al.*, 1969; Pietroni and Pietroni, 1989; van Dixhoorn, 1990). The lack of attention to these basic phenomena of human behavior is attested to by the fact that what is considered a "normal" rate of breathing has only recently been adjusted downward to 12 breaths per min in physiology textbooks from the traditional medical/nursing norms of 15 to 20 breaths per min. This change reflects recognition of the observation that patients in clinics or hospitals are breathing faster than relaxed, normal subjects. This new "norm," however, is still higher than 8 breaths per min, which is considered a truly relaxed rate by specialist physical therapists and is aimed at in their retraining programs (see Chapter 11 and Hough, 1991).

5.1. Psychophysiological Studies of Breathing Patterns

Some psychophysiologists have looked at features of breathing patterns in addition to rate. Clausen (1951) found that a sharp inspiratory–expiratory angle in recordings of abdominal movements consistently distinguished "neurotic" from normal subjects. Timmons *et al.* (1972) showed that abdominal-dominant

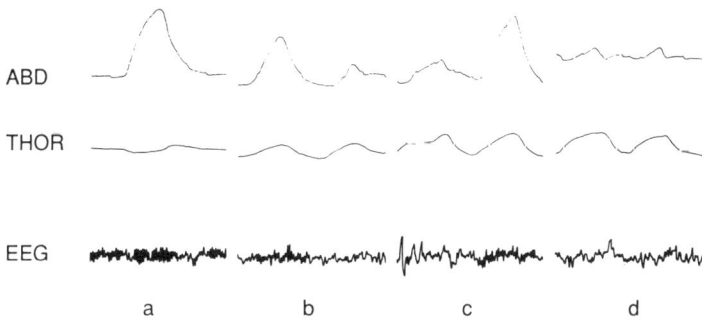

Figure 1. Breathing patterns, brainwave (EEG) patterns, and levels of arousal. From Timmons (1972), with permission.

breathing was associated with relaxed wakefulness (see Fig. 1a); equality of rib cage and abdominal movements (as measured by frontal strain gauges) with the hypnogogic state (Fig. 1b); and thoracic-dominant breathing with sleep onset (Fig. 1d). Svebak *et al.* (1981) found that abdominal circumference decreased and thoracic circumference increased during sustained mental tasks. Mador and Tobin (1991) measured breathing patterns during different forms of mental activity. Blanton and colleagues have investigated breath-holding span (Blanton and Alpher, 1983; Alpher *et al.,* 1986; Alpher and Blanton, 1991). Ancoli, Kamiya, and Ekman's studies of breathing patterns and emotional states were described in Section 2, above. Psychophysiological studies relating stress and emotion to breathing have also been described above and in Chapter 5 of this volume. Haas (1980) and Haas *et al.* (1980) have related behavioral traits to respiratory patterns. These authors have pointed out the significance of their findings for rehabilitation medicine; however, the potential therapeutic value of much psychophysiological such research remains largely unexplored.

Specialists in breathing retraining emphasize that clients with disturbed breathing should be helped to find their own "natural" abdominal breathing pattern, as Holloway calls it (see Chapter 11). The studies cited above suggest that it may ultimately be possible to define the "limits of normal" or even "physiologic norms" (Cheraskin and Ringsdorf, 1973) for breathing patterns and how these are related to psychological traits and behavior.

5.2. Physiological and Clinical Evidence

When one turns to the respiratory literature, one again finds a scarcity of documentation of phenomena that are routinely observed by clinicians. Peper, for example, made the interesting observation at the 1990 *Symposium on Respiratory Psychophysiology* that all asthmatic and postmyocardial infarction patients are rib cage breathers. One can, however, find evidence for the significance of breathing patterns in a variety of sources ranging from laboratory data to the anecdotal, and these are briefly described below.

5.2.1. Work of Breathing

Raising the rib cage and shoulders many times a day is an inefficient and tiring way to breathe (see Chapter 11). With proper use of the diaphragm, the work of breathing is reduced. The energy saved can be crucial for some patients with chronic lung diseases and is presumably beneficial for normal individuals as well.

5.2.2. Hyperventilation

Lum (1975) has described the typical hyperventilator's breathing pattern as an effortless heaving of the upper sternum and lack of lateral costal expansion, with little or no use of the diaphragm. He has emphasized that while increased thoracic breathing is normal during exercise or in the fight-or-flight response, such breathing at rest is almost always associated with overbreathing (Lum, 1977). Lum (1976) used impedence recordings to illustrate the striking differences between a hyperventilator's and a normal subject's breathing patterns. In one of the few attempts to document group differences in breathing patterns of suspected hyperventilators, Timmons et al. (1990) used physical therapists' ratings of breathing movements and found significantly more clavicular movement in patients with panic attacks than in matched normal subjects who had been carefully screened in order to exclude those with any tendencies to chronic hyperventilation.

While the pattern so typical of hyperventilators has received considerable attention in the literature, it should be emphasized that experienced therapists describe other patterns that are associated with physical and psychic complaints (see, e.g., Chapter 16). Holloway finds that a quarter of her caseload comprises patients with irregular, "apneic" patterns who respond equally well to her treatment as do hyperventilators (see Chapter 11). Patel, who describes an alternating pattern of *hypo*ventilation and *hyper*ventilation, claims that the latter type of breathing causes the brain's respiratory centers to switch off, resulting in "apneas" and, thus, "hypoventilation" (Patel, 1989, 1991). Using ambulatory monitoring, Anderson and colleagues (1992, 1993) identified an "inhibitory" breathing pattern—low frequency and low minute ventilation. This pattern was observed more often when subjects were in their workplace or in social situations. It was distinct from a fight-or-flight, hyperventilatory response, and may be associated with increased "sensory intake."

5.2.3. Chest Pain

In a convincing demonstration of the effects of breathing style, Friedman (1945) relieved chest pain of noncardiac origin by strapping patients' rib cages. When the straps were removed the pain returned. In addition, normal subjects developed chest pain after exercise when their abdomen and lower rib cage were strapped. However, as Bass comments in Chapter 10 of this volume, this experiment is unlikely to be replicated.

5.2.4. Sex

The effects of breathing patterns on sexual response have been most fully explored in the East by Tantric yogis (Eliade, 1958) and in the West by Reichians and bioenergeticists (see Chapter 16). Clinicians Kerr *et al.* (1937) suggested that orgasm may be the result of hyperventilation tetany (see also Bancroft, 1989). Kitzinger (1983) attributed some of the sensations women experienced with orgasm (faintness, numbness, dizziness, floating) to excited overbreathing. As sexual arousal is incompatible with anxiety and muscle tension, one might predict that chronically tense hyperventilators would be subject to difficulties in the sexual realm, but one finds surprisingly few references to sex-related complaints in the hyperventilation literature. In a rather histrionic paper that is rich in clinical detail, Schimmenti (1953) claimed that patients whom he labeled as "the hyperventilating type of human female" developed an aversion to sexual intercourse. Several factors contributing to this aversion are described, for example, respiratory alkalosis causing increased pH of the vagina, which in turn predisposes to reduced erotic sensation, chafing, and infection. Bradley (1991), who is apparently the first clinician to include sexual problems in a hyperventilation symptom list, argues that male as well as female hyperventilators may be at risk during sexual arousal. She states that the *normal* heavy-breathing that is necessary to achieve orgasm may lead to panic attacks. Clinicians caring for asthmatic patients confirm that overbreathing during intercourse can bring on asthmatic and then panic attacks. Nonasthmatic hyperventilators with panic attacks have apparently not been questioned systematically regarding sexual problems. Nixon comments that hyperventilators are often too tired to have sex (P.G.F. Nixon, personal communication, 1992).

Research in the respiratory aspects of sexual physiology could benefit many clients. Bradley is to be commended for bringing this subject to the attention of both clients and clinicians.

5.3. Performance and Breathing Patterns

The effects of hyperventilation on performance have been recognized by professionals in some fields for many years. Pilots' awareness of the hazards of overbreathing has led to a number of studies in aviation medicine (see Chapter 5). Actors have traditionally breathed into paper bags to relieve the "paralysis" of stage fright (Bradley, 1991).

Ley has recently shown that breathing is related to test anxiety and psychomotor performance (see Chapter 5). These studies seem to be among the most noteworthy of current research because they establish the importance of respiratory behavior in everyday life, in the workplace, and in school, rather than in the clinic or in elite athletic competition, as described below (see also, Wilson, 1992).

Other types of performance are also related to breathing patterns. One example described in this book is the improvement in voice quality after training in abdominal breathing (see Chapter 12). Finally, the effects of breathing retraining may soon be demonstrated in yet another way, namely, in athletic performance. Some breathing therapists have worked with Olympic competitors. While few published accounts of the results are available (e.g., Stough, 1970), there is an interesting anecdotal precedent. For many years, women involved in long-distance swimming or competitive athletics have believed that their performance has been improved as a result of childbirth. Currently, it is alleged that some world class athletes have "planned pregnancies" for the same reason. Lum suggests the following possible rationale for this purported improvement. Breathing against an enlarged uterus provides the diaphragm with about six months of "weightlifting" exercise. Also, it is known that both vital capacity and inspiratory capacity increase during the third trimester of pregnancy. Because descent of the diaphragm is hindered, the increase in inspiratory capacity must be due to increased thoracic expansion. Hence, through the last six months of pregnancy, the respiratory apparatus is progressively trained to work continuously at 30 to 50 percent above the nonpregnant workload. Lum also comments that it is well known that pregnant women are in a state of progesterone-driven hyperventilation and that they tolerate this state well. Hyperventilators, incidentally, normally lose their symptoms during pregnancy (L.C. Lum, 1991, personal communication).

6. Breathing Retraining

The above sections and other evidence presented in the previous chapters appear to justify one of the objectives of this book: to bring into awareness an easily observed but often overlooked phenomenon, how one's client is breathing. We have described a "natural" abdominal breathing pattern that is, as Bradley (1991) says, "the most energy-efficient and relaxing way to breathe." Deviations from this pattern can increase the work of breathing and thus cause fatigue and, in some persons, chest pain and other symptoms of hyperventilation. Disordered breathing apparently affects performance of psychomotor tasks and also, according to some, athletic performance, sexual arousal, and orgastic capacity. While breathing can be normalized by a reduction in arousal level induced by relaxation, reassurance, or other means as described above, these changes are unlikely to endure if the client has not been taught the neuromuscular skills involved in using the diaphragm correctly. This raises the question of whether clinicians in many fields have some responsibility to screen their clients' breathing. For example, Patel's (1989, 1991) advice to anyone teaching relaxation was unequivocal: *"until chest breathing is replaced by deep, even and steady diaphragmatic breathing, all efforts to relax the body, nerves and mind will be ineffective."* Bonn *et al.* (1984) provided behavior therapists with evidence that their agoraphobic patients could be put at risk of relapse unless attention was given to their breathing.

More recently, DeGuire *et al.* (1992) demonstrated to cardiologists that there is an alternative approach to the pharmacological treatments commonly used for hyperventilation-related functional cardiac symptoms. (Relapse is often reported when drugs are withdrawn from these patients.) In this study, frequencies of chest pain, palpitations, shortness of breath, and other symptoms were reduced in patients who had any of three types of breathing retraining, as compared to patients in a non-treatment group. Reduction in symptoms was associated with decreased respiratory rate and increased levels of $ETco_2$.

It is lamentable that there are as yet so few controlled studies of breathing retraining such as above. But it is also not surprising, given that even the long-observed benefits of breathing retraining for breathless patients (e.g., increased ability to walk and to climb stairs) have not been scientifically measured (Webber, 1991). Webber urges clinicians not to ignore obvious benefits to patients because measurement studies have not as yet been done.

Determining the role of breathing retraining when used as a component in multimodal treatments for breathing-related disorders will be more difficult. Bass comments in Chapter 10 of this volume that the contribution of breathing retraining "in pure form" is likely to remain controversial. [The effects, however, of instruction in slowing and pacing the breath, which might be called "pure breathing training," are described in Chapter 13 of this volume and in a review by Clark and Hirschman (1990).] Patel (as described in the Foreword) found at four-year follow-up that her subjects continued their brief daily breathing practices and cognitive strategies but not other relaxation or meditation techniques (Patel *et al.*, 1985). These findings seem highly significant, given the perennial problems of poor compliance and high dropout rates occurring in self-regulatory therapies. Patel agrees that it is unlikely that the contribution of breathing can be assessed separately, but readers may be persuaded by her comments and the substance of this volume that it is a key factor in these programs.

The reasons for retraining breathing thus appear to far outweigh minority opinions on the subject. Nonetheless, counterviews should perhaps be mentioned. For example, Howell (1990) has said that "attempts to influence breathing voluntarily should be avoided other than by relaxation," and Salkovskis (1990) claimed that retraining of breathing is "in no way essential" as a component in cognitive therapy for panic attacks. These authors have, it should be noted, provided no long-term follow-up data to support their assertions.

Garssen *et al.* (1992) have taken an extreme position, labeling breathing retraining as a "rational placebo," i.e., a treatment that is effective but the mechanisms of which are not those that are assumed to be operative. Garssen and colleagues suggest that the mechanisms by which breathing retraining *actually* works are not through reducing ventilation but through inducing the relaxation response; providing credible explanations of symptoms; prescribing distracting tasks to perform; and promoting a sense of self-control.

Garssen *et al.* (1992) identify two distinct components of treatments for hyperventilation and/or panic attacks: (1) "pure breathing technique" ("reduction of respiratory rate"), and (2) cognitive interventions. As their prime example of pure breathing technique, the authors cite a report by Lum (1983) on more than 1000 cases treated with his methods. The problem with this analysis is that, as explained above with regard to treatment of panic attacks, the Lum/Papworth and derivative methods comprise all the elements described above as efficacious in reducing ventilation, as well as breathing retraining. Thus the thesis of Garssen and colleagues seems unsupported and in fact lends confusion to an already complex field (see also Ley, 1993).

6.1. Problems in Retraining Breathing

Practices intended to alter human breathing patterns have existed for many centuries and have been applied to different subject populations for different purposes, whether spiritual or secular, ascetic or hedonistic, for self-realization or for medical treatment. A spectrum of methods developed by experts in various fields is presented in this book. At one end of the spectrum are the noninterventionist practices of Zen Buddhism, in which breathing is allowed to change by "just watching" it (see Chapter 18). At the other extreme are the vigorous interventions of those practicing Reichian therapy and bioenergetics. For example, these therapists may induce a client's gag reflex to "free the diaphragm" or bend the client backward over a "breathing stool" in order to "open the rib cage" (see Chapter 16).

Whichever method is used, it must be said that faulty technique or inexperience may lead to complications in treatment, as is the case, of course, in almost any clinical intervention. Lum's view on this subject is emphatic: "*It is better not to change a patient's breathing unless you know what you're doing*" (L.C. Lum, 1991, personal communication). The necessity for training and experience was referred to in Section 4.2.2, above. Younger or less chronically ill clients may learn and respond quickly to breathing retraining. Other clients, however, may present problems even for experts. Some contributors have for this reason appended guidelines and cautions where appropriate. Potential difficulties in retraining breathing may arise from one or more, or an interaction of the causes that are outlined below. Some ways in which these obstacles may be overcome are also suggested.

6.1.1. Learning Problems

Little is known about learning in the respiratory system, but in a recent series of publications, Gallego and colleagues have begun to investigate the relationship of voluntary, "controlled" breathing to spontaneous breathing, as well as the process by which controlled breathing can become automatized (Gallego and Perruchet, 1991a,b; Gallego et al., 1991b). Most significantly, recent clinical reports indicate that learning new breathing patterns is facilitated by integrating breathing retraining with counseling and other behavioral/cognitive approaches (Pinney et al., 1986; Hough, 1991; Bradley, 1992; DeGuire et al., 1992). DeGuire et al., for example, describe the "ease" with which their patients learned paced diaphragmatic breathing in six sessions.

Current evidence thus suggests that, for many hyperventilators, a shorter course of treatment may be adequate compared to that described in early reports by physical therapists. Those therapists' work, however, should be seen in the context of the British National Health Service at that time. Patients could be offered many more treatment sessions (and even hospitalization—see Chapter 11) than is now possible. Nonetheless, some hyperventilators are undeniably difficult to treat. According to Hough (1991), breathing *cannot* be reeducated in a person under stress. This observation supports Naifeh's conjecture described in "Stress and Breathing" (Section 1). When teaching clients to maintain abdominal breathing in stressful situations, one is working against a powerful unconditioned response.

There is accumulating evidence that presenting the client with respiratory parameter information obtained from electronic biofeedback instruments is another way to facilitate learning (Corson et al., 1979; Grossman et al., 1985; Kopp and Temesvary, 1990; Gallego et al., 1991; Peper and Tibbetts, 1992). A type of biofeedback simpler and less expensive than electronic instruments is now being used by some London and New York therapists. The subject is asked to recline with a light sandbag or large telephone directory placed on the abdomen while practicing abdominal breathing. This weightlifting is sufficient to strengthen the diaphragm and also to maintain the subject's awareness, thus providing continuous "feedback."

6.1.2. Symptoms Worsened by Retraining

Bass points out that it is possible to make some hyperventilators worse with breathing exercises, at least in the early stages of training (see Chapter 10 of this volume). In these cases, exacerbation of symptoms is probably occurring in what Lum and the British physical therapists have often referred to as the "get worse, get better" stage in treatment. Specialists have developed strategies to help patients through this stage (see Chapter 11 and van Dixhoorn, 1990). When patients begin to practice the new abdominal pattern, they may not as yet have learned to decrease their habitual rib cage breathing, especially under stress. Their ventilation, already excessive, can thus be further increased (especially if they have not learned to slow the rate), and Pco_2 levels can plunge. Overemphasis on slowing the rate without adequate attention to other parameters of breathing is another mistake in technique that can be disastrous for hyperventilators.

6.1.3. Hyperventilation-Induced Cerebral Hypoxia

Attention, memory, and thus ability to learn may all be impaired by the reduced blood flow to the brain that results from hyperventilation, as explained by Ley in Chapter 5 of this volume.

6.1.4. Lack of Awareness of Inappropriate Breathing

Few of us are aware of a properly functioning respiratory system; nor have we any need to be so aware in ordinary circumstances (see Chapter 4). The ease with which this continual rhythm recedes from awareness makes breathing an ideal object for the practice of concentrative meditation. For example, the basic Zen Buddhist practice of counting one's exhalations up to ten is very difficult for most persons to sustain without considerable practice. Retraining is another situation in which breathing must be brought into and kept in awareness in order to change it. And this, as Innocenti (1987) points out, is when the problems begin. Unless they are dyspneic, hyperventilating patients are often unaware of their abnormal breathing (Brodtkorb et al., 1990). Tavel (1990) explains that they may fail subjectively to recognize a respiratory problem because they are so obsessed with other somatic symptoms. This lack of awareness, which may be contributed to by cerebral hypoxia, is an obvious obstacle to learning and also has implications for prevention of hyperventilation (King et al., 1990).

6.1.5. Relaxation-Induced Anxiety

Anxiety and even panic attacks are commonly observed side effects of relaxation training, occurring even in normal subjects (see Chapters 5, 11, 13, 15, 16, and 18). The mechanism for relaxation-induced anxiety is the failure of hyperventilators to adapt their breathing to conditions of reduced metabolic need (Ley, 1988). Symptoms may also occur in analogous situations such as while driving, watching television, lying in bed, or during induction of hypnosis. Again, assured technique based on knowledge and experience is necessary.

6.1.6. "Obsession with Breathing"

Some clinicians have suggested that breathing retraining is contraindicated because patients can become "obsessed" with their breathing. This phenomenon is rare but well known to specialists, and failure to cope with it most likely reflects inexperienced management. If patients do not get on well with breathing practices, Holloway helps them to focus more on general relaxation in the early stages of training (see Chapter 11). In "Autogenic Training" (see Chapter 13), therapists have traditionally adopted a similar approach, avoiding areas of obsessive concern in the beginning of treatment. Practice of autogenic phrases such as "my heart beat is slow and regular" or "it breathes me" is delayed until the client has acquired some ability to relax.

6.1.7. Learning Impaired by Medications

Many psychotherapists consider it unethical to accept clients who are on tranquilizers or sleeping medications since it is held they are unlikely to learn while their feelings are blunted; the ability to learn new breathing patterns may be diminished as well. Severely anxious, panicky, or agoraphobic patients often need to continue medication in order to lower their arousal level sufficiently for them to be able to take on other treatment. Withdrawal from drugs, however, often allows symptoms of hyperventilation that have been suppressed by the drug to reemerge, thus complicating the problem in some cases.

6.1.8. Emotional Factors and Psychopathology

Reich stated that "changing the patterns of a person's breathing is tantamount to emotional surgery . . ." (see Chapter 16). While the effects of retraining breathing in normal or mildly anxious subjects may not be so drastic, clinicians should be aware of the complex interaction of breathing and psychopathology as discussed by authors of the psychodynamically oriented Chapters 9, 16, 17 and 18 of this volume.

6.1.9. Inappropriate Treatment

Sound judgment and experience are necessary to help clients find the therapy that is not only most likely to benefit them, but also will not make them worse or adversely affect their quality of life. Those who are experienced in treating hyperventilating or agoraphobic patients, or those patients with panic attacks, know how unhappy most of them are when obliged to take drugs in the absence of any alternative therapy. On the other hand, a minority of patients prefer drugs. Some clinicians now ask hyperventilating patients, after they have been fully informed of the options available, to choose which treatment they would prefer. Simply attending a relaxation or yoga class will benefit some clients, provided the teachers know how to prevent hyperventilation occurring as a result of their practices. Relaxation, including breathing retraining, is contraindicated for depressed patients unless done under the supervision of a therapist. Patients with chronic obstructive pulmonary disease, scoliosis, and other problems described in Chapter 11 of this volume should be treated at least initially by physical therapists. Some clients will accept *only* a somatic approach; for example, many cardiac patients (van Dixhoorn, 1990) and torture survivors (Hough, 1992). For others, breathing retraining integrated with behavioral–cognitive therapy may be appropriate. According to Pfeffer *et al.* (1982), symptomatic treatment may be adequate if hyperventilation is merely a residue of an earlier emotional problem that has been resolved. For most patients, however, these authors have found that treatment should be directed at underlying causes and usually will require some form of psychotherapy. If treatment is to be effective, hyperventilators and panic attack patients must have the opportunity to express their feelings or to learn to express them, according to Lum (1977), Pinney *et al.* (1987), Conway (see Chapter 17), and virtually all the psychotherapists and specialist physical therapists who have published in this field.

Some clinicians treating complex psychophysiological disorders are adopting other therapeutic strategies in addition to conventional onward referral and adjunctive therapy. Some are cooperating in interdisciplinary approaches such as the sharing of skills between physical therapists and specialist nurses. Some are acquiring further training themselves, for example, in accord with Gibson's (1978) suggestion that physical therapists be trained in behavior therapy. Some are adopting innovative approaches such as the integration of cognitive therapy with elements more often associated with humanistic or psychodynamic therapies (Evans, 1991; Ryle, 1990).

Ultimately, we may have answers to the questions, "*What* treatment, by *whom* is most effective for *this* individual with *that* specific problem, and under *which* set of circumstances?" which Paul (1967) suggested should be the key issues addressed by clinical outcome studies. Implicit in the chapters of this volume authored by our psychodynamically oriented contributors is the prediction that treatments involving "purely" somatic, behavioral, cognitive, *or* psychotherapeutic approaches will put some clients at risk of symptom substitution or "syndrome shifts." Only assiduous long-term follow-up of patients can test these predictions.

7. Breathing Measurements in Therapy

Observation of breathing is a traditional clinical skill in many professions: medicine, nursing, anesthesia, respiratory therapy, physical therapy, relaxation training, and hypnotherapy. One objective of this book is to bring to the attention of therapists in the behavioral disciplines the potential value of such observations. For example, a behavior therapist (Readhead) who had been trained as a nurse to count breathing rate inconspicuously, noticed that her agoraphobic patients breathed rapidly (sometimes more than 25 breaths per min) while at rest and filling out questionnaires. Her observation was one of the factors leading to the Bonn *et al.* (1984) study, one of the first trials to implicate hyperventilation in agoraphobia and provide evidence of the efficacy of breathing retraining for these patients.

Respiratory *measurement,* in contrast to clinical observation of breathing, is a topic alluded to relatively briefly in the preceding chapters of this volume. Since measurement is more in the realm of the lung function or research laboratory, behaviorally oriented readers may consider this omission appropriate. Recently, however, therapists have begun to supplement their skills with the use of instruments in office practice. What follows is a brief review of the rationale for, and potential importance of, some of these procedures to therapists.

7.1. Measurement of Breathing Patterns

Most of what we know about breathing patterns is from physiological and medical studies. In the past, these data were obtained primarily using face masks or mouthpieces and noseclips. Such apparatus changes breathing patterns and provides a prime example of the method of measurement influencing what is being measured (Western and Patrick, 1988). Jennett (see Chapter 4) points out that textbooks therefore need to be rewritten with studies based on noninvasive measurements.

In the few studies in which psychophysiologists have looked at breathing patterns, these researchers have most often used strain gauges or other noninvasive and nonintrusive measurement methods (reviewed in "Breathing and Emotion" and other sections of this chapter, above). The graphic recordings of breathing movements thus obtained can more accurately characterize abnormal patterns (irregularity, breath-holding, apneas, etc.) than can observation alone. The display and explanation of graphic records are also valuable aids in teaching clients new habits (see Chapter 13). One would think it might go without saying at this point that movements from *both* rib cage and abdomen need to be recorded, but psychophysiological publications which purport to characterize breathing continue to appear with only one of these measurements.

Although breathing movement is easily observable, it is, ironically, a difficult clinical measurement. Methods for obtaining accurate, calibrated recordings may not be practical outside a physiology laboratory. For example, the state-of-the-art instrument, the impedance pneumograph (Respitrace) must be recalibrated after any movement or postural change. Even more elaborate calibration and filtering procedures are needed during ambulatory monitoring of breathing (Patrick and Western, 1991). Anderson and colleagues (1992, 1993) used a portable microprocessor with the Respitrace while monitoring their subjects' breathing during 24 hours of normal activities.

An accurate, robust method of recording breathing which could be used easily by nonphysiologists is much needed, but to date has eluded the efforts of biomedical engineers (Timmons, 1982; Timmons and Meldrum, 1993, in preparation). Meanwhile, the strain gauges in respiratory biofeedback systems are adequate for office use (e.g., DeGuire et al., 1992).

7.2. Biofeedback of Respiratory Measurements

In common with standard behavioral practice, feedback of information such as data from chart recorders and capnographs may be invaluable in (1) demonstrating to the client that a physiological abnormality is present; (2) serving as an adjunct to breathing retraining; and (3) monitoring progress. Current models of capnographs incorporate features that make them well adapted to biofeedback of PCO_2 (Naifeh et al., 1982; Fried, 1987), as well as of rate and regularity of breathing (see also DeGuire et al., 1992).

7.3. Measurement of Other Parameters of Breathing

Other respiratory phenomena have been described in the chapters of this volume which may be proved to have clinical significance by future research. An example is the relative dominance or laterality of nasal airflow which is said to be related to autonomic nervous system function [see the review by Backon (1989), and Chapters 2 and 15].

7.4. Measuring the Effects of Hyperventilation

7.4.1. Measurement of Exhaled Carbon Dioxide

Measurement of end tidal (exhaled) carbon dioxide in subjects with normal lungs is technically a relatively simple procedure. The cost of capnographs for this purpose is now low enough to make them available for office or clinic use (see Chapter 6). In recent years capnographs have been in routine use in practices in London's Harley Street. These instruments provide accurate, nonintrusive measurement of $ETCO_2$ that can be used to aid the diagnosis of hyperventilation and monitor the progress of treatment.

7.4.2. Ambulatory Monitoring of Carbon Dioxide

Some patients with panic or chest pain are apparently overbreathing when picked up by the ambulance crew or admitted to the emergency room, but their Pco_2 is often found to be normal when measured later in the laboratory or office. Ambulatory monitoring of Pco_2 would seem to be the ideal method to determine whether their symptoms are caused by intermittent hyperventilation; however, the ambulatory monitors currently available which measure *transcutaneous* Pco_2 have as yet been used only for research and have been described by respiratory physiologists as problematic (see Chapter 6). The electrode's slow response time and insensitivity to small changes in Pco_2 make it inappropriate for assessing levels of Pco_2 during panic attacks. Results of research into the role of hyperventilation as a cause of panic attacks based on the use of these monitors are subject to considerable error and should therefore be viewed with caution.

7.4.3. The Voluntary Hyperventilation Test

While we await improved technological methods for diagnosis, the traditional procedure of asking the patient to overbreathe to elicit symptoms is still useful. Although voluntary hyperventilation (VHV) cannot be relied on solely for diagnosis of hyperventilation, practitioners who use this test routinely know how dramatically it can help patients to understand the connection between overbreathing and symptom production. Traditionally, patients have been asked to breathe deeply for 2 to 3 min at a rate of 20 to 30 breaths per min. There is no standard protocol for performing the test and but a few parametric studies to provide guidelines (e.g., Hornsveld and Garssen, 1990). Recent suggestions for improving and standardizing VHV are Howell's (1990) *20 Deep Breaths Test* and Folgering's "one minute of deep breathing" (Folgering and Colla, 1978), the latter based on the authors' findings that 1 min of VHV is as effective as 3 min in diagnosis of the hyperventilation syndrome. Because VHV can be a very unpleasant experience for some patients, Folgering's suggested modification seems to be an important and compassionate advance which is worth drawing to the attention of all therapists.

Bonn *et al.* (1984) have utilized an innovative approach to VHV, attempting to enhance the power of the test by asking patients to breathe predominantly with the upper chest, thus more closely simulating involuntary hyperventilation. Pacing at a fast rate (60 breaths per min) made it difficult for patients to breathe abdominally. Measurement of $ETco_2$ (see below) ensured that the patients were actually hyperventilating and not just "moving dead space."

In Chapter 6 of this volume, Gardner recommends that Pco_2 be brought down below 20 mmHg with 1 to 3 min of VHV; this criterion was achieved by

Bass *et al.* (1989). After 3 min of VHV, their panic patients' mean P_{CO_2} was down to 15.5 mm Hg, resulting in 59 percent of patients (13 of 22) experiencing familiar symptoms. Bass and colleagues point out that the results of such studies may vary because of the differences in hypocapnia attained, citing, for example, a paper by Gorman *et al.* (1988) who found that only 23 percent of their patients experienced symptoms similar to their usual panics, while their P_{CO_2} had only been brought down to a mean of 29 mm Hg. In contrast, in the study of Bonn *et al.* (1984), 95 percent (20 of 21) of the agoraphobic patients recognized symptoms; in addition, two-thirds of these patients experienced such severe effects, including panic, that they were unable to continue VHV for 3 min. More recently, Maddock and Carter (1991) required their subjects to maintain a P_{CO_2} of less than 20 mm Hg for 8 min. As a result, 7 of the 12 agoraphobic patients and 1 of 12 control individuals experienced panic.

As described above, several clinical researchers have already attempted to devise a protocol for the VHV test which would maximize its diagnostic and educational potential while minimizing its unpleasantness and risks. One must also ascertain, however, that overbreathing has been adequate in order for the test to be valid, as indicated in the discussion of research studies above. The adequacy of VHV cannot be determined by observation of breathing movements alone. Lum suggests that for therapists in office or clinic practice without access to capnography, a suitable alternative measurement for this purpose is *spirometry,* that is, measurement of the amount of air moved. He recommends that nonmedics and nonphysiologists use the small, inexpensive, and relatively accurate Wright spirometer to determine whether the client is overbreathing to a standard minimum *minute volume* (see Chapter 1) of, say, 30 liters per min (L.C. Lum, 1991, personal communication).

7.4.4. Assessing the Sensations of Hyperventilation

The assessment of the sensations produced by hyperventilation is, like pain, based on introspective reports. While it has generally been observed that these sensations are unpleasant, cognitive psychologists have emphasized the influence of beliefs on the interpretation of such sensations. For example, Salkovskis and Clark (1990) suggest that the effects are actually neutral and that subjects' experiences (pleasant or unpleasant) of these sensations can be manipulated with positive or negative suggestion. Their two groups, however, were hyperventilated down to means of only 32.1 and 31.2 mm Hg, respectively, well above Gardner's previously mentioned criterion of 20 mm Hg. Even then, the "positive" group's mean rating of pleasantness was not significantly different from the zero rating of neutral. In contrast, normal subjects in the Bass *et al.* (1989) study hyperventilated to a mean below 15 mm Hg and rated VHV as unpleasant.

Since Bonn *et al.* (1984) was one of the largest recent studies of healthy volunteers ($n = 47$), their unpublished measurement data merit attention. Voluntary hyperventilation was administered by this author, carefully avoiding suggestion except for the necessary control of expectancy bias. Forty of the normal subject's Pco_2s were brought down below the 20 mm Hg criterion. The mean for 47 subjects was 17 mm Hg ±0.45 immediately after 3 min of VHV. Unfortunately, hedonic scales were not used, but subjects were interviewed and rated on the effects of VHV, the results of which are as follows: 83 percent (39 subjects) experienced mild or slight symptoms of hyperventilation; 13 percent (6 subjects), moderate; and 4 percent (2 subjects) such severe symptoms they could not continue overbreathing for 3 min. In common with most studies of VHV in normal subjects, a small percentage reported pleasant effects—one spontaneously mentioned feeling sexually aroused and another that he felt intoxicated.

The tenability of the challenging suggestion that VHV results in hedonically neutral experiences thus awaits more rigorous testing. Meanwhile, the data presently available on normal subjects, in accord with clinical impressions, support the view that the affective responses to hyperventilation are predominantly unpleasant for all but a few subjects, especially if VHV reduces Pco_2 to levels lower than 20 mm Hg.

Aside from subjective effects, the physical risks involved in administering a VHV test need also to be considered. While the probability of inducing seizures in clients who have no history of this disorder is small, there are other hazards, particularly in patients with complaints of chest pain (see Chapters 6 and 11). For most hyperventilators, however, the potential benefits of VHV apparently far outweigh the risks, if the procedure is done with appropriate caution.

7.4.5. Psychological Stressing

Many clients who hyperventilate episodically and/or whose symptoms are not evoked by VHV may be positive to individually significant psychological challenges. Their exhaled Pco_2 drops below a criterion level when they imagine such stressors, as described above. Dudley et al. (1969) and Nixon and Freeman (1988) reported decreases in Pco_2 as a result of psychological stressing without the use of prior hypnosis. On the other hand, Bass et al. (1989) observed only small decreases in Pco_2 with Fear Talk.

More than any other current procedure, psychological stressing for hyperventilation provocation makes explicit the relationship between breathing and emotional states. Because it is a powerful intervention, its use raises ethical questions. Conway, who is one of the most experienced in the use of psychological stressing, has found that the results depend on a relationship of trust being established with the client preceding the test. In addition, back-up support and counseling should be available to clients (and normal individuals) to deal with disturbing issues that are likely to emerge during the procedure (A.C. Conway, 1992, personal communication). Every effort was made in Conway's studies (Freeman *et al.*, 1986a; Conway *et al.*, 1988) to "end on a note of helpfulness" for the client. As with any new procedure, the role of psychological stressing in diagnosis of hyperventilation and in research remains to be clarified.

7.4.6. Hyperventilation Symptom Questionnaires

At least one aspect of this field appears to be relatively uncontroversial, namely, the frequently described symptoms of hyperventilation. Holloway emphasizes that therapists should obtain a *full* list of these symptoms during initial assessment of their patients for accurate monitoring of subsequent progress and feedback to the patient (see Chapter 11). Gibson (1978), in exhorting physical therapists to incorporate the principles of behavior therapy in their treatment of hyperventilators, reminds them of the importance of keeping careful records. Several symptom lists have been used in clinical studies: Clark and Hemsley (1982); Grossman and de Swart (1984); Legg *et al.* (1984); van Dixhoorn and van Duivenvoorden (1985); and Timmons *et al.* (1990). Comprehensive, validated lists would expedite history taking (which can be very time consuming with these patients), and would also facilitate comparison of therapeutic trials and systematic investigation of symptom categories. Few if any studies have looked at the association of symptoms with age, sex, personality traits, and causal factors, but clinicians have provided interesting leads. Lum (1978/1979), for example, has reported that the symptoms of cerebral hypoxia due to vasoconstriction are seen in almost all young patients but are less common in older hyperventilators because of the latters' decreased cerebrovascular reactivity. Patients complaining of skeletal or muscular pain typically do not experience the above symptoms.

Therapists as well as researchers would benefit from guidelines on standards and procedures for all the psychorespiratory measurements and instrument-monitored procedures described above. It may be some time before we have such guidelines since agreement even on the definition and diagnosis of the "hyperventilation syndrome" was not reached at the 1984 and 1988 International Symposia on Respiratory Psychophysiology. Given recent advances, however, it may soon prove productive to convene a consensus development conference.

8. Future Directions

In the Foreword to this volume, Patel makes the point that the increasingly technological medicine of today badly needs to be balanced by a humanistic approach, and that a book on breathing is therefore particularly timely. Perhaps one of the most timely contributions of this book is that it provides an alternative to the use of drugs in certain breathing-related disorders. This is a crucial historical moment for hyperventilators in particular. Patients are currently being told by some British general practitioners that tranquilizers are the only treatment available for hyperventilation. And in the United States, as noted above, a physician has deplored the recent "inappropriate" recommendations of psychotropics for hyperventilators, rather than breathing retraining and "simple office psychotherapy" (Kaplan, 1992). Unless the effectiveness of the approaches described in this book can soon be more fully demonstrated, drugs could become established as the treatment of choice even for those breathing-related disorders without associated pathology. Patients who hyperventilate could be maintained indefinitely on new, so-called nonaddictive tranquilizers, and patients with panic attacks maintained on antidepressants. Asthmatic patients could continue to have limited access to behavioral management as an adjunct to their medical treatment.

Patel also emphasizes the enduring benefits that breathing retraining may contribute as a component in multifactorial treatments. Medical researchers are providing evidence that treatment of illnesses can be more effective when combined with psychosocial interventions, as, for example, in Patel's multimodal approach to hypertension and coronary artery disease (Patel et al., 1985; Patel and Marmot, 1988). Other examples are the programs for life-style change in cardiac rehabilitation (Ornish et al., 1990; van Dixhoorn, 1990) and group psychotherapy in conjunction with medical treatment for cancer patients (Spiegel et al., 1989; Greer et al., 1992). There are as yet, however, only a very few studies that suggest the possible benefits of combining two or more components in treatment of breathing-related disorders (e.g., Bonn et al., 1984; Pinney et al., 1987; Kopp and Temesvary, 1990; Fensterheim and Wiegand, 1991; and DeGuire et al., 1992). The development of more holisticially oriented treatment programs will surely be one of the most important future directions for therapists in this field.

Many possible further directions for researchers have been suggested throughout this book, some of the most interesting of which may be the investigation of the role of respiratory variables in task performance, sexual behavior, and placebo responses. Many other questions regarding breathing-related disorders remain unanswered, from the basic physiological mechanisms and etiology of these disorders to the efficacy of the multifactorial therapies used to treat them.

Throughout the chapters of this volume there has been an emphasis on the reciprocal interaction of breathing and consciousness. The implications of this reciprocity for therapy and for research have been described in all their diversity by the various contributors. Breathing-related disorders involve complex interactions of physiological and psychological factors. Of these factors, the emotional processes associated with disturbed breathing are perhaps of most interest to therapists, but for researchers to ignore these processes might now be said to be unscientific as well as inhumane.

9. References

Alpher, V.S., and Blanton, R.L. Motivational processes and behavioral inhibition in breath holding. *Journal of Psychology,* 1991, *125,* 71–81.

Alpher, V.S., Nelson, R.B., and Blanton, R.L. Effects of cognitive and psychomotor tasks on breath-holding span. *Journal of Applied Physiology,* 1986, *61,* 717–721.

Ancoli, S., and Kamiya, J. Respiratory patterns during emotional expression. *Biofeedback and Self-Regulation,* 1979, *4,* 242.

Ancoli, S., Kamiya, J., and Ekman, P. Psychophysiological differentiation of positive and negative affects. *Biofeedback and Self-Regulation,* 1980, 5, 356–357.

Anderson, D.E., Austin, J., and Haythornthwaite, J.A. Blood pressure during sustained inhibitory breathing in the natural environment. *Psychophysiology,* 1993, *30,* 131–137.

Anderson, D.E., Coyle, K., and Haythornthwaite, J.A. Ambulatory monitoring of respiration: Inhibitory breathing in the natural environment. *Psychophysiology,* 1992, *29,* 551–557.

Backon, J. Nasal breathing as a treatment for hyperventilation. *British Journal of Clinical Practice,* 1989, *43,* 161–162.

Bancroft, J. *Human sexuality and its problems.* Edinburgh: Churchill Livingstone, 1989.

Bass, C. *Somatization: Physical symptoms and psychological illness.* Oxford: Blackwell, 1990.

Bass, C., and Gardner, W.N. Emotional influences on breathing and breathlessness. *Journal of Psychosomatic Research,* 1985, *29,* 599–609.

Bass, C., Lelliot, P., and Marks, I. Fear talk vs voluntary hyperventilation in agoraphobics and normals: A controlled study. *Psychological Medicine,* 1989, *19,* 669–676.

Blanton, R.L., and Alpher, V.S. Experimental models for psychophysiological studies of breathing. *Biological Psychology,* 1983, *16,* 285–286.

Bloch, S., Lemeignan, M., and Aguilera-T., N. Specific respiratory patterns distinguish among human basic emotions. *International Journal of Psychophysiology,* 1991, *11,* 141–154.

Bonn, J.A., Readhead, C.P.A., and Timmons, B.H. Enhanced adaptive behavioural response in agoraphobic patients pretreated with breathing retraining. *Lancet,* 1984, *ii,* 665–669.

Bradley, D. *Hyperventilation syndrome.* Auckland, New Zealand: Tandem, 1991; Berkeley, California: Ten Speed Press, 1992.

Brodtkorb, E., Gimse, R., Antonaci, F., Ellertsen, B., Sand, T., Sulg, I., and Sjaastad, O. Hyperventilation syndrome: Clinical, ventilatory, and personality characteristics as observed in neurological practice. *Acta Neurologica Scandinavica,* 1990, *81,* 307–313.

Cheraskin, E. and Ringsdorf, W.M. *Predictive medicine: A study in strategy.* Mountain View, California: Pacific Press, 1973.

Christiansen, B. *Thus speaks the body.* New York: Arno Press, 1972.

Clark, D.M. A cognitive approach to panic. *Behaviour Research and Therapy,* 1986, *24,* 461–470.

Clark, D.M., and Hemsley, D.R. The effects of hyperventilation; individual variability and its relation to personality. *Journal of Behaviour Therapy and Experimental Psychiatry,* 1982, *13,* 41–47.

Clark, M.E., and Hirschman, R. Effects of paced respiration on anxiety reduction in a clinical population. *Biofeedback and Self-Regulation,* 1990, *15,* 273–284.

Clausen, O. Respiratory movements in normal, neurotic, and psychotic subjects. *Acta Psychiatrica Scandinavica,* (suppl. 68), 1951, 1–74.

Conway, A.C., Freeman, L.J., and Nixon, P.G.F. Hypnotic examination of trigger factors in the hyperventilation syndrome. *American Journal of Clinical Hypnosis*, 1988, *30*, 296–304.

Corson, J.A., Grant, J.L., Moulton, D.P., Green, R.L., and Dunkel, P.T. Use of biofeedback in weaning paralyzed patients from respirators. *Chest*, 1979, *76*, 543–545.

Cowley, D.S., and Roy-Byrne, P.P. Hyperventilation and panic disorder: A review. *American Journal of Medicine*, 1987, *83*, 929–937.

de Beurs, E., Lange, A., Van Duck, R., and Koele, P. Respiratory training prior to exposure in vivo in the treatment of panic disorder with agoraphobia. *Biological Psychology*, 1990, *31*, 285.

DeGuire, S., Gevirtz, R., Kawahara, Y., and Maguire, W. Hyperventilation syndrome and the assessment of treatment for functional cardiac symptoms. *American Journal of Cardiology*, 1992, *70*, 673–677.

Dudley, D.L., Holmes, T.H., Martin, C.J., and Ripley, H.S. *Psychophysiology of respiration in health and disease*. New York: Appleton-Century-Crofts, 1969.

Eliade, M. *Yoga: Immortality and freedom*. Princeton, New Jersey: Princeton University Press, 1958.

Evans, J. Cognitive therapy starts to think big. *The Psychologist*, 1991, *4*, 556.

Evans, D.W., and Lum, L.C. Hyperventilation: An important cause of pseudoangina. *Lancet*, 1977, *i*, 155–157.

Faulkner, W.B. Effects of the emotions upon diaphragmatic function. *Psychosomatic Medicine*, 1941, *3*, 187–189.

Fensterheim, H., and Wiegand, B. Group treatment of the hyperventilation syndrome. *International Journal of Group Psychotherapy*, 1991, *41*, 399–403.

Folgering, H., and Colla, P. Some anomalies in the control of $paCO_2$ in patients with a hyperventilation syndrome. *Bulletin Europeen Physiopathologie Respiratoire*, 1978, *14*, 503–512.

Freeman, L.J., Conway, A.V., and Nixon, P.G.F. Physiological responses to psychological challenge under hypnosis in patients considered to have the hyperventilation syndrome: Implications for diagnosis and therapy. *Journal of the Royal Society of Medicine* (London), 1986a, *79*, 76–83.

Freeman, L.J., Conway, A.V., and Nixon, P.G.F. Heart rate response, emotional disturbance and hyperventilation. *Journal of Psychosomatic Research*, 1986b, *30*, 429–436.

Fried, R. *The hyperventilation syndrome*. Baltimore: Johns Hopkins, 1987.

Friedman, M. Studies concerning the aetiology and pathogenesis of neurocirculatory asthenia: IV. The respiratory manifestations of neurocirculatory asthenia. *American Heart Journal*, 1945, *30*, 557–566.

Gallego, J., and Perruchet, P. Classical conditioning of ventilatory responses in humans. *Journal of Applied Physiology*, 1991a, *70*, 676–682.

Gallego, J., and Perruchet, P. Effect of practice on the voluntary control of a learned breathing pattern. *Physiology and Behavior*, 1991b, *49*, 315–319.

Gallego, J., Perez de la Sota, A., Vardon, G., Jaeger-Denavit, E., and Jaeger-Denavit, O. Electromyographic feedback for learning to activate thoracic inspiratory muscles. *American Journal of Physical Medicine and Rehabilitation*, 1991a, *70*, 186–190.

Gallego, J., Perruchet, P., and Camus, J-F. Assessing attentional control of breathing by reaction time. *Psychophysiology*, 1991b, *28*, 217–224.

Garssen, B., de Ruiter, C., and van Dyck, R. Breathing retraining: A rational placebo? *Clinical Psychology Review*, 1992, *12*, 141–153.

Gibson, H.B. A form of behaviour therapy for some states diagnosed as "affective disorder." *Behaviour Research and Therapy*, 1978, *16*, 191–195.

Gorman, J.M., Fyer, M.R., Goetz, R., Askanazi, J., Liebowitz, M., Fyer, A.J., Kinney, J., and Klein, D.F. Ventilatory physiology of patients with panic disorder. *Archives of General Psychiatry*, 1988, *45*, 31–39.

Greer, S., Moorey, S., Baruch, J.D.R., Watson, M., Robertson, B.M., Mason, A., Rowden, L.,

Law, M.G., and Bliss, J.M. Adjuvant psychological therapy for patients with cancer: A prospective randomised trial. *British Medical Journal*, 1992, *304*, 675–680.

Grossman, P. Respiration, stress and cardiovascular function. *Psychophysiology*, 1983, *20*, 284–300.

Grossman, P., and De Swart, J.C.G. Diagnosis of hyperventilation syndrome on the basis of reported complaints. *Journal of Psychosomatic Research*, 1984, *28*, 97–104.

Grossman, P., De Swart, J.C.G., and Defares, P.B. A controlled study of a breathing therapy for treatment of hyperventilation syndrome. *Journal of Psychosomatic Research*, 1985, *29*, 49–58.

Haas, S.S. Relationships between individual differences in personality and respiratory behavior: An exploratory study. *Dissertation Abstracts International*, 1980, *41*, (4), 1483-B.

Haas, S.S., Axen, H., Ehlichman, H.E., and Haas, F. Relationship between personality characteristics and respiratory behavior. *The Physiologist*, 1980, *23*, 74.

Hornsveld, H., and Garssen, B. Voluntary hyperventilation: The influence of duration and depth on the development of symptoms. *Biological Psychology*, 1990, *31*, 284.

Horowitz, M.J. "Some psychodynamic aspects of respiration" in *Hyperventilation and hysteria: The physiology and psychology of overbreathing and its relationship to the mind–body problem*. Lowry (Ed.), Springfield, Illinois: C.C. Thomas, 1967.

Hough, A. *Physiotherapy in respiratory care: A problem-solving approach*. London: Chapman & Hall, 1991.

Hough, A. Physiotherapy for survivors of torture. *Physiotherapy*, 1992, *78*, 323–328.

Howell, J.B.L. Behavioural breathlessness. *Thorax*, 1990, *45*, 287–292.

Innocenti, D.M. Chronic hyperventilation syndrome. In Downey, P.A. (Ed.), *Cash's textbook of chest, heart and vascular disorders for physiotherapists*, 4th ed. London: Faber & Faber, 1987.

Jongmans, M., Cox, N., Dekhuijzen, P.N.R., and Folgering, H. Physiotherapy and the hyperventilation syndrome. *Biological Psychology*, 1990, *31*, 284–285.

Kaplan, N.M. Anxiety disorders and hyperventilation. *Archives of Internal Medicine*, 1992, *152*, 413.

Kerr, W.J., Dalton, J.W., and Gliebe, P.A. Some physical phenomena associated with anxiety states and their relationship to hyperventilation. *Annals of Internal Medicine*, 1937, *11*, 961–962.

Kerr, W.J., Gliebe, P.A., and Dalton, J.W. Physical phenomena associated with anxiety states: The hyperventilation syndrome. *California and Western Medicine*, 1938, *48*, 12–16.

King, J.C., Rosen, S.D., and Nixon, P.G.F. Failure of perception of hypocapnia: Physiological and clinical implications. *Journal of the Royal Society of Medicine*, 1990, *83*, 765–787.

Kitzinger, S. *Woman's experience of sex*. New York: Putnam's, 1983.

Kopp, M.S., and Temesvary, A. Respiratory control treatment of panic patients. *International Journal of Psychophysiology*, 1991, *9*, 48.

Legg, C.R., Sheridan, K., and Timmons, B.H. The 'hyperventilation syndrome': A factor analytic study. *Proceedings of the Fourth International Symposium on Respiratory Psychophysiology*, University of Southampton, 1984 (unpublished).

Lewis, T. *The soldier's heart and the effort syndrome*. London: Shaw & Sons, 1918.

Ley, R. Panic attacks during relaxation and relaxation-induced anxiety. *Journal of Behaviour Therapy and Experimental Psychiatry*, 1988, *19*, 253–259.

Ley, R. The many faces of Pan: Psychological and physiological differences among three types of panic attacks. *Behaviour Research and Therapy*, 1992, *30*, 347–357.

Ley, R. Breathing retraining in the treatment of hyperventilatory complaints and panic disorder: A reply to Garssen, de Ruiter, and van Dyck. *Clinical Psychology Review*, 1993, *13*, 393–408.

Ley, R., and Walker, H. Effects of carbon dioxide–oxygen inhalation on subjective anxiety, heart rate, and blood pressure. *Journal of Behaviour Therapy and Experimental Psychiatry*, 1973, *4*, 223–228.

Lowry, T.P. (Ed.), *Hyperventilation and hysteria: The physiology and psychology of overbreathing and its relationship to the mind–body problem.* Springfield, Illinois: C.C. Thomas, 1967.

Lum, L.C. Hyperventilation: The tip and the iceberg. *Journal of Psychosomatic Research,* 1975, *19,* 375–383.

Lum, L.C. "The syndrome of habitual chronic hyperventilation." In O.W. Hill (Ed.), *Modern trends in psychosomatic medicine,* vol. 3. London: Butterworths, 1976.

Lum, L.C. Breathing exercises in the treatment of hyperventilation and chronic anxiety states. *Chest, Heart and Stroke Journal,* 1977, *2,* 6–11.

Lum, L.C. Respiratory alkalosis and hypocarbia: The role of carbon dioxide in the body economy. *Chest, Heart and Stroke Journal,* 1978/1979, *3,* 31–34.

Lum, L.C. Hyperventilation and anxiety state. *Journal of the Royal Society of Medicine,* 1981, *74,* 1–4.

Lum, L.C. Physiological considerations in the treatment of hyperventilation syndromes. *Journal of Drug Research,* 1983, *8,* 1867–1872.

Lum, L.C. Hyperventilation syndromes in medicine and psychiatry: A review. *Journal of the Royal Society of Medicine,* 1987, *80,* 229–231.

MacGregor, R. Why diaphragmatic breathing? *Biological Psychology,* 1990, *30,* 294.

Mador, M.J., and Tobin, M.J. Effect of alterations in mental activity on the breathing pattern in healthy subjects. *American Review of Respiratory Disease,* 1991, *144,* 481–487.

Maddock, R.J., and Carter, C.S. Hyperventilation-induced panic attacks in panic disorder with agoraphobia. *Biological Psychiatry,* 1991, *29,* 843–854.

Mooney, N.A., Cooke, E.D., Bowcock, S.A., Hunt, S.A., and Timmons, B.H. Hyperventilation is associated with a redistribution of peripheral blood lymphocytes. *Biological Psychiatry,* 1986, *21,* 1324–1326.

Naifeh, K.H., Kamiya, J., and Sweet, M. Biofeedback of alveolar carbon dioxide and level of arousal. *Biofeedback and Self-Regulation,* 1982, *7,* 283–300.

Nixon, P.G.F., and Freeman, L.J. The 'think test': A further technique to elicit hyperventilation. *Journal of the Royal Society of Medicine,* 1988, *81,* 277–279.

Ornish, D., Brown, S.E., Scherwitz, L.W., Billings, J.H., Armstrong, W.T., Ports, T.A., McLanahan, S.M., Kirkeeide, R.L., Brand, R.J., and Gould, K.L. Can life style changes reverse coronary heart disease? *Lancet,* 1990, *336, 1,* 129–133.

Patel, C. *The complete guide to stress management.* London: Macdonald Optima, 1989; New York: Plenum Press, 1991.

Patel, C., and Marmot, M. Can general practitioners use training in relaxation and management of stress to reduce mild hypertension? *British Medical Journal,* 1988, *296,* 21–24.

Patel, C., Marmot, M.G., Terry, D.J., Carruthers, M., Hunt, B., and Patel, M. Trial of relaxation in reducing coronary risk: Four year followup. *British Medical Journal,* 1985, *290,* 1103–1106.

Patrick, J.M., and Western, P.J. Monitoring of breathing in ambulant subjects using a mobile respiratory inductance plethysmograph. *Journal of Ambulatory Monitoring,* 1991, *4,* 13–26.

Paul, G.L. Strategy of outcome research in psychotherapy. *Journal of Consulting Psychology,* 1967, *31,* 109–118.

Peper, E., and Tibbetts, V. Fifteen month followup with asthmatics utilizing EMG/incentive in-spirometer feedback. *Biofeedback and Self-Regulation,* 1992, *17,* 143–151.

Pfeffer, J.M., Cohen, S.I., and Hughes, D. "The psychiatrist and the chest physician." In F. Creed and J.M. Pfeffer (Eds.), *Medicine and psychiatry.* London: Pitman, 1982.

Pietroni, P.C., and Pietroni, M. Respiratory mechanisms and clinical syndromes. *Holistic Medicine,* 1989, *4,* 67–79.

Pinney, S., Freeman, L.J., and Nixon, P.G.F. Role of the nurse counsellor in managing patients with the hyperventilation syndrome. *Journal of the Royal Society of Medicine,* 1987, *80,* 216–218.

Richardson, P.H. "Placebos: Their effectiveness and modes of action." In A.K. Broome (Ed.), *Health Psychology: Processes and Applications*. London: Chapman Hall, 1989.

Ryle, A. *Cognitive analytic therapy: Active participation in change*. Chichester: John Wiley and Sons, 1990.

Salkovskis, P.M. Panic attacks: Cognitive-behavioural treatment. *Psychiatry in Practice*, Spring 1990, 17–21.

Salkovskis, P.M., and Clark, D.M. Affective responses to hyperventilation: A test of the cognitive model of panic. *Behaviour Research and Therapy*, 1990, *28*, 51–61.

Salkovskis, P.M., and Clark, D.M. Cognitive therapy for panic attacks. *Journal of Cognitive Psychotherapy*, 1991, *5*, 215–226.

Salkovskis, P.M., Clark, D.M., and Hackmann, A. Treatment of panic attacks using cognitive therapy without exposure or breathing retraining. *Behaviour Research and Therapy*, 1991, *29*, 161–166.

Sargent, W. The hyperventilation syndrome. *Lancet*, 1940, *1*, 314–316.

Schimmenti, J.M. The hyperventilating type of human female. *Journal of Nervous and Mental Diseases*, 1953, *118*, 223–236.

Spiegel, D., Bloom, J.R., Kraemer, H.C., and Gottheil, E. Effects of psychosocial treatment on survival of patients with metastatic breast cancer. *Lancet*, 1989, *2*, 888–891.

Staeubli, M., Bigger, K., Kammer, P., Rohner, F., and Straub, P.W. Mechanisms of the haematological changes induced by hyperventilation. *European Journal of Applied Physiology*, 1988, *58*, 233–238.

Stevenson, I., and Ripley, H.S. Variations in respiration and in respiratory symptoms during changes in emotion. *Psychosomatic Medicine*, 1952, *14*, 476–490.

Stough, C., and Stough, R. *Dr. Breath: The story of breathing coordination*. New York: Morrow, 1970.

Suess, W.M., Alexander, A.B., Smith, D.D., Sweeney, H.W., and Marion, R.J. The effect of psychological stress on respiration: A preliminary study of anxiety and hyperventilation. *Psychophysiology*, 1980, *17*, 535–540.

Svebak, S., Dalen, K., and Storfjell, O. The psychological significance of task-induced tonic changes in somatic and autonomic activity. *Psychophysiology*, 1981, *17*, 403–409.

Tavel, M.E. Hyperventilation syndrome—hiding behind pseudonyms? *Chest*, 1990, *97*, 1285–1288.

Timmons, B.H. Breathing pattern measurement and monitoring: State of the art: A meeting report. *Journal of Medical Engineering and Technology*, 1982, *6*, 112–116.

Timmons, B.H., and Meldrum, S.J. Behavioral applications of respiratory measurements. 1993 (in preparation).

Timmons, B., Salamy, J., Kamiya, J., and Girton, D. Abdominal–thoracic respiratory movements and level of arousal. *Psychonomic Science*, 1972, *27*, 173–175.

Timmons, B.H., Somerville, S.E., and Bonn, J.A. Hyperventilation tendencies in patients with panic attacks: Psychorespiratory measurements and clinical assessment. *Biological Psychology*, 1990, *30*, 274–275.

van Dixhoorn, J.J. *Relaxation therapy in cardiac rehabilitation*. M.D. dissertation, Erasmus University, Rotterdam, ISBN 90-9003834-5, 1990.

van Dixhoorn, J., and van Duivenvoorden, H.J. Efficacy of Nijmegen questionnaire in recognition of the hyperventilation syndrome. *Journal of Psychosomatic Research*, 1985, *29*, 199–206.

Webber, B.A. Evaluation and inflation in respiratory care. *Physiotherapy*, 1991, *77*, 801–804.

Western, P.J., and Patrick, J.M. Effects of focusing attention on breathing with and without apparatus on the face. *Respiration Physiology*, 1988, *72*, 125–130.

Wilson, G.F. (Ed.) Cardiorespiratory measures and their role in studies of performance. *Biological Psychology*, 1992, *34* (2,3) (special issue).

Wood, P. Da Costa's syndrome (or effort syndrome). *British Medical Journal*, 1941, *1*, 767–772; 805–811; 845–851.

Appendix

Publications of the Symposia on Respiratory Psychophysiology

1981   Timmons, B.H. Breathing pattern measurement and monitoring: State of the art (A meeting report). *J Med Eng Technol*, 1982, *6*, 112–116.

1982   Richter, R., and Timmons, B.H. (Eds.), Abstracts of papers presented at the Second Annual Workshop on Respiratory Psychophysiology. *Biol Psychol*, 1983, *16*, 285–297.

1983   Third International Workshop on Respiratory Psychophysiology, Bordeaux, September. *Bulletin Europeen Physiopathologie Respiratoire*, 1984, *20*, 83–95.

1984   Lewis, R.A., and Howell, J.B.L. Definition of the hyperventilation syndrome. *Bulletin Europeen Physiopathologie Respiratoire*, 1986, *22*, 201–205.

1985   Folgering, H. (Ed.), Abstracts of papers presented at the Fifth International Symposium on Respiratory Psychophysiology. *Biol Psychol*, 1986, *22*, 173–197.

1986   Alwen, J.J., and Rosser, R.M. Abstracts of papers presented at the Sixth International Symposium on Respiratory Psychophysiology. *Biol Psychol*, 1987, *25*, 73–92.

1987   von Euler, C., and Katz-Salamon, M. (Eds.), Abstracts of papers presented at the Seventh International Symposium on Respiratory Psychophysiology. *Biol Psychol*, 1989, *29*, 61–89.

von Euler, C., and Katz-Salamon, M. *Respiratory Psychophysiology.* Proceedings of an International Symposium held at the Wenner-Gren Center, Stockholm. Wenner-Gren International Symposium Series, No. 50. Basingstoke and London: Macmillan, 1988.

1988   Gardner, W.N. (Ed.), Hyperventilation: Current controversies of defi-
        nitions and diagnosis: Abstracts of papers presented at the Eighth An-
        nual Symposium on Respiratory Psychophysiology. *Biol Psychol,*
        1990, *30,* 265–283.

1989   Nixon, P.G.F., Nixon, S., and Timmons, B.H. Therapeutic ap-
        proaches to hyperventilation and asthma. Abstracts of papers presented
        at the Ninth Annual Symposium on Respiratory Psychophysiology.
        Biol Psychol, 1990, *30,* 285–298.

1990   Garssen, B., Wientjes, C., and Hornsveld, H. Abstracts of papers
        presented at the Tenth International Symposium on Respiratory Psy-
        chophysiology. *Biol Psychol,* 1991, *31,* 271–286.

1991   No symposium held.

1992   Gallego, J., and Guenard, H. (Eds.), Abstracts of papers presented at
        the 11th International Symposium on Respiratory Psychophysiology.
        Biological Psychology, 1993, *35,* 255–271.

1993   Adams, L. (Ed.), Abstracts of papers presented at the 12th Internation-
        al Symposium on Respiratory Psychophysiology. *Biological Psycho-
        physiology,* 1994 (in press).

1994   Ley, R. (Ed.), The psychophysiology of breathing: selected papers
        from the twelfth international symposium on respiratory psychophysi-
        ology. *Biofeedback and Self-Regulation,* 1994 (Special Issue), in press.

Author Index

Subject Index

OUR OWN
LIGHT

Logan Sage Adams

CONTENT WARNING

This novel includes the following sensitive topics that may trigger reactions for some readers: period-typical homophobia; period-typical sexism; references to past rape (not by one of the MCs), which resulted in the birth of a child; child labor (period-typical occurrence); references to the loss of a loved one; PTSD/survivor's guilt; references to past childhood trauma/emotional neglect; references to past parental rejection; and explicit sexual content involving consenting adults.

To my husband: Thank you for your unwavering support as I pursue my passion.

To my daughter: I hope that by watching me chase my lifelong dream, you will have the courage to someday chase yours, whatever it may be.

To my friend Tori: Thank you for encouraging me to start writing again.

To my beta readers and developmental editor: Thank you for your encouragement and suggestions. I couldn't have crafted this story without your help.

CHAPTER ONE

FLOYD

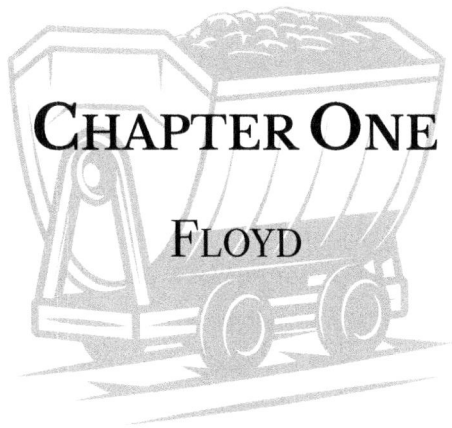

FLOYD BENNETT WAS BUSY trying to choose between peach and strawberry jam when a few beads of sweat trickled down his brow and mixed with the coal powder on his skin, clouding his eyes and burning his vision. For the next couple of seconds, Floyd's eyes continued to sting, and he squeezed them shut to try to stop the pain. Saying it was hot for May would have been an understatement. It was a scorcher.

When Floyd moved to wipe his face with the sleeve of his coal-stained shirt, someone slammed into him from behind, knocking him forward a little.

"Oh, Jesus, I'm sorry."

Arching an eyebrow, Floyd turned toward the unfamiliar voice. Someone he'd never seen before was looking up at him with what looked to be an earnest, if not slightly apologetic, smile. Floyd couldn't help but notice the man's eyes—both brown and green at the same time—and feel a little fascinated by them.

He watched those eyes flit over to the shelf behind him.

"Peach jam," the man said, wrinkling his nose. "Never cared for it. It's a little too sweet, in my opinion. Strawberry's not bad, though."

Without even waiting for a response, the man walked away, leaving Floyd to consider this stranger's opinion, one he hadn't even asked for. He turned back to the jam jars. Strawberry. Peach. He reached for the peach but hesitated and chose strawberry instead. Unsure whether or not he was even happy with his choice, Floyd left to find the stranger again.

Tall enough to see over the rows and rows of shelving, Floyd spotted the man easily a couple of aisles over. Pretending that he was browsing, Floyd followed and stopped in front of a section of canned soups a few feet away. He took notice of the way the stranger stuck out like a sore thumb in that fine clothing of his—a nicely tailored beige suit, complete with a brown silk tie and matching fedora—and wondered if he was from the city.

Could be that the fella was one of Don Chafin's men trying to sniff out folks who were trying to unionize. Floyd hadn't heard of that happening in Rock Creek yet, but still, his muscles tensed at the thought. Because the last thing Floyd needed was for that kind of uncertainty to make its way to Logan County—miners striking, families being forced out of their homes, folks losing work, fights breaking out. Unionizing seemed like it'd lead to a whole heap of trouble. Faced with that kind of chaos, Floyd would probably need to move his family elsewhere. Golly, he could barely even stomach the thought.

While Floyd was pretending to study the selection, the man moved to the next aisle. After placing a couple of cans of soup in his basket—the cheapest ones he could find—Floyd rounded the corner so that he could keep an eye on the stranger with the fancy-looking clothes. Lingering in front of the coffee tins, Floyd once again tried to look like he was working out which one to buy.

Out of the corner of his eye, Floyd watched the stranger walk up to the counter.

"Uhm, hello," the man said, catching the attention of Charlie Williams, the elderly fella who ran the company store. "I need to speak with Mister Donohue. Frederick, I mean. Frederick Donohue? I met with him in Charleston last week. We spoke about me starting to work for his coal company. He told me to come to the store today so that I could be set up with the proper housing and tools and, well, whatever else I might need. I kind of assumed he'd be the one to—"

"Oliver Astor?"

"Yes, that's me."

"Mister Donohue came here from Charleston yesterday to tell me 'bout you. We got room for you in the boardin' house."

Oliver would have to learn that everyone went to Charlie for everything, not Fred. Charlie had worked for Fred Donohue ever since the beginning. Whether you were converting currency or taking a loan or buying food from the store, Charlie was the one to talk to.

"Oh . . ." Oliver scrunched up his nose. "Frederick never mentioned a boarding house. I'd much prefer one of the single-family homes."

He'd prefer one of the single-family homes? Floyd wanted to tell this Oliver fella that he'd have to live wherever they told him to live. Housing was up to the company, not a miner.

"Do you got a family?" Charlie asked.

"Well, no."

Charlie crossed his arms over his chest, his patience clearly waning.

"Then I suppose you'll be livin' in the boardin' house."

Oliver let out a long sigh.

"Where's your telephone?" Oliver asked. "I'm sure I can clear this up with Frederick."

"We ain't got a telephone yet," Charlie said. "You can catch the train back to Charleston. I reckon they have a bunch in the city. You can call Mister Donohue's house from some business there."

Throwing his head back, Oliver let out a groan. Floyd had the impression that Oliver was someone who had never even had to share a closet, much less a bedroom, and certainly not with a bunch of other people. Floyd wasn't sure that Oliver'd even survive the boarding house.

"Aren't there over two hundred people living here? Why wouldn't there be a single fucking—" Floyd was already wincing from the swear word when Oliver seemed to catch himself, pausing for a moment before clearing his throat. "Why wouldn't there be a single telephone in the entire town?"

Floyd ran a hand over his face. Gosh, Oliver seemed lost. Floyd couldn't help but feel a tad sorry for him. Hadn't he ever been in the mountains before?

While Charlie and Oliver picked up bickering over the housing situation, Floyd considered how to help. He couldn't take listening to this no more.

"What about Fred's son?" Floyd asked, cutting in as he approached. "Ain't James got a telephone over at his place?"

Charlie sucked on his teeth, thinking this over.

"Can't say."

"Might as well check. He's probably home. He ain't never leave Rock Creek except on weekends. Not that I seen, anyway." Floyd came up next to Oliver. "I can take you."

"Oh, I wouldn't want to inconvenience you," Oliver said.

Floyd wasn't exactly in the mood for taking some uppity city fella across town, but he hated to think that Oliver might keep on bothering Charlie otherwise.

"It's a short walk."

"Oh, thank God," Oliver said, his shoulders relaxing and face brightening a little.

"Just need to pay for these," Floyd said before setting his basket on the counter.

While Charlie totaled the prices for the groceries, Floyd rocked back on his heels and tried not to think about the fact Oliver was staring—probably eyeing the coal powder coating near every inch of Floyd's skin and clothing. It felt strange to be looked at like that—like he was some sort of museum oddity. Floyd wondered whether Oliver had ever even seen a coal miner before.

After Charlie totaled the food items, Floyd reached into his pocket for some scrip—the currency issued by the coal company—and counted out the coins to pay.

Groceries paid for, Floyd took his poke from the counter and said, "Well, we better head out."

"Fine, yes," Oliver said, adjusting his hat. "Lead the way."

"Take care, Floyd," Charlie said after them.

Floyd held up his hand. "You, too, Charlie."

On the way out, Oliver stopped to study the hats on one of the hat racks.

"You know, these are pretty nice, considering," he said.

Considering what? Floyd wanted to ask but stopped himself. He wasn't exactly keen on listening to whatever Oliver would have to say on that subject. So, Floyd simply stood by while Oliver studied the selection for a bit before plucking one of the flat caps off its hook.

The moment Oliver removed his fedora, Floyd found himself mesmerized by Oliver's hair—blond like the color of wheat stalks. Not many men had light hair like that. Some kids, maybe, but not men. Just as Floyd started thinking on how soft it looked, Oliver fit the flat cap on his head and Floyd was left wondering where his own head was at.

"Why're you trying to be a miner?" Floyd asked, feeling the need for conversation.

"Just, you know, starting a new life," Oliver said before turning to face him. "What do you think? Not bad, right?" Floyd started to fumble through a response, but then Oliver plowed on like he had no real interest in Floyd's answer. "I noticed that people seem to be wearing flat caps here, not fedoras or bowlers. Maybe I'll fit in better if I buy one. I might have one already, come to think of it. I honestly can't remember. I'll have to check my bags before I purchase one."

"Bags?"

"They're scheduled to arrive sometime tonight," Oliver said, putting the hat back. "Christ, I hope I won't need to stay in the boarding house. I haven't a clue where I'd fit everything. It was a real chore to pack so much in so little time. I'm sure I'll have trouble sorting through the clothes I stuffed into various—"

It was clear by now that Oliver was talking to hear himself talk, not because he wanted to have a conversation. As Oliver prattled on about clothes and hats, Floyd thought back on what he had said about starting a new life. Oliver coming to Rock Creek was a curious thing. Even though Donohue Coal and Steel employed plenty of men who had come from other countries and neighboring communities—farmers who had recently sold their land, young men starting out in life, that sort of thing—not once had Floyd seen someone who looked like Oliver come to Rock Creek to look for work. Someone with that much money—a person who had too many hats to keep track of—ought to have been able to find work elsewhere, like in the city. Why Oliver would want to come to Rock Creek, well, that was a real puzzle.

Floyd couldn't resist the pull to try to solve it. He thought on it for a while. Oliver was still talking, but Floyd had stopped listening. Could be that Oliver was running away from something. Running away could make people act funny—move to faraway places, take whatever work they could find, try something new. If that was the case, Floyd supposed he couldn't fault Oliver for not knowing left from right.

"Come on," Floyd said, interrupting Oliver's babbling. "If I'm late for supper, my wife'll nail my ears to the wall."

Floyd continued toward the entrance, hoping Oliver would follow.

"Ah, was she the one Ivan Karamazov was referring to, then?" Oliver asked, catching up and chuckling like he had said something funny.

"What?"

Oliver pursed his lips and hummed. "Or maybe it was Dmitri?"

"Who are these people?"

"Oh. Sorry. I was trying to make a joke. *The Brothers Karamazov?*" Floyd silently cocked an eyebrow in response. "Obviously, that only works if you've read the book I was trying to reference. Of course, I may not have even had character right, so there's a chance that still wouldn't have been very funny even if you had read it." Oliver smiled sheepishly. "So, I take it you're not familiar with Dostoevsky, then?"

"I never heard of him."

"He's, uh, he's a Soviet novelist," Oliver said, a kind of reluctance in his tone. "I read his work in college. Well, some of his work."

If Oliver had been to college, why was he trying to work as a miner? Couldn't he be working in the city somewhere?

As though Oliver had magically read Floyd's mind, he said, "I never finished college, though. I was bored. Or something *like* boredom, anyway. I couldn't manage to keep my mind on the material. So, I stayed home for a while after that, but I needed to leave. You know how life is, or maybe how I should say how family is, or can be, with their expectations and obligations and everything." Floyd watched him blow out a long breath. "Anyway, I needed a change."

Floyd was staring at Oliver, thinking on how strange it was to meet someone else who had felt forced to leave home, when Oliver removed his hat again. Right away, the sight of Oliver's soft-looking blond locks wiped Floyd's mind plum clean. Oliver raked a hand through his hair, nervous-like, and Floyd was nearly overcome with the sudden urge to reach out and touch it.

Quickly, Floyd forced himself to look away. Wanting to touch Oliver's hair was a reminder—a swift kick in the behind—to hurry up and rid himself of this newcomer.

He started walking again, his feet kicking up little puffs of dirt with each step.

"True enough," Floyd said. He knew what it was like to feel the weight of family obligations. He had felt that way plenty helping out on his family's farm as a kid. "You still never really explained your comment, though. About my wife."

"Well, it wasn't about your wife, really, but what you said about her nailing your ears to the wall. Dostoevsky had a line like 'a tiger would never think of nailing people by the ears, even if he were able to.'"

"What's it mean?"

"It's . . . well . . . people are cruel. Uniquely cruel. Worse than tigers, worse than beasts," Oliver explained. "Or that's the point of the view of the character who said it. I'm not sure if Dostoevsky believed it himself."

Well, that was a sad sort of belief, wasn't it? Floyd hadn't never thought that people—people as a whole—were beastly. Even when he had been forced to leave McDowell County, he hadn't never felt that way. Did Oliver feel like this Dostoevsky fella?

"Do you believe it?" Floyd asked.

Oliver shrugged. "I think so. Sometimes."

It seemed peculiar that someone like Oliver had such a hard-bitten attitude about other people. He was dressed in Sunday's finest on a weekday, and his "Sunday's finest" looked nicer than most any outfit Floyd had seen for some time. Oliver must have had his secrets. Which was fine. Floyd had his, too.

Floyd realized that he must have been wearing a sour expression when Oliver started chattering on like he felt the need to explain himself for that remark about people being cruel.

"Not like my opinion is an enlightened one, though. I'm pretty sure I was supposed to have some kind of revelation about the inherent goodness of mankind or the importance of faith or something, but I never felt any of that. Maybe because I never finished the book."

Floyd saw an opportunity to lighten the mood.

"Sounds like you tend not to finish things."

Oliver smiled at that. "Yeah. Apparently not."

Floyd couldn't make himself keep up the conversation. He couldn't really talk about Soviet novelists. Or most novelists. By now, Oliver had stopped talking, too, which meant that they could enjoy the sights and sounds of nature.

While they walked the path that ran alongside the train tracks, Floyd noticed Oliver looking beyond it, his eyes fixed on the mountainside, which was really something to see in the springtime—near every inch of the hills covered in lots of shades of green. Seeing Oliver captivated by the sight had Floyd's chest swelling with pride. Wherever Oliver was from, he likely hadn't seen the kind of beauty that nature had to offer out here in the mountains.

Minutes passed. As Floyd was listening to the chirping of birds in the surrounding forest, like the high-pitched *cheep-cheep-cheep* of the song sparrow, he was happy to realize that Oliver could, in fact, keep quiet for a while. Not that there was nothing wrong with Oliver's rambling, but Floyd had become comfortable with silence, especially when on his walks through town or in the woods. Most of the time, Floyd kept to himself. He had come to like it that way.

As they neared Donohue's place, Floyd could hear children playing over in the fields, and soon, there was a sudden series of whistles, one after another after another, like everyone was singing in a round. It continued on and off for a bit.

"What's that?" Oliver asked.

"Dinner time. Moms whistling to call their children home."

"Ah, that's nice. Wholesome, even," Oliver said. "I was never permitted to roam like that. Farthest I had ever been was our backyard. So I spent a lot of time inside reading. I still read a lot, though I tend to abandon books when I'm three-quarters of the way through. I mean, I can typically sense how they end by that point, so . . ." He shrugged, and there were a few seconds of silence. Floyd was wondering whether Oliver wanted him to say something in response to that when Oliver picked right up talking some more. "Reading is my favorite activity, I think, aside from piano, though sometimes I wonder if I really enjoy piano or if I only like that I'm not too terrible of a pianist. I'm inclined to say that I like it, though. It's only been a week since I left home, and I find myself missing it already." Talk, talk, talk. Oh well. At least Oliver had a nice voice, one that wasn't bad to listen to. "What about you, Floyd? Did your mom whistle for you to come home when you were little?"

Oliver's question caught Floyd by surprise, both because Floyd was impressed that Oliver could even remember what they had been talking about before his mouth had taken off like a racehorse and because no one had asked him about his family for a long time. Suddenly, a handful of bittersweet memories were resurfac-ing—moments that managed to make Floyd smile even though they were painful—like little heart-shaped bruises of the mind.

"Yeah," Floyd said. "In her own way."

"What do you mean?"

Floyd supposed sharing a story couldn't hurt.

"She couldn't hardly whistle. Still, she expected me to come home on time. If I listened real close, I could hear this right pathetic attempt of hers, one so quiet it sounded more like wind moving through tree branches. Sometimes, when I really wanted to keep playing, I'd pretend I never even heard her." Floyd laughed to himself. "When I'd come home, she'd say something like, *'Why're you so late? Ain't you hear me whistling for you?'* and I'd lie right to her face saying, *'No, ma'am, I swear I never heard a thing.'*"

Despite the twinge of pain that nearly always accompanied thoughts of his mother, Floyd found himself happy to have shared the memory with someone.

"I love that," Oliver said with a warm laugh. "It's sweet."

Floyd noticed, then, that Oliver had a real nice laugh. It was a kind one, the type of laugh that made others happier for hearing it. Suddenly, it was like the memory hurt a little less.

Floyd kind of wanted to share some more with him. Oliver talked a lot, but the man hadn't been born without listening ears, it seemed.

"I like to think that my mom's poor whistling is the reason I can hear better than most folks I've met. Made me a real sharp hunter."

"Wow. I've never even shot a rifle in my entire life."

"Now I *know* you must be from the city," Floyd said. "I been hunting since I was a kid."

"Lucky," Oliver remarked, which was a nice thing to hear. Floyd hadn't expected that from someone like Oliver. "I've never spent much time in nature, mostly because of my parents. Honestly, I've always been fascinated by places like this—little towns tucked away in the mountains. It's one of the reasons I wanted to move here."

"Well, there's plenty to like out here—birds and wildflowers and such."

"I can tell," Oliver said, still beaming. "Thank you for taking me to find a telephone so that I can try to talk to Frederick. Or maybe James will be able to help. I can't imagine myself staying in a boarding house. Trust me, it'll be better for everyone if I have my own space. I know what I'm like. Someone would probably smother me in my sleep before the week is out."

Floyd nearly choked on his spittle. What kind of person would talk like that about themselves? And to someone they'd only known for fifteen or twenty minutes? What a funny thing.

Oliver seemed to take some kind of offense to Floyd's non-response.

"Uh, you know, because of my mouth?" Oliver clarified, as though Floyd needed the explanation for him to properly appreciate the humor.

Sure enough, something in the eagerness of Oliver's expression, coupled with the words he had said, made Floyd laugh.

"Are you referring to your constant talking or the swear words you seem to like peppering in from time to time?" Floyd had to ask.

Oliver answered without hesitation. "Both. Definitely both."

Floyd snorted and shook his head. "Funny man."

"Thank you."

They came to the long dirt drive at the end of the road, the one that led up to James Donohue's mansion.

Floyd pointed to it and said, "Well, that's the house. Good luck trying to figure out your situation."

"Thanks," Oliver said. "I hope your ears are intact the next time I see you."

Floyd smirked. "Yeah, we'll see."

After the two of them parted, Floyd started for home. He only made it a few paces before having to contend with the urge to look over his shoulder. Floyd felt some strange kind of pull toward Oliver. He wasn't sure why. Just an interesting fella, Floyd supposed. Oliver wasn't really like anyone else Floyd had ever met. For one thing, no one else in Rock Creek ever prattled on like Oliver, which made him pretty interesting to talk to. For another, Oliver was funny. His sense of humor was a little off, but Floyd was surprised to find that he kind of liked it. Last, but certainly not least, Oliver was handsome. He had that nice smile and that soft-looking yellow hair and those eyes that were a real unusual color. He was tall, too. Not that much shorter than Floyd was, which was really saying something, and had been wearing that fine-looking clothing. Yup, Oliver was a handsome fella, for sure.

Jeez, what in the world was wrong with him? It had been years since he had let himself think about a man's looks like that.

When Floyd looked over his shoulder for the third time (Lord help him, he was counting), Oliver was quite a ways away, nearly at the front door of Donohue's house, and so Floyd paused to watch him for a bit. While Floyd was busy thinking 'bout that friendly sounding laugh Oliver had, Oliver looked over his shoulder, too. And then their eyes met, and Floyd's stomach tumbled. After a quick wave, Floyd turned back around and continued home.

It wasn't long before Floyd reached his house. It was a near duplicate of the other homes closest to the train tracks—a single-story dwelling with white siding and a front porch. As soon as he stepped inside, Josephine came running toward him, her long blonde hair swishing back and forth with each step. Kneeling, Floyd set his poke by his feet and held out his arms for her to barrel into. It made him so happy that she was still so excited to see her daddy every evening.

"Josephine May," he said, wrapping his arms around her. "I missed you."

"I missed you, too," she said before pulling away. "Want to see a new trick I learned?"

"Sure, pretty lady."

Josephine planted her palms flat on the floor and proceeded to kick her legs up in the air. For a split second, she balanced perfectly, but then tumbled sideways and crashed into the rocking chair to her right, making it topple. Even though she'd landed with a loud thud, she only cackled. Floyd couldn't remember the last time she so much as whimpered from falling, let alone cried from it. Stubborn and feisty, Josephine was a force to be reckoned with.

"I had it earlier, I swear."

Her comment—"I swear"—made Floyd think of Oliver and that big mouth of his.

Floyd wagged his finger in a playful manner. "No swearing in this house."

He looked up to see his wife, Effie, watching with a hand on her hip, her short honey-brown hair hidden beneath the white silk scarf she had tied around her head. Gosh, she was beautiful. In the eight years they had been married, she had only become prettier. Not only was Effie's new, shorter haircut flattering for her heart-shaped face, but the crow's feet that now lingered in the corners of her eyes were nothing if not becoming. In moments like these, Floyd nearly found himself wishing he could feel something more than friendship toward her.

"If she's swearing, I promise she hasn't picked it up from me," Effie teased.

Floyd picked up the poke and pushed himself to stand. "Jo was showing me how she can balance on two hands."

"Josephine, if you keep this up, you're fixing to break your neck," Effie scolded in a light-hearted manner before pointing over to the hallway. "Now that you're covered in coal dust, you better wash up."

With a pout, Josephine skulked off to wash her hands in the basin. Effie narrowed her eyes at Floyd in a jokey manner, and Floyd feigned innocence in return, shrugging his shoulders and looking away.

"You and her are so alike," Effie said. "If Josephine was a boy, she'd be trying to work right alongside you in the mines."

"She's only seven."

"You think that'd stop her? I'm pretty sure she'll chop off that hair of hers and follow you to work soon enough," Effie said with a sigh. "She's a tomboy, alright. Always climbing trees and learning new stunts. I caught her with a slingshot yesterday."

"What can I say, Effie? Guess she takes after me."

Effie pursed her lips, an obvious attempt to contain her smile.

"I'm no scientist, but I'm pretty sure that ain't how it works."

"Mmm . . . I disagree." Floyd lowered his voice to a whisper. "I may not be her father, but I am her daddy. I learned her everything she knows."

He wrapped his free arm around Effie, who immediately elbowed him in the side.

"Are you trying to ruin my clothes?" she asked.

Before Floyd could answer, Josephine called out as she returned.

"All clean!" she said. "Can we eat now?"

Effie looked up at Floyd. "You better wash up, too."

"Yes, ma'am."

Once Floyd had finished washing up and had changed out of his work clothes, the three of them sat at the table for supper—cornbread, baked beans, and coleslaw. It was one of their most frequent meals, but Floyd still loved it. He eagerly dipped a hunk of cornbread into the bean sauce. Josephine copied him.

"You were later than usual today," Effie said, poking at her coleslaw with a fork. "Something happen at the mine?"

"No," Floyd answered. "I met a strange fella at the store. He's from the city. Or *a* city. Dressed all fancy and such. He wants to be a miner. Was trying to convince Charlie that he was owed a single-family home even though he ain't a family man. I took him over to James Donohue's place. Maybe the two of 'em will work something out."

"That was nice of you."

"Yeah, well, he wouldn't last in the boarding house. Trust me."

"Why do you allow he's here? Sounds like he has money."

"Coming out of his ears, I suspect," Floyd confirmed. "I wonder if he was forced to leave home. He kind of made it sound that way. Said he wanted to start a new life."

"Ah, so *that's* why you stepped in to help him."

Floyd shifted uncomfortably. "Nah, I was helping him before that," he said, though he knew that Effie was on to something.

Josephine piped up. "What do you mean by that, Mama?"

"Nothing, baby," Effie said, petting Josephine's hair. "Make sure you eat your coleslaw."

Floyd returned his attention to the food in hopes that Effie wouldn't keep pressing, especially now that Josephine had reminded them both that she was listening. While Floyd had initially only helped Oliver because he was feeling sort of bad for him (and for Charlie), he couldn't pretend that Effie's comment was empty of truth. Oliver saying that he had come to Rock Creek to start a new life had caught Floyd's interest for certain.

Thinking back on it now, Floyd's stomach started to feel a little fluttery. Who'd have thought that someone like Oliver might show up in their little coal town?

Over the next couple of minutes, Floyd started thinking of his hometown and how he and Effie had been forced to leave. Sadness came over him—one so heavy it was making his body feel heavy, too. Moving the coleslaw with his fork, Floyd started wondering about his folks—how they were, whether they still owned their farm, whether they had been forced to sell their land to one of the coal companies—and heaved a sigh, forcing the memories away. Within a heartbeat, his thoughts returned to Oliver instead.

CHAPTER TWO

OLIVER

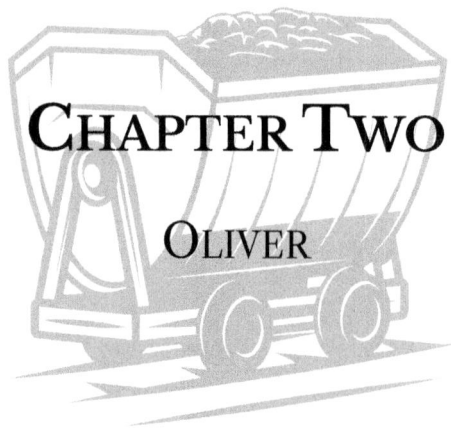

OLIVER WOKE UP LATE. Well, not late, really, but much later than he had intended for his first shift at the mines. Glancing at his watch, Oliver supposed he could still make it to work on time if he left without eating breakfast. But that wouldn't be smart, would it? He needed the energy. Especially since he hadn't ever worked before. Helping his father with finances barely constituted a job. Not when compared to something like coal mining, anyway.

Sitting up, Oliver stretched his arms over his head and looked around the bedroom—mostly bare, save for the full-size bed, a small desk, an empty bookcase (which he had every intent of filling sooner or later, even if it required a couple of trips to Charleston), and half of his luggage (the other half was still piled up in the main room).

As Oliver walked to the living space, he remembered that he'd have to venture outside to relieve himself. He'd had indoor plumbing back in New York City, but there weren't many homes like that in Rock Creek. Well, even if his home was lacking in plumbing, it was still probably better than the boarding house. Good thing James Donohue was a businessman. Oliver hadn't been able to reach Frederick, but James had been able to be convinced, with the help of a bit of money, to follow Oliver back to the company store and have Charlie set him up in one of the recently vacant single-family homes.

After Oliver finished relieving himself, he fetched some water from the water pump to wash up in the basin and then changed into what would have to be his temporary work clothes—an old pair of tan slacks and his least favorite button-up shirt.

Even though Oliver had remembered to buy everything else he'd need for his first shift—blasting caps and powder, a pickaxe, an oil lamp, and a shovel—he had forgotten to purchase more suitable work clothing. He'd have to visit the company store later to find a pair of overalls, maybe, and some better work boots. He still had plenty of money left. Too much, probably, for him to need to be a miner, but he liked the idea of earning money for a change. Coal mining would be such an adventure, too. And Rock Creek was the perfect place for him to try it. Since the town was unincorporated, his parents would have a harder time ever finding him. God, he couldn't stomach the thought of his father someday contacting him, only to shame him for not wanting to follow in his footsteps.

After eating a simple breakfast of puffed rice cereal—sans milk—Oliver packed up his work tools and headed toward the mine. During his short walk, Oliver tried to enjoy the wildflowers—sporadic patches of blueish-purple flowers and bright yellow ones behind the rows of houses.

Unfortunately, Oliver's pleasant walk was followed by a very *un*pleasant elevator ride into the mine. It was so rickety, his entire body vibrated the entire time. It felt like his brain was being scrambled. God, the shaking was frightening. Oliver kept wondering whether or not it was actually safe.

Once Oliver reached the bottom, he was surprised to see that no one else was around. Well, no one except for a boy who was manning the tunnel entrance, one who couldn't have been more than ten, which was kind of strange. Wasn't the legal working age fourteen? Or maybe thirteen? Whatever it was, it sure as hell couldn't have been *ten*. Oliver put on his friendliest smile and approached the boy, who was eyeing him with suspicion.

"Hi," Oliver said, feeling woefully unprepared for this interaction. "I thought I might find a fellow miner or two out here, but it seems like everyone is already hard at work. Not that you aren't a miner, too, of course. Shit. Sorry."

"You ain't one of Chafin's men, are you?"

"Who?"

"Good," the boy said, seemingly satisfied with Oliver's non-answer. "You need to take your tab off the brass board."

"Tab?" Oliver asked before suddenly remembering. "Oh!" Frederick had mentioned the brass board when Oliver had eaten lunch with him in Charleston. Oliver tried to remember his number. One hundred thirteen? Thirteen was a fairly unfortunate number to have been assigned, especially since Oliver knew he'd need all the luck he could find to make a life for himself out here, but hopefully the "one hundred" would make the "thirteen" matter less. He walked over to the board and found the hook with brass circles numbered 113, but for some reason, there were two little tabs, not one. He walked back over to the entrance. "Why are there two?"

When the boy subsequently smacked his forehead head with his palm, Oliver realized what a monumentally naïve question that must have been.

"Before you head inside, you take one tab with you. When you come back, you match it with its twin."

"Oh, I see. Clever. Gotta keep *tabs* on everyone."

Silence.

Feeling a little silly for what had apparently been a misplaced attempt at humor, Oliver walked back to the brass board, took his tab, and shoved it into his pocket. After the boy opened the door, Oliver crept inside. Anxious excitement buzzed beneath his skin. As soon as it shut behind him, he realized that he had no idea where he was supposed to go or what he was supposed to do. Hopefully, he could find someone who would be willing to show him the ropes.

Touching one hand to his shoulder strap to reassure himself that his pack was still present, Oliver started down the corridor. It was fascinating the way it was laid out like a little city. Some roads were wider than others, some branched off in one direction only to circle back to the main avenue, and some were occupied while others were empty. Oliver passed several men who were hard at work shoveling coal into cars, which looked like something he would be capable of, even on his first morning, but for some reason, he couldn't bring himself to try to talk to them.

Remembering how helpful that man Floyd had been the previous evening, Oliver tried to find him instead, but even after a half hour of searching, he wasn't able to.

Determined not to be completely useless, Oliver continued to traverse the underground city, exploring the various caverns and corridors, all the while trying to find someone who could teach him how and where to extract the coal. He wondered when everyone else had learned. Perhaps as children?

The thought entered Oliver's mind like a revelation. Children! Back at the entrance, the boy manning the door had been helpful (though a bit of a bastard about it). Maybe there were other children working in the mines, too. Oliver felt a little nauseated thinking about that. Mining wasn't exactly safe. He hoped none of the children were ever forced to participate in tasks that could lead to serious bodily harm.

After a moment, Oliver forced himself not to linger on those thoughts. He needed to fit in here, not criticize these people.

Holding tight to the horrible hope that other children might be working somewhere, Oliver continued to search. Sure enough, Oliver soon came across a whole room filled with children, most of whom looked to be between eight and twelve, seated on wooden benches near the coal chutes, their legs stuck inside piles of coal. One of the oldest boys was walking between the rows. He seemed to have some kind of authority.

"Hello," Oliver said, coming closer. "I'm new." He paused to consider if it would be possible for him to say what he needed to say without sounding completely inept. Probably not. "And I have no idea how to mine coal yet. You see, it was kind of impromptu, me moving here, and, well, I think Frederick—the, uh, coal company operator—only hired me because . . . well, probably because he thought that I'd lost my mind and, so, you know, maybe he felt sorry for me. Or maybe he thought it would be funny if I failed. I paid his son James, too, which I realize now sounds pretty strange, because you're not supposed to pay your employer, are you? But uhm . . ." The boy was looking at Oliver like he had sprouted an extra head. He'd better jump to the point. "Anyway, I want to be useful while I'm waiting for someone to show me what I need to do in there. Maybe I can work here for now instead? Do you need some help?"

"Can you sort coal?"

"Probably," Oliver answered. "Uhm, how, though?"

"Just make sure you remove the rocks and slate and such. Break up some of the larger chunks, too."

Oliver answered with more confidence than he actually possessed. "I can do that."

When Oliver sat at one of the benches, it was immediately apparent to him that he was much too large for the spot. In order to reach the coal, he had to hunch over in a ridiculous way. Besides that, his knees were sticking out far enough to intrude on the spaces of the boys beside him. He probably looked very silly. Worse, he would probably be uncomfortable soon. Oh well.

For the next couple of minutes, Oliver watched the boy next to him. He came to the conclusion that he could, in fact, sort coal. It looked easy enough.

Within the hour, Oliver realized he had been mistaken.

It wasn't that the task was particularly complicated, but holy hell, was it tiring. Not only tiring, but painful, too. By lunchtime, Oliver's hands were completely cut up, his fingers swollen, his skin a fiery red. He supposed this was why most boys had been wearing gloves.

When it was finally time for a break, Oliver realized that in his morning haste, he had completely forgotten to pack something to eat. He wondered what the other miners even brought with them to the coal fields. Back in New York, Oliver's favorite lunch had been pineapple upside-down cake, which his mother liked to have their cook bake every couple of weeks. Remembering the tangy-sweet taste was making his mouth water.

Deciding that it might be best to head home early, Oliver left the mine. At the surface, he spotted Floyd sitting in the shade of a sugar maple with two other men. Before Oliver could figure out whether or not he wanted to approach, Floyd laughed a big, boisterous laugh, one that was so enthusiastic Oliver found himself smiling a little. Yes, he would try.

When Oliver reached the edge of the tree shade, Floyd looked over and the two of them locked eyes. Oliver found himself admiring the way that the light sparkled in Floyd's baby blues.

"Hello," Oliver said. "Do you mind if I sit with you?"

"We're finishing up, but I can stay and keep you company while you eat your lunch," Floyd said.

Oliver let out a little puff of air. "Well, funny thing, I forgot to bring one."

"Do you want the last bites of my sandwich?" Floyd offered.

One of the other miners spoke up, too. "I ain't eating the rest of my strawberries. You can have 'em if you want."

"Thank you," Oliver said, the rush of gratitude making his chest swell as he settled next to them. "That's very kind of you." He held out his hand to the middle-aged man who had offered him the fruit. "I'm Oliver."

"Roy Johnson."

When Roy took Oliver's hand, a tiny zip of pain shot up the length of Oliver's arm, causing him to wince, though he tried his best to hide it behind a smile.

As soon as Oliver released Roy's hand, the other miner offered his. At least Oliver would be prepared for the sting this time.

"John Straub."

"Nice to meet you."

Oliver couldn't stop himself from looking longingly at the ripe red fruit resting on a cloth at the bottom of Roy's copper-colored lunch pail. Roy scooped up the cloth, folded it closed, and handed it to Oliver.

"Strawberries are my favorite," Oliver said, hoping to communicate how thankful he was, except, as usual, he couldn't seem to stop himself from babbling. "Or boysenberries. Or blueberries. All fruit is delicious, really. Except pears." He suddenly became worried he might have inadvertently insulted one of the others. "I'm not trying to offend anyone who likes pears, of course. I'm sure it's only me who thinks they're terrible."

Everyone laughed. Oliver forced a laugh, too, though he was worried about whether or not these men found him funny in a ha-ha way or funny in a *wow, take a look at this fellow* kind of way. Embarrassed by his rambling, Oliver started on the strawberries.

"We'll see you inside, Floyd," Roy said, turning to leave.

Floyd responded with a wave and then reached for the scraps of his sandwich.

"I only eat the crust if I skip breakfast," Floyd explained, placing the pieces on the cloth next to the strawberries. "Don't tell Effie. She'll poke fun of me for it. I like to throw the leftovers to Roy's pigs on the way home."

"Is Effie your wife?"

"Yup, she is."

"How long have you been married?"

"Almost eight years."

"I can't even commit to a favorite fruit, and you've been married for eight years."

"You were plenty certain about your least favorite."

"Oh, I have no trouble identifying things I *don't* like," Oliver said. "I only have trouble figuring out what I *do* like. I've always been that way." He tossed the strawberry stem into the bushes. "I'm sorry if you enjoy pears, by the way. Right after I said they were terrible, I realized that I probably sounded like an ass."

"Mmm, a little."

"I think I came across that way yesterday, too. At the store, I mean, when I was looking at hats."

"Yeah, you did," Floyd confirmed, though he shrugged like he wasn't bothered by it.

Oliver was surprised that even though Floyd was agreeing with him so readily and openly about his previously horrible behavior, he hadn't tried to make Oliver feel bad about it, nor had he reassured Oliver that it was fine. It was like Floyd had only been stating a fact. Strangely enough, there was some comfort in that—in honesty for honesty's sake.

When Oliver moved to pick up one of the sandwich crusts, Floyd sucked in a breath through his teeth and the sound startled Oliver out of his thoughts.

"What?"

Floyd's face was screwed up with what looked like revulsion. Oliver realized that Floyd was staring at his hands.

"Red tips," Floyd answered.

Which was probably what this lovely ailment was called. Oliver's face warmed. It had probably become even redder than his pathetic, swollen fingers.

"I spent the morning sorting coal."

"Is that what Fred Donohue told you to do?"

"No, but I couldn't find anyone to show me what else I was supposed to do. For some reason, I thought that when I came in today, there would be someone who would be paired up with me or something," Oliver said. "Very naïve, I'm sure."

"You ought to have come found me."

"I walked around for a while, but I couldn't really tell Dick from Harry in the mine."

Floyd continued to look at Oliver's hands, and Oliver's face continued to burn. Oh, he was so embarrassed about them.

"Goose grease'll help," Floyd said. "If you can come over to my house later, I'll make sure Effie fixes you up."

Floyd's offer made Oliver's stomach feel a little funny. He wasn't used to being cared for. Even in small ways.

"Thank you."

"If you want, you can be my shadow from here on out. I won't mind. I was working with a kid named Billy, but now that I been with him for a couple of weeks, I think I'm realizing that he ain't really ready to work with me yet. Still too young."

"So, can you teach me how to be a proper miner then?"

Floyd smiled in what looked to be a playful manner. "Well, maybe not a proper miner, but I can learn you how to be a regular one."

"Regular is fine," Oliver said, now smiling, too. "Preferable, even."

Oliver marveled at how wonderful it was to connect with someone so easily. He hadn't expected that when he'd set up the meeting with Frederick in the city. He had only been hoping to escape from his past. And his future.

Truthfully, Oliver had assumed that he'd never really bond with anyone in a coal town, which had been part of the appeal. He was tired of rejection. Over the years, Oliver had been rejected by his parents so many times, in so many ways, whether they had been cold to him when he had needed comfort, even from something as simple as a skinned knee, or whether they had been completely unsympathetic to the struggles he'd sometimes faced with his schoolwork, like his inability to finish his assignments.

Oliver's heart simply hadn't been able to take it anymore.

But maybe he'd been wrong about not bonding with anyone here. Floyd seemed to be friendly enough, at least. And Oliver was plenty happy about that.

Floyd tapped Oliver's foot with his own.

"Hurry up, slow poke."

"Right." Oliver picked up another strawberry. "Sorry."

Throughout the afternoon, Oliver followed Floyd around the mine. Floyd showed him how to blast the coal seams (though Oliver hadn't touched the blasting powder himself) and break the coal. While they worked, Floyd taught Oliver about some of the other roles that were fulfilled by children, too—like spraggers, who controlled the speed of the coal cars, and mule drivers, whose task was obvious from their title.

By the end, they hadn't collected much coal—maybe only half a car's worth—which had Oliver worried, especially when Floyd informed him that they weren't paid by the hour, but by the weight of their coal car, but Floyd told Oliver that it was fine. Still, Oliver's stomach sank when he saw everyone else's coal cars and compared them to Floyd's. He offered that they not split the money and instead, Floyd could keep the entirety of their earnings, but Floyd refused.

While walking to Floyd's house, Oliver's stomach continued to feel full in a nauseating sort of way, though he tried not to let it show. He couldn't help but feel horrible that Floyd had taken the time to train him and had made less money as a result. Having someone show him such kindness still felt so foreign.

Around ten minutes later, they arrived, and when they walked through the threshold, Oliver's heart practically leapt up into his throat from the surprise presence on the other side. Oliver was very much not prepared to be confronted with a little girl's high-pitched shriek.

"Baby girl!" Floyd exclaimed, throwing his arms around her. "How was school?"

Seeing the way she beamed up at Floyd had Oliver's heart melting, even while he was still frozen in fear from having been completely frazzled by the child's scream. While Oliver was listening to Floyd's child tell him about school, a very pretty woman approached.

"Hi, I'm Effie," she said. "Are you Oliver?"

"Oh, Floyd already told you about me?"

Effie smiled. "Yes, last night."

"I must have made an impression. Hopefully not a bad one."

Floyd pushed himself to stand. "I had to explain why I was late coming home."

"So, yes, a bad one," Oliver lamented in a playful manner.

"Effie already started on the 'Wanted' posters," Floyd teased.

Before Oliver could respond, Josephine piped up.

"What happened to your hands?"

Oliver looked at them. God, they really were nasty looking, weren't they? They were still hurting, too—throbbing uncomfortably, warmth radiating from the skin.

"I hurt them when I was working," Oliver explained.

"I thought you could fix him up, Effie," Floyd said.

Oliver said, "Floyd said you might have—"

"Goose grease," Effie finished before turning toward the kitchen. "I remember Floyd's mama treating his hands with it when we were kids."

Oliver smiled at Floyd. "You were a breaker boy?"

"Uh-huh," Floyd confirmed. "I started work when I was ten."

"Christ," Oliver said, inadvertently letting the profanity slip, which he then swiftly tried to cover up with more commentary. No one else in Rock Creek seemed to curse or take the Lord's name in vain. "Before this, I had never even had a single callous."

"Well, that's . . . something," Floyd said with a simpering smile.

Likely translation: Well, that's pathetic.

"Very something," Oliver agreed, shame coloring his cheeks.

Effie returned with the goose grease—off-white in color, like the pork fat he had seen his family cook save from time to time. Even though the thought of rubbing it on his skin made his stomach turn, Oliver knew he had to soothe his hands somehow, which only seemed to be worsening the more time passed without care.

"Thank you," Oliver said, taking the jar. "I'll try to be quick."

"No need," Floyd said.

"Do you want to stay for supper?" Effie asked. "I'm serving breakfast foods tonight. Corned beef hash and peas. Well, the peas ain't really a breakfast food, but we had a can."

"Are you sure?"

LOGAN SAGE ADAMS

"I wouldn't have asked otherwise."

"Alright, yes, I'd love to."

After Oliver washed up, he came back out to the living room to smear some goose grease on his injured hands. Effie and Josephine set the table while Floyd sat on the sofa nearby, looking a bit lost in thought. Oliver thought he should try to make conversation with him even though he hadn't the slightest idea what the two of them might have in common.

"So, what'd you end up buying yesterday? Strawberry or peach?"

Floyd cocked an eyebrow. "Uh, strawberry."

"Good choice," Oliver said before realizing that it seemed like he thought Floyd needed his approval or something. "I've never liked either that much, to be honest. Fresh fruit is tastier. Have you ever had frozen fruit?"

"Frozen fruit?"

"Yeah. We had a Domelre where I lived before."

"What's a . . . Domellery?"

"Domestic Electric Refrigerator. Just a new kind of appliance. Keeps things cold." Oliver wondered if he was sounding like a pretentious asshole. "It wasn't that impressive, honestly." Did that make it better or worse? "But it had a little compartment for people to make ice, if they wanted to. I thought making ice seemed a little boring, so I liked to stick fruit in there instead. Strawberries and blueberries mostly. Cherries once, but that was a mistake, what with the pits and everything."

"Oh."

Jesus, what a flop that was. While Oliver was busy trying to think of something else to say about it, Floyd stood up and clapped him on the back on the way to the kitchen.

"You're an interesting man, Oliver Astor."

Well, it was a compliment at least, which was better than the "oh."

Oliver followed Floyd to the kitchen table. Halfway through their meal, he remembered that he should have complimented their home.

"I like the wallpaper," Oliver said, looking over at the closest wall. All of them were lined with newspapers. "I haven't seen that before."

"Effie likes to put up the happy stories," Floyd explained. "Like if someone has a baby, she'll paste up the newspaper clipping. Lots of families hang up newspapers for insulation. But Effie is picky about which stories she chooses."

Effie tucked a lock of hair behind her ear. "It's probably silly."

"Not at all," Oliver said. "I should try that, too. Or maybe the opposite. Lining my kitchen with the obituaries wouldn't ruin my appetite, personally, but perhaps other folks could benefit. If someone wanted to feel sad, they could simply come over and read my walls." Floyd snorted a laugh, cocking one eyebrow in a curious manner and looking at Oliver like maybe his head had fallen off. "Sorry. I've been told that I have an interesting sense of humor."

Josephine cut in. "Can I have some cake? I ate my peas."

Effie and Floyd looked at one another, both of them pursing their lips to temper their burgeoning smiles. Effie flashed two fingers, and Floyd flashed one back. Effie raised both of her eyebrows, and Floyd flicked his wrist. It was incredible. Oliver couldn't even fathom what it would be like to be that close with someone—to communicate vaguely complex ideas without even speaking a single word.

Watching the scene unfold, Oliver's chest twinged with a sense of longing, one he hadn't let himself feel for many years. Oliver had never liked someone else romantically. It seemed impossible that he'd ever find what Effie and Floyd had with each other.

"One more bite of corned beef first," Effie finally said.

Josephine's face lit up. "Yay!"

Both Floyd and Effie shook their heads as they watched Josephine practically inhale her last forkful of supper, and then Effie cut a slice of pound cake while Floyd reached over to playfully tickle Josephine's side.

And all the while, Oliver's chest continued to ache.

Chapter Three

Floyd

It was nearly two o'clock in the morning, and Floyd couldn't sleep. For hours, he had been listening to Josephine's soft snores beside him, occasionally checking to see if Effie had woken up, too, either from the snoring or something else. But she hadn't even stirred. Not that he wanted her to sleep poorly or nothing, but he would have liked the company. Five more minutes passed before Floyd couldn't take lying awake no more. He walked out of the backroom to waste some time on the couch. He crept over to the faded-brown sofa—its long cushion saggy in the middle—and sat.

Once he was settled, he lit a candle and took out a stack of playing cards. He was close to finishing the setup for solitaire when Effie crept out into the living room, her slippers shuffling against the floorboards with each step.

"Can't sleep?" she asked, her voice soft.

"Nope," Floyd said, placing the final card on the table.

She placed a hand on his forehead. "Are you feeling sick?"

"Nah," he said, a smile pulling at his lips as she smoothed back his brown locks. "I can't switch my brain off tonight."

She took a seat next to him. "What are you thinking about?"

Floyd only shrugged. Effie probably thought that Floyd was thinking 'bout the same thing—the same *person*—he ought to have been thinking 'bout, the man with the reddish-brown hair who he had lost all those years ago. After all, Floyd had spent many other sleepless nights thinking of him over the years. But tonight, Floyd hadn't been able to stop thinking 'bout Oliver instead.

After a moment, Effie wrapped her arms around Floyd's shoulders and pulled him in for a sideways hug. They rested their heads together.

"Do you want to talk about it?"

"I'm fine."

"What'd you think of Oliver?"

Floyd nearly heaved a sigh but kept it in. Effie was only trying to be nice. She had no way of knowing that Oliver was what was bothering him, thoughts of his soft yellow hair and handsome face rolling around inside Floyd's head and messing up his brain.

"He's nice enough."

"I think so, too," she said. "Do you think you'll spend a lot of time with him?"

"Probably. He's new. Miners need someone to work with."

"What happened to Billy?"

"Billy needs to wait a year or two, in my opinion. He'll stay a spragger for now."

"Well, I hope you like working with Oliver. He's welcome for supper anytime."

"Thanks," Floyd said before realizing he wasn't sounding too thankful. "Appreciate that."

As Effie rubbed Floyd's shoulder, pieces of the evening started replaying in his head like a movie picture, and when watching it back, Floyd couldn't help but see how much fun he'd had with Oliver, whose stories and comments had been making him laugh.

Guilt coiled in his stomach like a copperhead, causing him to shift uncomfortably on the couch. Why couldn't he stop fixating on this city boy who owned too many hats?

Effie stood and said, "I think I'll try to catch some more sleep. Unless you need me to stay?"

"Naw," Floyd said. "I'll be fine. I'll be here beating myself at cards."

"Alright. Night, then."

"Night."

After that, Effie left for the bedroom and Floyd continued to think about how much fun he'd had with Mister Frozen Strawberry.

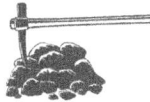

After spending most of the night wide awake, except for the two hours of shut-eye he had caught on the couch, Floyd woke up feeling both sore and irritable. And, frustratingly enough, as soon as he opened his eyes, he started thinking of Oliver—of his nice laugh and his nice head of pretty blond hair and that nice beige suit he was wearing when they had first met. Nice. Jeez, why was the only word his tired brain could come up with such a plain and boring one? Oliver was far from either plain or boring. Especially with that sense of humor he had. It had been nice to laugh with him. Dang, there was that word again. Nice this. Nice that. What Floyd really needed was a *nice* night of sleep.

While Floyd rubbed the sleep from his eyes, his stomach tightened from unease. Guilt was not an uncommon feeling for Floyd Bennett, but experiencing it because some random man was invading his thoughts every waking moment? Now that was another story.

On his way to work, Floyd made up his mind that even though he had promised to let Oliver shadow him, it would be best for Mister Frozen Strawberry to learn from someone else. Floyd wanted to be alone. Or, well, as alone as he could be in the mines. He considered staying by the brass board to tell Oliver this his own self, but the thought of talking to him while his insides were still knotted together was only making him feel worse, and so, Floyd took his tab and left to find Billy. He had to hope that Oliver would figure out on his own that Floyd had changed his mind.

All morning, Floyd continued to feel off. Guilt came in waves. If Floyd wasn't feeling bad for having this fixation with Oliver, he was feeling bad for turning his back on him, with little reprieve in between. Floyd supposed he ought to have seen it coming. Exhaustion had never once failed to make his upset even worse. Hopefully, Oliver had found someone to work with.

By lunchtime, Floyd was plum tired. Carrying his lunch to his usual spot underneath the sugar maple, Floyd expected to spot Oliver nearby eating, too. But Oliver wasn't there. Floyd took his time munching on his sandwich, thinking he'd see Oliver eventually, but Oliver never came out of the mine.

At the end of Floyd's shift, he headed over to the company store, hoping to splurge on some Tootsie Rolls or Hershey's Kisses or, heck, whatever else might sweeten his sour mood, only to see Oliver browsing one of the men's clothing aisles. As soon as Floyd caught sight of him, a little shudder of excitement rolled through his body, causing his heart to race.

One aisle over from Oliver, Floyd crouched low so that he could pretend to study the items on the bottom shelf—pairs of work boots and bundles of cotton socks. Gosh, what was wrong with him? He had never let someone rile him up like this before.

Floyd took a breath. Oliver was nothing more than a talkative man with an odd sense of humor and a nice head of hair. Nothing special. Just a handsome man from the city.

Determined to overcome this odd pull toward a man who was more or less a stranger, Floyd stood back up to leave. And locked eyes with Oliver.

Suddenly flustered, Floyd whirled around and walked right into a hat rack, knocking the fedoras and flat caps to the floor.

"Dogonit," he muttered, heat blooming on his cheeks.

While Floyd picked up the hats, every single muscle in his body tensed, bracing for Oliver's presence. Seconds passed without Oliver pitching a verbal lashing over Floyd's abandonment, and so, Floyd forced himself to look up. Oliver was no longer there. Confused, Floyd stood to look around the store and spotted Oliver heading outside empty-handed. Floyd realized, then, that Oliver was probably avoiding him, and that realization settled heavily on his chest, momentarily making it hard to breathe.

Floyd hurried to catch him.

"Ain't you buying something?" Floyd asked.

"No?" Oliver responded, his voice hitching up as though he was confused as to why Floyd was asking. Or, heck, why Floyd was even talking to him, considering the fact that he had broken his promise and left him to find someone else to help him in the mine.

Oliver continued out of the store. Floyd found himself following. He wondered why in the world he was bothering to. Wouldn't life be easier if he let Oliver walk away?

After two painfully awkward minutes of this, Oliver stopped and turned to face him, his eyebrows lowered and knitted together, lips pressed into a thin line.

He took a breath and asked, "Where were you today?"

Floyd fumbled for a response. "Work."

Which, he knew, was a right stupid answer.

"Yes, I know that," Oliver said. "You're covered in coal dust. But, I mean, what happened?"

Oliver said this a little loudly, which had a few people staring. Oliver, though, wasn't embarrassed. While Floyd stayed silent, Oliver plowed on, clearly too mad to care.

"Did I upset you or something? I mean, I thought we had a nice meal together yesterday. Two meals! And I thought you said I could be your work shadow. I still have no idea what I'm supposed to do in there. I wandered around the mine like a chicken without its head for over three hours before I went home. At this rate, I'll bleed through every penny I have by the end of summer."

Once Oliver finally stopped ranting, Floyd couldn't seem to make himself do anything except stare. What was he supposed to say? *"I slept bad because I felt like I had snakes strangling my insides"*? Of course not. *"I kept thinking 'bout you, and it bothered me a lot, so I thought I'd ignore you for the rest of my life"*? He couldn't say that neither.

As Floyd was racking his brain for some kind of response, Oliver crossed his arms over his chest and tilted his head in a way that said, *"Ain't you fixing to apologize?"* or however the heck someone like him would phrase it, and Floyd knew he needed to say something, even if that something wasn't the truth.

"Yeah, I know I ought to have kept my word. But I felt kind of sick this morning."

"Sick?" Oliver scoffed. "Clearly you still went to work."

"Not too sick to work. Just too sick to . . . to talk to you."

Oliver's face fell, the fire he seemed to have had inside of him becoming extinguished instantly.

"Oh, I see," Oliver said, his voice was so much softer now. "Oliver's too strange. Oliver's too irritating. I've heard it plenty of times before. Guess I shouldn't be surprised. I'll try to work with someone else."

"What?" Floyd sputtered. "No, that ain't what I meant."

"Alright, so, what is it, then?"

Floyd's heart sank. He couldn't stand how upset poor Oliver looked now. Floyd liked him. He hadn't meant to make Oliver sad. It wasn't Oliver's fault that he had been feeling too bothered by his own feelings to keep his promise.

"I felt like I needed some time to myself, is all. I can't really figure out how to explain it." Oliver turned to walk away, but Floyd caught his arm. "But it won't happen tomorrow. I promise."

"Tomorrow?"

"I still want to work with you. I . . . well . . . Billy's too young and you need someone to help you with everything. I been a miner for 'bout twenty years, if you count the time when I was a kid. I reckon you could use a teacher with a lot of experience. And I'd like to be the one to learn you. If you want, that is."

Oliver started chewing on his bottom lip, and then he narrowed his eyes a bit like he was studying Floyd's face, maybe for insincerity. Oliver was probably having a hard time believing him, which made Floyd's chest feel even heavier, especially when Oliver's earlier words flitted into his mind. *Oliver's too strange. Oliver's too irritating.* Gosh, maybe Oliver had been rejected for them kinds of things in the past. Before Floyd could try to make sure that Oliver knew that it wasn't that he had messed up or nothing, Oliver spoke.

"Really?" he asked.

"Really." Floyd tried to smile through his lingering upset. Gosh, he still felt so bad. He hoped he could let Oliver know how much he really *had* been enjoying his company. "Besides, no one else ever tells me strange stories about frozen fruit. Stories like that, I reckon they'll make the time pass faster while we work."

Oliver's face relaxed a little as he let out a long breath, one that seemed to blow away some of Floyd's upset over how horrible he had behaved.

"Alright," Oliver said. "I'll still work with you."

After a moment, Floyd nodded back toward the store and said, "Do you want to buy whatever it is you wanted to buy before you tried to run away from me?"

"Not really. I was upset about you avoiding me, so I thought maybe I'd buy myself a shirt or a hat or something."

"I thought you said you were worried about bleeding through your money."

"Don't throw logic in my face," Oliver said with a fake-sounding scoff. "Besides, I was exaggerating about that. I have too much money, really. Or, uhm, sorry, I'm not trying to boast. Oh God, I really can't blame you for avoiding me."

Oliver insulting himself made Floyd realize that he still hadn't mended things enough.

"I wasn't avoiding you," Floyd said. "I promise."

But Floyd knew it *still* wasn't enough. He wondered if maybe he ought to invite Oliver out for some fun. His stomach rumbled a bit, like there was a part of him that wasn't too happy with that idea, but the feeling would probably fade with time. Or, if not, Floyd supposed he'd better learn how to live with it, especially since he'd be spending time with Oliver every day in the mine.

"How about you come with me to the pool hall later?" Floyd offered. "I've never been, but I been told it's nice there."

"Wait, you're telling me there's no telephone in this town, but there's a pool hall?"

"Why's that odd?"

"Never mind," Oliver said with a slight shake of his head. "Yes, I'll play pool with you. What time?"

"Seven?"

"Sure, seven. Uh, where is it?"

Floyd pointed down the road a bit.

"Over yonder—that big brick building. Before 1913 or there-abouts, it was a saloon, too. Or so I heard."

Oliver tilted his head, looking puzzled. "1913?"

"Prohibition?"

Oliver's eyes widened. "Oh my God, I completely forgot about that! While we were all still getting zozzled up in New York, alcohol was already illegal here, wasn't it?"

"New York, huh?"

"Shit, I let that slip, didn't I? Yeah, I'm from New York."

"Is that what that accent is?"

"Not really. It's how I was taught to speak in school. Elocution classes." Floyd raised both of his eyebrows. He hadn't never heard of something like that. "As far as where I'm from, well, I was raised in Ohio, mostly, in Cleveland, and then my parents moved to New York when I was in secondary school. Which is how I eventually ended up at Princeton."

"So, you're from everywhere."

"Guess you can say that."

"Hm."

Oliver was becoming more and more interesting by the minute. Maybe friendship wouldn't be so bad.

"Seven, then?" Oliver asked.

"Yup. Seven."

Not long thereafter, Floyd arrived home. After he finished washing up, he came out to the living room area to relax in his favorite armchair. Effie was cooking supper while Josephine was out back with one of the neighbor boys.

Floyd chewed on his fingernails, trying to work out how to tell Effie that for the first time in more than eight years, he had the urge to make a friend. It wasn't that Floyd was worried that she would mind or nothing, but Effie would probably look at him funny. Maybe ask a bunch of stuff, too. Even though Floyd had played pool back in their hometown, he hadn't never been to the pool hall since moving to Rock Creek. Everybody in town probably thought it was because Floyd was simply a family man—someone who wanted to spend his spare time with his wife and kid. Which, he supposed, was true enough, though the real reason for him not caring to be close with the other miners wasn't one he'd ever let on about. Effie knew the reason, of course. But she knew him better than anyone.

"Effie?"

She kept on stirring the beans on the stovetop. "Hm?"

"I reckon I might head to the pool hall tonight."

Effie stopped stirring. When Floyd heard the sound of the metal spoon clanging against the metal stovetop, near every muscle in his body tensed in anticipation of her reaction.

"Really?" Effie asked, leaning back against the counter to face him. "Why?"

"I wasn't very nice to Oliver today. Left him to fend for himself in the mine."

"So you invited him to play pool with you?"

"What's wrong with that?"

"Ain't nothing *wrong* with it, Floyd. I'm surprised, that's all. You know I been wanting you to make friends ever since we moved here."

"I know."

"What's so special about Oliver?"

"Nothing. I like him."

"Ah, I thought so."

The teasing edge in Effie's voice made Floyd's ears turn hot. "Not like *that*, Effie."

Floyd might have found Oliver interesting, but that was the extent of it. Acknowledging that a person was funny or attractive or such was a normal thing to do. Even though Oliver had been taking up space in his head and making him feel strange, it wasn't like that. Not like Effie was implying. Floyd only wanted to be Oliver's friend, which was unsettling enough without complicating it even more. He had only been thinking about Oliver so much because the man was so unusual. What kind of man has blond hair?

"I wouldn't fault you," she said in a sing-song voice, turning back to tend to the beans. "Oliver is a handsome man."

"He ain't bad," Floyd said, knowing that Effie would likely poke him even more if he tried to pretend that he hadn't noticed Oliver's looks. "But you know that I try not to think about that sort of thing no more."

"Whatever you say."

"It's the truth."

"Alright, so, what makes Oliver special, then? Roy and John and plenty of other folks are nice. You like them, too, but you never want to spend time with them outside of work."

"Oliver is new in town. Seems like he could use a friend, is all."

"Well, that's true. And you could use one, too," she said before turning off the stove. "Supper's ready. Mind fetching Josephine?"

"I'll call her in," Floyd said. He stood up and placed a hand on the small of Effie's back. "I already have a friend, you know."

"I'm your wife."

"We been friends since we were six."

Effie smirked. "Go call our daughter in for supper, Floyd."

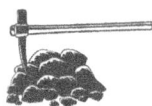

Floyd arrived at the pool hall fifteen minutes early. It was smaller than he'd imagined—with three pool tables lined up in a row in the center, cues stacked up in the corner, and a line of chairs from one end of the room to the other. On the far end, there was a bar, but of course, that hadn't been in use for years. No one else was there except for a man with a long mustache, probably someone employed by Fred Donohue to watch over the place.

Floyd walked over to the bar counter wringing his hands—both because he had some worriment that the other men might wonder why he had come out for the first time and because the thought of spending time with Oliver was making his heart race. Effie's comment about Oliver's handsomeness kept coming back into his head, hovering like some kind of specter.

Watching the minutes tick by on the wall clock, Floyd tried to remind himself that there were plenty of other handsome men around—men he had noticed over the years in a passive sort of way. He had always been strong enough and smart enough to resist the kinds of thoughts that came with noticing such a thing. Oliver's handsomeness was neither here nor there.

Neither was Oliver's unique sense of humor or the funny way he peppered in swear words from time to time or the fact that he liked to freeze strawberries before eating them. Neither here nor there.

Finally, at 7:05 p.m., Oliver strolled into the pool hall wearing a fancy plaid suit and a matching gray fedora, looking every bit as stylish as the men in the pictures. For those first few seconds, Floyd could think of nothing else except how doggone nice looking he was. Darn. He really did like Oliver, huh? He stood there, staring wordlessly, imagining Effie rolling her eyes as though to say, *"I knew it,"* and Floyd had to take a moment to reorient himself.

"Hi," Oliver said, smiling an uneasy smile as he approached. "I'm overdressed, aren't I?"

"Just a smidge."

"I thought . . . oh, hell, I'm not sure what I thought. I wanted to look nice."

Oliver took off his hat and raked a hand through his hair. Golly, it looked soft. So, so soft. Floyd had to curl his hands into fists to resist the urge to touch it. Gosh-darn-it, Effie!

"Why are you staring like that?" Oliver asked. "Does my hair look funny?"

Unsure how to respond, Floyd snatched Oliver's hat and placed it on his own head.

"Now I can look nice, too."

"Oh, well, I've never seen you not look nice," Oliver said. He cleared his throat and shifted his stance. "Not that I've known you for very long."

Time seemed to stop, like projector film suddenly becoming caught in the reel. Floyd's brain stalled, and he could feel the heat rising to his cheeks. Oliver's face flushed, too, which made Floyd's heart pitter-patter a little.

Finally, Oliver said, "Wow, that was odd of me, wasn't it?"

"Yeah," Floyd said because what else was he supposed to say?

Floyd's face was still on fire when Oliver asked, "Can we play pool now?"

"Uh-huh."

And Effie was laughing it up inside his head.

Floyd and Oliver chose the closest table and set up the balls. Floyd broke. He sank the blue number two, which meant that he was solids, and then shot for the six but missed.

Oliver proceeded to sink six balls in a row.

"Shit!" Oliver exclaimed upon missing the seventh.

Which was when Floyd realized that his mouth had fallen open, probably some time ago.

"What in the heck was that?" Floyd asked.

"What?"

"You sank six in a row."

"Oh, well, I had a pool table in New York."

Oliver said this like it was completely normal. Completely uninteresting. But it *was* interesting. Worse, it was infuriating. Embarrassment and irritation flooded Floyd's veins, making his blood run hot. Now Floyd felt silly for inviting Oliver to play pool. He hadn't played in years. Even when he'd played as a kid, he hadn't been very good at it. Pool was one of the few things Floyd couldn't seem to pick up too easily.

"I ain't in the mood to play no more," Floyd said, placing his cue on the table. Not only was he not impressing Oliver, but he was practically making a fool of himself, too.

"Don't be like that," Oliver protested. "Lucky shots. That's all."

"Lucky? I know luck, and that ain't it."

"Come on, keep playing with me. Or are you a chicken?"

"Just not in the mood," Floyd said curtly. "Like I said."

Oliver made a couple of chicken noises—sputtering a bunch of fast *bok-bok-boks*—and started to flap his pretend wings. Floyd clenched his teeth in response. When Oliver continued teasing him—making a few more sounds that were even louder—Floyd couldn't hold back anymore.

"Oliver, you're a—" Floyd started to say but caught himself before he might have said something he'd likely regret.

Oliver wiggled his eyebrows up and down. "I'm a what?"

"Never mind."

"I nearly upset you enough to make you finally utter some profanity, didn't I?" Oliver asked with a smirk. Gosh, he was so fun. Floyd couldn't even manage to be mad no more. "Honestly, Floyd, I had no idea you'd be so bad at pool."

Floyd reached out and lightly shoved Oliver back a step.

"I ain't bad," Floyd said defensively, now unable to keep himself from smiling, too. "I'm rusty, is all."

"Alright, then, practice," Oliver said. "We won't play a real game. Just take a few shots. I'll take some, too."

Floyd hesitated before ultimately relenting. Over the next half hour, the two of them went back and forth with their shots, with Oliver making nearly all of his, no matter how hard they looked to be. Floyd wanted to be more irritated than he was. Truthfully, he liked watching Oliver play. It was pretty dang impressive. While they were practicing, Oliver offered up a constant stream of funny commentary, too. Floyd sure was enjoying spending time together. He hoped they'd come back to the pool hall again sometime.

When Floyd had finally had enough practice to make three shots in a row immediately after poor Oliver had somehow only made one, Oliver sputtered something like, *"you Goddamned lucky lunkhead!"* with such seriousness that Floyd burst out laughing.

By the time Floyd composed himself, he realized that Oliver was staring, wearing a lopsided grin.

"What?" Floyd asked.

"Nothing." Oliver shrugged. "I'm having fun."

"Yeah. Me, too."

Their conversation was interrupted when Roy and John came into the pool hall.

"Hey, Floyd. We ain't seen you in here before," Roy said, sounding pleased rather than accusatory, which made Floyd realize that his work buddies probably wouldn't prod him about his seemingly inexplicable outing too much; they were simply happy to see him. "Who won?"

"We only took some practice shots," Floyd answered.

"Oh yeah? Why?"

"Oliver's too good a pool player."

Oliver cut in with a dismissive wave of his hand.

"I'm only so-so."

Roy smiled wolfishly. "How about we play each other then?"

"Yeah, sure," Oliver said.

Floyd had half a mind to cut in and say that Oliver was being too modest, but he sort of liked the thought of Oliver wiping the smug smile off Roy's face for some reason.

Over the next half hour, Oliver and Roy played each other, and even though Floyd had been upset about Oliver's talent earlier in the evening, he now felt a sense of pride watching Oliver make Roy look like he'd never even played pool before.

After some time, John tapped Floyd on the shoulder.

"Did you hear the latest from Mingo County?"

John wasn't the type to talk for the sake of talking. He wasn't someone who liked to spread rumors neither. But John had been real interested in the talk of unionizing lately, probably because he thought the trouble might bring him a better life. He was struggling to make enough to provide for his family—four kids, three of them girls. His boy, Richard, was only seven, like Josephine. Not yet old enough to help earn more money.

"No, what?"

John answered in a hushed voice. "Some sort of skirmish between the union and non-union miners. And the sheriff deputies and members of the National Guard, too."

Floyd's heart started beating faster. He hated these stories. Because it was a struggle to keep his emotions hidden well enough whenever he caught wind of them. What if that sort of violence came to Rock Creek someday? Thinking of the possibility of being forced to leave—either to flee from the fighting or to simply look for new work—was making his palms sweat.

"Was anybody hurt?" Floyd asked, shoving his hands in his pockets to hide the evidence of his upset.

"I reckon so."

"Mmm . . ." Floyd hummed, trying to choose his next words carefully. Even though he was none too happy about the prospect of potential fighting in Logan someday, he never wanted to let the other miners know his opinion, especially John, who he knew would welcome the change the United Mine Workers of America might bring. Even if that change wouldn't come easy. "Do you think we'll see some issues over here?"

"What, the fighting?"

"Yeah."

"Probably not. Not so long as Chafin's men are watching our trains. Ain't no way the UMWA will ever take hold here." John nodded toward Oliver. "I'm surprised they even let him come here looking like that. He looks like one of them union fellas, like one of their leaders."

Floyd huffed a laugh as though the notion was silly, but he'd had the same thought back when he had first seen Oliver in the company store. He had to wonder whether Oliver had been properly checked by Chafin's people or not.

Turning back toward the pool table, Floyd tried to pay attention to the balls moving across the felt but kept thinking back on John's comments instead. If the United Mine Workers of America—the UMWA—ever tried to recruit folks from Rock Creek, Floyd knew he'd feel a lot of pressure to support them. But if Fred Donohue ever threw him and his family out of their home, Floyd knew, too, that he couldn't let them stay holed up in some tent colony. He reckoned he'd have to come up with the money they'd need to move somewhere else—to another coal company, probably, but one that was far, far away. Or, heck, what if he'd have to leave the coal industry completely? Unease continued to claw at Floyd's insides, making it harder and harder to breathe.

All of a sudden, Roy tossed his cue onto the table.

"God dang it!" Roy shouted. "He beat me!"

"Sorry, Roy," Oliver said with a simpering smile. "Just luck."

Roy turned to Floyd with his hands on hips. "You ought to have warned me!"

"I told you he was good," Floyd said, some of his earlier upset falling away. He was thankful that this silly squabble had interrupted his nervous thoughts. "What more do you want?"

After that, John and Oliver played for a bit, while Roy and Floyd talked about their families. Roy's wife was pregnant with their third. Floyd wondered if folks ever questioned why Effie had never fallen pregnant after Josephine. No one ever said nothing to him, though. Throughout their conversation, Roy never brought up the problems over in Mingo County either, which was a relief.

Not much time passed before Oliver and John were finished playing. Oliver had won. Again.

Afterward, Floyd and Oliver started toward home. They walked side by side through the town as the sun started to set, passing the company store and coming to the first houses—the smallest ones in town, more like shacks than houses, all lined up in a row. Soon, they came to the larger houses, ones like the home that Floyd lived in, homes that had both a combined living room and kitchen area as well as a back room or two. When they came to the bottom of the road, Floyd ought to have veered right while Oliver turned left, but instead, Floyd took the left road, too. He wanted to spend some more time with Oliver.

"You really won't mind me shadowing you tomorrow?" Oliver asked. "I promise I'll try not to be annoying."

"Don't talk like that. You ain't never been annoying."

"Good." Oliver started wandering a little closer. Floyd pretended not to notice. "I had a lot of fun tonight. It's nice to have a friend. I sometimes had trouble making friends back in New York. I'm not sure if you've noticed, but I'm a little odd."

Before Floyd could catch himself, he said, "Odd can be nice."

"Yeah?" Oliver's eyes brightened. He seemed to like that comment a whole lot. "Do you want to come over sometime? I can try to cook us something." He asked this in a heartbreakingly sweet way, one that sent Floyd's heart a-flutter.

"I, uh, I eat with my family, typically," Floyd said, hating his response a bit as he said it. "But you can come back to my house sometime. I'm sure Effie and Jo would love it."

"Really? I'd like that."

And suddenly, Floyd couldn't fathom waiting longer than he absolutely had to.

"Tomorrow?"

"Oh, well, you see, I'll have to check my very busy schedule. Didn't you watch me shoot pool back there? Roy and John will probably spread the word. Why, I'm practically famous. Everyone will be lining up to watch me play soon enough."

"Be careful with that head of yours. Pretty soon you'll float away like one of them hot air balloons."

Oliver chuckled. "Ah, if only I *really* had that kind of confidence."

Even though Oliver was laughing, the fact that he was poking fun of himself again reminded Floyd of the comments Oliver had made earlier outside the company store. He couldn't have Oliver continuing to feel bad about himself.

"I reckon you ought to," Floyd said. "Really, I ain't never seen someone shoot pool like that before."

Oliver's expression softened, his eyes becoming hopeful.

"Thanks, Floyd."

And Floyd's heart suddenly felt so full. It was nice to make Oliver feel better about himself, if only for a moment.

"So, supper?" Floyd asked.

"Right, yes, sorry. I'd love to come to supper tomorrow."

"I'd like it, too," Floyd said with a nod.

"Oh, that's a relief. I thought only Effie and Jo would be happy to see me."

"What do you mean?"

"Nothing."

"No, tell me."

Oliver scrunched up his nose and said, "I'm nitpicking because I like teasing people, which is probably one of the many reasons for me never holding onto friends for very long." Floyd kept looking at Oliver, hoping he'd say some more. Floyd was still feeling confused. Oliver sighed. "Earlier, you invited me and you said that your wife and daughter would love my company, but you didn't say that *you'd* love my company, so I was poking at you for the hell of it. And, selfishly enough, I needed to hear you say that you wanted to spend time with me, too. Because even though we spent the entire evening together shooting pool, I'm still stupidly mad about you abandoning me today."

"I never really apologized for it, huh?" Floyd looked at his shoes, his face reddening with shame over how much he had hurt his new friend. "It was wrong of me to abandon you today, Ollie. I'm sorry about that."

"Ollie? Do I have a nickname now?"

Floyd reached up to scratch the side of head so that he could hide his face, which was only becoming hotter by the second. Though he had no idea whether Oliver could see the color of his cheeks in the low light of the moon, he still felt vulnerable enough that his first instinct was to try to hide a bit.

"If you want one," he said.

"Yeah, I like it. I'll have to think of one for you, too. You seemed to like lunkhead earlier. How about that?"

Floyd bellowed a laugh. "You're real strange, Ollie." He realized Oliver might take that the wrong way. Before he could think better of it, he said, "I like that about you."

As soon as the words left Floyd's mouth, his heart started fluttering like mad. But luckily, Oliver held himself back from commenting on the bluntness of that statement.

Floyd and Oliver continued their walk, though neither of them said much else for a while. Seemed like Floyd could make Oliver stop talking if he sputtered something awkward enough. He tried not to beat himself up for how risky it had been to say that he liked Ollie's strangeness. Who knew what Oliver thought of him now.

After a while, Floyd heard a night bird calling in the distance. Its familiar high-pitched *woop-woo-woo* comforted him, even though he wasn't exactly sure what type of bird it was. He kind of liked not knowing, though, because it meant that his little old coal town still had some mystery for him. He might not have been well-traveled like Oliver, but that was fine. There was still plenty to discover in the mountains of West Virginia.

Sometime later, Oliver stopped walking and Floyd realized that they had probably reached his house.

"Well, this is me," Oliver said. "It looks like your house from the outside, but it's way more depressing on the inside. No newspaper on the walls or children running about. I haven't even bought any books yet. Speaking of which, where could I find some?"

"We got a few over at the company store."

"I must have missed them. I'll look harder next time."

Floyd wondered what kinds of books Oliver would buy.

"I'll see you tomorrow," Oliver said with a half-smile. "Bright and early."

"Bright and early," Floyd confirmed.

As Floyd walked home, he couldn't stop thinking 'bout Oliver. His entire body was burning with a new kind of energy, one that was making him feel like running and jumping and maybe even skipping, as ridiculous as that was. It had been eight long years since Floyd had felt anything even close. He reminded himself that nothing could come of these feelings he was having for Oliver because Oliver surely wasn't like him. Not many men were.

Instead of that reminder making him sad, it somehow had the opposite effect. If Oliver wasn't likely to feel a romantic kind of way in return, Floyd felt like he could be free to enjoy his crush. Suddenly, the strange swirl of energy was less terrifying, and the copperhead in his stomach stopped writhing. Floyd carried the happy Oliver-energy with him the entire way home, holding onto it with care, pleased that he could enjoy the sensation for a while.

When Floyd reached home, he found Effie rocking back and forth in the rocking chair, mending a hole in one of Josephine's skirts. She looked up at Floyd with a little knowing smile. And he realized, then, that he was still wearing Oliver's hat.

CHAPTER FOUR

OLIVER

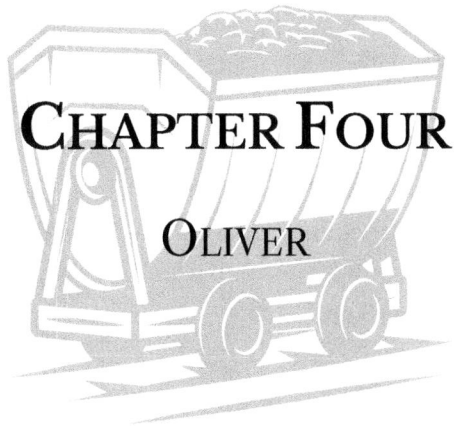

WHEN OLIVER ARRIVED AT the brass board, Floyd was already there waiting for him. Following Floyd through the mine, Oliver noticed that many men, especially those who were older than either Floyd or Oliver, had boys working with them—kids who looked to be between the ages of fourteen and eighteen. Floyd said that they had essentially been hired by the miners themselves. Sometimes they were relatives, sometimes neighbors, sometimes kids who had previously been working as a spragger or a breaker boy. Oliver wondered if Floyd would have stuck it out with Billy if it hadn't been for him. He kind of hoped so. Because that would mean that Floyd had chosen him, in a way, which was a really touching thought. He really liked Floyd so far. It'd be a Goddamn miracle if Floyd liked him back even half as much.

For safety reasons, everyone in the mine needed someone to work with. Some men worked in clusters of four or six, but many worked in pairs, oftentimes with a friend, rather than with a child.

"Whoever you're working with, we call 'em your butty," Floyd said very matter-of-factly, enunciating the *t*'s.

It was clear that the potential silliness of the term had never even occurred to him.

"I'm sorry, my what?"

"Butty," Floyd repeated in the same serious tone.

"Like B-U-T-T-Y."

"Yeah."

Oliver started chuckling, which soon changed to full-blown laughter.

"Oh my God," he said.

"What's funny?"

"I am one hundred percent sure you will not appreciate what I'm laughing about."

"Why not?"

"Because I have the sense of humor of a twelve-year-old. Actually, twelve-year-old kids around here seem to be more mature than me. Clearly none of them are laughing about this."

"Ollie, tell me. I want to know."

"It's . . . well . . . the term 'butty' has the word 'butt' in it, right? So, it . . ." Oliver snickered. "Jesus Christ, it'll sound even more demented when I say it out loud, but to me, the word makes it sound like we're . . . like we're friends who like each other's butts."

Floyd's subsequent facial expression was one of the funniest that Oliver had ever seen—his mouth hanging open and eyes wide. Oliver couldn't tell whether Floyd was horrified or amused or merely in a state of shock from the comment. Just when Oliver thought he should probably apologize for his clearly inappropriate humor, Floyd started to laugh, and then Oliver watched this behemoth of a man—one who couldn't have been a hair shy of six foot three—slowly but swiftly lose his composure, eventually laughing so heartily and loudly that Oliver found himself wondering about the chances of a cave in.

"I feel like I broke your brain with that comment," Oliver said.

Through a happy sniffle, Floyd replied, "Jeez, Ollie, I can't remember the last time I laughed like that. Not even from that lunkhead comment of yours yesterday."

Oliver grinned. "You're welcome." He clapped Floyd on the back. "Come on, butty, let's pick up our long, steel rods and—"

Floyd shoved his elbow into Oliver's side, cutting him off.

"You'll be run out of town with that mouth of yours," Floyd scolded in a friendly way.

"Don't people like raunchy humor around here?"

"No."

"Oh, come on, yes, they do. Everybody does. People are reluctant to admit it, that's all."

"Ollie, hush up before people think there's something wrong with you. Or with me."

"Ah, that's what this is about. You're worried that since we're friends, people will think you're as strange as I am."

Floyd seemed to have no response for that other than to shove Oliver sideways.

"Alright, I surrender," Oliver said. "You can show me how to mine now."

"Well," Floyd said with a big, heaving sigh. "Lord help me, but we need to . . . to . . . ."

"Drill the long, steel rod into the coal seams?"

Floyd leveled a look. "Yes, Ollie."

But Oliver could see the faintest hint of a lingering smile on Floyd's face, and so, he threw Floyd a wink, which made Floyd smile even more, even though he was rolling his eyes a little.

Oliver and Floyd worked side by side to extract and shovel the coal, traveling up one of the newer coal arteries—a little "road" in their underground city that had been named Sycamore Street—and even though Floyd wouldn't let Oliver handle the blast powder or light the fuses, he tried not to let it bother him. He was still learning.

All in all, it had been a really nice workday.

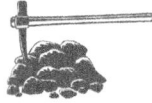

By the end of May, Oliver and Floyd had become friends. Every morning, Oliver would wake up bursting with energy, eager to spend time with Floyd. Even though spending hours swinging a pickaxe and shoveling pounds of coal wouldn't have been fun otherwise, being with Floyd made it so. Especially since they spent a lot of the time teasing each other. Becoming so close to someone, it was wonderful. Floyd never minded his rambling. In fact, he seemed to enjoy it. And Oliver never minded Floyd's comparative shyness.

Well, not *never*.

Even though Floyd had previously informed Oliver that he had once been a breaker boy, he hadn't shared more about his past otherwise. Despite Oliver having inquired about Floyd's upbringing a few times, Floyd had stayed stubbornly tight-lipped. His secrecy was becoming a little upsetting. After all, friends should be open with each other, shouldn't they? Sure, Oliver had never really had a proper friend before, so he wasn't *exactly* certain how close the two of them should be by now, but . . .

He really wanted them to be close. He had never felt this kind of kinship, this kind of pull, toward another person before.

Craving to know more about Floyd's life, Oliver thought he'd try pushing Floyd a little. Not by making him uncomfortable, of course, but by reminding Floyd that they could trust one another.

While they were both resting up against the rocky black wall, taking a break from shoveling, Oliver turned to Floyd and said, "So, tell me more about the time you spent as a breaker boy."

Floyd let out a long breath.

"I can't talk about that part of my life with you."

"Why not?" Oliver asked. "I thought we were friends. You can trust me."

"Ain't about trust."

"What is it, then?"

"Just can't."

"Don't be silly. Of course you can."

Floyd only responded with one word. "Ollie."

And the way Floyd said it—stern yet pleading—it made Oliver want to crumple in on himself.

"Sorry," Oliver said, self-loathing twisting inside of him. God, why was he so nosey?

For the rest of the workday, Oliver continued to mentally pummel himself for being the world's biggest bastard. After their coal car was weighed, Floyd and Oliver parted ways. While Floyd hadn't seemed upset in the end, Oliver continued to feel horrible.

Halfway home, Oliver spotted Roy, who lived one house over. He hurried to catch him, hoping he could take his mind off his earlier blunder somehow.

"Hi, Roy," Oliver said, slightly out of breath. "How are you?"

"Not bad. Just looking forward to relaxing a little."

"What would you say to playing some pool?"

Roy sucked on his teeth, thinking it over, and then said, "I'll need to tell my wife first, but I reckon it'll be fine."

"Great!"

While Roy left to talk to his wife, Oliver hovered outside near the picket fence. Not everyone's houses had fences, but Roy's had a nice one. He had probably put it up himself. Gripping one of the posts, Oliver tried to wiggle it back and forth. It seemed sturdy. Oliver couldn't help but be impressed.

Not much later, Roy flung open a window and stuck his head through the opening.

"Gotta clean myself up first, but I can meet you there," he hollered.

"Perfect!"

Oliver looked at his clothes. He really was filthy. While he was itching to play pool to take his mind off how badly he had messed up with Floyd, he knew he should probably bathe first, too.

Over the next half hour, Oliver took a sponge bath in the basin, and then he chose some clothes to wear to the pool hall. Even though he enjoyed looking nice, he found he wasn't as keen on wearing one of his better suits this time. Not like he had been when he had met up with Floyd. After choosing a simple beige suit and brown fedora, Oliver threw everything on and rushed over to the pool hall. Roy was already there practicing.

"Sorry I took so long," Oliver said.

"Not a problem." Roy nodded toward the table. "I'll re-rack the balls while you find a cue."

Oliver left to find a cue. Resting next to the others on the wall, Oliver spotted the one that Floyd had used last time. It was the only one with a blue wrap, rather than red. He chose it immediately.

While Roy and Oliver took turns with their shots, Oliver's thoughts kept finding their way back to Floyd. Probably because of the stick. He wondered when the two of them might spend some more leisure time together. Maybe he'd see if Floyd wanted to come with him to the company store soon. Oliver needed some more work pants.

When they were nearly finished with their first game, the man who seemed to run the pool hall—a middle-aged man with an impressive mustache—left to fetch some more chalk from the company store. After he left, Roy shot the seven ball into one of the corner pockets and then turned to Oliver, planting the butt of his cue on the floor.

"Did Floyd tell you about the violence over in Mingo County?"

"No," Oliver said. "What happened?"

Roy proceeded to explain to Oliver what was happening in some other areas of West Virginia, how coal companies were resisting coal miners unionizing, sometimes even responding with violence, which had resulted in many pro-union miners being forced out of their homes. Miners who continued to support the UMWA were living in tent colonies, and the previous summer, militiamen employed by Mingo County itself had raided colonies, supposedly over suspicion of bootlegging, though Roy suspected they had wanted to send a message to the striking miners, too.

Oliver wondered how people could survive in colonies like that in the mountains. Where did they find food? What about medical care? Picturing the families and their broken lives had Oliver's stomach roiling. Finally, Roy informed Oliver that there had been some sort of skirmish recently, resulting in bloodshed. Oliver could hardly believe events like these were happening only a short ways away.

"I thought I'd try to find out if you had already heard about all this stuff happening," Roy said. "John and me have been saying that you kind of look like one of Chafin's men in those fancy clothes you keep wearing."

"Oh . . ." Oliver wrinkled his nose. "I think I've heard of Sheriff Chafin, maybe, from Fred Donohue. He's the one who keeps the UMWA from coming here, right?"

"Yep. I reckon Fred Donohue pays him a pretty penny to keep watch. Chafin has a whole lot of people working for him—watching the trains, threatening those who try to come here to organize us. We probably ain't supposed to know as much as we do. But some of us got families in other counties. We find out everything that's happening. Sooner or later."

"No one has ever really challenged Chafin on that?"

"Couple years back, yeah, but . . ." Roy shrugged. "Nothing came of it. I heard thousands of miners were trying to come here some years back, but the Governor at the time—Governor Cornell—stopped them. Nothing since."

"Hm." Oliver thought for a moment, twirling his cue. "Would you want to unionize? If you could?"

"Better pay, shorter hours, better safety. Don't see why not." Oliver nodded.

Just then, the man with the mustache came back with a box of chalk. Oliver and Roy turned back to the pool table. Oliver supposed that was the end of their conversation. He bet a lot of miners would want to be members of the UMWA if they could. He wondered how Floyd felt. Would Floyd want to fight for the changes? Why hadn't Floyd talked to him about any of this? Surely they could have kept their voices low enough in the mine.

For the rest of the evening, Oliver couldn't stop thinking about everything Roy had told him.

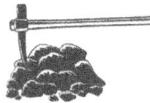

Later in the week, Oliver and Floyd were walking through the company store together. Floyd was having Charlie sharpen his pickaxe. While they waited for it to be finished, Floyd accompanied Oliver to the men's section so that Oliver could find a new pair of overalls. Oliver took two wildly similar pairs off the rack.

"What do you think? Grayish blue or blueish gray?" Oliver asked playfully, holding up one and then the other. "You know, the array of choices here will never not impress me."

"Whatever you choose, it'll be stained tomorrow."

"Well, not permanently. I mean, coal dust washes out."

"Yeah, when you got a strong woman like Effie to scrub it."

"I'm stronger than Effie!" Oliver sputtered, pretending to be offended, which had Floyd chuckling. "Jesus." Oliver looked back and forth between the two pairs of overalls before settling on the blueish-gray ones. He set the other back on the rack. "I should ask James or Frederick to order some other colors. Brown or beige. I mean, those are more my colors than blue. I look nicest in them. Do you want to know yours?"

"Mine?"

"Yeah, sure. Everyone has colors."

Oliver studied Floyd's face, only intending to try to figure out the man's colors, but instead, noticing so much more—his thick eyebrows, his chiseled jaw, and the light shadow of stubble. Last, Oliver's eyes found Floyd's—sky blue, the prettiest eyes Oliver had ever seen. Wow, Floyd was handsome. What a strange thing this was, to focus on someone else's features so closely.

"What are mine?" Floyd asked, which reminded Oliver that he was supposed to have been thinking about the colors Floyd would look best in, not how handsome he was.

"Uhm, yours are . . . hm . . . blue, probably, because of your weirdly pretty eyes, and . . . oh, maybe black and dark gray."

By the time Oliver finished his sentence, Floyd had started to look a little queasy, like a spoonful of ipecac had been shoved in his mouth. Oliver wondered if it was the comment about his eyes that had upset him. Christ, he needed to stop sharing every little thought that popped into his head.

"Don't look at me like that," Oliver said. "Sometimes I can't control the things I say."

Floyd continued to look slightly nauseated.

"Oh, take the compliment and move on," Oliver said, unsure why he was stubbornly trying to force Floyd to be fine with what he had said, rather than apologizing for it. "I like your eyes. I'm allowed to like things, aren't I?"

Finally, Floyd sighed and said, "Yeah, you are."

When Oliver turned to head to the register, he noticed a couple of well-dressed men loitering around the canned food aisle. Briefly, he wondered whether either of them was friends with James, but then he remembered what Roy had told him about Don Chafin's men—the people who supposedly spied on the townsfolk.

"Hey," Oliver said in a hushed voice, leaning in closer to Floyd. "Do you think they work for Chafin?"

Floyd's eyes widened. "How do you know about Chafin?"

"Doesn't everybody know about him?" Oliver continued to watch the men. "No chance they're men from the UMWA, right? If so, I'd be interested in talking to them."

"Shh!"

"What?"

"Don't talk about the UMWA in here! Where's your head?"

"What, is it illegal to even talk about the United Mine Wor—"

Floyd's hand flew to cover Oliver's mouth.

"Ollie, if you keep this up, I'll carry you out of here!" Floyd whisper-yelled in a manner that was, admittedly, a little funny.

Even though Oliver wanted to press Floyd on it—he was curious to learn how Floyd felt about the UMWA—he could tell by the intensity behind Floyd's eyes that he was serious. Oliver held up his hands, one of them still clutching tight to the pair of overalls he had chosen, in mock surrender.

"Go pay for those," Floyd said, taking his hand away. "I'm finding my pick."

When Oliver met up with Floyd outside, he took Floyd by the sleeve and pulled him farther away from the store, both of them kicking up dirt as they moved across the footpath and over toward the railroad tracks.

"Alright, now that we're out of earshot, what's your opinion on the UMWA?"

"I . . ." Floyd huffed. "I'm not in the mood to talk about this."

"Why not?"

"I'm tired from work."

Oliver narrowed his eyes, scrutinizing Floyd's reaction. After a moment, Floyd looked away, and then Oliver noticed how Floyd had started nervously wringing his hands.

"Do you . . . not want to unionize?"

"Change would be hard, Ollie. Let's leave it at that."

God, why was Floyd being so tight-lipped? First, he wouldn't tell Oliver more about his past, and now, he was refusing to have an honest conversation about the benefits of the UMWA? It wasn't like Oliver would be upset with him for his opinion. Oliver was still new. He was still figuring out how everything worked.

He couldn't resist pressing further.

"Well, what would be hard? Maybe you should enlighten me."

Floyd let out an irritated-sounding sigh.

"Did Roy tell you about the tent colonies?"

"Well, yeah, but—"

"Then you know what could happen."

"But—"

"I won't put Effie or Jo through something like that."

"Don't you want a better life for your family?"

Floyd's eye twitched, nostrils flaring. "I like our life!"

Jesus Christ, why was Floyd becoming so irate? Oliver was only trying to have a conversation with him!

"Doesn't your family deserve—"

Floyd took a step forward, closing the distance between them.

"Don't you talk about my family, Ollie," Floyd hissed through clenched teeth. "You know nothing about where I come from or how hard I worked to make a life for us here."

Irritation zipped through Oliver's veins faster than lightning.

"Of course not! You won't talk to me! You won't even tell me about your childhood!"

Floyd curled his lip. "I talk plenty."

"Bullshit!" Oliver yelled before remembering not to be so loud. "You refuse to tell me anything real about your life."

"What's wrong with you? I've known you for less than a month."

Floyd's words hit Oliver like a bucket of cold water, cooling every ounce of his fury instantly. With the flames of upset snuffed out, Oliver could see his request for what it was: selfish and child-ish, a misplaced expectation of a fool who had never had a friend before.

Without waiting for Oliver's response, Floyd turned to leave. And Oliver stayed fixed to the spot, wondering how the hell he could ever come up with a sufficient enough apology.

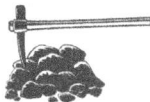

That evening, Oliver was standing in front of Floyd's house, ner-vously shifting his weight from one foot to the other as the soft late-spring breeze whipped through his hair and rustled the fabric of his worst-looking suit—a rust-colored, ill-fitting atrocity. Earlier, while Oliver had been stewing in his remorse back home, he had started to feel that all-too-familiar itch—the itch to cut his losses, either by simply ignoring Floyd and finding a new butty or by reaching out to Frederick to inquire about employment with the steel mill instead.

But Oliver had never felt such a strong connection before. He had been having so much fun with Floyd. And Floyd was so, so sweet. Oliver couldn't explain it, exactly, but Floyd had a sickly sweetness about him sometimes. It seemed as though he truly cared about Oliver, even though they'd only met earlier that month. Ever since Floyd had made Oliver his butty, he had been such a patient teacher, always looking at Oliver with kind eyes and speaking to him like he wasn't ever frustrated, even when Oliver had made a mistake. No one else had ever really treated Oliver like that. Not family members. Or teachers. Which, Oliver realized, was probably why Floyd's random bouts of secrecy had bothered him so much. In some ways, it felt like the two had known each other for much, much longer.

Floyd seemed to like Oliver's playfulness as well. He had never once scolded him for his strange humor. He listened to Oliver babble, which was really sweet of him, especially since most people either stopped listening or made excuses to leave the conversation whenever Oliver veered off into one of his tangents. But not Floyd. Not since they had started to become friends. All of these things together—they made Oliver realize that he had to try to fix things.

So, Oliver smoothed out the fabric of his terrible suit (mostly out of habit, because, God, there was no way to make it look less hideous) and started up the porch stairs. With a slightly trembling hand, Oliver rapped his knuckles on the wood.

Floyd answered with a scowl, and Oliver smiled sheepishly.

"Uh, hi," Oliver said. "Can we talk?"

"I never talk."

"Right." Oliver blew out a breath. "I'm sorry I said that. I'm sorry for, well, everything."

Floyd simply crossed his arms over his chest. He looked like he was waiting for Oliver to elaborate, which made Oliver's stomach creep up into his throat from nervousness.

"Do you mind if we talk inside? Or outside?" Oliver asked. "Anywhere else, really. Just not, you know, with you standing in the doorway like that. You're making me worried that we'll let your cat out or something."

"Cat?"

"Yeah, uhm, I had a cat in New York—a sweet little fellow I found by a dumpster when he was only a teeny tiny kitten. I brought him home with me, and then, once he was big, it became clear to me that I shouldn't keep letting the poor fellow outside. It wasn't that I was worried about him running away or anything, but I realized that he was the type of cat who would run into the street and try to fight other cats and even try to fight squirrels sometimes. After that, we had to be careful not to keep letting him out, and so, now I end up feeling nervous whenever people leave their doors open for too long." Oliver took a pause. He couldn't stand how Floyd was just staring at him, not making a single comment of his own. Instinctively, Oliver continued to ramble. "I kind of miss Colonel Whiskers—that was what I'd named him. Which I know is a strange name for a cat. It's not like he was in the military. Obviously. I mean, he was a cat, for Christ's sake. Or *is* a cat. He's probably still alive. Jesus, I sound like a fucking lunatic."

Just like that, Floyd was laughing that perfect, melodious laugh of his. With a flick of his wrist, he pointed toward the other end of the porch, and so Oliver took a few steps back, the floorboards creaking beneath his feet. Floyd followed and shut the door. Then they stood around awkwardly for what felt like a year but was probably more like four minutes.

Floyd cocked an eyebrow. "Colonel Whiskers, huh?"

"He might be General Whiskers now. I have no way of knowing."

Floyd's face broke into the nicest smile—one that made his eyes crinkle at the corners and dimples etch into his cheeks like little parentheses. And, God, Oliver loved seeing him smile like that. Suddenly, Oliver couldn't stop thinking about how nice of a smile Floyd had and how badly he wanted to keep making it happen. He hadn't ever experienced something like this before.

"I'm really, really sorry," Oliver said. "Sometimes, when we're together, it feels like I've known you for a long time, and then I realize I know next to nothing about you and—" He ran a hand through his hair. "Anyway, I'm sorry."

After a moment, Floyd leaned against the porch column, looking a bit lost in thought, tilting his head and furrowing his thick brows. Oliver had to force himself to look away so he wouldn't ruin everything by talking at him. He wished Floyd would say something.

Floyd heaved a sigh and said, "I'm from McDowell County. My family had a farm there."

I thought you worked in a coal mine, Oliver wanted to say but stopped himself. Instead, he forced himself to wait so that he could hear what else Floyd might want to share on his own.

"Coal companies were buying up a lot of the land around us. I'd been working on the farm since I was little—helping out here and there—but when I was ten, I started as a breaker boy for the closest coal company. Just wanted to earn some money."

Floyd became quiet again. His eyes had a faraway look about them as he stared off into the night. Oliver tried to focus on the high-pitched chirping sound of the spring peepers coming from the woods so that he wouldn't feel the need to fill Floyd's silence with commentary of his own.

Floyd eventually continued, "Years later, some events happened and . . . we had to leave. Me and Effie. I chose Logan for us since I knew there were some big coal companies here. Effie was pregnant with Josephine then, and I knew I had to take care of them both."

Oliver tried to imagine what had happened to make them have to leave but couldn't come up with much. Floyd and Effie were probably the kindest people in the entire world.

"Our lives ain't perfect, but I like to think I made the right choice," Floyd said. "Don Chafin may be a bully, but I'm thankful we're here, not over in Mingo. If we'd had moved there, I'm sure I'd have felt the need to strike with my work buddies, too. We'd have probably ended up in one of them tent colonies." He clicked his tongue once, shaking his head. "I couldn't put Effie and Jo through that. We're lucky that, well, if it happened here, if we were forced out of our home, I think I'd have the means to help start our lives over somewhere else. I'd have to sell something first, but I could come up with some money. Not much. Just, you know, maybe enough to move to another coal town. But I like our life here. I can't . . . I can't never start over again."

"I understand," Oliver said, trying to keep his voice soft and kind. He hoped he could make Floyd see that he really hadn't meant to upset him. "I'm sorry for pushing you about it earlier. I couldn't understand why you wouldn't want to better your lives and—" He realized he was putting his foot in his mouth again. "Sorry. I respect your choice."

Floyd nodded. Oliver nodded back.

Seconds passed. Both men stayed silent. Oliver chewed on his bottom lip while Floyd seemed to be studying his boots. After a minute or two, Floyd looked Oliver up and down.

"What in the heck are you wearing?"

Oliver grinned. "This is my worst suit. I thought that by wearing it, I'd be able to prove to you how terrible I feel about how I acted earlier. You know, because I made myself *look* terrible. I tried to make my outsides match my insides. Does it look horrible?"

Floyd's mouth twisted up into a half-smile, and he raised one of his eyebrows. "Yeah, pretty bad."

"Alright, well, pretty bad isn't nearly horrible enough." In rapid succession, Oliver loosened his tie, popped the top button of his shirt, and yanked one of the buttons clean off his suit jacket. And then, as the final touch, he mussed up his hair. "Better? Worse?"

Floyd snorted a laugh. "Worse."

"Good," Oliver said, feeling relaxed and content once again.

And Floyd looked plenty relaxed now, too. His shoulders weren't tensed up anymore, and he had finally uncrossed his arms.

He said, "We had supper earlier, but you can come in if you want. Effie and Jo would be happy to see you. Sorry, I meant *I'd* be happy to see you."

"You haven't seen too much of me already?"

"Not at all," Floyd said, a sweetness in his voice.

"I'd love to come in, then."

As soon as they were inside, Josephine skipped over to them. She stopped a handful of paces short of Oliver and tilted her head to the side.

"Why's your hair like that?"

"I thought I'd try a new style tonight. What do you think?"

Josephine pursed her lips for a moment as she thought.

"Too messy," she said.

"Yeah, I thought so, too."

Oliver noticed Effie sitting on the sofa, kneading the sole of one of her feet with her thumbs, and Floyd went to sit beside her. Even though Oliver knew what was coming, seeing the scene unfold still made his stomach drop like a rickety old coal elevator.

"Let me help," Floyd said, pulling Effie's feet on top of his lap, which made Oliver have to turn away for some reason. "I told you not to bother washing clothes today. You spent too many hours on them feet of yours yesterday."

Oliver's heart fluttered at the way Floyd said the word "wash," which sounded more like "warsh" because of his accent. It was so . . . God, it was fucking adorable. What a peculiar thought that was. But it was so true. Water was wet, and Floyd was adorable. Facts were facts.

"I can't let Josephine run around in rags," Effie said. "All her nice clothes were filthy."

Oliver looked back to see Floyd massaging Effie's feet.

"So, uhm . . ." Oliver looked around, eager to focus on something other than the way that the sight of Floyd massaging Effie's feet was making his neck burn and his ears feel hot. His eyes found Josephine, who was sitting on the floor cross-legged, fiddling with the dress of a very well-loved doll. "How was school, Josephine?"

Before Josephine could answer, Effie cut in.

"Floyd, stop massaging my feet. You're making poor Oliver uncomfortable."

Floyd looked like he wanted to protest but released Effie's feet anyway.

"School was boring," Josephine answered before looking up at her parents. "Can Mister Oliver play with me?"

Floyd chuckled. "I reckon Mister Oliver is a little old for toys."

"Well, he certainly looks like a schoolboy with his hair mussed up like that," Effie teased. "He reminds me of you, Floyd, messing around near the mines when we were kids."

Oliver knelt down to talk to Josephine. "I'd love to play, but I'm afraid I forgot to bring my own dolly."

"What about checkers?" Josephine asked.

"I can play checkers," Oliver agreed.

"Mama, will you be on my team?"

"Josephine is still learning. We only started playing earlier this week," Effie explained. "Yes, Josephine, I can help you."

While Josephine scrambled to her feet to find the board and pieces, Floyd pulled the coffee table closer to the couch and then made his way to the burnt orange armchair. Oliver looked over to the bookcase, which was mostly filled with knickknacks and other board games, and saw that they had a chess set, too.

"So, which of you is better at chess?" Oliver asked.

"Effie," Floyd said without hesitation. "Because she won't learn me how to play."

Oliver laughed. "Why's that?"

"Floyd always picks things up so quickly. If I teach him, I'll lose my title."

"Title?" Oliver asked, arching an eyebrow.

"It's not a real title, but—"

"Effie is the best chess player in the entire town," Floyd said, his voice filled with unmistakable pride.

It pulled at Oliver's heart.

"I learned when I was little. I was only a couple of years older than Josephine."

Josephine plopped the board and pieces onto the table. She and Effie started setting them up. Oliver scooted over to sit across from Effie, sitting back on his heels. Floyd nudged him with his foot from behind.

"Want my chair?"

Oliver smiled up at him. "Nah, I'm fine."

For the next half hour, Oliver played Effie and Josephine in checkers while Floyd looked on. It was so strangely calm. Blissful, really. Oliver had sometimes imagined that there were families like

Floyd's—ones who spent time together, who laughed with one another, who enjoyed each other's company—but he had never expected that he might become close with one of them. His own family was nothing like this.

On the surface, the Bennetts looked like every other family that Oliver had ever spent a small amount of time with, but now that he had spent time with them, he could see that they were something truly special. He could sense the tightness of the bond they shared.

It reminded Oliver of the time he had broken open one of those special rocks—the ones that were sparkly inside. At first look, the thing was utterly unimpressive—an ordinary rock, like every other rock—but once he had broken it open, Oliver had been completely taken aback by its beauty.

God, how incredible Floyd's family was.

When Oliver sighed, Floyd nudged him again, and Oliver turned to see Floyd looking at him with one eyebrow raised inquisitively, perhaps to check on him. Oliver nodded, silently reassuring Floyd that he was fine, but as soon as he turned back around, Floyd nudged him again, more forcefully and playfully this time, which made Oliver chuckle.

"King me!" Josephine suddenly cried.

"You only say that when you reach the last row on Oliver's side," Effie said with a laugh.

"Well, then, what do you say when you win?"

Oliver answered, "Whatever you want."

"Queen me!"

Oliver reached across the table and tapped each of Josephine's shoulders.

"Oh. I think I knighted you instead," Oliver said. "Sorry."

"Good enough, Oliver," Effie said. "Now it's time for the Queen to go to bed."

Josephine threw her head back and groaned. "Why?"

"Because it's late, and you got school tomorrow morning."

"Fiiine," she relented before hopping off the couch.

Without even a parting word, she ran toward the back room.

"Want to me put her to bed?" Floyd asked.

"You stay with Oliver," Effie said.

"I should head home anyway," Oliver said.

Floyd pushed himself to stand. "I'll walk you out."

"Yes, I mean, your front door is so far away," Oliver said, hopping to his feet. "How ever would I make it on my own?"

Floyd responded by shoving Oliver forward a step.

Once the two of them were outside, Oliver paused at the edge of the porch and said, "I really liked spending time with all of you tonight."

"Why'd you seem sad earlier?"

"Hm?"

"You were sighing and such."

"Oh. I was thinking about my terrible parents. We never spent time with each other like that," Oliver said. "In fact, they rarely ever wanted me around when I was a kid. God, I can't even fathom what it would have been like to play checkers with my mother."

"I'm sorry, Ollie," Floyd said, and the sweetness in his voice made Oliver's stomach tumble. "Was there really no one you were close to?"

"Well, I suppose I had my Aunt Betty for a bit. We weren't close, exactly, but she was kind to me. Actually, I've been considering visiting her. She lives in Charleston. And, well, she isn't in contact with my parents anymore. I tried to visit her when I first came here, but I was too nervous."

"Why?"

Oliver shrugged. "Just was. Everyone in my family makes me nervous."

Letting out a soft hum, Floyd nodded in response. Oliver was thankful that Floyd was respectful enough not to press him for more information. He wished he possessed that kind of willpower himself.

After a moment, Floyd asked Oliver to wait while he fetched something from inside. Floyd returned a short time later with Oliver's hat.

He held it out and said, "Here, Ollie. I plum forgot I was wearing this when we played pool. Kept it on the whole way home."

"I know," Oliver said. "Keep it."

"It's your hat. I can't take it from you."

"You're not taking it. It's a present." Oliver took the hat from Floyd's hands and placed it atop Floyd's head. "Gray is *definitely* one of your colors."

"Ain't it a little depressing?"

Oliver's voice softened. "Not on you."

When Floyd reached up to adjust his hat, Oliver's chest warmed in the most wonderful way. He loved seeing Floyd wear it.

Even though they'd see each other in less than twelve hours, it pained Oliver that he had to leave. He wanted to keep spending time with Floyd. He'd honestly spend every second with him if he could. Which was a strange feeling. Oliver had been his own best friend for as long as he could remember. Now things were different, though. Oliver liked Floyd way more than he liked himself. He liked Floyd more than he had ever liked anyone.

"Oh, I've been meaning to ask you, how does everyone spend their leisure time around here? Like on weekends?" Oliver asked. "I've mostly been reading, myself. I found a few books at the company store like you said I would. Just Dickens and Poe. I played pool with Roy once, too, which was fun. I think he's a little sour that I keep beating him. But, uhm, what else?"

"Well, a lot of people work in the mines on Saturdays, especially if they need to make some extra money to pay what they owe at the store. Settle their debts and whatnot. Sundays, though, most people attend church."

"Do you?"

"Yep. All three of us."

"I'm not . . . I mean, I . . ." Oliver cleared his throat. "I'll probably stay home on Sundays. Unless . . . uhm . . ."

"If you change your mind, you can sit in our pew."

"Thank you."

"You know, I'm not one to work on Saturdays."

"Oh?" Oliver's heart started beating a little faster.

"You and me could do something."

"Sure!" Oliver exclaimed before intentionally reigning in his excitement. "What?"

"I can show you how to shoot a rifle gun."

"Yeah?"

"Yeah."

"Wow, that would be wonderful. I have to warn you, though, that I'll probably be a terrible shot. I mean, I'm shit even with a slingshot."

With a snort of amusement, Floyd shook his head.

"I might have to sew my mouth shut before I come to church, huh?" Oliver teased.

"Nah, I like listening to you. Even those silly remarks of yours and the obscenities you seem so fond of."

Oliver's stomach fluttered as Floyd's compliment made his face tingle, his cheeks heating up from Floyd's unexpected praise. God, he had never felt this way before. About anyone.

"Alright, well, I'll see you tomorrow for work, Floyd."

"Goodnight, Ollie."

Oliver was so Goddamn excited for the weekend.

CHAPTER FIVE

FLOYD

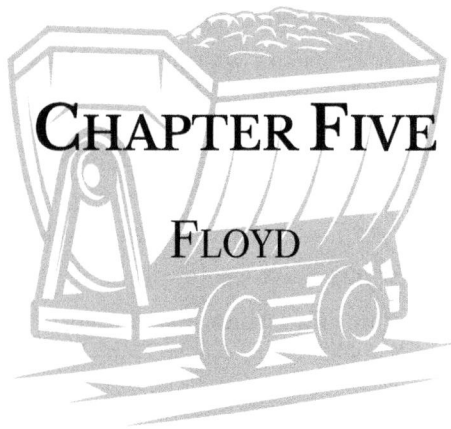

ON SATURDAY, FLOYD WAS pacing back and forth in the living area, counting the minutes until Ollie was supposed to arrive. He kept fiddling with his shirt, unbuttoning the second and third buttons from the top, only to refasten them moments later. He wasn't sure why he was fretting so much about his appearance. It wasn't like Ollie hadn't seen him like this before. He had worn nearly the same exact outfit to work many times.

Except that this particular shirt was a plaid pattern of sky blue and steel gray rather than a single muted color like most of his work ones. Floyd had chosen it on purpose since Ollie had kind of implied that he thought Floyd would look nice in these colors. And, well, as such . . .

Floyd blew out a forceful sigh, one that had him puffing out his cheeks. After a moment, he settled on leaving the top three buttons of the shirt unfastened, telling himself that it looked more casual that way. Besides, it was hot outside. He wouldn't want to be uncomfortable.

He continued to pace. Josephine was out with their neighbor's boy, William, probably playing in the woods, while Effie was scrubbing the stove. Earlier, Floyd had urged Effie to see one of her friends instead. It was only fair that she have some fun, too. But Effie was Effie. If she had set her heart on scrubbing the stove, then that's what she would do.

"You're about to wear a hole in our floor," she said.

Floyd stopped. "Sorry."

"Don't worry about it. I know how you can be."

"What do you mean?"

"When you're sweet on someone."

"What?" Floyd asked, feigning surprise, though both Effie's bluntness and the truth in what she had said sent the blood rushing to his cheeks. "I ain't sweet on Ollie."

"It's sweet that you got a nickname for him already."

Floyd scoffed and said, "We're friends."

But he knew that Effie would see right through him.

"Uh-huh. You know, I swear I seen Oliver making eyes at you, too."

"Don't start. Ollie ain't like that."

"He might be."

Floyd's heart sped up—*a lot*. Ever since the pool hall, Floyd had come to accept the way Oliver could make his heart pitter-patter with all that handsomeness of his. But that had been the extent of it. He hadn't never allowed himself to consider the possibility of Oliver liking him back. It made no sense to entertain silly fantasies like that. Men liking other men wasn't exactly common. Or, if it was, no one ever seemed to talk about it. Besides, the thought of maybe starting something with Ollie, it was enough to wake that copperhead in his stomach. Somehow, the snake had been calm ever since the pool hall. But if Ollie and him ever . . .

No. Ollie and him could never be more than friends. He had a family.

"So what if he is? Did you forget that we're married?"

Effie said, "We could figure something out," like it would be the simplest thing in the world.

Her words sent little tremors of fear rolling through Floyd's body. For years, he had been keeping his heart safe. Ever since he had lost his most important person all them years ago, Floyd hadn't never allowed himself to even consider being romantic with someone else. His palms started to sweat, painful images flashing in his mind—thick black plumes of coal powder and the enormous pile of rubble.

"Effie, stop," Floyd shot back, unable to let himself think of a relationship with Ollie right now. He had to steady himself. Ollie was supposed to arrive any minute.

Effie held up her hands innocently. "Alright, I won't bother you no more."

Floyd startled from the knock at the door.

"Go ahead," Effie said with a playful chuckle.

Floyd tried to ignore the strange new fear he was feeling, but with every step toward the door, his heart was hammering a tiny bit faster, his worriment becoming so intense that he had to pause and take a few breaths to calm himself before turning the knob.

Thankfully, as soon as Floyd opened the door, Ollie's silly smile and even sillier outfit tempered some of his nervousness, calming his racing heart and releasing some of the tension in his muscles.

"What in the tarnation?" Floyd laughed. "Why are you dressed like that?"

"What do you mean?" Ollie asked, looking down at his own outfit. "I look nice, right?"

Of course, Ollie looked nice. He looked so nice, in fact, that if Floyd let himself think about it too hard, he'd have to steal some private time in Effie's little sewing room (which was more like an oversized closet) later, probably in the middle of the night, but *nice* wasn't what Floyd was reacting to. Ollie was wearing a slightly off-white suit, paired with a brown vest and a blue-and-yellow striped tie. And, typical for Ollie, he was wearing a hat, too—a straw boater, one with a silky brown ribbon encircling the base, the color an exact match for the shade of his vest.

"I thought I was learning you how to shoot," Floyd said. "You look like you're heading to the pictures."

"We could?" Ollie suggested, which made Floyd roll his eyes.

"We could what? See a picture? In *Charleston*?!"

"Yeah, maybe we'd have had to plan that better. Oh well. I'm sure I can shoot in these, though. I mean, you're wearing a nice shirt yourself. Don't think I haven't noticed the colors."

Ollie smiled in a flirtatious way, tipping his head slightly, one side of his mouth twisted up higher than the other. It was playful and sweet and knowing—like he knew *exactly* why Floyd had chosen that shirt; like he knew *exactly* why Floyd had left the top buttons unfastened; like he knew *everything*.

Floyd swallowed against the rising fear of being seen.

Did Ollie know of Floyd's feelings for him?

"Leave your suit jacket here," Floyd said, purposefully ignoring Ollie's comment or compliment or whatever it was. "Your hat, too."

Even though Ollie started to shrug off his suit jacket, he said, "But I like my hat. It'll protect my head from the sun."

"Fine. Bring your hat."

"What about your hat?" Ollie asked, handing Floyd the jacket, which Floyd then tossed over the back of the rocking chair.

"Why would I wear my hat?"

"I'll look less silly if you wear yours, too."

"No, if I wear mine, *I'd* only look more silly." Floyd pointed outside. "Get."

"Sheesh," Ollie said, turning around.

Floyd looked back to wave to Effie. "Be back for supper."

"Have fun," Effie called in a sing-song voice that made Floyd's cheeks flush.

Out on the porch, Floyd picked up the poke he had packed earlier with a whole mess of empty Coke bottles. Then, he went around back to fetch his rifle from the shed. Afterward, he and Oliver started into the woods.

While they walked, Ollie kept tripping on various rocks and tree roots. To keep himself from chuckling too much about Ollie's plight, Floyd focused on telling the story of when he had first learned to shoot. Floyd's father had learned him when he was twelve. At that time, Floyd had been working as a breaker boy for the coal company, and as such, he and his father hadn't been spending as much time together, not like back when Floyd had been helping out on their farm every single morning. And so, his father had learned him to shoot so that they could have something to share on the weekends when there wasn't too much farm work. Floyd had taken to it immediately.

While Floyd was telling the story, Ollie kept looking over at him. It was like Ollie wanted to keep his eyes on Floyd even at the expense of his own safety. This had Floyd's body buzzing with energy, each of Ollie's sweet smiles sending little blips of electrical current through him, making his heart pound.

When they were nearing the area Floyd wanted to use for Ollie's lesson, Floyd breathed a sigh of relief. Finally, something else for them to both focus on.

Oliver tripped over another tree root.

"Why'd you dress so fancy?" Floyd asked, looking at Ollie's brown leather shoes. "Did you really want us to see a picture?"

"No, not really. Just, well, I like clothes. I like looking nice." Ollie scrunched up his face. "I'm sorry if that's strange."

"Nah, everyone has their own things they like."

Truthfully, Floyd really liked Ollie's outfits, but he couldn't make himself say that.

"Are you coming to church tomorrow?" Floyd asked. "It won't be strange to wear a suit there."

"Yeah, I think so. I hope that's alright?"

"Of course."

Which meant that, if Ollie kept coming to church, Floyd would see Ollie near every day. The possibility of being with Ollie so often filled Floyd's chest with the most tender warmth.

Once the two reached the spot Floyd had picked out—a clearing free of trees and shrubbery, save for some stumps here and there—Floyd instructed Ollie to line up the Coke bottles atop a stump some one hundred yards away while he took out his 1870/87/15 Vetterli and checked it over. Floyd was finishing up loading the bullets when Ollie came up beside him.

"I can't believe you're teaching me how to use that," Ollie said. "I want to ask if it's safe, but it's a weapon, so . . ."

Ollie's unease tugged at Floyd's heart. It was strange, in some ways, how Ollie could seem so worldly, and yet so innocent, too.

"It's safe enough." Floyd said reassuringly. "You know, a lot of folks around here like a Winchester. It's a newer type of rifle gun. I heard some not-to-nice stuff about it, though, like that it ain't easy for loading and unloading the bullets. Couple of men have lost their fingers. Sometimes, I catch myself thinking I'd be too smart to maim myself like that and consider buying one, but it ain't worth chancing. Not when I have this here Vetterli, which is plenty safe. Accurate, too." Floyd clapped Ollie on the shoulder. "You'll be safe, Ollie. I won't let you blow your fingers off."

"Thank God for that," Ollie said, his voice still sounding a tad unsteady.

Ollie's innocence was making Floyd feel tingly inside. Little bursts of protective energy were rippling over his skin, and Floyd had to force himself to ignore it.

"Mind if I impress you before I move on to the lesson?" Floyd asked.

"Definitely not."

Floyd brought the rifle up to his shoulder, lined up the shot, and fired, shattering one of the bottles.

"Not bad, huh?"

"Jesus."

Floyd laughed. "Not the name I'd expect someone to say after watching me obliterate a Coke bottle."

"Yeah, well, you're—wow," Ollie said, as though he couldn't think of a response. "Can I try now?"

"Yep. But first, let me explain how it works."

Floyd pulled up and back on the extractor to expel the spent casing and launched into his lesson on the mechanics, telling Ollie how the Vetterli worked the best he could, and once he was finished, he handed the rifle over to him. Next, Floyd tried to explain to Ollie how to aim properly, but Ollie eagerly lifted the rifle and fired before Floyd could say much. He missed the target by a mile.

"Damn," Ollie sighed.

"What'd you expect? It was your first shot."

"Yeah, I suppose. You made it look easy, though."

"Well, it ain't."

"I can see that now."

Ollie struggled to ready the rifle for the next shot. Floyd opened his mouth to try to explain how he could hold it better, but Ollie fired again. Floyd could tell that Ollie's pride was hurting a little bit, which seemed kind of silly to him, especially since Ollie couldn't seem to hold still long enough for a proper lesson. Floyd considered reminding Ollie that learning something new takes both time and patience, but in the end, he thought that maybe Ollie wouldn't like that.

So, Floyd stood back and watched Ollie struggle. He watched him struggle with dislodging the casing. He watched him struggle with firing the next shot. And the next. And the next. And when it came time for Ollie to reload, he watched Ollie struggle with the clip.

After one more round of this, Ollie still hadn't hit a single bottle. His cheeks had become a pinkish red, whether from shame or anger, Floyd didn't know, but either way, Floyd could sense what was about to happen before Ollie even turned away from the targets.

"Alright, let's head back," Ollie said, holding out the rifle. "Here."

Looking at the Vetterli, Floyd's mouth set to a frown. He thought about how Ollie tended not to finish things. Like college. Or books. Which was a shame. Because Ollie had a real potential inside of him.

"Nope," Floyd said. "We can head back once you hit one of them bottles."

"Well, then I hope you like living in the woods," Ollie said, sarcastic-like.

"It takes practice, is all."

"I've been practicing."

"You only fired a couple of rounds."

"More than a couple," Ollie said, starting to raise his voice. "I'm shit at this, Floyd. I can't aim right."

"You ain't sh—" Floyd caught himself. "You ain't that. Like I said, you need practice. Look how fast you're taking to mining. Don't sell yourself short, Ollie." Floyd came up beside him. "I can help you. Ready your shot."

Ollie brought up the rifle, and Floyd came up behind him. Floyd helped adjust Ollie's positioning, lifting the butt a little higher so it would rest closer to his shoulder, rather than the fleshy part near his armpit, where he'd been steadying it before. Next, Floyd pressed Ollie's elbows in and instructed him to keep them that way.

All the while Floyd's heart was hammering ferociously in his chest again, and the intensity of it—the pure *energy* of it—made him think of an old Model T. It was like every touch between the two of them was one more turn of the hand crank, each one building upon the other 'til a spark of fierce yearning had roared to life inside of him. Desire continued to rumble, the force of it nearly causing Floyd's body to shake.

"Alright, now you need to relax your body," Floyd said, as much to himself as to Ollie. Backing off, he said, "Try to control your breathing. Slow and steady."

Ollie fired. And missed. He lowered the rifle.

Before Ollie could protest, Floyd came up behind him and forced Ollie to lift it by raising his arms.

"Ollie, you can do this," Floyd said close to Ollie's ear, his voice low and stern. "I want you to try one more time."

Ollie turned his head slightly, locking eyes with Floyd, and the two of them were close enough that Floyd could feel the warmth of each of Ollie's exhales. He fought to keep his expression neutral, though on the inside, he was feeling what somehow seemed like two hundred crazy emotions at once.

"Alright," Ollie finally said. "One more time."

Floyd nodded curtly and backed away. Ollie took his time readying himself for this one. Floyd could feel a change in him, a tiny flame of determination, one that hadn't been there before. He prayed to God that Ollie would succeed. Golly, how he wanted the two of them to celebrate together.

Ollie pulled the trigger, and then one of the bottles exploded.

"Holy Moses!" Ollie looked excited enough to leap out of his own skin. "I hit one!"

"Nice shot," Floyd responded with a proud smile.

"Thank you," Ollie said before holding out the rifle. "Can we head back now? I'm starving. All that success really worked up my appetite."

"Yeah, we can. Go fetch the rest of them bottles. We can use 'em next time," Floyd said, taking the rifle from him. "Be careful not to cut yourself."

And Floyd's still-hammering heart was happy that Ollie was happy too.

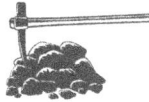

Later that evening, Floyd and Ollie were sitting together on the couch while Josephine and Effie finished cooking supper. Josephine liked to help in the kitchen sometimes, which was nice, though sometimes it meant that the food might be either a little too salty or too sweet, depending on what they were making. Floyd hoped that Ollie wouldn't mind. It was just one of them things about having kids, especially when you're someone like Effie, who liked encouraging Josephine's independence and creativity, even at the expense of her taste buds.

"Supper's ready!" Effie called.

They all sat together for some bean stew, which, surprisingly enough, wasn't too overly seasoned, and Floyd was happy to see that Ollie seemed to like it, too. When Josephine caught Floyd's eye, he threw her an appreciative wink, which had her giggling.

Throughout the meal, Ollie talked a little bit (or, well, Ollie was Ollie, so "a little bit" was maybe underselling the amount) about his life in New York City, mostly about the entertainment they had up there, not so much about his home life. He told them about music lounges and baseball games and vaudeville shows. It sounded real magical. Floyd had never been in the habit of coveting somebody else's life, but it was hard not to feel a tad envious of Ollie's time in New York. He had experienced so much in life already. It was a wonder that he had chosen to leave that style of living behind.

Josephine seemed a little bored of the conversation for a while, her eyes wandering to this and that, her shoulder slumping. But then Ollie started talking about the circus he had seen in Charleston, and once that happened, Josephine was visibly buzzing with energy—her eyes brightening and her face lighting up with excitement. Ollie was painting such an incredible picture of the circus with his words, telling them about people flying through the air and elephants performing tricks and even a man who could bend his body into the shape of a pretzel (Ollie had to explain what a pretzel was, which, once he had, made Josephine real eager to try one someday). Apparently, Ollie had seen the performance shortly before meeting with Fred Donohue.

"Daddy, can you take me to the circus someday?" she asked, excitement radiating off her as she wiggled around in her chair.

Floyd's smile faltered. "Uh . . ."

Josephine's eyes widened. "When, when, when?!"

Shame pricked at Floyd's insides. He wasn't too sure how much the circus was, but it probably wasn't cheap. It wasn't something you could keep neither, like a toy or a piece of clothing. It might not be the best use of the savings they had. Not unless Floyd could try to make a little more money to offset it somehow.

Effie answered for him. "We can't afford that right now, baby. Probably not for a while."

Josephine's shoulders slumped forward again, the excitement and happiness rushing out of her in an instant, leaving her looking like a limp balloon.

"I'm sorry, Jo," Floyd said.

"It's fine," she said, even though it was painfully obvious that it was very much not fine. "It sounded magical, is all."

"I know."

Everyone was quiet for a few ticks of the clock. Suddenly, Ollie snapped his fingers.

"Josephine," Ollie began, "you can see magic right here in Rock Creek. There's no need to catch a train to Charleston."

Josephine looked skeptical. "What do you mean?"

Ollie fished around in his pocket and pulled out a quarter, which he then held up for Josephine to see.

"I have magical powers," he said. "Do you believe me?"

Josephine was clearly fighting a smile now. "No."

"I'll prove it to you," Ollie said. "I can make this coin disappear."

"No, you can't!" Josephine protested, her voice playful and happy once again.

"Let's see your magic, Oliver," Effie said. "I believe in you."

"Ah, what a supportive family," Ollie said, looking over at Effie in an affectionate sort of way before shooting a look of mock disapproval over at Josephine. "Most of you, anyway."

Which made Josephine giggle.

Ollie proceeded to balance the coin on the top of one of his index fingers. Next, he closed his free hand over both, squeezing tight. When he uncurled his fingers, it seemed like the coin had vanished.

"Oh, my word!" Effie shouted, sounding immensely pleased.

Josephine's mouth had simply fallen open.

Ollie repeated the motion, but this time, when he uncurled his fingers, the coin had magically reappeared.

"Wow!" Josephine exclaimed.

"See, there's plenty of magic here already," Ollie said, handing Josephine the quarter. "You can have this for your circus fund, though. I'm sure you'll make it to one someday."

Without even taking the time to thank Ollie, Josephine leapt out of her chair.

"I need to put it somewhere safe!"

Floyd called after her. "What do you say to Mister Oliver?"

"Thank you!" she called from the back room.

Arching an eyebrow, Floyd looked over at Ollie.

"Magic?"

"I know plenty of useless stuff."

"Clearly that wasn't useless," Effie said. "Look how happy you made her."

"I suppose that's true."

"Yeah, it is true," Floyd said. "That was real kind of you, Ollie."

Floyd and Ollie smiled at each other for a few long seconds. Effie cleared her throat.

"Oliver, you had speakeasies in New York?" she asked.

"Um, yeah, why?"

Effie stood up from the table and walked over to the counter. "Well, if y'all are finished with supper, maybe you ought to have a treat."

"What, like a cocktail?" Ollie asked through a confused-sounding laugh.

"Not exactly," she said, opening a cabinet and pulling out a very old bottle of clear alcohol. "We got this, though."

Floyd made a face. "Effie, come on, Ollie ain't gonna try moonshine."

"Yes, I will," Ollie sputtered. "Of course I will. Where'd you even find that?"

"Floyd bought it last year over in Mingo County. We barely ever drink it ourselves."

"Mingo, huh?" Ollie asked, raising his brows in a teasing manner.

"Yeah, I wanted to be nice, is all," Floyd responded, trying to keep his voice level even though his heart was starting to hammer a little thinking of the striking miners and the fight he'd had with Ollie in front of the company store. "Some of them strikers were selling bottles, so I bought one."

Effie set the bottle on the table.

"You left out the best part," Effie said. "Floyd bought it with stuff the families needed—a bunch of food and some blankets and a couple of oil lamps."

"It was probably a strange thing for me to do," Floyd said dismissively, wondering why Effie was embarrassing him like this.

"Why would it be strange?" Effie asked, turning to fetch a couple of tumblers. "You heard about what had happened and so you wanted to help."

"That's admirable," Ollie said in earnest. "Really fucking admirable."

Which was probably the nicest and most vulgar compliment Floyd had ever received. Suddenly flustered, Floyd busied himself with counting the little scuff marks that were etched into the wood of the kitchen table, waiting for the feeling to pass.

Besides only feeling flustered by Oliver's compliment, Floyd was starting to feel uneasy about the striking too. Suddenly, it was like he was back in Mingo County seeing the tent colonies in person. He couldn't never put the people he loved through something like that. And the thought of leaving coal mining behind instead? No. He couldn't never.

He knew the kinds of things the UMWA wanted to help with. All of these worries together, they were making his palms sweat. Over the next couple seconds—seconds that seemed to stretch on into eternity—Floyd started thinking 'bout the changes those families were fighting for. Changes that might have helped the man he had lost. Floyd's heart clenched.

By the time Floyd forced himself to look up, Effie had finished pouring both him and Ollie a couple of fingers of moonshine.

"You boys can take these outside," she said, moving the drinks closer. "Me and Josephine will clean up. Or maybe I'll let her play for a while. She's probably taking her paper dolls to the circus or something."

Floyd wasn't really one to consume alcohol, not outside of special occasions. It wasn't as though he had purchased the moonshine because he'd been hankering for it. As such, Floyd considered protesting, but he figured it probably wouldn't work. Because when Effie had an idea, especially one she was particularly proud of, pushing back against it rarely ever ended up yielding the sought after result. And she seemed to be pretty proud of this one.

"Thanks, Effie," Floyd said, standing up and taking his tumbler.

Floyd and Ollie walked to the porch together and sat down on either of the two rocking chairs. Floyd took a small sip of the moonshine while Ollie continued to inspect his. Floyd watched him smell it and then wrinkle his nose. Dang, that was adorable.

"Smells . . . uhm . . . interesting."

Floyd hid a burgeoning smile behind his tumbler. "Drink up, city boy."

"Wow, one sip and you're already insulting me."

"'City boy' is an insult?"

"If 'Jesus Christ' is a swear word, then 'city boy' has to be an insult."

Floyd snorted. "Whatever you say," he paused and raised his tumbler back up to his lips before slyly tacking on the supposed insult. "City boy."

With a shake of his head, Ollie clucked his tongue in mock disapproval.

"Here I thought you were a perfect gentleman," he said before swiftly throwing back a huge swig of his moonshine, which immediately had him making one of the most bizarre faces Floyd had ever seen. After Oliver swallowed, he started sputtering and coughing. "Jesus, Mary, and Joseph!"

"All three, huh?"

"Yes, all three." Ollie smacked his lips. "Why'd you let me have half of it all at once like that? It feels like my stomach is on fire."

Floyd started cackling. "Sorry."

"Phew," Ollie shook his head kind of violently. "I need some time to recover now."

If Ollie wanted time to recover, Floyd had no problem sitting back and relaxing. Ollie could relax, too. Or talk. Or continue to make funny comments about the moonshine. Whatever he wanted. Floyd was just happy that they were spending time together.

Ollie cleared his throat in a very showy manner. Floyd cocked an eyebrow in response. Knowing Ollie, he was probably fixing to say something funny.

But then Floyd watched Ollie sit forward to rest his forearms on his knees, and his expression turned serious. Floyd crossed one leg over the other, waiting to hear what he had to say.

"Floyd, I want to talk to you about something," Oliver said.

"What is it?"

"Nothing bad. Or nothing bad about you. Just . . ." Ollie paused for a while, which wasn't really like him. It had Floyd a little worried. "I really appreciate that you told me so much about your life in McDowell. I've talked about New York a little, but I've never really talked about anything . . . real. Like my family."

"Doesn't bother me."

"No, I know I shouldn't feel obligated to tell you, but I, well, I want us to be honest with each other." Ollie set his tumbler down on the porch floor and married his hands together. "I left home because I wasn't interested in a future that was planned for me. I mean, maybe there were other reasons, too, but they'd probably seem silly to you. Anyway, I was supposed to take over my family's railroad someday. Or network of railroads. Our family owns a few small lines out in Ohio. It was the plan that I'd move back there once I finished college. But, of course, I never completed my coursework. I couldn't make myself want it. So, yes, before you ask, I have a lot of money. I'd have had even more if I had stayed in New York or had moved back to Cleveland—you know, from taking over the railroad lines. Still, I have plenty, so if you ever need my help—"

"Don't," Floyd said. "I won't ever be borrowing from you, Ollie."

Floyd tried to smile to let Ollie know he wasn't upset by the suggestion but had a bit of trouble looking happy. It was strange to learn that Ollie had come from that kind of money. Jealousy started burning inside him, making Floyd feel like maybe his stomach juices had spilled out somehow, and so he tried to force the feeling away with some more moonshine, which thankfully burned even stronger, vanishing that silly envy in seconds.

Ollie said, "I know you probably think that I'm . . . that I've lost my head coming out here. But, Floyd, it is so nice to be somewhere new, to have moved to a place where no one knows who I am or who my family is, or who I was supposed to be." Hearing those words—that sentiment—from Ollie, Floyd was finding it a bit hard to breathe. "Well, you know what that's like, right?"

Floyd managed a nod. He knew it well.

Oliver picked up his tumbler and smelled the moonshine again.

"I'll try a smaller sip this time," Ollie said before bringing it to his lips and taking a swig. "Jeez, that's strong. At least the cocktails I had in New York were watered down. Probably to cheat me out of money, but, Jesus, I kind of appreciate that now."

Thankfully, Ollie's humor had lifted the weight that had come to settle on Floyd's chest earlier. He could breathe easy again.

"Well, me and Effie would never cheat you, Ollie. If you ask for moonshine, we'll serve you moonshine. Ain't my fault you can't pace yourself."

"It's one punch after another with you tonight, isn't it?" Ollie teased. "God, it's like you're Jack Dempsey and I'm Bill Brennan."

"Am I supposed to know them people?"

"Do you not like boxing?"

"Is that the sport where two men try to beat each other sense-less?"

"More or less. It's not as lawless as you're making it seem. Well, sometimes it is, like in a few of the neighborhoods in the city, but it's a real sport, too, with rules and everything."

"Well, I never watched it. Or listened to it."

"Really? Haven't you ever had a . . . a pretend fist fight with someone? That would be kind of like a boxing match."

"Can't say that I have."

"Not even when you were a kid? When we moved to New York, I'd see kids fighting each other once in a while, but they never looked like real fights. Just kids being kids, having fun."

Floyd shook his head. When he was a kid, he had been busy on the farm and then eventually he'd been busy in the coal mine too.

"Nope."

"Really?" Ollie set his tumbler by his feet and stood. He closed both hands into fists. "Let's try one."

"Try a boxing match?"

"Come on, put up your dukes or whatever it is boxers say."

"Ollie, no."

"Why not? We'll only tap each other." Ollie uncurled his fists. "If it'll make you feel better, we can fight like this instead—open palms. Even though you're, what, two or three inches taller than I am, I'd put money on me slapping better than you."

"What's wrong with you?" Floyd asked through a laugh. "Moonshine takes longer than this to work."

Ollie took two steps forward and swung his arm, smacking Floyd on the shoulder, the movement surprising Floyd enough to cause him to fumble with his tumbler, sending some moonshine sloshing over the brim. With an irritated sigh, Floyd bent down to place his tumbler down on the porch, figuring he might as well put Oliver in his place. He stood and held up his hands.

"Alright, so, on the count of three, we'll see who can smack the other first," Ollie said. "Are you ready to cry, lunkhead?"

"You become odder every day," Floyd said, though he still readied himself by adjusting his stance to match Ollie's.

"One . . . two . . . three!"

It was over very quickly. Ollie took two pitiful swings, both of which Floyd blocked with ease, and then Floyd smacked Ollie clear across the face. Ollie shouted an expletive and turned away, covering his cheek. Floyd offered a sympathetic clap on the shoulder.

"Sorry about that."

"It's fine," Ollie said, rubbing his face and laughing. "I kind of forced your hand."

"Why'd you want to fight each other?"

"I'm not sure." Ollie touched his cheek with his fingertips. "When I was in New York, I wanted to try it, but of course, I'd been a smidge too old by then. I thought this would be fun."

Ollie seemed to have been trying to take back a little piece of childhood, one he hadn't never been fortunate enough to experience before. Floyd felt a warm tenderness flicker to life inside of him, happy that he could provide Ollie with a bit of childhood merriment. Even if their boxing match *had* been kind of silly.

"Yeah, it *was* fun," Floyd said, sitting back down before throwing Ollie a teasing smile. "For *me*."

After a playful scoff, Ollie staggered back to his chair, too, though he was intentionally walking in a way that suggested he might need medical attention, stumbling this way and that.

"Sometimes, I think you ought to be in the pictures," Floyd said.

Ollie collapsed onto his chair in a dramatic fashion and sighed. "What, like an actor?"

"Yeah."

"Ah, no one wants to see my ugly face on screen."

Floyd couldn't have held back his response if he'd tried. "You're far from ugly, Ollie."

His own cheeks instantly started to burn. It looked like Ollie's were, too.

"Oh . . ." Ollie said. "Thank you."

All of a sudden, Ollie was looking at Floyd like he ain't never been complimented before—like he was touched and shocked and confused all at once—which made Floyd want to say something else nice to him. Or maybe he'd make sure to say a whole lot of those somethings to him over the course of their friendship. Because Floyd really wanted Ollie to like himself. Ollie was wonderful. Before Floyd's brain could think of something else to say, Ollie was talking again. Like always.

"Well, you, too," Ollie said. "You're far from ugly, too."

Just like that, Floyd's entire body caught fire, burning hotter than hotter than a kiln, hotter than a blast furnace, heck, maybe even hotter than the sun. He couldn't even make himself thank Ollie for the compliment. He was too busy trying not to melt.

"Or, uh, sorry," Ollie said. "Was that not something I should have said for some reason?"

"It was a fine thing to say," Floyd forced himself to say before stupidly adding, "I know I'm not ugly."

Ollie sputtered a laugh. "Gee, Mister Modesty over here."

And Floyd felt so thankful that Ollie had the sense to tease him about that.

"Yeah, sorry," Floyd said, laughing, too.

At the same time, they both took sips of their moonshine. After, they sat in a comfortable silence for a while, watching the sunlight fade into darkness, and once the sky was awash with stars, Ollie set his tumbler down and walked to the stairs. After he cleared the porch, he looked up at the sky. Floyd soon followed.

"It's incredible out here, isn't it?" Ollie said.

"Did you not have stars in the city?"

"Did we not *have* them?" Ollie asked with a snort. "Of course we had them. We couldn't always *see* them, that was the problem. Not like this, not the whole open sky. How do you think stars work, exactly?"

Floyd's stomach churned. Ollie hadn't never really insulted him before. As silly as it probably was, Floyd couldn't help but wonder whether his fancy, supposed-to-be-running-a-whole-railroad, wealthy-as-sin friend honestly thought that little of him.

"You know what I meant," Floyd sneered, crossing his arms over his chest. "I know how stars work."

"Hey," Ollie said, touching Floyd's forearm. "I'm sorry."

Ollie's touch reignited that spark of yearning in Floyd's heart—the one he had felt flare to life while he had been learning Ollie to shoot—and he tried to extinguish it by looking away. He wanted to be mad at Ollie for thinking he was less, not to be thinking of him in this romantic sort of way.

"I was only trying to be funny. I wasn't . . ." Ollie squeezed Floyd's arm. "Jesus Christ, Floyd, I like you. *Of course* I wasn't trying to insult you. I was teasing."

As soon as Ollie said those three words—*I like you*—Floyd's lingering upset vanished. He couldn't force himself to stay mad no more. Slowly, Floyd let his eyes fall to where Ollie's hand was resting—right near his own. He wanted so badly to hold it. Instead, he shifted his own hand the slightest bit, moving it in such a way that his pinky touched Ollie's, but only barely.

Because the word "like" could mean all kinds of things.

Floyd braced himself for rejection. But Ollie shifted his hand closer, linking their pinkies together. And it was the tiniest, silliest, most wonderful thing.

They stood there like that—holding hands but not—for what felt like a long time.

"You lunkhead," Ollie finally whispered. "I can't believe you thought I was insulting you."

Floyd couldn't fight the smile. Gosh-darn-it, he liked Ollie so much. He liked how funny he was and how smart he was and how he could brighten a whole room with that big, sparkling personality of his.

As Floyd prepared to respond, the front door clattered open, and Floyd instinctively moved back a step, pushing Ollie away.

"Floyd, your daughter is asking for you to read her a bedtime story," Effie called.

Oliver and Floyd locked eyes. After a moment, Ollie nodded, maybe like he was trying to remind Floyd to answer.

Floyd called back. "Be right there!"

Once Effie was back inside, Ollie reached up to rub the back of his neck. Floyd wondered if he was feeling ashamed of what they had done.

"Sorry," Ollie said. "I'll head home now."

"Yeah," Floyd said, now unsure how to act. "Church tomorrow?"

"Yeah. Maybe."

"Goodnight, Ollie," Floyd said.

"Goodnight, Floyd."

And Ollie walked away.

When Floyd came back inside, he was feeling all kinds of ways—wondering if Ollie was embarrassed about having held hands, worrying that their friendship could be coming to an end, and confused as to whether Ollie really liked him or not. All this uncertainty had Floyd's skin itching. It was like the very act of being a person had suddenly become uncomfortable.

As Floyd tried to force away the strangeness of it all, his eyes fell upon the little black book in the bookcase, the one that held the coin collection of the man who had once been Floyd's most important person—Matt.

Exactly then, the copperhead came back, twisting and turning in his stomach. For the rest of the evening, Floyd could think of nothing else except the man he had lost.

CHAPTER SIX

OLIVER

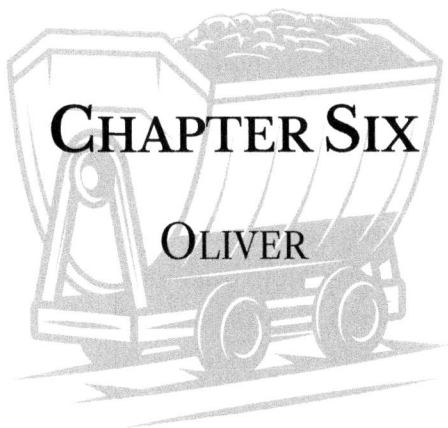

OLIVER LIFTED A STEEL frying pan into the air and held it an arm's length away from his face so that he could scrutinize his appearance in the reflection. He couldn't believe he was so forgetful, so incompetent, that he hadn't yet purchased a proper mirror. How pathetic.

More pathetic, though, was the fact that Oliver had confessed his fucking feelings to Floyd—a married man, a *happily* married man, an endlessly sweet happily married man who deserved to *stay* happily married. And yet, here was Oliver, the eternally broken misfit, trying to ruin everything. Over the last twelve hours, Oliver had mentally beaten himself so mercilessly that the memory of Floyd's friendly smack seemed as soft as a loving embrace.

And yet, Oliver couldn't seem to stop himself from preparing for church.

Because even if it meant another sleepless night of internal anguish and mental pummeling, Oliver wanted to see Floyd again. He wanted to see him and to smell him and to hear his low, beautiful voice. He wanted to be near him every second of every day.

God, it was so terrifying. Oliver had never liked anyone before. Not sexually. Not romantically. From time to time, Oliver could recall maybe experiencing a small bit of attraction toward another person, but there had never been any real intensity to it. Or consistency. Sometimes, that person had been a man, while other times, that person had been a woman. By the time Oliver had reached the age of twenty-five, he'd thought for certain that he must have simply been incapable of experiencing whatever the hell everyone else must have been experiencing for them to want to write love letters and fuck each other and be married.

Oliver took a moment to smooth down his hair. After placing the frying pan back onto the counter, he turned to retrieve a hat from the bedroom, but then vaguely remembered that it was frowned upon to wear hats in church. Or maybe even illegal? He couldn't be certain. Either way, he'd have to leave it behind. He wondered what Floyd would be wearing. It would be a suit, obviously, but Oliver had never seen Floyd in a fancy suit. He'd probably look fucking magnificent in one, though. Oliver may have told Floyd that certain colors worked well on him, but truth be told, that man would look stunning in anything. Or nothing. Maybe *especially* nothing.

Holy hell.

With that thought in his head, Oliver left for church.

Shortly before the top of the hour, when most people were already in their pews, Oliver arrived. Looking around the nave, Oliver spotted Floyd easily. He was taller than nearly everyone else. Thankfully, Floyd seemed to have saved him a seat, but he and his family were all the way on the far side of the room. Oliver hoped that the sound of the pipe organ would hide the noises he'd make heading over there. Trying his best to stay silent, Oliver started over. He was successful for a while. Until he tripped over a bump in the carpet and then his only saving grace was that he had spluttered a surprised yelp instead of an expletive.

By the time Oliver reached his seat, Floyd was very clearly fighting back a smile.

"Do you always got to make a big entrance?" Floyd whispered.

Oliver whispered back, "Believe it or not, that was me attempting to be inconspicuous."

Effie sat forward and caught Oliver's eyes. "Glad you could make it. Floyd said you might come."

"Do you mind that I'm here?" Oliver asked, as though by asking Effie if he could sit next to Floyd in a house of worship, he was also somehow asking her for permission to steal away her stupidly beautiful husband right out from under her Goddamned nose.

"Of course not," Effie said. "It's church."

Church. Oliver exhaled a long, nervous breath.

All of a sudden, the volume of the music swelled, the entire room filling with the organ's reverent-sounding notes, and then, in tandem, everyone stood. Oliver scrambled to his feet.

"What's happening?" he whispered to Floyd.

Floyd arched an eyebrow. "Uh, it's a hymn."

"Him who?"

As soon as the words left Oliver's mouth, the townsfolk started to sing.

"Oh, Jesus, a hymn," Oliver said under his breath.

Somehow, everyone knew the words. It made Oliver feel very silly. He wasn't sure whether he should move his mouth and pretend to know them or stand there like a Goddamned heathen. Probably the latter.

During the song, Oliver realized something terrible: Hymns were very, very long—so long, in fact, that more time had likely passed from the start of the hymn to the current note than from the time that Moses had parted the sea or walked on water or whatever it was that he had accomplished until Oliver had rolled out of bed that morning.

Once everyone sat down, Oliver leaned over to whisper to Floyd, "Can I say 'Jesus Christ' in here or is that still considered a cuss word?"

Because humor tended to make him feel less inadequate somehow.

Floyd responded by elbowing him. Which, Oliver supposed, was a pretty clear answer.

For the rest of the service, Oliver floundered worse than a fish out of water. He was, at best, a fish flopping around on Mars. He clearly hadn't thought this through. By the time everyone was shuffling out of the pews, Oliver was feeling so disoriented, it seemed as though he must have somehow soaked his breakfast cereal in moonshine.

Outside the church, Floyd, Effie, and Oliver congregated in a circle while Josephine ran off to play with her neighbor, William. Oliver watched her sprint away with her friend.

"So, Oliver, what'd you think?" Effie asked. "Floyd said you ain't much of a churchgoer."

"It was lovely," Oliver lied.

"Aw, I'm so happy to hear that," Effie said before a friend called to her from a few yards away. "Be right back."

Once she left, Floyd looked at Oliver with an expression that suggested he would not be fooled so easily.

"Lovely, huh?"

"Yeah, you know, lovely," Oliver said. "Like a slow, painful execution."

Floyd was kind enough to laugh at that. Even though it was wildly insulting—a stupid comment that poked fun of beliefs and traditions that were probably both cherished and important to him. Realizing this, Oliver suddenly wished he *had* found it lovely.

Floyd asked, "Do you not believe in God? Or Jesus?"

Oliver's heart quickened. His answer would probably be important to Floyd. He had better make it a good one. More importantly, he had better make it an honest one, too.

"I'm not sure. I think that . . . well . . . I'm not sure what I think." Oliver looked away, unable to stomach looking Floyd in the eye while he attempted to put his feelings into words. "Sometimes, I try to talk to God. I'm never sure if anyone is listening when I do. I figure that . . . if someone really is out there . . . they'll hear me wherever I am. I hope that's . . . acceptable."

"Yeah, it is," Floyd said. He caught Oliver's eyes. "Ain't a problem for me, Ollie."

"Really?"

"Really."

"Could I still come to church with you from time to time? I like being around you," Oliver said, immediately feeling his cheeks warm. "And your family, too. I mean, it won't offend you if I sit with you in your pew, will it? Especially now that you know that I think it's . . . lovely."

Floyd's smile blossomed like the most beautiful fucking altar flowers.

"I'd like that."

Effie returned with a big smile of her own.

"Good news! Frank and Martha's pig died this morning."

Oliver wasn't certain whether or not that was some kind of joke.

"Ha, wow, yeah, death is always happy news, isn't it?"

Effie laughed. "Well, she was old, and now we're all invited over for some smoked meat. What do y'all think? I can fetch Josephine."

"Let her play with William. She seemed excited about that today," Floyd said.

"I reckon that means they're up to no good," Effie said.

"Yeah, probably not," Floyd answered. "Margaret'll watch them, though."

Oliver cut in. "Is she William's mom?"

"Yup, we'll take her a plate of pork later," Effie said.

"Well, I could eat," Oliver said.

"Me, too," Floyd said.

Effie's face brightened. "Come on, then. Let's head on over."

When Floyd reached for Effie's hand, Oliver tried not to show his envy. While the three of them walked to Frank and Martha's house together, which wasn't far from Floyd's, Oliver kept his mind occupied by spotting the differences among the near-identical houses, like noticing that one house had a small flower garden in front of the porch, the purples and whites brightening up the view, while another's shutters had been painted a bright shade of red. Focusing on the land around him helped the time pass without issue. Once they arrived at a house that looked like every other house, save for the mass of people chatting outside, Oliver breathed a sigh. Now, instead of focusing on how badly he wished that he could hold Floyd's hand, he could fixate on how scary it was to partake in his first town-wide event.

Effie made the introductions. Oliver met Frank and Martha and Jonathan and Eleanor and many, many couples whose names he would likely not remember, and then, eventually, Oliver met a few other unmarried men, most of whom were very keen to talk about how they liked to travel to Charleston with some frequency, with the hope that they might meet a beautiful woman with whom they could settle down. Oliver, on the other hand, inadvertently confessed that he had no intention of marrying. Some cad had the fucking audacity to verbalize the very obvious fact that this was peculiar. Oliver hadn't been able to stop himself from squirming uncomfortably when the fellow had said that. By the time some of the men left to help Frank finish preparing the meat, Oliver had lost most of his appetite. He wasn't in the mood for pork, no matter how fresh. He wasn't really in the mood for conversation, either. Instead, Oliver wanted to go home.

But, for the moment, he couldn't seem to tear himself away from Floyd's side. Effie had followed some women into the house to assist with the preparation of a couple of side dishes—coleslaw and strawberry salad—and now that Floyd wasn't holding her hand, Oliver couldn't make himself pass up the opportunity to be near him for as long as possible. It was horrible. He *knew* it was horrible of him. And twisted. And wrong. And any number of negative-sounding adjectives he could pull out of his ass. But, oh God, Floyd was so perfect. How could he resist?

"So, Oliver, where'd you say you were from?" a stout man whose name was either Marvin or Melvin asked.

"New York."

"Do them men up there not like women or something?"

If Oliver had been sipping on water, this would have been the moment when he'd have inadvertently spat it in the other man's face, making the two of them look like they were performing a silly scene for one of Chaplin's films. Instead, Oliver simply stumbled through a response.

"Uh, what? No, they like women. Don't all men like women?"

What a stupid comment to make, especially in front of Floyd. He couldn't even bring himself to look over and see Floyd's reaction.

"Hm."

That was it. Hm. Two measly letters. And yet, those two stupid letters said so much. *"What about you, then? Why aren't you interested in finding a woman to sire your children? Is there something wrong with your pecker? Are you out of your head?"* Not that any of these people talked like that, but still.

Some other unmarried man—one named Harry—cut in to say that he had traveled to New York once, which diverted the attention away from Oliver momentarily. He'd had just enough time to mentally recover when everyone started on the trials and tribulations of married life, which made Oliver feel terrible all over again, and the more time that passed, the more broken Oliver started to feel. He tried telling himself that none of it mattered, because he was happy to be unmarried, especially since it seemed to mean that he could covertly hold pinkies with a handsome man like Floyd beneath a sky filled with stars. Maybe Floyd hadn't *verbally* confirmed that he reciprocated Oliver's romantic feelings, but men tended not to be physically intimate with other men for the hell of it, right?

As Oliver was busy trying to make himself feel less horrible, Effie came by and stood next to Floyd, who immediately wrapped an arm around her. Effie whispered something to him, and Floyd whispered something back, and then the two of them laughed. God, they were together! What the hell was Oliver doing? Seeing Effie and Floyd be playful with each other was enough to open Oliver's eyes and reveal to him how screwy this whole situation was. Floyd was married. He was married to a wonderful woman. Just like every other man in Rock Creek either was or wanted to be. Every other man except for Oliver.

Why had he thought that he could make this work? He wasn't a coal miner. He wasn't a West Virginian. He wasn't any of the things he was supposed to be. Like always, Oliver didn't belong. Why had he thought Rock Creek would be different? He and Floyd had shared a few nice moments together, but Floyd was taken. Jesus Christ, what was wrong with him?!

Effie smiled up at Floyd. "Would you mind coming out back to help Frank for a bit?"

"I'd be happy to," Floyd responded. He looked over at Oliver. "You can come, too, Ollie. If you want."

"Um, yeah," Oliver said. "In a minute."

And as soon as Floyd was out of sight, Oliver turned and left. He walked away without so much as uttering a word to anyone, no longer seeing the need for performances. Or for continued politeness. Because Oliver wasn't heading home. He was heading to Charleston.

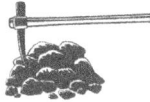

Hours later, Oliver was standing on the sidewalk on the outskirts of the city, in front of his Aunt Betty's home—a canary yellow mansion with black shutters and a large, well-kept porch. He wondered if she would remember him. He hadn't seen her for . . . God, had it been over ten years?

While the two of them hadn't been especially close back in New York, Oliver had still enjoyed her presence, especially since she was the only other person in his family who never seemed to meet the expectations that had been placed on her. Aunt Betty had never married. Not only that, but she had been more interested in education than homemaking. Her peculiarity must have played into her leaving. At the time, Oliver had thought it strange that Aunt Betty had followed him and his immediate family to New York from Cleveland only to vanish less than a year later.

But now Oliver understood the urge to run from those people. Perhaps that was something they could bond over.

Oliver raked a hand through his hair. Though he was terrified of potential rejection, he needed someone to talk to—someone who might understand him a little, someone who might make him feel like he wasn't alone. Sure, Oliver had Floyd, but Floyd had Effie. While Oliver had played pool with Roy and had chatted with John sometimes, Roy and John were married to women, too. All Oliver wanted was to talk to someone who might help him feel less strange.

Mustering every last scrap of courage inside him, Oliver walked up the stairs and knocked. Twenty or thirty seconds later, Aunt Betty answered. She was somehow both taller and smaller than he remembered. When he was a child, she had towered over him, but now she was several inches shorter than he was. While it made sense, it was still strange. It served as an unsettling reminder that Oliver was supposed to be an adult, even though he scarcely ever felt like one. Aunt Betty looked the same otherwise but with more wrinkles. Also, her previously blonde hair was now mixed with shades of white and light gray, and she wore it piled high atop her head. It made her look regal. Like the fucking Queen of Charleston.

"Hi," Oliver said, putting on his best smile.

"I'm not interested in whatever it is you're selling," she said, turning right back around. God, she had barely even looked at him!

"Oh, sorry, I'm not selling anything," he sputtered, stopping her in her tracks. "It's Oliver!"

Aunt Betty whirled around, and the moment their eyes met, she sucked in a breath.

"Oliver?!"

He couldn't yet tell whether or not she was happy about it.

"Yes, that's me. Henry's son. Not that you want to be reminded of him. Probably."

Shock transformed into scrutiny. She narrowed her eyes at him. "Why are you here?"

Ah, so, she maybe wasn't exactly happy to see him, then.

"Just, you know, to say hello."

"Did my brother send you?"

"God, no. I left. Permanently."

She hummed a little, seeming to think this over.

"Come in."

Oliver followed her inside. Her home was beautiful, the walls decorated with stunning flower wallpaper and furnished with tasteful cherry oak furniture. Oliver was immediately taken aback by the charm it had. Even though Oliver knew that his home in New York had probably been beautiful, too, he remembered it having such an ugliness about it. Perhaps every horrible event that had ever transpired within its walls was preventing him from thinking anything nice about it now. If Floyd were here, Oliver would have probably said that his house in New York had been *lovely*.

Thinking of Floyd had Oliver suddenly feeling lightheaded. Because he simultaneously never wanted to see Floyd again and wanted to see Floyd that very second. It was wildly disorienting.

"Are you well?" Aunt Betty asked as they took a seat in what looked to be her own private library.

"Not at the moment," Oliver answered truthfully, panic and regret swirling inside him, the sensations making it harder to breathe.

"Did you just arrive from New York?" she asked. "Where are your bags?"

Pushing past his rising upset, Oliver said, "No, I, uhm, I live in Rock Creek now."

"Why on earth would you have moved there?"

"Because I wanted to . . . to move to a place where my parents wouldn't find me, where they wouldn't bother me anymore."

"Oh. I see."

"And, well, I knew you lived here in Charleston. I thought it might be nice to reconnect." Aunt Betty only nodded thoughtfully in response. "Besides, who better to help me find work than our old family friend Frederick Donohue, right?"

Oliver's statement hung in the air for a few seconds. Uncomfortable with the subsequent silence, Oliver tucked his hands beneath his thighs to keep himself from biting his fingernails. Aunt Betty smoothed out her dress.

"Well, it's very nice to see you, Oliver," she finally said. "I hope you're enjoying Rock Creek."

"Mostly." Oliver chewed on his bottom lip. "Aunt Betty, have you ever fallen in love with someone who you're not supposed to fall in love with?"

It was probably too intimate of a thing to ask, and especially too intimate of a thing to randomly sputter forth in the middle of a conversation, but he couldn't make himself care anymore. He needed someone to talk to.

"Why are you asking me that?" she asked in a biting tone.

Aunt Betty's sudden show of hostility had Oliver wondering the reason for it. Perhaps the two of them were more alike than he had previously thought.

Looking up, Oliver asked, "You have, haven't you?"

"What did Henry say about me?"

"Nothing. He never said anything. He never even talked about you."

It was only *slightly* a lie. His father had voiced his upset over their relationship on several occasions.

Her expression softened, and Oliver had to bite his tongue to keep himself from obliterating whatever tiny smidgeon of affection she might still have for him.

"Oliver, I came here to start a new life. It sounds like you're trying to do the same." She folded her hands in her lap. "If that's the case, I suggest you forget about the 'supposed to's' because, in truth, you're *supposed to* take over your father's railroad someday, if I'm not mistaken, and I'm sure you aren't planning on running it from a shanty in rural West Virginia."

Her comment would have been funny had it not been so painfully true.

"You're right," Oliver said. "I'm sorry to bother you."

"You're welcome to visit, but I would appreciate some notice next time. I have to warn you that I will not always be so amenable to entertaining. Depending on the circumstances, sometimes I simply can't be."

"May I ask why?"

"No, you may not."

"Wow, that's some honesty."

"I live my life as honestly as I can," she said. "And I hope the same for you, Oliver."

"Thanks. I think." Oliver blew out a breath. "Are you free to chat some more right now? I had a hard morning. It would be nice to talk for a little while."

Aunt Betty looked over at the mantlepiece clock.

"I have time."

Oliver's shoulders relaxed, long-held tension falling away.

"Thank you."

For the next half hour, the two of them talked. And, God, it was nice. Oliver was suddenly so comforted to have her nearby—to have someone in his life who'd been connected with his past and was now connected to his present, too. Even though the two of them only spoke about superficial matters—pictures they had seen and books they had read—every word of their conversation still helped Oliver let go of some of the unpleasant thoughts he had been having earlier.

Eventually, Oliver noticed Aunt Betty looking at the clock again. He realized he'd better leave. After all, he had come by without a formal invitation. Aunt Betty probably had other plans.

"Well, I think I should catch a train home, then," Oliver said, pushing himself to his feet. "And try to figure out how to muddle through the mess I've managed to make of my new life in less than a month."

"You'll figure it out. You've always been a smart boy."

Her compliment pulled at his heart.

Before they parted, Oliver considered extending his hand, but that wasn't proper etiquette, what with her being a woman and him being a man. Since an embrace seemed too familiar, especially since Oliver's family had never been too keen on physical affection, Oliver only waved. Aunt Betty seemed mildly charmed by this, at least. Surprisingly enough, she waved back.

As Oliver made his way to the train station, he thought back on her advice to him. At first, Oliver thought she may have been encouraging him to insert himself into Floyd's love life like a stick of dynamite and blow it all to hell. But the more he ruminated on it, the more he realized that she had only been advising him not to fight his feelings because of the "supposed to's," not offering him wisdom about what to do with those feelings.

So, if Oliver let himself fall in love with Floyd, where did that leave him? Hopefully, Floyd would still have him as a friend, though probably nothing more. Which, Oliver supposed, was fine, in a way, since he hadn't even thought he could ever fall in love with someone else, let alone fuck them. Could he settle for friendship? Maybe? Probably?

Oliver really liked Floyd. God, they had only known each other for a short while and already Oliver couldn't imagine life without him. What a mess.

By the time Oliver was nearing the train station, he was mentally worn out. Since the train wasn't supposed to arrive for a little while, he sat on one of the nearest benches. Listening to the sounds of the city—the hustle and bustle of the folks walking past—Oliver's thoughts kept returning to Floyd—his sweet dimples and his big laugh and the way they liked to be playful with one another.

Oliver's thoughts were interrupted when someone caught his eye. Less than a block away, there was a little girl with long blonde hair who was wearing the very same pink and white dress that Josephine had worn to church that morning. Oliver squinted to try to see her better. It *was* Josephine!

Without a second thought, Oliver leapt to his feet and started toward her. She continued meandering farther from the station.

"Josephine!" Oliver cried out.

Why was Josephine here? Where were Floyd and Effie? Had they come looking for him or something?

"Josephine!"

Josephine stopped and turned toward him. God, the sight of her took Oliver's breath away. Her eyes were pink, her cheeks were puffy and red, and her pretty blonde hair was a complete mess.

As soon as Oliver was close, he knelt in front of her.

"Mister Oliver, can you take me home?"

"Home? Josephine, how the hell are you here? Where are your parents? Why were you crying?"

Tears started to pour from her eyes. "I don't want to go to the circus no more."

"Circus?!" Ah, Jesus Christ, of course, this was Oliver's fault, too. Why'd he have to crow about the fucking circus? And to a child who had probably never even left her tiny unincorporated mining town, too. "Where's William?"

"Home."

"So, you came here by yourself?" Oliver asked, and Josephine nodded, tears pouring from her blue eyes. "How?"

"I took a train."

"They let you on a train? By yourself?!"

But that only made Josephine cry more.

"I'm not . . ." Oliver sighed. "Jesus Christ, Josephine, I'm not *scolding* you. I'm trying to understand how Don Chafin's men supposedly have time to scrutinize each and every person who hops on a train to Rock Creek, but they can't be bothered to . . ."

Ah, but she hadn't been taking a train to Rock Creek, but to Charleston. And she was no union man. She was a tiny little thing. It was possible they hadn't even seen her. Or, worse, they *had* seen her, but they hadn't cared. If coal operators were happy to let boys only two years Josephine's senior toil away in the mines, risking their lives, then why would anyone care about a well-dressed little church girl stowing away on a train heading toward the city? It was very possible that it simply hadn't been of interest to them.

"Alright, Josephine, you can stop crying now," Oliver said, reaching inside his suit jacket for a handkerchief and handing it to her. "Dry your eyes. I'll take you home."

Josephine wiped her face and blew her nose. "Thank you."

After she handed the now-wet handkerchief back to Oliver, he took her hand, and they walked to the train station together, where they sat on one of the free benches. Watching Josephine swing and kick her legs back and forth as they dangled over the side of the bench, Oliver was reminded of how Goddamn young she was. He had to fight the urge to make a comment about it. Floyd probably wouldn't appreciate Oliver calling his missing child "brave" for hopping on a train. He *was* curious, though, how she had known what to do.

"Why a train?"

"What?"

"How did you know to take a train?"

"Well, you said, 'take a train to Charleston.'"

"I *told you* to take a train to Charleston?"

"You said I ain't have to because of your magic."

"Oh. Right."

And yet she had anyway. Oliver wondered if that was a trait from Floyd or from Effie. When Oliver looked over, he noticed that another tear had trickled down her cheek and thought back on his own childhood, wondering how he'd have felt in her situation.

"Are you nervous about how much trouble you'll be in?"

"No."

Oliver smiled a little at that. Was it because they wouldn't punish her too much? Or because the punishment she knew would be waiting for her simply wasn't very scary? Either way, he liked her answer.

"Are you sad because you think your parents will be mad at you?"

"I'm sad because of how much they miss me."

Her seemingly simple answer immediately stirred something strong within him—a sorrow for his childhood self—and the fierceness of the sudden swirl of sadness compressed Oliver's heart, squeezing it like a vice. What it must be like to be missed. And to know that you are missed. And loved.

Josephine was so very lucky in that way. Oliver realized, then, that he could never live with himself if he ever played a part in breaking up her happy family. He would settle for friendship. And friendship would be enough. Because it had to be.

CHAPTER SEVEN

FLOYD

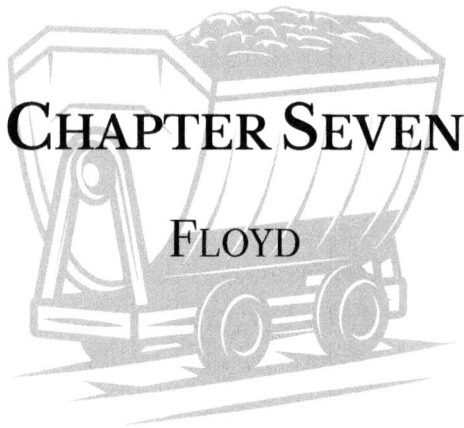

FLOYD STORMED UP THE porch stairs and threw open the front door, his empty oil lantern swinging wildly in his left hand. Effie hurried across the room, her wide eyes scared and pleading.

"Why're you back without her?"

"I need more kerosene," he said, struggling to keep his voice steady even though with every passing second, fear was swirling harder and harder within him, fast and furious like the wind. "Can't believe it got dark so fast."

"I know. I thought she'd be home by now. I can't hardly believe that she left William's house hours ago. What if she's hurt?"

"She's fine, Effie, you'll see."

"What if she went into the woods? Where else would she be?"

"Josephine's smart. She knows how to navigate them woods better than boys twice her age."

It was an exaggeration. But it was a needed one.

"Maybe I ought to come look, too."

"Naw, you need to stay here. What if she came back and couldn't find nobody?"

"You're right," Effie sighed. "Are Margaret and Leonard still out there looking?"

"Yep. With William and Grace and Carl and all the rest of their kids. Some of the other families are starting to look, too." The worry lines that were etched into Effie's forehead deepened, and Floyd wondered if maybe that comment had been a mistake on his part. "Now, she's only been missing for a few hours. You and me liked to run off into the woods plenty when we were little."

"We came home once it got dark."

Floyd couldn't figure out how to respond to that, because Effie was right, and so, instead of fumbling through empty reassurances, he simply held out his arms and let Effie fall into them. He pulled her close and kissed the top of her head.

"I'll find her," he said with conviction. "You know I will."

There was a small pause, heavy and heartbreaking.

"I know."

Suddenly, the front door flew open. Floyd released Effie and turned to see Josephine bounding into the house, her face a strange mixture of elation and sadness, like she wanted to laugh and cry and scream all at once.

"Oh, my stars, Josephine," Effie said, tears welling up in her eyes in an instant. Josephine barreled into Effie's waiting arms. "Where were you?"

"I'm so sorry, Mama. I tried to find the circus."

Floyd's eyes found Ollie waiting in the doorway with a remorseful-looking half-smile.

"I believe this was my fault," Ollie said. "I shouldn't have blathered on about the circus like that. It was inconsiderate of me."

Effie looked back and forth between Josephine and Ollie.

"What do you mean you tried to find the circus?" she asked Josephine.

Ollie took a tentative step into the house. "Josephine told me that she took a train to Charleston. That's where I found her, incidentally. Near the train station."

"Josephine May," Effie sighed, her face reddening. Floyd could tell she was trying hard not to lose her temper in front of Ollie. "We were so worried."

Floyd knelt down and placed a hand on Josephine's back.

"Jo, you can't run off like that. You nearly put your mother in an early grave." He said this in a harsh tone, the harshest he could muster, hoping it might knock some sense into her, even though he knew she probably felt as sorry as she looked with her puffy pink eyes and trembling bottom lip. "I spent over two hours searching the woods for you. Wasted a whole lot of kerosene."

Which was a cold thing to say. But Floyd couldn't seem to tell her how worried he had been when she hadn't come home, how the sweat soaking his shirt was from the fear he had been feeling, rather than from how physically tired he was. He couldn't find the words to tell her how terrifying it had been when the sun had set and the woods had become black and every little sound suddenly seemed to have come from a monster, one that had taken his little girl.

It was easier to talk about the kerosene.

"I'm sorry, Daddy," Josephine said, choking back a sob. "I'm real, real sorry."

"I know," he said, holding back the comfort he wanted to give.

He needed her to learn her lesson. Even if her sadness made him sad, too.

Floyd looked over his shoulder to thank Ollie but saw that he had already left. He'd have to find Ollie later. It was a right miracle that his friend had found Jo in Charleston. Floyd suddenly remembered that he still needed to tell everyone else that the search was over, and so, he promised Effie that he'd leave in a bit and spread the word so that no one would continue looking through the night. Before leaving though, Floyd spent a little more time with both of his girls, making sure they were good, reassuring *himself* that they were good, and then refilled his lamp with kerosene.

Once Floyd had made good on his promise to call off the search, he started toward Ollie's house. As he walked, the chaos of the day's events continued to hum beneath his skin, making him anxious. First, Ollie had vanished from the pig roast and then Josephine had missed supper. Floyd had gone from worrying about his friend to plum near losing his mind over his missing baby girl. All in the span of a few hours. He still couldn't understand how Ollie had been the one to find her. Why had he been in Charleston? Why hadn't he talked to Floyd before leaving Frank and Martha's house?

When Ollie had acted so funny right after the two of them had kind of held hands in a really strange way, Floyd had convinced himself that their friendship was over. But then Ollie had shown up at church and, well, Floyd had been so happy about that. He hadn't even minded Ollie's humor about religion. Or the fact that somehow, the man hadn't known what a hymn was. All that had mattered was that they were spending time together.

But then, Ollie had left Frank and Mary's so suddenly . . .

Was Ollie still feeling strange about them holding hands? Floyd wondered if maybe telling Ollie the truth about his marriage would help. But, well, probably not. Ollie was probably thinking that two men being together was wrong, and with how that sort of thing was seen by plum near everyone else in the world, Floyd supposed he couldn't really fault him if he really was feeling bad.

When Floyd arrived at Ollie's house, Ollie was already outside. He was sitting on his porch, not on a chair, but on the floor of the porch itself with his back resting against the house, probably because he hadn't bought any kind of chair for it yet.

"Hey, Ollie."

Oliver skipped right over the salutation and said, "God, Floyd, I can't imagine what that was like for you today."

"Yeah, well, she wouldn't be home if not for you," Floyd said, walking up the porch stairs. He sat beside Ollie without even confirming that he wanted the company. He figured they were beyond simple pleasantries like that now. He hoped so, anyway. "Thank you for bringing her back."

"Of course," Ollie said. "I'm surprised, you know, that she knew to take the train. I mean, I think I only mentioned it once."

Floyd nodded. "Jo's a smart one. But, well, I figure she kind of knew about the trains to Charleston before. Some other families here take one on occasion to shop in the city. We're lucky in that way. Plenty of trains because of the coal."

"It's a miracle that I spotted her."

"I know. Poor Jo. She seemed to think the circus would be there waiting for her."

"Like once the train stopped in Charleston, she'd see the circus from the station?"

"More like she thought Charleston *was* the circus." Floyd shook his head. Josephine's mind sure was interesting. "We ain't never been there before. As a family."

"Oh, I see," Ollie said. "Well, she wasn't entirely wrong about Charleston. It's a little like a circus. All cities are."

Floyd could tell by now when Oliver was fixing to say something funny.

"How's that?" he asked, happy to indulge his friend.

"They're run by clowns," Oliver said with a silly smile. "Or wait, circuses aren't run by clowns, are they? Sorry, I hadn't really thought this through."

"I like it."

"So, for Logan County, is Don Chafin a clown, then?"

Floyd tried not to let on how funny he thought this was. He pursed his lips to keep himself from chortling.

"I reckon so."

"You've never met him?"

"No," Floyd said. "I met a couple of them people he has working for him, though. I had two over for supper once. Not intentionally. We had a bunch of train delays. I saw the men milling around the company store and knew they probably hadn't eaten a proper meal since breakfast."

"So you invited them, these horrible men, into your home and served them supper."

Floyd shrugged. Oliver had a way of twisting things. No wonder he liked them pretzels.

"They weren't that bad, considering."

Oliver sighed. "You're too nice, Floyd."

Floyd wasn't sure how to respond to that.

"Why were you in Charleston?" he asked instead.

"I went to see my Aunt Betty."

"How was it?"

"It was fine. I can't tell whether she likes me or not."

Floyd snorted. "I ain't sure how anyone couldn't like you, Ollie."

Ollie smiled wider, but only for a moment. Quick as the wind, he started to have a sadness about him, his smile falling away and shoulders slumping forward. Maybe Floyd had said something he ought not have.

Minutes passed. Floyd waited for Ollie to respond, but Ollie only sat there, silently staring off into the night. Normally, Floyd liked silence. But this silence was hard. It made him understand why Ollie often liked to fill up the air with conversation.

During this time, Floyd thought about how much he liked Ollie. And how much that liking had taken him by surprise. Before

Ollie had come to town, Floyd had promised himself that he'd never again let himself like someone in this way. He had spent *years* cultivating a big barrier between that part of himself—the part that found men attractive—and the rest of him. But, funnily enough, Ollie had mowed into Floyd's life like that sulky-type plow they'd had back at the farm, the one made by the Oliver Company, and he had cleared away each stalk of Floyd's defenses. Now, thanks to Ollie, new seeds of affection had been able to sprout, and even though it was probably foolish, Floyd wanted those saplings to thrive. He wanted the two of them to *be* something, even if them being something meant that the stupid copperhead would keep writhing around in his stomach, making him feel sick sometimes.

He'd tolerate the sick feeling for Ollie.

After another few moments, Ollie spoke.

"Do you think we could forget about what I said yesterday? About me liking you?"

It took Floyd a moment to accept what Ollie had said. It seemed to Floyd that maybe he had been right about Ollie feeling ashamed on account of them both being men.

"Yeah," Floyd forced himself to say. "We could."

But how could he ever forget something so special?

Heartache rose inside of him, stronger than the rain shower, or even a summer thunderstorm, and Floyd knew, then, that if he stayed, he'd probably start to cry. And he hadn't cried for a long, long time.

"I need to head back," Floyd said, standing quickly. "See you tomorrow, Ollie."

"Bright and early."

Floyd kept walking, unable to even look back.

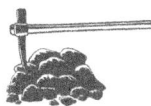

By the time Floyd was back home, Josephine had already fallen asleep. Effie was sitting on the couch knitting, probably still too rattled to sleep herself. Floyd sat next to her.

"Did you thank Oliver?" she asked.

He nodded.

"I still can't believe he found her."

Floyd nodded again. This time, Effie looked over at him.

"What's wrong?"

Floyd had to concentrate on keeping his voice even.

"Ollie asked me to forget what he said."

"What do you mean?"

Floyd swallowed thickly. "What he told me. Last night. About liking me."

"Oh, Floyd. I'm sorry." Effie placed a hand on his knee. "I thought you told me that you held pinkies or something sweet like that."

"Yeah, well, it must not have meant that much to him."

"Are you alright?"

Floyd shook his head. "Not right now, no."

Effie looked at him thoughtfully—her eyes kind and her brow furrowed. Floyd could tell that she was trying to figure out what to say or how to help. That was very Effie. For her to be content, she had to know that she was taking care of the people around her.

"Here," she said, handing over the knitting needles. "I'm teaching you how to knit."

Floyd blew out a breath. "Why?"

"Because you need something else to focus on right now."

"Can't we play checkers?" he asked. "Or chess?"

"Nuh-uh, you ain't pitiful enough for me to teach you how to play chess."

"Worth a try."

"Now, here, I'll show you how to make the basic stitch," she said, placing her hands on top of his and adjusting his fingers. "But first, I need you to hold them needles right."

And so, Effie and Floyd spent the next hour knitting together. It wasn't easy to learn. For Floyd, the whole thing felt frustrating and pointless and mind-achingly boring. During their lesson, there were a few times when Floyd's thoughts flitted back to Ollie. Whenever it happened, Effie must have noticed a change in him because she'd work to take his mind off him somehow.

When the two of them were finally ready to head to the backroom, Floyd was too busy being mad at them stupid knitting needles for never working right to think too much about Ollie.

He was so stinkin' thankful for it.

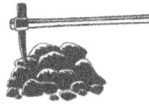

By eleven o'clock the next workday, Floyd was exhausted. Practically every time he looked at Ollie, he felt like his heart was cracking in two, and once that happened, he had to concentrate on repairing it, even while trying to wield the pickaxe or shovel mounds of coal. Floyd tried reminding himself that he had spent all them years walling himself off for a reason. He ought not to have been trying to be with Ollie in the first place. Because of Matt. Floyd still loved Matt. Ever since Ollie had put a stop to the romance, the copperhead in Floyd's stomach hadn't been fussing. Guilt wouldn't be a problem no more, and Floyd could carry on in life like he always had.

But then, every time Floyd was finished reminding himself of these things, Ollie would smile sweetly or say something funny or even act a little flirtatious, and Floyd couldn't figure out how he was supposed to feel. All this back and forth was confusing. Worse, it was making him mad.

When lunchtime came around, Floyd's muscles were tense, hot irritation simmering beneath his skin. While he and Ollie were eating together under the maple tree, he had to focus on not snapping like a twig.

"So, Floyd," Ollie said through a mouthful of food, which was a habit that had been strangely endearing before but was on its way to becoming annoying. "How about the two of us visit Charleston sometime? Could be fun."

"Maybe."

It was all Floyd could muster.

"I know you said you've never been there as a family, but have you ever taken Effie?"

"Mm-hmm. Long time ago."

"Aw, that's sweet. What'd you two do in the city?"

"Saw a picture."

"Oh yeah, I love the pictures. I went all the time when I was living in New York. By myself, typically, but I still had fun. One time, I tried to take Colonel Whiskers with me, though. I thought that might have been nice. I even bought a cage for him. Well, it was a birdcage, so it hadn't been a *perfect* fit. I figured it would hold him well enough, though. Do they make cages for cats, you think? I haven't ever seen one. Anyway, when I tried to buy a ticket—"

"Hey, uhm, Ollie, would you mind closing that mouth of yours?" Floyd asked, even though saying that made him feel sick. He really did want to hear the end of that story. He liked Ollie's stories. He liked near everything Ollie had to say. But he was still feeling upset about Ollie's rejection, especially since Ollie was being so lovable, telling such a funny story that was making Floyd like him even more. "I ain't feeling too good right now."

"Yeah, of course. I'm sorry."

"Not your fault."

Ollie managed to keep quiet for the rest of lunch. Floyd's chest hurt a bit—sadness tugging at his heart—because he knew Ollie was probably itching to talk to him. And Floyd was itching to listen.

By the time they started for the elevator, Floyd couldn't stand how much he was missing Ollie's voice, and so, Floyd let him know that he could talk again. For the rest of the afternoon, listening to Ollie was kind of bittersweet, like sucking on a lemon while eating a spoonful of sugar. Ollie was still sending Floyd mixed up messages. Trying to figure out whether Ollie still liked him or not was like trying to make sense of the foreign languages Floyd heard some miners speaking from time to time.

One time, when they were shoveling coal, Ollie turned to Floyd and said, *"Jeez, lunkhead, you're so strong,"* in this playful sort of way that made Floyd think about how fun it would be to lift Ollie up and carry him off somewhere. But then he thought that maybe Ollie had only said it because they were shoveling, and Floyd was lifting a whole lot more than he was. Like maybe Ollie had only been making an observation. But no one else Floyd knew ever made comments like that. No one else ever said those kinds of things in fun, playful voices. So, then Floyd was left wondering whether or not Ollie was thinking about his strength in a romantic kind of way, too.

When the workday was finally over, Floyd felt a huge rush of relief. As soon as the two of them entered the elevator, it seemed like the tension Floyd had been feeling left his entire body in one, fast *whooosh*. Once Ollie and him reached the surface, the company weigh boss—a curt but even-tempered man named Stuart—weighed their car and stamped each of their pay envelopes with the tonnage. Since it was only Monday, neither of them could collect their pay until the end of the week, and so they each put the envelopes back in their pockets. After uttering a fast "see you, Ollie," Floyd started toward home. He needed a nap.

"Do you want to come by later?" Ollie asked, catching up with him moments later. "I need to wash my clothes. I thought maybe you'd have fun watching me struggle with the washboard."

"I reckon I'll eat with my family."

"Well, yeah, of course, but maybe you could stop by later?"

Struggling to resist the offer, Floyd bit his tongue. Dang, he really wanted to spend time with Ollie.

"I'm sorry if you noticed my smelly clothes, by the way," Ollie said. "I should have washed some last night. I'm over here being smelly and you, well, you always smell nice."

Enough was enough.

Letting out a breath, Floyd stopped walking.

Lowering his voice to a whisper, he said, "Ollie, I can't do this no more. Do you like me or not?"

Ollie started rubbing his forehead, like Floyd's question was making his brain hurt. "Can you come over so that we can talk in private?"

"Yeah, that's fine."

They walked the entire way in silence. Floyd thought this probably meant that Ollie was fixing to smash his heart again, only he was busy working out how to do it.

Once they were inside, Ollie made his way over to the couch—a ratty old one with faded black upholstery, probably been left behind by the previous tenant—and sat down. Floyd wasn't sure whether or not he was supposed to sit, too. Yesterday, he wouldn't have hesitated. But so much had changed since then.

"I feel like I'm about to receive a lecture," Ollie said.

"What?"

"You towering over me like that," Ollie said with the flick of a wrist. "Can you sit? You're making me nervous."

"Oh." Floyd shifted his weight from one foot to the other. "Where?"

"What do you mean 'where'? On the couch, lunkhead." But Floyd still hesitated. Finally, Ollie stood, took Floyd by the sleeve, and yanked him onto the couch. "There. Christ."

There was another stretch of silence, itchy and uncomfortable like a new woolen scarf, and Floyd couldn't manage to keep himself from fidgeting. Neither could Ollie. They sat there like that—silent and awkward, shifting this way and that—before Ollie finally let out a small, frustrated scream.

"Will you stop moving like that?" Ollie nearly shouted. "Are your clothes filled with ants?"

Floyd sputtered, "Ain't like you're keeping still neither."

"Because of you! You're making me crazy, moving like that!" Ollie exclaimed. "And, yes, I know this couch is pathetic, but it's not that bad, is it?"

"It's kind of lumpy."

"Well, where else are we supposed to sit? On my *bed*?" Floyd's face immediately turned hot. He must have been redder than an overly ripened strawberry. Ollie probably noticed because he buried his head in his hands and said, "Don't think too hard about that."

"I wasn't," Floyd lied.

Ollie huffed a laugh, one that made him sound tired, rather than happy, and then he came out from hiding behind his hands. "Oh, fuck, Floyd, what's wrong with me? I can't stop liking you."

Floyd's stomach pulsed and squeezed and fluttered, but he wasn't too bothered by the sensation, not enough to keep his own feelings to himself. On the night when he and Ollie had held pinkies, Floyd had promised himself that he'd tolerate his stomach feeling sick if it meant that the two of them could be together. And, so, he said, "I like you, too, Ollie."

"You like me, too," Ollie repeated under his breath. "Great, Floyd, that's perfect."

"We won't tell no one," Floyd said cautiously, thinking maybe that would help.

"Don't you understand how horrible that is?" Ollie asked, and Floyd stayed quiet.

It was horrible *not* to tell people? Floyd had to wonder what kind of life people like him were living up in New York.

Ollie fell backward to rest against the cushion and sighed. "Floyd, you're married."

Floyd's eyes went wide. "Oh!"

It suddenly occurred to Floyd that Ollie wasn't aware of the peculiar nature of his marriage. Somehow, in letting Ollie into his life, Floyd had forgotten that Ollie only knew what everybody else in town knew. He only saw what everybody else saw. Gosh, he had been fixing to tell Ollie about his marriage, but then when Ollie had rejected him, Floyd had plum forgotten. He'd been busy thinking that Ollie had rejected him on account of them both being men!

"Oh, my God. Did you *forget* that you have a wife?!"

"No," Floyd said quickly. "My marriage ain't like that, is all."

"Your marriage isn't like what?"

"Me and Effie are friends."

Ollie stared for a few seconds, his brow creasing like he was thinking this over.

"Are you trying to tell me that you and Effie aren't really married?"

"Well, no, we are. We were married in the courthouse."

"But it's not a real marriage, then?"

Floyd wasn't too happy with the way Ollie was making it sound—black and white. But it seemed real important for him to hear Floyd answer in a specific way.

And so, Floyd cringed and said, "No, it's not."

"What's that look for?" Ollie asked.

"Ollie, my marriage to Effie is real. It ain't romantic, but I love her. I care about her. She's my best friend."

"I know you care about her, Floyd," Ollie said, his voice much softer. "I'm sorry for upsetting you." He let out a breath and continued on, "So, you love Effie. Were you ever *in love* with her? I mean, why are you two married?"

Floyd stayed quiet for a few moments while he thought it over. It felt wrong to tell Ollie the reason without first checking with Effie. It was a shared secret. Not his secret alone.

"I can't say more without talking to her."

"But, alright, what we're trying to establish here is that you like me. And that it's not a problem for you to like me. Yes?"

"Yeah, I suppose."

"Does Effie know you like me?"

"Effie knew before me, even."

"Well, that sounds very Effie. I barely know her, and yet you saying that is not the least bit surprising to me."

Ollie moved his hand toward Floyd's, stopping when his fingers were a couple of inches away. Floyd supposed it was up to him to close the space between them. Studying Ollie's hand—his smooth skin, long-since healed from the cuts he had received from the slate—Floyd readied himself for that snake nip at him, for it to make him feel even worse than it had on the night the two of them had held pinkies, but nothing happened. Even though Floyd was still thinking 'bout Matt, even though his insides were still a tiny bit knotted together, he still wanted to hold Ollie's hand. Pushing past the mild nausea, Floyd took Ollie's hand in his.

"Holy Moses, Floyd," Ollie said as their fingers laced together and his reaction was so stinkin' sweet it somehow calmed every bit of Floyd's remaining unease. "Sorry. I've never held anyone's hand before."

Once again, Ollie had surprised him by being so innocent.

"Do you want to stop?" Floyd asked.

Ollie squeezed his hand. "Never."

Floyd couldn't resist a tease. "Well, I *will* need to see my family at some point."

Oliver wasn't too fond of that comment, though.

"I can't believe you have a family," he said. "Actually, I can't believe any of this. I'm holding hands with a man. With a married man. With a married man who still loves his family. And that's fine, somehow. Completely normal. Nothing to worry about."

"Have you ever liked a man before?"

"Floyd, I've never liked *anyone* before. I'm still trying to accept that I'm capable of it."

That was an interesting thing, one that made Floyd feel special. He hadn't never met someone like that before.

"I haven't liked anyone in a long time," Floyd said, wanting Ollie to feel special, too. "Since before Josephine."

"Wow, that is a long time," Ollie said. "So, uhm, what now?"

"Whatever you want," Floyd said with a shrug.

"Whatever *I* want? God, Floyd, don't put that on me! I told you, I have no idea what we're supposed to be doing. It's not even like I can try to think back on whatever the hell I learned about courtship all those years ago because, like I said, you're a man. And you're married!" Ollie raked his free hand through that nice hair of his. Floyd sort of wanted to reach up and touch it. Before he could, Ollie was talking again. "How are you so calm, Floyd? Unless that means you must have . . . well . . . none of this is new to you, is it?"

"No," Floyd said. "Not to say that I'm some kind of expert, though."

"So, you've been with, what, more than zero men, but less than fifty? Fifty would make someone an expert, I'd think."

Floyd supposed he had to be honest, even if he wasn't too keen on talking about Matt much yet. He couldn't have Ollie thinking he'd somehow held hands with forty-nine other men.

"One."

"You've been with one man?" Ollie asked, and Floyd nodded. "Did you kiss him, fuck him, what?"

Floyd winced. Why'd Ollie have to be so colorful about it?

"Don't make it sound so . . ."

"Crass?"

"Yeah."

"Sorry." Ollie's cheeks reddened. "So, can you tell me more?"

Floyd could see how badly Ollie wanted to know. But he had barely ever talked about his love for Matt before. Not even with Effie. Effie only knew everything because she had been right there when Floyd and Matt had started seeing each other. Talking about Matt was still too painful. Floyd had yet to make it more than a week without a nightmare about what had happened to Matt, one that hurt so badly it'd rouse him awake and leave him with the feeling that there was something heavy sitting on his chest. How could he ever even begin to talk about the man he had lost?

"Me and him only ever kissed," he said, purposefully leaving it vague.

"I can live with that."

"But you couldn't have lived with it if it had been more?" Floyd asked, trying to lighten the mood with some playfulness.

"No, of course I could have." Ollie sighed, sounding exasperated. Obviously, Floyd hadn't yet managed to figure out how to tease Ollie correctly when he was in one of these nervous, insecure moods. "But I wasn't sure what else I was supposed to say. I'm trying my best."

Floyd rubbed the back of Ollie's hand with his thumb.

"I know. I was trying to be funny."

"Oh. Well, that's where you went wrong. I'm the only one allowed to be funny."

"Yeah, Ollie, whatever you say."

"Don't mock me."

Floyd playfully nudged Ollie with his elbow.

"I got to head home soon."

"I know. And I have to struggle with washing clothes." Ollie squeezed Floyd's hand harder, making Floyd's stomach flip-flop. "Can we hold hands again tomorrow?"

"I can come here after work."

"I'd like that. I'd love it. But I have to be honest. I'm still not sure how to be right now. Like I said, I've never liked anyone before and I still feel a bit funny about it."

"Because I'm a man?"

"Yes, and no. I mean, yes, a little, but it's . . . Floyd, I'm scared out of my head right now. You could break my heart into a million little pieces."

"I won't."

"Sure, you say that *now*, but—"

"I won't," Floyd repeated, trying to make his voice as warm as possible to reassure him. He knew Ollie still wasn't too confident sometimes. After squeezing Ollie's hand once more, Floyd let go. "Except to leave for supper. I told you what'll happen to my ears if I'm late."

"Yes, yes, I remember," Ollie said. "But you're right, my heart is a *smidge* broken right now."

"I'll come back," Floyd said. "We'll see each other at work tomorrow. As soon as it breaks daylight."

"Breaks daylight," Ollie repeated. "I will never not love every single adorable thing that comes out of that handsome mouth of yours."

Floyd's cheeks turned hot. He wasn't used to these sorts of compliments.

"Take care, Ollie."

"You, too, Floyd."

All the way home, Floyd kept looking at his still-warm hand.

CHAPTER EIGHT

OLIVER

THE INITIAL THRILL THAT Oliver had been feeling from holding Floyd's hand had long since passed, leaving him with the sudden, terrible fear that Floyd might not really like him back enough to want to keep their agreed-upon arrangement. Not that Floyd had acted in a way to suggest that this might be the case, but . . .

But Oliver had never liked someone in this way before.

Oliver's worry was resulting in some regrettably strange behavior. For hours, Oliver had been bouncing between talking way, way too much, even for him, which was certainly saying something, and clamming up entirely. Worse, he kept leaping from one work task to the next, completing each of them in a hurried sort of way, the result of which was unbearably sloppy work. By noon, Oliver had already dropped his shovel over ten times. Thank God Floyd had yet to let him handle the explosives.

Throughout it all, Floyd was so, so forgiving. Even after hours of witnessing Oliver's blunders, Floyd still hadn't made even one teasing remark.

One of the most torturous facts of the workday was how incredibly attractive Floyd had suddenly become. Or, well, he had always been attractive, but now Oliver couldn't seem to watch the man bend over to lift a pickaxe without wishing he could be alone for a little while to take care of himself. Jesus Christ, how had Floyd become so . . . so delectable? Oliver had never, in his entire life, wanted to devour another person, but holy hell, Floyd certainly looked scrumptious enough to eat. Oliver was busy silently musing on the strangeness of this urge when Floyd caught him staring.

"Ollie, you're making it hard for me to work today."

God, Floyd probably hadn't even caught the potential filthiness hidden inside that stupidly tantalizing statement.

"Yes, well, same to you."

"I ain't the one staring. I can't focus with you looking at me all the time."

"Floyd, even if you're not the one staring, you're the one who . . ." Oliver took a couple of steps toward Floyd to close the space between them and lowered his voice to a whisper. "I'll put it this way: you look very nice in those pants."

"I have no idea what to say to that," Floyd remarked with an amused snort. "Look, we only got one more hour or so left. Let's focus on filling up this here car. I need money to feed my family."

"And money for more nicely tailored pants, too, I hope."

"Whatever makes you focus on helping me shovel coal, city boy."

So Oliver tried to concentrate on shoveling the last heaps of coal into the car. But once their playful banter ended, Oliver's niggling fear of rejection started percolating once again, first only manifesting a small rumble, but soon, becoming as powerful as an earthquake, causing Oliver's hands to tremble enough that he ended up dropping the shovel. Again.

"Unbelievable," Oliver muttered under his breath.

"Something wrong?"

"I'm fine. Probably had too much coffee this morning."

Oliver picked up his shovel and returned to the task. He still kept looking over at Floyd, though he tried not to be quite so obvious about it, and nearly every time, Oliver's eyes inevitably wandered to find Floyd's hands. He really liked Floyd's hands. They were beautiful. Large and strong and calloused and a perfect fit for his own.

Still shoveling, Oliver kept on worrying about whether or not he'd ever be able to hold them again, his mind continuously circling back to the possibility that Floyd might want to cancel their unconventional arrangement. Because why wouldn't he? Oliver wasn't special. He was a loudmouth who made too many silly jokes and took the Lord's name in vain. Besides, maybe Floyd wasn't as excited about their budding relationship as he was. Floyd hadn't been staring and tripping over lunch pails and forgetting not to shovel too many regular rocks in with the coal.

For the next while, Oliver busied himself by mentally listing out the many reasons why Floyd shouldn't like him, and by the end of it, he was feeling incredibly lousy about everything. So lousy, in fact, that he thought he should tell Floyd that he was no longer interested in romance or sex or strangely intimate hand-holding sessions. After all, he could avoid the pain from Floyd's eventual, inevitable rejection by rejecting Floyd first.

Pondering over this, Oliver bent to pick up his lunch pail.

And was met with a rat.

With a surprised yelp, Oliver leapt backward, crashing into Floyd, who had been shoveling the last bit of coal into the car. Floyd, being as large as a fucking house, barely even stumbled. He set his shovel on the car and turned to Oliver.

"Oh my God, oh shit, oh fuck," Oliver kept cursing, his heart thundering in his chest. "I think there's a rat in my lunch pail."

Floyd chuckled softly. "Maybe it opened when you tripped on it earlier."

"Well, that's the end of that particular lunch pail, then. I hope it's alright if I stop at the company store later. I'll have to purchase another one."

"Why would you do that?"

"In case you haven't noticed, the vermin is still in there, probably slathering himself in honey from my leftovers." Oliver shuddered. "I feel like I might vomit."

"Ain't you never seen rats in here before?"

"Yes, I have, but they typically stay far, far away from me and my lunch." Oliver cringed. "I nearly touched him!"

"It's only a rat," Floyd said, walking over to the lunch pail. "I'll shoo him away."

"Don't let him bite you. I'm sure you'll upset him by taking away his treat."

Oliver looked on nervously as Floyd kicked the pail, knocking it over and sending the rat scurrying into the darkness. He bent down and picked up the scraps.

"Mind if I toss these to him?"

"I thought we weren't supposed to feed them."

"Well, like you said, he was already eating these."

Floyd tossed the sandwich remnants into the darkness and wiped his hands on his pant legs. Oliver was still too shaken to retrieve the pail himself. Floyd probably realized this because he replaced the lid and set the pail on top of the coal pile in the car.

"Happy?" Floyd asked.

"Not really."

Floyd moved in close, close enough that Oliver's heart had started beating wildly again, though this time, not from fear of rodents.

"You're sweet, Ollie," Floyd whispered, his low voice sending shivers up Oliver's spine.

"Yeah?"

"Yeah. I can't wait to be alone with you later."

Oliver felt as though he might faint.

"Can we leave now?" Oliver found himself saying. "I promise I will make up whatever money we lose as a result of heading out early."

"Yeah, we can. Don't worry about the money, though. Our car's about full now."

Moving their car to the weigh station, Oliver was no longer thinking about ending their arrangement. Nor was he thinking about all the ways in which he was inadequate. All Oliver could think about was how much he liked Floyd and how much Floyd seemed to like him, too. His heart stuttered at the thought. God, how excited he was to hold Floyd's hand.

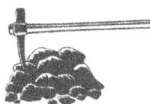

As soon as Oliver and Floyd were inside, they each flung their work bags to the floor, both of them sort of relishing the opportunity to be a little showy about it, and then, when they collapsed onto the couch next to one another, they immediately found each other's hands. It was only then that Oliver realized how magnificently filthy both of them were. Floyd's face was still caked with black coal powder. His clothes were a mess. Oliver knew he probably looked even worse himself (mostly because Floyd was so handsome, there would never be a time when Oliver *wouldn't* look worse; Oliver could be wearing his nicest suit while Floyd was wearing tattered, blackened overalls, and Floyd would still be the more handsome one).

"How are you so handsome?" Oliver asked.

"Just am," Floyd responded, ever-so-modestly. "Ain't more handsome than you, though."

"I wouldn't have taken you for a liar, Floyd Bennett."

"Because I ain't no liar, Oliver Astor," Floyd replied playfully. "You're a handsome man. I want you to know that about yourself."

"You need me to accept your compliment before you allow us to move on, huh?"

"Yup."

"Fine. I accept it. Begrudgingly," Oliver said before sighing very loudly, hoping to make a point about how tricky it was to internalize such things. "I'm sorry about earlier, by the way. I was in such a sorry state."

"Ollie," Floyd said, his voice suddenly so much softer. His thumb rubbed the back of Oliver's hand and the feel of Floyd's calloused skin sent little tingles up Oliver's arm. "Don't insult yourself so much."

Floyd's warm words wrapped around Oliver like a blanket, comforting and protective. Oliver squeezed Floyd's hand.

"I'll try not to."

For the next little while, they sat in a comfortable silence. Oliver was still enjoying the way that Floyd's continued kindness was making him feel so cared for and safe. Dazed, Oliver let himself become lost in Floyd for a bit. When his eyes settled on Floyd's lips—pinkish and plump and oh-so-kissable—he couldn't hold back his next series of comments.

"I'm not sure if we're supposed to kiss now. Should we? I mean, I'm not sure if it's what you were expecting, but we could if you wanted to. Of course, it's fine if you aren't interested in kissing, too. It's not like we *need* to kiss. I've made it twenty-six years without kissing someone. I'm sure I could make it however long I have left to live."

Floyd was silent for a few terrifying seconds, and then, finally, he said, "I ain't ready to kiss you, Ollie."

Shit.

"Oh."

Floyd's rejection curdled in Oliver's stomach like sour milk. Oliver had to look away. Why had he thought Floyd would want to kiss him? *Of course* Floyd wasn't as invested in all of this as he was. He had a family. He had a whole pre-established life, in fact. One that was perfectly lovely. In the real sense of the word.

Oliver felt Floyd release his hand, eliciting a tiny prick of pain in Oliver's heart. But then Floyd's hand cupped his chin instead.

"I will be ready one day," Floyd said, forcing Oliver to meet his bright blue eyes. "I promise."

"Did I . . ." Oliver's nausea was preventing him from formulating a proper response. He closed his eyes so that he could try to pretend that Floyd wasn't looking at him. "Is it me?"

"No," Floyd said, his tone tender. "Ain't about you, Ollie."

Oliver swallowed. "Alright."

"I want to kiss you. I *will* kiss you."

He opened his eyes again and managed a timid, "Alright."

"Ollie, remember the other man I told you about?" Floyd asked, and Oliver nodded. "I lost him, and I'm still . . . hurting. I can't . . . I can't figure out how to make myself tell you too much right now, but me not kissing you, that's about me, not you."

Hearing that soothed some of Oliver's pain. It wasn't him. Oliver repeated that to himself a few times in his head. Before Oliver could thank Floyd for the reassurance, Floyd took Oliver's hand and started to massage it with both of his.

"I like you, Ollie," Floyd said. "Don't forget it."

"I won't." He looked at their hands and watched Floyd's fingers press into his skin, each touch massaging away some of Oliver's insecurities. "I like you, too, Floyd. I can't believe I've only known you for a little over a month. I feel like I've known you my whole life. Only . . . not. Because then I'd have probably been a lot happier a lot earlier."

"I feel that way, too."

"I can't believe you have to leave soon."

Floyd tapped Oliver's knuckles a few times with his thumb.

"Do you want to come over for supper, then?"

"Jesus, that sounds terrifying," Oliver sputtered.

"Why?"

"How am I supposed to face Effie?"

"Effie ain't scary. She likes you."

"I still feel like I'm ruining your family."

"I'd never let you ruin my family."

"And I'd never want to. But, God, Floyd, what if she starts to resent me?"

"Look, Effie knows about you. About us. She knows where I am right now. And she's happy for us. Happy for me. She'll probably ask me all sorts of uncomfortable things later, not because she's worried or nothing, but because she wants me to be happy. She's always been like that."

"Are you sure it's not a problem?"

"Yeah, I am."

"Alright, then, let me wash up and change. I want to look nice."

Oliver had to practically pry himself off the cushions. He'd have happily continued to marinate in coal dust and sweat if it meant that he and Floyd could have kept holding hands until their filth-riddled bodies eventually fused with the cushions of his off-putting couch. Though, he supposed, wearing a moderately expensive suit to impress his new hand-holding butty would be fun, too.

While Floyd waited in the living room area, Oliver filled a tin bath with some water from the outdoor water pump and brought it inside to the bedroom. He refused to waste time heating up the water. Since it was summertime, the water wasn't too cold, though it wasn't one of Oliver's more pleasant sponge baths.

Once Oliver finished bathing, he picked out an outfit: a brown tweed suit with undertones of light blue, which he paired with a navy-blue tie and a simple white button-up shirt. He considered whether or not he should wear a hat. He liked hats. It was more proper, more fashionable, to wear one. But no one else in Rock Creek really seemed to wear hats much outside of their work hats. He supposed he'd leave it up to Floyd.

Oliver returned to the living room with a flourish.

"What do you think?" Oliver asked. "Blue and brown."

Floyd's eyes widened, a smile stretching across his face. He clicked his tongue once. "Golly, you're handsome."

"Alright, well . . ." Oliver paused and snatched a tan fedora off of the coat rack before placing it atop his head. "Hat or no hat?"

"Either."

"No, no, you have to pick."

Floyd pursed his lips, looking thoughtful. After a moment, he came over and removed Oliver's hat.

"No hat," Floyd said. He reached up to touch Oliver's hair, running his fingers through it, and the sensation had Oliver feeling momentarily lightheaded.

"Jeez, Floyd," Oliver said, letting out a breath. "I like that."

"Good."

"Alright, so, no hat." Oliver took his hat back from Floyd and tossed it aside, sending it over to the God-awful couch. Oliver couldn't care less that this would probably cause the fabric of his hat to be smudged with coal dust. All he wanted was for Floyd to touch his hair again. "Do you hate my hats? Because if so, I will burn each and every one of them, especially if it means that you'll keep touching me like that."

Floyd smirked. "I like your hats. Just not tonight. I want to touch that soft hair of yours whenever I can."

"Won't Josephine wonder why you're fixating on another man's head?"

"She'll be in bed at some point." Floyd reached up and fluffed up Oliver's hair once more, humming sweetly while his fingers threaded through Oliver's blond locks. "I been wanting to do that ever since we met."

"I think we need to leave now or I swear to God I might lose consciousness."

Floyd burst out laughing. "You say the strangest things, Ollie."

"I try." Oliver nodded toward the front door. "Come on. Let's head out."

Oliver and Floyd walked through the neighborhood together. Being side by side in public, now that they had confessed their feelings for one another, was turning out to be a uniquely upsetting experience. Halfway to Floyd's house, Oliver started thinking about how desperately he wished he could hold Floyd's hand. It occurred to him, then, that even if Floyd hadn't been married, the two of them still wouldn't have been able to hold hands in public, even in a cozy little community tucked away in the mountains.

Ruminating on this, hot fury settled in Oliver's stomach, making his blood boil. It infuriated him to think that most people would have a problem with the fact that he and Floyd had romantic feelings for each other. He hadn't ever had to think about such travesties before. Which was pretty egotistical of him, wasn't it? How was it that he had never thought about—*really* thought about—the hatred society had for men who fancied other men? God, he couldn't believe how shortsighted he was sometimes, like he was so self-absorbed it was a miracle he could even see past his own nose.

"You look sad," Floyd said, his brow furrowed with concern. "Do you not want to come over no more?"

"It's not that," Oliver said. "I can't tell you what it is, either. Not out here."

"Are you sure?"

"Yes," Oliver said. "Don't worry about it."

Floyd stayed quiet for the rest of the way.

After they went inside, Floyd left to wash up from work. Effie had already prepared a wash basin with water for him. Meanwhile, Oliver stayed out in the living room and played jacks with Josephine. Effie, who was finishing up a bean and vegetable stew over the stove, kept looking back and smiling, which was making Oliver so nervous that he kept messing up his moves. Which was fine. Because playing poorly was proving to be an effective way to further win over Floyd's adorable little girl.

Sometime later, Floyd came out of the bedroom wearing a pair of tan slacks, a light blue button-down shirt, and brown suspenders. Seeing this picture-perfect outfit, Oliver reached up to shield his mouth with his hand in a pathetic attempt to conceal the size of his embarrassingly large smile.

Floyd smiled shyly in response, shoving his hands into his pockets.

"Is supper ready?" he asked.

And this was when Effie saw him.

"Oh my word, you look so handsome!" she said, her eyes sparkling with fondness. "Don't he look handsome, Oliver?"

Oliver had only just managed to reign in his stupid smile. And now it had come back.

"Exceedingly handsome," Oliver admitted with a lovesick sigh, one that had seemingly come out against his will.

"You hear that, Floyd? *Exceedingly* handsome."

Effie said these last two words like this compliment was the pinnacle of all compliments. Now blushing madly, Oliver looked away. He heard Josephine hop to her feet.

"Daddy, you look like you're going to church," she said. "Is it a church night?"

Effie laughed softly. "No, baby. Daddy wanted to look nice for his friend, is all."

"Oh. Can I wear my Sunday dress, then? I want to look nice for Mister Oliver, too."

"Sure, why not?"

Josephine shrieked and ran into the bedroom, so excited to change that she slammed the door behind her. Effie and Floyd looked at each other and shrugged.

"She never wants to wear nothing fancy, normally," Effie said. "I have to beg her to put on her Sunday dress *on* Sunday. Guess you must be special, Oliver."

"Oh yes, I'm even more special than Jesus," Oliver said, realizing his social faux pas the moment the words tumbled out of his mouth.

To Oliver's relief, Effie laughed. Floyd laughed, too, of course, but that wasn't nearly as surprising anymore. Floyd had probably become accustomed to Oliver's proclivity for socially unacceptable humor by now.

"Well, I ain't sure about *that*," Effie said. "But Floyd seems to worship you."

"Effie!" Floyd scolded. He picked up the nearest piece of paper, rolled it up, and smacked her in the arm with it. "Hush up!"

Effie kept laughing. "Look, if y'all want to be whatever it is that you're trying to be, you best let me have some fun with it."

Floyd whacked her again. But Effie was stubborn.

"Floyd is so smitten with you, Oliver. He talks about you like a preacher on a mission."

Another whack.

"I think you need to surrender," Oliver said. "I have a feeling Effie is tenacious enough to keep embarrassing you with these clever comments, no matter how many times you pummel her with two ounces of paper."

With an irritated-sounding grunt, Floyd dropped the roll of paper onto the table, though he was smiling a lot, if not a tad red in the face. Josephine skipped into the kitchen wearing a pink and white dress, the same one Oliver had seen her wear to church.

"Ready!" Josephine squirmed. "It's still a little wet."

"I washed it this morning," Effie explained. "How was I supposed to know you'd want to wear it so soon?"

Oliver smiled. "Well, I think you look very pretty, Josephine. Like a little Ethel Clayton."

Despite the fact that Josephine very likely had no idea who the film actress was, she nevertheless looked pleased with Oliver's compliment.

Now that everyone was very nicely dressed, they sat down for supper, and as soon as Oliver took the first bite, he intentionally let out what he hoped would be an appreciative-sounding moan. He really liked Effie's cooking. And he needed her to know it. It tasted like there was a lot of love in it. Like the care she felt for her family was somehow baked right into the cornbread. In New York, Oliver had been privileged enough to try all sorts of exotic dishes, but that food had tasted like . . . well, maybe like obligation. Not that it had been their cook's fault, he supposed, but he would have taken Effie's bean and vegetable stew over the soft-shell crab with remoulade of his childhood any day. He told Effie as much, which made her smile in a really sweet, really heartbreaking sort of way, like she might melt into a puddle and spill onto the floor. Floyd winked at him afterward, too, which was so wonderful it made Oliver's stomach flutter.

Once everyone was finished eating, Oliver volunteered to help Effie clean up, but then Floyd offered to help, too, and of course, Josephine wanted to be part of the fun. This meant that there ended up being way too many people in the little kitchen area at once. Oliver thought he was probably in the way more than he was helping, and so, he stood off to the side, nodding approvingly and offering occasional encouragement like some sort of misplaced baseball coach.

Dishes clean, everyone retired to the living room to relax. Or maybe relax wasn't the right word, really, especially for Josephine, who still had a lot of energy. Ricocheting from the couch to the floor and back to the couch again, she talked and talked and talked. Adorable, but a bit tiring to watch.

"You know what we need?" Effie said when the sun started to set. "Some music."

"I like music," Oliver said, which was probably silly, because everyone liked music. "What do you have? A Brunswick?"

"Oh, our phonograph broke last year. We haven't replaced it yet," Effie said. "But Floyd plays the banjo."

"Ah, Ollie don't want to hear me play," Floyd said with a dismissive wave.

"Are you insane?!" Oliver exclaimed, practically leaping off the couch with excitement. "Of course I want to hear you play!"

"Yeah?"

"Yes!"

Cheeks tinged with pink, Floyd walked off to the bedroom to retrieve his banjo. Though Floyd had looked a tad uneasy—perhaps nervous—when he left, he had a little knowing smile on his face by the time he returned, like maybe he knew he was about to knock Oliver's socks off, which made Oliver even more excited to listen to him play.

Josephine curled up in her mother's lap on the rocking chair while Floyd sat on the couch beside Oliver. As Floyd tuned the banjo, his face slowly started to redden again, and holy hell, it was so amazingly adorable. Floyd couldn't have looked more endearing if he tried.

Moments later, Floyd started to play. And, oh, it was beautiful. Oliver had only ever heard a handful of songs played on the banjo before—lively ones, fast ones, ones that made people want to move their feet—but the tune Floyd was playing was so magnificently different, slow and sweet and beautiful. Each pluck of the banjo strings produced a lovely sound, one that softly thrummed against Oliver's tender heart and awakened a longing inside of him. For love. For closeness.

Listening to Floyd's music, Oliver let himself pine for Floyd to know him—to *really* know him—and to someday even love him, *all* of him, even the parts that he believed weren't the least bit lovable. Oliver imagined what it might be like to one day be nestled in Floyd's arms and what it might be like to hold Floyd in his arms too. While Floyd played on, Oliver became lost in this longing for intimacy, and he wondered if such closeness might somehow help him mend the wounds from his childhood. Oh, what would it be like to be healed and happy and whole?

Midway through the song, Floyd started to sing. Though his voice was low and shy, it was still so powerful, and its beauty brought tears to Oliver's eyes. It was a sweet song, one with lyrics about love and loss, and Oliver had to fight to keep his tears from falling. When Floyd finished playing, he looked up and met Oliver's waiting gaze, his blue eyes a tad misty too. While it hurt Oliver's heart to see Floyd's sadness, he welcomed the twinge of pain. Because it felt like Floyd was finally letting Oliver see him.

Oliver wondered, then, how it was that he could feel so happy and so sad at once.

"Beautiful," Oliver said.

Because Floyd was beautiful.

"Just a song I heard a long time ago."

Effie chimed in. "Floyd is very talented. He can hear a tune and play it right back to you. He remembers notes and words and things so easily."

"Thanks, Effie," Floyd said.

Oliver noticed then that Josephine had nodded off.

"I'll take her," Floyd said, setting his banjo on the couch.

Floyd scooped Josephine up in his arms and carried her off to the bedroom. Oliver and Effie smiled at one another as Effie's hands twisted in her lap.

"I want to tell you about Josephine," Effie said. "Floyd told me I could."

"Alright," Oliver said, already feeling the weight of the secret he was about to hear.

"Josephine ain't Floyd's. He's her Daddy, but . . ." She trailed off and looked down at her still-moving hands. "Floyd ain't the man who got me pregnant. Another man did that. One I never even wanted to be with in that way, but, well, you know how these things go sometimes."

Oliver's muscles tensed against his fast-rising anger. He tried not to let it show, keeping his expression soft.

Effie continued, "Floyd was working in one of them mines in McDowell back then, living in the boarding house. When I told him what had happened, he told me he'd take care of us. Of me and the baby, I mean. We couldn't stay out there, though. By the time I'd told Floyd about Josephine, everybody had already heard what had happened. Or, well, they heard the untrue version. Everybody had already made up their minds about what kind of woman I was. I was afraid for Josephine. I was worried that someone would tell her that Floyd wasn't her real daddy. And so, we left. Floyd brought us here, far away from everybody who knew our history."

"I'm so sorry that happened to you."

Effie nodded sadly. "Thank you. Floyd has been a treasure, though. He works so hard for us. He loved Josephine right away. Even before she was born, he loved her. Because he loves me. That's why I ain't worried about you and him. I know he loves me. It ain't the kind of love you see in the pictures or in storybooks, but it's real love. It's forever love."

"Haven't you ever wanted more? You know, romance?"

"Maybe someday. I'm not too interested in it, to be honest with you, but if it ever happened, I know Floyd would support me. Just like I'm supporting him now. Whoever it was would have to understand, though, that Floyd ain't going nowhere. If they couldn't accept that, well, then they wouldn't be the man for me."

"Sounds sensible."

"Our family comes first. Always."

Oliver tilted his head inquisitively. "How'd you know that you could trust me?"

"Floyd," Effie said simply. "I think he could tell. Ever since we been married, he ain't never liked another man. He told me that sort of thing was behind him. So, when I saw the way he was looking at you that first night you came over for supper, I figured that Floyd must have known that you had a kind heart. Otherwise, he'd have never let himself start falling for you."

"That's very sweet," Oliver said, scooting closer. He looked into Effie's eyes, trying to wordlessly communicate his sincerity before saying what he wanted—no, *needed*—to say next. "Floyd was right, you know. You can trust me. I won't tell anyone about any of this. No matter what happens between me and Floyd, I won't ever hurt your family, Effie."

"Thank you."

Oliver turned toward the sound of heavy footsteps.

"Effie told you everything?" Floyd asked, approaching.

"Yes," Effie confirmed.

Floyd nodded once. "Good."

Effie stood and smoothed out her skirt. "I'm a bit tired. I think I'll try to sleep."

"Goodnight," Oliver said. "Thank you for sharing your story with me."

"Of course." Effie looked at Floyd with a teasing smile. "You two have fun. Not *too* much fun, though."

Floyd rolled his eyes. "Night, Effie."

Effie walked off to the bedroom, laughing softly while she did.

Floyd and Oliver looked at each other. Finally, they were alone. As soon as Floyd plopped onto the couch beside Oliver, he reached up and threaded his fingers through Oliver's hair.

"I been wanting to do that for hours," Floyd said with a low hum.

Oliver closed his eyes and sighed.

"It's heaven," he said.

Floyd kept playing with Oliver's hair. "So, you liked my song?"

"I loved your song. It nearly made me cry. I would have hated you a little for it."

"I like slow, sad-sounding songs," Floyd said. "Effie and Jo like when my music sounds a bit happier, but more often than not, I play songs like that one."

"I'm pretty sure I'd like anything you wanted to play."

Oliver turned, tucking his legs underneath him, and rested the side of his head against the back cushion of the couch. Floyd continued to play with his hair.

"I've never experienced this before," Oliver said. "I know you probably have, but Floyd, it's so special to me."

"It's special to me, too, Ollie."

"Will you come by after work tomorrow?"

Floyd's hand briefly brushed Oliver's cheek before he lifted it to thread his fingers through Oliver's hair again.

"I'll come by every day if you want."

"Yes, I want that."

Oliver shut his eyes and let himself become lost in Floyd's soft touches. Each minute felt like an eternity. In the very best possible way.

"Ollie?" Floyd asked.

"Mmm?"

"Why were you so sad before?"

"Oh . . ." Oliver opened one eye to see Floyd looking at him with so much sweetness that he couldn't not be honest with him. "I was thinking about how horrible it is that no one would ever accept us. Outside of Effie, I mean, which is really saying something."

Floyd's face twisted up like he was struggling with some sudden rush of upset from the comment, but then, in seconds, his brows relaxed and his frown lifted like he had managed to force that bit of fury away.

"Dang, it's been a while since I thought 'bout them kinds of things," Floyd said. "What you said about us not being accepted, it's true. How the world is, well, it's harder for people like us."

"How do you make yourself . . . feel at peace with it?"

"I been living with it for a long time. It bothered me more when I was a kid. Sometimes, it bothers me now, but not a lot."

"Wow, I . . . I can't even imagine trying to understand all of this as a kid. I mean, when I was a kid, I thought I was, well, I thought I was strange, but I was strange in all sorts of ways, so this was just one more thing to add to the pile of eccentricities, you know? Besides, I thought I'd eventually figure it out, but then, by the time I realized that I probably never would, I was an adult, one who was too busy hating his predestined future to worry too much about whether or not he'd ever kiss someone." Oliver reached for Floyd's free hand and squeezed it. "Sorry. We were talking about you. Was it hard for you, then, when you were younger?"

"It was," Floyd confirmed. "I had Effie, though, and . . ."

"And what?"

Floyd was silent for a few seconds. His eyes became misty again. Finally, he choked out, "I had my friend, too."

Probably whoever Floyd had kissed. Oliver wanted to pry. God, how he wanted to know more about this mysterious man who Floyd had kissed, but with the way Floyd was clamming up, Oliver knew that he wasn't ready to talk about it. He wondered if Floyd would ever be ready. He really hoped so.

"I'm sorry, Floyd," Oliver said. "For . . . whatever happened."

He kneaded Floyd's hand, hoping that his touches could soothe some of Floyd's pain. Floyd took a couple of breaths.

"Thanks, Ollie," Floyd whispered.

"Of course." Oliver continued to massage Floyd's hand for a bit before saying, "Did your parents know?"

"I confessed to them when I was eighteen," Floyd confirmed. "After that, they sent me to live in the boarding house."

Oliver's chest tightened. Holy hell, it pained him to hear how Floyd's parents had treated him. Floyd was such a sweet man, one who had deserved so, so much better.

While Oliver tried not to be so upset with what Floyd had told him, Floyd continued to stroke his hair, which was really Goddamn nice, but a little infuriating, too. Why was Floyd comforting him through this? It wasn't right. Oliver should have been the one comforting Floyd. He had to fix it.

Over the next few moments, he racked his brain for ideas. Jeez, the only thing he could think of to try to help Floyd feel better was to try to make him laugh.

Oliver said, "Actually, that was kind of silly of them, wasn't it?"

"Silly?"

"Well, think about it," Oliver said. "When you told your parents that you liked men . . . you were essentially telling them that you wanted to sleep with men. Sexually. And, Floyd, they sent you to *sleep with* a bunch of men."

Floyd snorted.

Oliver continued, "So, on second thought, it sounds like they were very supportive people."

He said this with as straight a face as possible, which luckily had the intended effect of making Floyd laugh, though he was obviously trying to hold back because of how late it was. Watching Floyd's body silently shake from barely-contained laughter was . . . oh, God, it was everything.

"Thank you, Ollie," Floyd said once he calmed himself.

And, thank God, Floyd had the biggest smile, one that was so large, his beautiful blue eyes were nearly closed from the size of it. Oliver's chest warmed from the sight. He felt so incredibly proud of himself for helping Floyd through that painful memory.

"You're welcome."

"It'll be easier for you one day," Floyd said. "I can always listen to you if you need me to. If you're ever upset about how we have to be or what people think about us, I can listen."

"I really appreciate that," Oliver said. "Can I ask you one more thing, though?"

"Yeah, sure."

"What about church? How can you make yourself sit there like that?"

"I like church."

"Even though—"

"Yeah," Floyd said, cutting him off. "Even though."

"Why?"

Floyd shrugged. "All of this—it's between me and God," he said, as though it was the simplest thing in the world. "I like the rest of the teachings. Or, most of them."

"Does part of you attend because of the, uhm, the role you're playing?"

"Yep," Floyd admitted. "I need to keep an image."

"Smart," Oliver said with a nod. "Thank you for talking to me, for being honest with me."

"Anytime." Floyd's fingers trailed lower, caressing Oliver's cheek. "It's late."

"I know," Oliver whispered in response. "But this is so nice."

"It is. We have tomorrow, though."

Oliver smiled wistfully. "Tomorrow and tomorrow and tomorrow, creeps in this petty pace from day to day, to the last syllable of recorded time."

Floyd shook his head, confused. "What's that?"

"Shakespeare."

Floyd hummed and repeated, "Tomorrow and tomorrow and tomorrow."

Oliver reached up to catch Floyd's hand and then brought Floyd's knuckles to his lips.

"To the last syllable of recorded time."

CHAPTER NINE

FLOYD

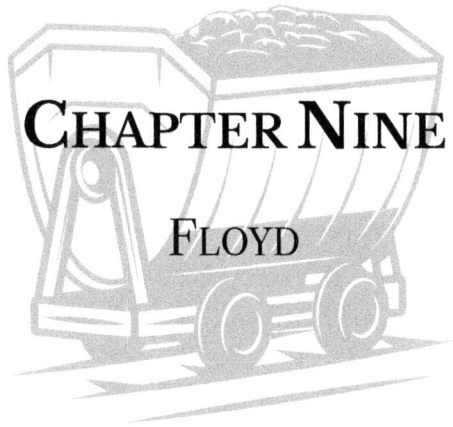

ON A SATURDAY TOWARD the end of June, Floyd and Ollie walked together to the company store. Ollie wanted the two of them to take a train to Charleston, have an adventure. Normally, Floyd would have resisted the urge to travel to the city, mostly because it was too much of a hassle, especially when it came to converting scrip over to United States currency. It was a pain in the rear end to figure out how much you'd need to change over at the company store in order to buy whatever it was you wanted to buy out there.

Complicating matters, the exchange rate wasn't too good. If a miner was feeling bold (or foolish), he might want to borrow from his future self—to request a loan, of sorts, from his future paycheck, and exchange that money over so that he could spend it in the city. If a fella kept this up, he'd end up in debt. Floyd had seen it happen a few times. Coal companies were probably happy when it did. Miners who owed the company money couldn't very well leave, could they? Luckily, Floyd had never needed to borrow money from his future self, even to cover necessities, which also happened to folks sometimes. He never borrowed for entertainment purposes neither, even taking it so far as to avoid changing scrip over entirely. He thought it best to stay away from all that. But . . .

Lord help him, how could he say no to spending time with Ollie? If Ollie wanted to explore the city, Floyd supposed he'd have to explore it, too.

Floyd and Ollie approached the counter where Charlie was reading a newspaper.

"Morning, Charlie," Floyd said. "I need to change some scrip over."

"*You?!*" Charlie asked, raising an eyebrow. "Now that's new." Floyd prepared himself to receive some sort of lecture, but instead, Charlie held up a finger and walked away toward the windows. After resting his hands on his hips, Charlie looked up like he was searching the sky. For what, Floyd didn't know. After another few seconds of this, Charlie returned to the counter. "Strange. There ain't no pigs flying out there."

Floyd snorted. "You're worse than Effie."

Ollie arched an eyebrow. "Jeez, you weren't exaggerating when you told me you never leave Rock Creek, were you?"

"Nope." Floyd tossed a little cloth poke onto the counter. "In there's twenty in scrip. How much is that in dollars?"

Charlie dumped the tin-colored coins out onto the counter to count them.

"Yep, twenty." He opened the register and proceeded to count out paper bills. "That'll earn you an even fifteen."

"Wait, wait, wait," Ollie said in rapid succession. "Floyd, no, keep your scrip. I hadn't realized you would lose that much money for the exchange. I have plenty to cover both of us."

Charlie whistled. "Wow, that's some friend you got there."

Floyd ignored Charlie's comment.

"I ain't taking your money, Ollie."

"You lose five dollars!" Ollie protested. "I've been told that's nothing to sneeze at."

Through a brief flash of envy, Floyd had to fight to keep a straight face. Of course Ollie been *told*, because Ollie wouldn't know otherwise. He had come from money. He still *had* money. Sometimes, it felt like Ollie was a little boy playing pretend out here in the mines.

"Well, fortunately, I ain't sick," Floyd said before turning his attention back to Charlie and holding out his hand. "I'll take the fifteen."

Floyd heard Ollie let out an irritated huff beside him.

"What are you planning on buying?" Charlie asked.

"Probably a phonograph or whatever it is they got in the stores nowadays. We need a new listening device. Effie's sick of my sad banjo playing."

"Good luck to you. I know them things are expensive."

"Fifteen should cover it. Ollie and me want to see a picture, too. Maybe I can pick up a new toy for Jo if there's extra."

Ollie tugged on Floyd's sleeve. "Come on," he said, voice rife with irritation. "I think the next train will arrive soon."

Floyd shoved the empty cloth poke back in his pocket and folded up the bills.

"Have a nice Saturday, Charlie," Floyd said, sliding the paper money into his wallet.

After that, Floyd and Oliver walked across town to catch the train. Floyd could still sense some tension between them. He knew Ollie wasn't very happy with him for refusing his offer. But Floyd took care of his family his own self. If they needed a new listening device, *he* would be the one to buy it. Ollie could keep his money, maybe buy more of them fancy suits he liked so much.

Minutes into their train ride, Ollie still looked pretty mad—his brows furrowed slightly and a scowl on his face. Meanwhile, most of Floyd's earlier upset had since faded away. Now, instead of feeling bitter about Ollie's expensive suits, Floyd found himself thinking 'bout how nice Ollie looked in them. He wondered if a compliment might lift Ollie's mood.

Floyd tapped Ollie's foot with his own.

"I know what you can spend your money on," Floyd said before leaning in close, hoping to sound playful. "How about another one of them fancy suits? I like seeing you in those."

Ollie pursed his lips, hopefully to keep himself from smiling. Feeling confident that his plan was working, Floyd tried again.

"You look real nice today, Ollie. I ain't mention that to you yet."

Ollie's cheeks flushed. "Floyd, I know what it is you're trying to do."

"What is it you think I'm trying to do?"

"You're trying to make me forget about the fact that you snubbed my offer back there."

"I wasn't trying to snub you."

"Why wouldn't you let me pay for you today? I mean, I'd even prefer to buy you the phonograph myself, especially if it would mean that the two of us could listen to music together."

"I wasn't raised to take charity."

"It's not charity." Ollie lowered his voice to a soft whisper. "I wanted to treat you. Especially now that I'm aware of the fact that you're being taken advantage of by the coal company like this. I can't believe I had never really paid much attention to the exchange rate before."

"Not like we'll be heading to Charleston every weekend."

"Not if Donohue Coal and Steel has something to say about it."

Floyd tried not to react to Ollie's tone. He hated when Ollie talked about life in the coal town like he actually knew something about it, like he was really living it. Because Ollie *wasn't* living it.

He'd never really be living it, not like everybody else in Rock Creek. Because Ollie had plenty of money. He was still an outsider. Still new to mining, too.

Which was one of the reasons why Floyd always made sure to take care of him in the mines. Whenever they needed their blast powder, Floyd took it upon himself to handle it, making sure Ollie wouldn't be in harm's way. Whenever they were assigned a new tunnel, Floyd ventured in first, test lamp in tow, to check for the so-called asphyxiant gasses and confirm that it was safe. He needed to keep Ollie safe. Like he ought to have kept Matt safe all them years ago.

Floyd's chest tightened at the thought of Matt.

Ignoring the upset, Floyd scooted closer to Ollie. He wanted them to have fun in the city. He couldn't let Ollie keep sulking about the money, and he couldn't let himself start to sulk about Matt neither.

"Just have fun with me today," Floyd said. "Don't worry about Donohue Coal and Steel. Worry about spending time with me."

Floyd waited for Ollie's response. He hoped Ollie would let it go.

"Fine. I'll *try* not to worry about Donohue," Ollie relented. "Can I at least pay for the pictures?"

"Mmm . . . yeah, I suppose."

"Thank you." Ollie's face lit up, the wrinkles on his forehead finally fading while his eyes brightened. "And thank you for the compliments. You look very nice, too. Fantastic even."

"Yeah, I like this suit." Floyd studied the light gray sleeves. "I wear it to church a lot."

"Well, I think it's officially too tainted for church now."

Floyd smiled, already aware of what was a-coming.

"Why's that?"

"Because it has me thinking some very *un*holy thoughts."

Floyd let out a puff of air. "You're really something, Ollie."
"So are you, Floyd."

Floyd tapped Ollie's foot again. Ollie tapped his back.

Soon, they arrived in Charleston. Floyd and Ollie spent the majority of their time doing something Ollie called "window-shopping," where they walked by a bunch of stores real slow-like and talked about what they seen on display and whether or not they'd ever buy any of it. It was a little strange since Ollie could probably buy every single item if he wanted to, but it was fun, too. A couple of times, Ollie made comments about the prices of some of the items—boots and men's shirts and the like—and seemed keen to point out that they cost less in Charleston than in Rock Creek. More evidence, he said, that the company was taking advantage. Comments like that had Floyd's heart hammering, fury about the past and worry over the future swirling in his chest like a storm, but Floyd managed to fight the feelings back. He really wanted their special day to stay special.

At one point, they walked past a toy store, and Floyd seen something Josephine might like—a box of building materials called Lincoln Logs—but thought that he should make sure he'd have enough left after the phonograph before trying to buy it. They passed a hat shop, too. Floyd could tell that Ollie was fighting the urge to go inside. He wished he could sneak away and buy Ollie one of them hats. He'd have loved to see Ollie's face light up when presented with a new one. But, of course, he'd never have that kind of money, especially not after buying the phonograph.

Around noon, they had lunch in a restaurant, which Floyd hadn't never done before. It was a real treat, especially since it was with Ollie. They had the same sandwich—brisket, mustard, and pickles—which they both really liked. After that, they saw a picture called *The Kid*, and it was a thrill to spend so much time laughing like that. Being in the dark with Ollie was romantic, too, even if the film wasn't a romantic one.

Finally, once the movie was over, they found a music shop, one that sold phonographs and records and even instruments, too. Unfortunately, none of the models they had cost less than twenty dollars, which was something Floyd had not expected.

"How can they be so expensive?" he wondered aloud, scratching his head. "Last one we had cost me fifteen. I thought they might be even cheaper now."

Ollie touched his arm. "Let me ask the owner. Maybe they have more in the back."

While Ollie talked to the owner, Floyd stood there staring at the little white price tags. Twenty. Twenty-two. Thirty! How could people afford these?

Ollie returned, wearing a frown.

"He says they stopped carrying some of the cheaper models last year."

"Why?"

"I'm not sure," Ollie said. "I'm sorry, Floyd."

"Guess I'll have to save up some more."

Ollie huffed in irritation. "You'd have had enough if it hadn't been for the exchange rate," he muttered.

Anger zipped through Floyd's veins, hot and fast like lightning. Why was Ollie so keen on talking about Donohue Coal and Steel? Every comment Ollie was making kept reminding Floyd of the past—of the conversations he'd had with Matt about them needing to leave the coal industry. Floyd was already aware of the problems with these coal companies. Ollie wasn't telling him nothing new. But no matter how bad things were, Floyd couldn't never leave. Not when Matt hadn't never been able to. Thinking of the fact that Matt hadn't never made it out, Floyd's heart started beating wildly. Pretty soon, it was pounding so doggone ferociously

that he couldn't keep himself from showing how flustered he really
was.

"I thought we weren't talking 'bout the coal company no
more," Floyd spit, his voice stern.

"Jesus Christ, Floyd, why are you so upset every single time
I mention the many, many ways in which the coal company is
cheating you? It's not like I'm saying it's your fault. It's Frederick
fucking Donohue's! And Don Chafin's, too."

"Hush up, Ollie!" Floyd said, the volume of his voice startling
even to him.

Ollie looked unfazed by it.

"You're being so . . . so ridiculous about this!" Ollie exclaimed,
and Floyd's hands started to shake. "Look, Rock Creek is a fine
place to live, but I know there have to be better towns out there,
towns where companies can't fucking mandate that you work
past lunchtime even if you've filled your car early, towns where
companies can't short you because they *feel like* your car has too
much rubble, towns where companies aren't charging miners an
arm and a leg to replace a broken carbide lamp!"

Floyd's nostrils flared. "I like Rock Creek! I worked hard to
build a life there!"

"But there are better—"

"So, what, Ollie, you want me to up and leave? Are you saying
I chose wrong? Are you telling me that I ain't taking care of my
family?"

"What?! No! Of course not!"

"After everything we been through in McDowell, me and Effie
are happy to have a home in Rock Creek. Donohue's nicer than
some of them other coal operators out there, *trust me*." Thinking
of the man who had hurt Effie, Floyd's stomach tightened, and
he swallowed hard, fighting the bile that was rising in his throat.
"Effie . . . Effie knows that, too."

"Floyd—"

"You think you're so smart because you been to college, but I *know* we got it better than a lot of other miners in West Virginia. Did you know that Donohue only stocks them short-range explosives in the company store now? He came by a couple years ago and made a big speech about it, saying it was safer, saying he wanted to make things better for us," Floyd said. "And we got them test lamps now, too. And plenty of other things. I'm not risking what I have—what my *family* has—by moving somewhere else. I can't move somewhere else. I can't leave the coal industry. I can't—"

Floyd's breath shook, and suddenly, the world started to spin. Squeezing his eyes shut, Floyd had to hold back tears. Not only were his hands starting to tremble, but his whole body was shaking too. He couldn't stop thinking of poor Matt. Smart, caring, loyal Matt who had never made it out, who had never realized his future. Who had never realized *their* future.

While Floyd was lost in his upset—trapped in visions of the past—Ollie took him by the forearm and led him outside. Dazed, Floyd let Ollie take him far from the store and over to a bench. Floyd's breath was still shaking when he sat.

"Floyd," Ollie said softly. "Deep breaths. Slow."

It took a whole bunch of breaths before Floyd could calm himself. Once his body stopped trembling and thoughts of Matt and the coal companies finally faded, Floyd was left feeling completely and utterly embarrassed about how fast his emotions had spiraled out of control. Shame trickled up the back of his neck, turning his ears hot, and he leaned forward to bury his head in his hands. Ollie rubbed his back.

"I never meant to upset you like that," Ollie said softly.

"I know," Floyd managed to say in return.

He wanted to tell Ollie what had him so flustered, but the shame he was feeling had wrapped itself around his throat, strangling him and preventing the words from coming.

"How can I help?" Ollie asked.

"I need . . . I need some time," Floyd choked out.

"Do you want me to go, then?"

After a pause, Floyd managed a nod. But only barely.

"Should I wait for you at the train station?" Ollie asked.

Eyes tearing, Floyd shook his head.

"I feel so bad leaving you, but if that's what you need . . ." Ollie rubbed his back a couple more times. "I'll see you back in Rock Creek, then?"

Floyd stayed hidden behind his hands as Ollie walked away. He waited on the bench for a while—maybe a whole hour—feeling horrible for losing his temper with Ollie. Poor Ollie hadn't meant no harm. He was only trying to help. Golly, what a mess this was. Why hadn't he been able to keep himself from falling to pieces like that?

After Floyd spent some time wallowing, he started toward the train station. On the way, he purchased the Lincoln Logs for Josephine and a summer dress for Effie. Last, Floyd stopped at the hat shop and bought the nicest, most expensive hat he could afford.

Traveling back to Rock Creek, Floyd kept bouncing his leg and shifting in his seat on the train. He hoped Ollie would forgive him for yelling and for saying that he needed some time to himself.

Shortly before supper, Floyd arrived home. After presenting his family with their gifts, he told Effie what had happened between him and Ollie back in Charleston and asked her if he could head over to Ollie's once they were finished eating so that he could try to patch things up. Effie was supportive, as she always was, and even told Floyd not to worry about tucking Josephine into bed. But then, when it came time to leave, Floyd suddenly felt too nervous to follow through. He needed a little more time to himself, a little more time to come up with the right words to say. So, he read Josephine a bedtime story and stayed with her until she fell asleep.

By the time Floyd came back to the living room, Ollie had come over his own self and was sitting on the sofa.

"Hi," Ollie said with a half-smile that pulled at Floyd's heart.

Floyd tried to smile back. "Hi."

Effie excused herself and left for the sewing room, saying she had to patch up one of Josephine's dresses. Floyd sat beside Ollie on the couch.

"I'm so sorry for everything I said earlier," Ollie said. "It wasn't my place to criticize the town like that."

"It was your place. It *is* your place. You live here, too."

"I'm not a real miner."

"You are a real miner," Floyd said. "And I'm a real lunkhead."

"You're not a lunkhead. I only call you that because I'm . . . well because *I'm* a lunkhead. I shouldn't have kept hounding you about the coal company. You're content with your life here and I have to respect that. God, I knew that already. But I couldn't stop myself."

"You were only trying to look out for me. I know that now. I was too thick to see it before."

"I would *never* try to suggest that you made the wrong choice for your family. Ever. I can see how hard you work to take care of Effie and Josephine. I know you want what's best for them. I want you to be happy, Floyd, that's all."

"I am happy." Floyd took Oliver's hand and kissed it. "Especially now that you're here." He shifted closer to Ollie on the couch, shuffling over until their thighs were pressed against each other's. "And I need to tell you why I reacted like that."

"Oh, Floyd, I can tell that whatever it is must be hard for you to talk about. It's fine to keep it to yourself. Really."

"Nah, I want to tell you. I want to make sure you know why . . . why talking 'bout the coal company can be so hard for me." Floyd took Ollie's hand and kissed it one more time. "I've mentioned the man who I was with before you. But I never told you . . ." Floyd inhaled a shaky breath. "I never told you that the two of us were planning on leaving the coal industry together, but then he . . ."

Floyd couldn't even make himself say it.

"Did he pass?" Oliver asked, his voice warm and kind.

Floyd swallowed. "Yeah." He kissed Ollie's hand a couple more times. It was like having Ollie close was keeping him tethered to the present. Without Ollie's touch, Floyd thought he might slip into the past and become lost in those horrible memories again. Golly, it was still so hard to talk about Matt. "I can't never leave the coal industry. Because my friend . . . well, he wasn't never able to leave."

"So, me reminding you of how much better you might have it if you ever left is making you feel like I'm . . . like I'm pushing you to leave, maybe?"

"Something like that."

"Oh, Floyd, I'm sorry."

"It's fine, Ollie. I know you never meant no harm." After a moment, Floyd squeezed Ollie's hand and stood. He started toward the hat rack. "I bought something for you." He took the brand-new navy-blue fedora off the rack and sat back on the couch. "Here."

Slowly, Ollie reached for the hat.

"You bought this for me?" Ollie asked, his soft voice filled with wonderment.

"Yeah. I wanted to say sorry for everything—for losing my temper and for making you come back to Rock Creek by yourself."

"Oh my God." Ollie turned it around and around in his hands, running his fingers over the wool. "It's perfect."

Floyd took it and fit it atop Ollie's head.

"You look real handsome, Ollie," Floyd said with a smile. "You always do."

"Thank you."

Ollie snatched Floyd's hand and squeezed it. They sat there for a while, playing with each other's hands. Floyd wanted so badly to kiss him, to kiss this wonderfully sweet man who he cared about so much. And who cared about *him* so much, too.

But somehow, he still wasn't ready. Even though he wanted to be.

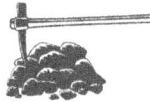

One week later, Floyd was building a little miniature log cabin on the floor with Josephine while he was waiting for Ollie to stop by. Ollie and him had been spending time together every single day after work, sometimes over at Ollie's house, where they'd hold hands and talk, sometimes over at Floyd's house, where they'd play checkers with Josephine and Effie. It was nice to see each other so much. Only problem was they hadn't kissed yet. And it was all Floyd's fault. Ollie had been real patient, too. Floyd could tell how much Ollie wanted them to kiss. Heck, Ollie probably wanted them to try other things, too.

But every time Floyd considered kissing Ollie, he'd think about Matt and then his stomach would start feeling funny—like the copperhead had come back—and he hadn't managed to push past the upset to make himself kiss the man he liked so much. Whenever Floyd let himself imagine what Ollie's lips would feel like on his own, whenever he thought about how nice it would be to pull Ollie onto his lap and be intimate with him, the snake would writhe in his stomach to torture him some more, making him feel sick.

Finally, close to Josephine's bedtime, Ollie came over. After Floyd put Josephine to bed, he and Ollie and Effie talked for a little while. At one point, Effie and Ollie took to arguing about chess strategies, which was fun to listen to, but when Floyd told them they should play, Effie protested, claiming that Floyd would pick up the rules simply by watching, which he thought was a bunch of hogwash. He'd seen her play a little here and there over the years. He still couldn't make heads or tails of it without her explaining more about the pieces and how they moved. More likely, Effie knew that chess took a while to play and wanted to make sure Floyd and Ollie had some time to themselves before it got too late. Sure enough, after only a little while longer, Effie excused herself to the bedroom.

And Ollie and Floyd were alone. Ollie tip-toed his fingers across the couch toward Floyd's waiting hand, and when their fingers laced together, Floyd hummed happily to himself. Ollie hummed back, too, and the sweet sound made Floyd's breath catch. Golly, Ollie was so sweet and so fun.

After a couple of minutes of them talking 'bout work and smiling big, silly smiles at each other, Ollie asked Floyd if he could have some coffee. While Floyd was busy in the kitchen grinding up some coffee beans Effie had roasted earlier, Ollie called to him from the couch.

"Hey, Floyd, what's this?"

When Floyd turned to face him, it was like the whole world stopped, and had it not been for the constant ticking of the nearby clock, he would have thought that maybe time itself had ceased to exist, too.

Because Ollie was holding Floyd's most treasured possession—Matt's old coin-collecting book. Floyd's throat tightened.

"Am I not supposed to see this or something?" Ollie asked, a playful edge to his voice. When Floyd only managed to stare wordlessly in response, Ollie's small smile fell away. "I'm really *not* supposed to see this, am I? Jeez, I'm sorry."

Before Floyd could tell Ollie what it even was, Ollie scrambled to set it on the coffee table, and then he folded his hands in his lap. Floyd tried to swallow.

"It was under Dog Race," Ollie said, pointing accusingly at the board game box.

Seconds ticked by.

Finally, Floyd managed a soft, "It was Matt's."

Golly, he hadn't said Matt's name in what felt like forever. Not outside the confines of his own head.

"Oh . . ." Oliver looked back at the book. "Was Matt the man who you, uhm, the man who—"

"Yeah," Floyd interrupted. "Matt Parsons. He was my . . . my best friend. He was . . . my everything."

Saying Matt's name had somehow caused the earth to start turning again, so Floyd crossed the room to sit next to Ollie.

"He collected coins," Floyd said, picking up the book. "Before . . ." He paused, the words catching in his throat. Even though Ollie knew the truth now, Floyd still couldn't manage to say it himself.

"Before he passed," Ollie finished for him, his voice filled with empathy. "Gosh, Floyd, I'm sorry for bringing him up."

"Nah, it's fine," Floyd said, forcing himself to flip open the book and face the rows of silver and bronze. "He was real proud of these."

Ollie looked on, his hands twisting in his lap.

"I can see why. Not that I know anything about coin collecting. But, you know, coins are supposed to be valuable. I think. Sorry. I'm nervous."

Floyd tried to smile. "Don't be."

"I think I've seen that one before," Ollie said, pointing, but clearly taking care not to get too close. "Is it an Indian Head penny?"

"Mm-hmm."

"Which one was Matt's favorite?"

Ollie's words rang in Floyd's ears. *Which one was Matt's favorite?* Tears sprang to his eyes, clouding his vision. He couldn't yet tell whether it made him happy or sad to hear Ollie ask about Matt so openly. He thought maybe it was both. Regaining composure, Floyd tapped the Flying Eagle penny.

"He liked this one a lot."

"Do you know much about it?"

"Not really. I think someone in Bramwell sold it to him. Some wealthy fella."

"He must have paid a bundle for it."

"Well, he might have traded something instead. Matt collected other things, too—stamps and pocket watches."

Ollie's tentative smile broadened. "It sounds like he was an interesting person."

Floyd inhaled deeply, breathing in Ollie's words. He let them expand in his chest, their warmth comforting him and calming him and settling that nervousness in his stomach.

"He was. He was a real interesting person," Floyd said, smiling back. "Like you, Ollie. You're real interesting, too."

"Well, that's . . . Floyd, that's probably the nicest compliment I've ever received." Ollie scooted closer and looked back at the book. "Which one is *your* favorite?"

Floyd had never thought about that before. He turned this over in his head for a bit before pointing to one that was so old, so faded, there was no sort of picture left anymore, only what looked to be the number 1754, but even that was sort of unclear.

"Probably that one."

Ollie's warm laughter clutched at his heart. "Why?"

"It's sort of mysterious."

"Mysterious? Floyd, it looks like trash," Ollie said, still laughing, but even more than before.

And that laughter bubbled up right inside Floyd's body, making him laugh, too.

"Yeah, a little."

"Oh God, it's a near-perfect metaphor for us, isn't it? You think I'm this mysterious and interesting person, but really, I'm trash."

Floyd snorted and shoved Ollie with his elbow. "Stop."

But that only prompted Ollie to keep poking at himself. If only Floyd could make himself stop laughing, he'd have told Ollie not to talk about himself like that.

"I'm an obscure, silver-colored, unreadable coin," Ollie continued. "I came into town looking exactly like that coin there. Don't tell me that thing belongs in the coin book. I mean, there are real fucking coins in there, coins worth money. But, you, Floyd Bennett, took one look at me and thought, 'Gee, there's something wrong with that fellow. He's clearly running away from some kind of cushy life, behaving like a pompous windbag and clamoring about the proper housing for a man of his stature, a stature which was . . . let me see . . . an unmarried, childless man, so, yes, clearly someone who deserves the best of the best, and oh Jesus, he has so many hats! Oh well. Guess I'll keep him.'"

Holy heck, Ollie was so stinkin' funny. He was witty and smart and unique and strange and so many other words, words that only Ollie would think of because Ollie knew a lot of them. And Floyd loved that about him. He loved that Ollie was different. So, yeah, maybe Ollie was a little like that silly, unreadable coin. But Floyd loved that coin. And Floyd thought that, well, maybe he was starting to love Ollie, too.

"Ollie," Floyd said, snapping the coin book shut and setting it on the coffee table. "Don't insult yourself like that. I know you're trying to be funny, and you *are* funny, but you're so many other things, too. *Wonderful* things."

Ollie let out a long breath. "Thank you, Floyd. I know I'm not supposed to say things like that anymore, but, well, I've been saying them for what feels like my whole life. It's a hard habit to break."

"I know, but you're wonderful, Ollie. You're funny and fun and kind and handsome. And I like you so much." Floyd reached up to cup Ollie's cheek. "Can I kiss you now?"

"Yeah?" Ollie said, raising both of his eyebrows in surprise. "Alright, yeah, of course."

Heart pounding, Floyd leaned in close, stopping when their noses only barely touched. He waited, silent and still, for the snake to bite him. But there was nothing. Only Ollie's soft breathing. Floyd was close enough that he could feel the little puffs of warmth with each of Ollie's exhales. He could smell the sweet smell of sweat clinging to Ollie's skin, too. Closing his eyes, Floyd waited for fear or shame or sadness. But still, there was nothing. Nothing except want. He wanted to kiss Ollie. He wanted it so much.

Slowly, Floyd nuzzled Ollie's nose, savoring every moment of this beautiful closeness. Ollie sighed sweetly and that little sound provided the nudge Floyd needed to touch their lips together.

So he did.

They kissed. And kissed. And kissed. And when their tongues brushed against one another's, Ollie sighed again, and Floyd thought that he could listen to that tiny sound forever, like it alone would fill him and keep him whole and happy and alive.

Ollie's hand found Floyd's thigh, sending little tremors of want coursing through his body, making him shudder.

"Oh God, Floyd," Ollie murmured between kisses. "I want you."

Ollie saying those words was like him igniting a blasting cap. Without a second more hesitation, Floyd let his other hand fall to Ollie's waist, and then, in a flash, he pulled Ollie onto his lap. As soon as Ollie was settled, he started to rock his hips. Feeling Ollie's hardness pressing up against him, Floyd's own cock stiffened too.

With a needy whimper, Ollie continued rolling his hips and said, "I can't tell you how many times I've thought about this."

Floyd's cock twitched, and only a few thrusts later, it was practically throbbing with need. He knew that they ought to stop. He knew they ought to wait—for real love confessions, maybe, or, heck, even only for more privacy—but he couldn't make himself stop. He couldn't make himself wait. Floyd moved backward to lie back on the couch, pulling Ollie with him. Once Ollie settled on top of him, he started rolling his hips some more, and Floyd moaned into his mouth.

Breaking their kiss, Floyd whispered, "Ollie, you made me so hard."

"Can you come like this?" Ollie whispered back, continuing to rock against him.

"Yeah. You?"

"God, yes," Ollie said, and Floyd could feel him pressing more firmly with each thrust. "I'm so close."

Floyd had to fight to contain a moan, his body burning for release. Each thrust of Ollie's hips was bringing him closer to the edge, and soon, there came that familiar tingling sensation, the one that meant he was close.

"Almost," Floyd rasped, his voice low and husky.

Ollie clutched onto Floyd's shoulders. His thrusts became harder, rougher. Feeling Ollie's strong hands pressing against him, firmly holding him in place, Floyd let out a pleased grunt. He was surprised to find that he liked the way Ollie was on top of him like this. Liked the way Ollie was in control. Gosh, it felt so right.

He'd let Ollie keep thrusting with whatever pace and intensity he wanted.

That's it, Ollie, Floyd wanted to say, but embarrassment held him back. He hadn't never been this intimate with someone before.

More and more strange comments flitted into Floyd's mind, but he couldn't make himself say none of them out loud. Still, Floyd said them in his head, enjoying the fantasy of it.

That's right, I'm yours. Show me I belong to you.

Ollie kept thrusting.

Make me finish for you.

With Ollie's next thrust, Floyd bucked his hips and came. One low, hushed moan escaped his lips.

"Jesus, Floyd," Ollie whispered, moving his hips faster.

Seconds later, Floyd felt Ollie's body shudder and cut off Ollie's accompanying moan with a kiss. They continued to kiss for a while longer, love-drunk and spent and happy. Overcome with a fierce tenderness, Floyd reached up and ran a hand through Ollie's beautiful, soft hair. Ollie smiled against his lips. And Floyd smiled too.

But their untroubled bliss was short-lived. Because finally Floyd had the sense to remember where they were. Carefully, he pushed against Ollie's shoulders, breaking them apart. They sat up.

"We can't never let that happen again," Floyd said, a little more sternly than intended, mostly upset with himself, not with Ollie. "Not here."

"You're right," Ollie said. "I'm sorry." He nuzzled Floyd's nose. "I lost myself in you."

Floyd turned these words over in his head. He liked the comfort they brought with them. He really had lost himself in Ollie. With their truth, Floyd found he could forgive himself a little.

"I lost myself in you," Floyd repeated. "I like that."

"I won't let it happen again."

Ollie's apologetic tone awakened a sympathetic sadness in Floyd's heart. Because they had both been lost in each other's touches. Ollie hadn't acted alone.

"Ain't your fault. I enjoyed myself too. I thought I was making that clear when we were in it." He kissed the tip of Ollie's nose. "We got to be respectful of my family, is all. Can't have Effie or Jo walking in on that kind of sinful behavior."

"I know." He climbed off of Floyd's lap. "I understand."

As soon as Ollie settled next to him, Floyd pulled him in for a short kiss. He couldn't hardly believe he hadn't even kissed Ollie yet a few hours ago. It felt so natural now, like they had been kissing for years.

Ollie pulled back and said, "I had so much fun, sweetheart."

Floyd's stomach fluttered in the most wonderful way.

"Sweetheart?"

"What do you think? I can alternate it with lunkhead."

"I like it."

"I know it's not exactly the most unique nickname, but you're my sweetheart, Floyd. You're the sweetest person I've ever met."

Floyd laughed a little. "You're too nice to me sometimes, Ollie. I'm sorry I ain't thought of a better nickname for you yet."

"I love the way you say 'Ollie.' It's the only nickname I need." Ollie shifted and tugged at his pants. "Yeesh, I'm not looking forward to my walk home."

"Do you want to borrow some clothes? I can sneak into the bedroom and find some."

"Nah. It's a short walk."

"Yeah, that's true."

"I should head out."

"Are you coming to church tomorrow?"

"How are you asking me about church right now? Did you forget about the fact that we finished fucking each other? Or, kind of fucking."

"Well, I'll be there. Even though we . . . effed each other through our clothes."

Ollie laughed. "Jeez, that's adorable. One day, though, sweetheart, I will coax some very naughty words out of you."

"You can try."

"I will." Ollie smiled wolfishly. "I can't wait."

Blood rushed to Floyd's cheeks. He couldn't wait neither.

CHAPTER TEN

OLIVER

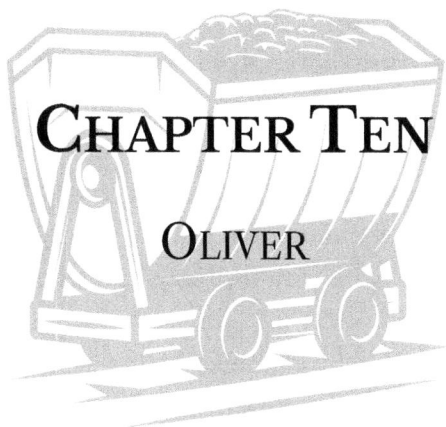

ON A THURSDAY, OLIVER was working with Floyd in the mines, looking on while Floyd poured the black powder into a paper casing. Even though Oliver was trying his best not to focus on the fact that Floyd had yet to let him help with the explosives, he wasn't able to keep himself from constantly wondering why that was. Floyd had yet to let Oliver take on any *real* responsibility in the mine. Oliver had been Floyd's butty for weeks, and *still* Floyd continued to insist on being the only one to prepare the explosives. Hell, Oliver had even suffered some trouble convincing Floyd to let him shimmy into tight spaces from time to time with his pickaxe. Luckily, Oliver had been able to reason with him on that front. Oliver liked to be the one to carve the "V" into the coal wall underneath where they'd be blasting. And *still* Floyd had pushed back a few times. God, Floyd was so stubborn. All Oliver wanted was to feel like they were equal partners.

Later, when the two of them were shoveling coal, Oliver thought he'd try to push the subject. Gently.

"So, uhm, how long had you been working in the mine before you felt, you know, competent?"

"Can't remember."

"Well, was it long before you felt like you were a real miner?"

Floyd scooped up a shovelful of coal and tossed it into the coal car. "Breaker boys are miners."

"Yes, that's true." Oliver paused shoveling to catch his breath, equal parts nervousness and manual labor taking the wind out of him. "But I mean, you moved up to excavating, eventually. Who taught you how to work with the black powder and the clay and everything?"

"Matt's father. See, I had known Matt's whole family for forever and so, his father was happy to show me."

"Oh. Interesting."

"Matt was working with one of his brothers," Floyd said next, as though he had anticipated Oliver's next question. "But once we'd both learned enough, we paired up."

"Ah," Oliver said, suddenly feeling as though his organs were being smushed together, envy bursting to life inside him and taking up too much room in his chest. Still, he tried to keep his voice even so as not to let it show. "Matt was your butty."

Floyd tossed some coal into the car. "Yup."

"You were partners."

"Uh-huh."

"Equals."

All of a sudden, Floyd stopped shoveling, and then he planted his shovel in the coal pile and leaned against it, looking up at Oliver like he was completely exasperated by this nonsense.

"Ollie, what are you trying to say?"

"Nothing," Oliver sputtered. "Sorry. Not important."

So Matt had been Floyd's partner. His *butty*.

Jealousy continued to twist his organs together, but Oliver tried his best to ignore it. Once Floyd and Oliver were finished with lunch, they were assigned to work somewhere else, in a section

of the mine that the miners liked to call Timber Alley because
of the sheer number of pieces of timber that had been placed to
help prop up the ceiling. Many of those logs had already begun to
bend and crack, too. Consequently, a few miners had recently been
instructed to install new pillars with the intention of extending the
life of this particular section of the mine, but it was evident even
to Oliver that the company would have to leave it soon enough.

"Just wait out here for a while," Floyd told Oliver at the entrance. "I'll collect as much as I can over the next hour or so my
own self. Why, I ought to march over to James Donohue's house
right now and tell him that his father is plum crazy to keep asking
folks to work over here, but we might as well try to make a little
money before complaining. It'll hold for a while yet."

"I'm not standing here twiddling my thumbs while you exert
yourself in there."

"Ollie, it ain't safe enough for you."

"But it's safe enough for you?"

"I been a miner for near twenty years. You, on the other hand,
are still learning."

"I know how to shovel coal."

"No," Floyd responded firmly. "I ain't arguing with you about
this neither."

"Fuck, Floyd, first you won't let me handle the powder, and
now you won't even let me work next to you? Do you even want
me around?"

"What? Of course I want you around."

"You're treating me like a child."

"No, I ain't."

"Yes, you are. I've seen fifteen-year-olds with more responsibility than me."

Even in the relatively poor lighting, Oliver could sense that
Floyd was upset. Through the tense silence, Oliver heard Floyd

let out a long breath through his nose. Still, Floyd had yet to respond to what Oliver had said. Christ, that man was so stubborn sometimes.

"No wonder you like working here. You're even more stubborn than the mules," Oliver said, half-expecting Floyd to be upset with him for the insult.

But Floyd cracked a smile and said, "Yeah, I suppose you ain't wrong about that. Though right now, it seems like you're trying to compete with me on stubbornness. Look, I won't let you work in there, and if you won't let me work in there neither, then I reckon we ought to head over to James's house to complain."

"What about the money?"

"Guess I'll have to be more careful at the store this week since our paycheck won't be as big."

"Well, you *could* borrow from next week's paycheck."

"I told you, that's how you end up in a hole you can't claw your way out of."

"Can I buy some of the things your family needs this week, then?"

Floyd rubbed his chin, thinking it over, and the fact that Floyd was even hesitant made Oliver scoff.

"Please?"

"Yeah, I suppose. We're running short on corn and peas and such. Shouldn't cost too much. I'll return what I owe."

"Don't be like that."

"Be like what?"

"Don't pay me back." Oliver leaned in close and whispered, "Let me treat you a little."

Floyd whispered back, "You want to treat me to some canned vegetables?"

"Only the best for you, sweetheart," Oliver teased.

Floyd snorted. "Fine, Ollie, you win."

So, the two packed up their tools and left the mine. First, they stopped at the company store. Oliver bought Floyd a whole two brown bags' worth of food, not only canned vegetables, but beans and fresh fruit and a loaf of bread, too. He could tell that Floyd was a little unnerved by it. Floyd still had trouble accepting Oliver's help. Or "charity" as he liked to call it. Oliver tried not to let Floyd's reaction upset him, but he had to wonder if Floyd would have let Matt purchase a couple of cans of lima beans without making a whole to-do about it.

After Oliver and Floyd stopped at Floyd's house to drop off the food, the two of them started walking to James Donohue's. Perturbed by the lingering tension between them, Oliver intentionally bumped Floyd with his shoulder.

"What was that for?" Floyd asked.

"If you keep stewing about me purchasing three dollars' worth of food for you and your family, I'm afraid I'll be forced to beat the upset right out of you."

"Uh-huh, sure you will." Floyd rolled his eyes in that adorable way of his. "You're a fair bit smaller than me."

"Yeah, but I'm scrappier." Oliver held up his fists and grinned. "I'm from New York."

"You're too sweet to be scrappy. Besides, remember what happened with our so-called boxing match?"

Now Oliver had to roll his eyes. "First, I'm not trying to look sweet. I'm trying to look threatening. Second, I was zozzled. I can be plenty threatening when I need to be."

Oliver moved his fists in a little circle, but Floyd only laughed.

"Real scary, city boy."

Playfully irate, Oliver thumped Floyd's biceps. Even though he'd put some muscle behind the blow, Floyd's only reaction was to cock one of his eyebrows, which was stupidly adorable, but also a little maddening.

"Come on, that must have hurt a little."

Floyd held up his thumb and index finger millimeters apart. Oliver let out a puff of air.

"That is very offensive."

Without warning, Floyd took hold of Oliver's sleeve and pulled him close, the force of the movement making him stumble.

"You show me how scrappy you are later," Floyd whispered, the timbre of his voice causing the hair on Oliver's neck to stand on-end.

"You lunkhead," Oliver whispered back, wrestling his shirt out of Floyd's hand. "Now I'll be walking around with a half-hard piece in my pants."

In response, Floyd flashed a wolfish smile.

"Jesus, stop that," Oliver said with a warning look.

Oliver expected Floyd to relent, but instead, he said, "Maybe we ought to visit your place first."

"Can we really?"

Floyd made that incredible half-hum, half-growl sound he made sometimes when he was aroused. "Don't see why not."

Holy hell. Suddenly, all Oliver wanted was to feel Floyd's hard cock rocking against him. Every one of Floyd's touches had become a confirmation of their ever-strengthening bond.

Oliver took off, walking with long, purposeful strides, while Floyd trailed behind.

"Hurry up!" Oliver called over his shoulder.

With a chuckle, Floyd picked up the pace.

After only a few minutes, they were inside Oliver's house, and as soon as Floyd shut the door, Oliver shoved him up against the wood and pressed their lips together. Soon, Floyd's hands were unbuttoning Oliver's shirt and Oliver's hands were unbuttoning Floyd's, and holy hell, it was wonderful. Both of their work shirts fell to the floor, and when Oliver's head started to swim from seeing Floyd's broad, beautiful chest, the hair of which was only barely visible through the thin cotton of his sleeveless union suit, Floyd hoisted Oliver up into the air to carry him into the bedroom.

"God, sweetheart, you're so strong," Oliver breathed, wrapping his legs around Floyd's torso. "I love it."

Floyd's reply was to capture Oliver's mouth in another kiss. Their frenzied, hungry kisses continued on the way to the bedroom, only ceasing for a moment as they crashed onto the bed. Lying beside one another, they both worked to remove each other's pants, and then they were in the last bits of clothing. For Oliver, that meant his custom-made silky drawers, and for Floyd, it was his sleeveless union suit. Oliver's hands found the top buttons on Floyd's undergarment.

"Do you want to?" Oliver asked, tugging on one.

Even though Oliver had plenty of fun fucking Floyd through his own silk underwear, he still craved so much more. He wanted to see what Floyd's cock looked like, to feel him, to *taste* him.

"Not yet," Floyd said, pulling Oliver on top of him. "Soon."

Floyd wasn't ready. *Of course* he wasn't ready. Self-doubt wrapped around Oliver's nearly naked body, making him feel as though his skin was on fire. Aware of the mortifying blush that had probably come to color his face, Oliver lowered himself to nuzzle Floyd's cheek, hoping to hide the embarrassing evidence of his shame. But Floyd must have sensed it.

"Ollie." Floyd caught Oliver's chin and tried to force Oliver to look at him. "Soon."

"No, I know," Oliver said, still not able to meet Floyd's gaze. "I know."

"Look at me," Floyd said, his tone tender but stern. Oliver's face was still burning as he forced his stupidly teary eyes to look at Floyd's. "I want you."

"I know."

Somehow, fourteen years of schooling had resulted in Oliver only being able to say two fucking words. Shame twisted inside of him. Why was he so upset—so *tore up*, as Floyd would say—about this? He knew Floyd cared for him. But God, Oliver couldn't rid himself of the feeling that Floyd was still holding part of himself—part of his *heart*—back.

"I want you," Floyd repeated, the urgency in his voice nearly enough to coax Oliver out of this pathetic spiral of self-reproach until Oliver's eyes found the still-fastened buttons of Floyd's union suit and insecurity started clawing at him again. Floyd continued to try. "I want to feel you rub up on me, to make me come for you."

"I know," Oliver said, cringing. Floyd's broken phonograph would have been a better conversationalist.

"Let me see your hand," Floyd said. Oliver held it up, and Floyd took it, bringing it low and pressing it to his erection. "Do you feel that? Do you feel how bad I want you?"

All of a sudden, Oliver's stomach was no longer twisting unpleasantly, but somersaulting in an exciting sort of way, his yearning for sexual contact finally overtaking his sense of shame. Even though Oliver wanted to stay upset and wallow in his inadequacy, Floyd continued to move his hand, stoking the fire of yearning.

"I like you so much, Ollie. I'm so hard for you."

Oliver's cock began to throb, but still, he had trouble forming a response, unable to stand to repeat the only two Goddamn words he had been capable of saying before.

Seconds passed until finally Floyd paused and asked, "Do you still want this right now?"

God, the way Floyd's voice was thick with sadness, it nearly broke Oliver's heart. Thankfully, the heaviness of Floyd's sadness managed to shatter Oliver's verbal blockage along with it.

"Of course I want this," Oliver said. "Just, well, I'm embarrassed."

"About what?"

"About how much I want this. About how much I want *you*."

"Are you worried you want me more than I want you?"

"Yes," Oliver said, shame warming his cheeks once more. "It's silly, I know."

"It ain't silly," Floyd said, moving Oliver's hand up and down. "That's for you, Ollie. *Only* for you. I barely even touched myself for *years* before I met you. I want you *just* as bad as you want me. I promise."

"Really?"

"I wouldn't lie to you about that. Having you . . . eff me through those nice silky drawers of yours is real exciting to me." Floyd smiled up at him. "I like you a lot, Ollie. I want to take our time with these kinds of things, is all."

Oliver tried to let Floyd's words sink in. Over and over, he repeated them to himself, chiseling them into his mind, hoping to sanctify them, to etch them onto a stone tablet, for Floyd's words seemed more precious, more important than even the word of God.

"Are you feeling better now?" Floyd asked.

"Yes. Thank you," Oliver said. "Sweetheart, there are so many things I want to try with you someday."

Floyd hummed appreciatively. "Can I hear some of them fantasies?"

"Of course," Oliver said, nuzzling Floyd's nose. "I want to lick you. No, better, I want to *devour* you. I want to make you finish with my mouth, to consume every drop." Oliver started peppering kisses along Floyd's cheek and jaw. "Do you ever think about that? About me using my mouth on you?"

"Mm-hmm." Kissing Floyd's neck, Oliver could feel him swallow. "When I touch myself, I imagine you making me come like that. I want to make you come like that, too."

Oliver's half-hard cock began to stiffen again. He shifted his weight and rocked his hips.

"I want to fuck you, Floyd. God, I want to fuck you so bad."

"I want that, too."

"Yeah? You wouldn't rather be inside of me instead?"

"No," Floyd said with a certainty that sent shivers up Oliver's spine. "I want you to take me, to show me I'm yours. I want you to *make me* yours."

"Jesus Christ, sweetheart," Oliver said, moving his hips. "I will."

He moved faster, pressing his erection against Floyd's thigh with each thrust, the sensation momentarily making his breath catch in his throat. Imagining what it would be like to feel Floyd's muscles clenching around his cock, Oliver clutched tight to Floyd's shoulder, steadying himself so that he could thrust harder, and in doing so inadvertently sunk his fingernails into Floyd's skin, his mistake then making Floyd suck in a breath through his teeth.

"Sorry," Oliver said, only then realizing that by focusing so much on massaging his own cock against Floyd's thigh, he had been neglecting to focus on Floyd at all. "Do you want me to shift my position?"

"Nah, I want to watch you finish yourself."

"I want you to come, too."

"We'll worry about me later. You take what you need, Ollie."

Floyd's words brought with them a tremor of pleasure, one that caused Oliver's body to shake. *You take what you need, Ollie.* Oliver couldn't remember the last time someone had shown him such tender care. Despite its vulgarity, that statement was one of the most beautiful that Oliver had ever heard in his life. It was so selfless, so raw, so sweet, leaving Oliver wondering how he could have ever doubted Floyd's feelings for him.

"Fuck, Floyd, you really are a sweetheart," Oliver rasped, still thrusting.

Floyd reached up to thread his fingers through Oliver's hair, and the soft benevolence of Floyd's touch coaxed an impassioned moan from Oliver's lips. He rocked his hips harder, faster, rougher, taking exactly what he needed, what he *wanted*, and finally climaxed.

Still panting, Oliver lifted himself up to kiss Floyd on the lips.

"Now you, sweetheart," Oliver said in between kisses. "I need to take care of you."

Once again, Floyd took one of Oliver's hands and moved it over his cock. Oliver could feel a little spot of wetness that had soaked through the cotton fabric. It had his stomach flip-flopping, renewed desire percolating low in his belly. Had his cock been willing to cooperate, Oliver would have happily *effed* Floyd's thigh to completion once more. Jesus, only Floyd could manage to make himself even more irresistible by leaking pre-ejaculate onto his undergarments.

Running his hand up the length of Floyd's shaft, Oliver yearned to wrap his hand around it. God, he wanted to see Floyd's naked member, to feel the softness of his skin. Losing himself to the fantasy, Oliver started moving his hand faster and was rewarded with the most tantalizing moan. Dipping lower, Oliver kissed Floyd's chest and continued to move his hand.

Oliver asked, "How's this?"

Floyd answered by pushing Oliver's hand away. For a moment, Oliver thought that Floyd was rejecting him, but then Floyd began unfastening the buttons of his union suit, the ones closest to his erection, clearly rushing to free himself. After unfastening three buttons, Floyd snatched Oliver's hand and slipped it inside.

"Will you touch me?" Floyd asked, closing Oliver's hand around his cock.

Oliver's breath caught. "Yeah."

Floyd must have already been teetering on the precipice because Oliver only needed to stroke him for twenty or thirty seconds before—

"Oh, fuck, Ollie," Floyd moaned.

And Oliver was so Goddamn taken aback from hearing Floyd utter the F-word that it took him an extra second to register the sensation of the warm liquid spilling over his fist.

Once Floyd's cock ceased to pulse, the two looked at one another, and it seemed that they were both temporarily stunned. Oliver's wet hand was still resting on Floyd's flaccid cock. He couldn't bring himself to remove it. What if Floyd never let him touch it again? He had been so hesitant for them to be physically intimate like this before.

After another few seconds, Oliver cleared his throat.

"So . . ." Oliver tried to think of what he should say. "I'm fairly positive I heard you say the word 'fuck.'"

Floyd made a sound in between a laugh and groan. "Yeah, I know."

"What was that about?"

"Guess I lost myself in you."

"Will that be your excuse for everything now?" Oliver teased. "What about you shoving my hand inside those undergarments of yours?"

"I needed your touch, Ollie. I couldn't finish otherwise. I . . ." Floyd flung one of his arms over his face, covering his eyes with the crook of his elbow, as though he needed to hide from whatever it was that he wanted to say next. "I touched myself twice before work this morning."

"*Twice?!*" Oliver sputtered a laugh, excited to tease Floyd about this. "Jesus, Floyd, you're a family man. How did you have the time?"

"I woke up at four."

"On purpose?!"

Floyd uncovered his face and laughed. "Shut up."

"Oh my God!" Oliver exclaimed. "Did you really just tell me to shut up? First, you're spewing expletives and now this?! I am thoroughly and completely appalled, Floyd Bennett."

"I'd whack you, but your hand is on my cock."

"Yeah, I'm too scared to remove it."

"Why?"

"Well, what if you never let me touch you again?"

"Of course I'll let you touch me again."

"Promise?"

"What if I say no? You want to keep it there forever?"

"Probably."

"What about work?"

"I'll tell everyone I've been promoted," Oliver said, barely able to keep a straight face to say the next part, "from butty to front-y."

He had burst out laughing by the end of it. And then Floyd was laughing, too. God, he felt so incredibly lucky.

Finally, Oliver had the confidence to remove his sticky hand.

"Let's wash up," he said.

So, Oliver and Floyd took turns washing themselves with water from the basin out of view from one another, though Oliver wished that the two of them were washing each other instead. He loved the idea of the two of them tending to each other like that, cleaning the coal powder off each other's skin and being vulnerable in a new and unexpected way. He wondered if they would ever make it that far.

When they were finished, Floyd needed to borrow a pair of Oliver's silk drawers. Oliver thought he might inquire as to whether Effie had noticed that Floyd had accumulated a few of them by now.

"Has Effie said anything about your—sorry, *my*—drawers?"

Floyd let out a puff of air. "Yup. Effie ain't shy about these kinds of things."

"What do you tell her?"

"I tell her that we're having fun. I'd never tell her the specifics, but she knows we're together. She knows how much I like you. And, well, she sees these fancy silky pants of yours, so I'm sure she knows what's happening. Don't worry, she's fine with it."

Oliver came closer and placed his hands on Floyd's waist, and then Floyd planted a soft kiss on Oliver's lips, one with so much love and sincerity that even once Floyd pulled away, Oliver could still feel its affection blooming there.

After they both put on their boots, they started walking together to James Donohue's house, and within a half mile or so, Oliver started thinking about work again, about how Floyd was still hesitant to let Oliver take on the tasks he should have been responsible for by now. Halfway there, Oliver began wondering whether Floyd had ever treated Matt this way.

"Floyd," Oliver began, "Did Matt ever work with the black powder?"

"Of course."

Of. Course.

All of a sudden, there was a sinking feeling in Oliver's chest. Fuck, his fast-beating heart seemed to have plummeted all the way into the pit of his stomach, leading him to wonder how the hell it was even still working. Shouldn't it have been obliterated by his stomach acid?

Through his pain, Oliver sputtered, "So, you two split the work pretty evenly, then."

"Yeah, I suppose," Floyd said before tilting his head slightly. "Why're you asking these things?"

Oliver stayed silent, embarrassed that he was still so Goddamn insecure.

"What is it?" Floyd asked, his voice tense with worry. "Are you feeling torn up about Matt or something?"

Oliver managed a nod, though he hated himself for it.

"Ah, Ollie, I'm sorry."

"It's . . . fine."

"Don't be upset 'bout Matt."

"But he was your *butty*," Oliver said, the words coming out with more venom than he had intended. "Sorry, I—"

"Yeah. He was," Floyd confirmed, his tone now low and soft and filled with so much sorrow. "We won't talk about him no more. How's that?"

Oliver wasn't sure that he wanted Floyd to stop talking about Matt, but . . .

God, he was still struggling to believe Floyd was here to stay.

Before Oliver could protest, Floyd continued, "And, Ollie, I only keep the harder tasks from you for now because they're . . . well, because they're hard. I want to keep you safe. I care about you."

Floyd's beautiful words brought tears to Oliver's eyes. Quickly, he blinked them back and then, very softly, he said, "Thank you, sweetheart."

In a measured and sincere tone, Floyd said, "I'll learn you everything one day, Ollie. I promise."

"I know. I believe you."

Or well, he wanted to.

CHAPTER ELEVEN

FLOYD

FEET PLANTED AT THE edge of the stream, Floyd cast his fishing line into the water while Ollie knelt nearby, scowling at the can of worms. Squinting from the hot late-summer sun, Floyd looked over his shoulder with the intention of teasing Ollie somehow, only to be knocked with a whole heap of fondness instead. Using the heel of his boot, he made a little cavity in the mud and stuck the butt end of his fishing pole in it, not particularly concerned about catching a bite already, and walked over to Ollie.

"Are you upset about the worms?" Floyd asked, crouching.

"Not upset, exactly, though I feel a bit bad." Ollie made a face. "How am I supposed to just *stab* one of them? It seems cruel."

"What about the fish?"

"Well, I feel sad for the fish, too, but I like eating fish, so it sort of makes it easier to stomach for some reason."

"Don't you need the worm to *catch* the fish?"

Ollie sighed. "Yes."

"Well, then, why's it worse?"

"It's not, really, but . . ." Wearing an apologetic smile, Ollie held out the hook to Floyd. "Will you help? Please?"

With an affectionate roll of his eyes, Floyd took the hook in his hands.

"Give me a worm," he said.

"Oh, uhm, no, see, that's part of the reason why I couldn't do this myself. I can't be the one to choose which one meets his end."

"Oh, Ollie," Floyd said, cracking a smile. He took a worm from the can. "You're too sweet sometimes."

As Floyd pierced the worm, he couldn't help but notice Ollie's face out of the corner of his eye—nose wrinkled, eyes squeezed shut, lips tight—and it really was about the most endearing thing he had seen in weeks, though every other contender was Ollie, too, just other versions of him.

"Here you go," Floyd said, handing Ollie the pole.

"Thank you, sweetheart."

"Am I still a sweetheart even though I stabbed that poor worm?"

Ollie pursed his lips, thinking. "Yes. Somehow. It's complicated."

Once Floyd had picked up his pole, Ollie tried to cast his line. He succeeded. Kind of. It had barely made it beyond the edge of the water.

"If there are any fish stupid enough to swim right up to the shore here, they'll be in for a surprise," Ollie remarked.

Floyd liked that Ollie could tease himself, but sometimes, he wished Ollie would compliment himself more, too.

"For a first cast, that was pretty decent."

"Yeah?" Ollie perked up a little. "Guess I'm a natural, then."

Gosh, now *he* couldn't resist a tease, either. "Yeah, as soon as you learn how to touch a worm, you'll be the second-best fisherman for miles."

"Hmmm . . . we're miles away from civilization, aren't we?"

"Just about."

"Wow, so I'm not currently second best even though there are only two of us out here, huh?"

"Nah, I think the worm has you beat. He's working *way* harder than you are."

"Floyd!" Ollie scolded through a laugh. "Don't make me feel even worse for him!"

Now Floyd was laughing, too. "Sorry." He came closer to Ollie and bumped him with his elbow. "I was only trying to be funny, by the way. I hope you know I think the world of you."

"Yeah," Ollie said, beaming up at him. "I know."

For the next half hour, the two of them relaxed near the stream's edge, sometimes sitting, sometimes standing, listening to the burbling water and the intermittent croaks of bullfrogs.

Eventually, Ollie started talking about the kinds of activities he had enjoyed back in Cleveland and New York. Other than reading, Ollie liked playing instruments, mostly piano, like he had told Floyd before, but cello, too. Floyd liked to listen to him talk about music. He wished the two of them could play together someday. Ollie was probably a talented piano player, especially since it sounded like he had practiced so often for so long. It'd be nice to play music with someone. Matt had never been interested in all that.

As soon as the thought entered Floyd's head, it felt like a battering ram had struck him in the chest. He couldn't believe he had thought such a terrible thing. It was like he was saying that Ollie was better than Matt, but Ollie wasn't better. He wasn't worse neither. Ollie was Ollie. Matt was Matt. Comparing them wouldn't lead nowhere.

A faint roar of thunder rumbled overhead, rolling in from miles away. Floyd looked up to see some clouds coming in. Even though it would probably be a while before the storm arrived, it was a nicely timed excuse for heading back. After having caught himself comparing Matt and Ollie, Floyd wasn't really in the mood for fishing no more.

"Hey, Ollie, I reckon we ought to head back," he said, pointing up at the sky. "Storm clouds are a-coming."

Ollie frowned. "Neither of us caught anything."

"Oh well. I was plenty excited for beans and cornbread," Floyd said. "I like fish, but mostly, I like being out here, listening to the water."

"Well, I mucked that up, too, by rambling about my music lessons."

"I liked listening to you talk about all that," Floyd said, setting his pole by his feet so that he could pull Ollie close. "I hope I can hear you play sometime."

"Maybe I'll look into buying myself a piano, then."

Floyd kissed Ollie softly on the lips. "I could put some money toward it. Just need me some time to save up."

Ollie nuzzled Floyd's nose. "See? You're a total sweetheart. Even though you murdered a poor worm for no reason."

"Not *no* reason."

"Did we catch any fish?" Ollie asked, and Floyd leveled a look. "See? No reason."

"Come on, silly," Floyd said. "Let's head back."

Floyd ripped his dead worm off the hook and tossed it into the stream. While the water was still rippling from the tiny splash, Floyd turned to see Ollie carefully removing his own worm from the hook.

"I'm sorry, buddy," Ollie said to the worm. "We tried."

Watching Ollie gingerly set the worm atop the nearby patch of bluestem grass, Floyd's breathing turned shallow, the sudden heaviness in his chest preventing him from more. He had to close his eyes for a few seconds, to muster the strength to lift the weight of tenderness that had settled upon his shoulders. Ollie's niceness was still too heavy for him sometimes.

"Alright, ready," Ollie said, pushing to stand, his brow creasing the moment their eyes locked. "What's wrong?"

"Nothing," Floyd said softly, wiping his hand on the side of his pants and lifting it to cup Ollie's chin. "You're real special, Ollie. I hope you know that."

"Oh. I, uhm, thank you, sweetheart," Ollie said, stumbling over his words.

Floyd kissed him, putting more passion behind it this time, and Ollie smiled through it. After they parted, they started the long walk back to town.

Floyd's head was still swimming when they reached his house. Even throughout supper, Floyd's thoughts stayed far away, like he had left his brain back at the burbling stream. He couldn't seem to stop thinking about how kind Ollie was and how much he liked him.

After everyone finished eating, Ollie volunteered to clean up. Josephine was eager to help him. She was really liking spending time with Mister Oliver lately, even when that time was spent helping Effie clean the kitchen. Floyd wandered over to his favorite armchair and sat, his mind too muddy to remember that he ought to have volunteered to help too.

Once Ollie and Jo were settled with the water that they brought in from outside, Effie came over and sat on the armrest.

"Where's your head today? Did you lose it in the woods somewhere?" she asked.

"Yeah, maybe."

"What's wrong?"

"Ollie was nice to a worm."

Effie hummed and nodded. "I can see how that would be hard."

"Hush," Floyd said, pinching her leg, which elicited a little "eep" sound. "I like him a lot, Effie. I never thought I'd ever like someone this much."

"Is it scary?"

"No, not scary, really. It's . . . heavy, though. It feels heavy."

Effie squeezed his shoulder.

"Now I feel bad for what I wanted to come over here and tell you."

Floyd cocked an eyebrow. "What?"

"Before you two left on your fishing outing, Oliver mentioned how much he wished he could spend the night with you. I took the whole afternoon to think about it, and I wanted to tell you that it'd be fine with me."

"Are you sure?"

"Yeah, I'm sure. I can't imagine how hard it must be for him for you to sleep here every single night." Effie smiled warmly. "So, what do you think?"

Floyd rubbed his chin. He really liked the idea of waking up next to Ollie. Even though Floyd still felt a sickly sort of sadness about Matt sometimes, he still loved plum-near every second he and Ollie spent together. How could he say no to letting them be close for the night?

"Yeah, I'd really like that, Effie. Thank you."

"Of course."

Suddenly, there was a big splash of water followed by Ollie saying "whoa!" and Jo cackling in a mischievous sort of way. That was the end of their conversation, Floyd supposed. Effie and Floyd both started toward the kitchen area to help with the mess.

Later, once everything was cleaned up, Ollie and Floyd left together to head to Ollie's house. Midway there, the sky finally opened up, pouring buckets of rain over them. They had to run the rest of the way. Ollie was cackling the entire time, which made

Floyd burst out laughing, too. By the time they reached Ollie's house, they were both soaking wet. Luckily, it seemed that the rain had washed away some of Floyd's earlier unease about Matt. Standing inside Ollie's living space, dripping water all over the floorboards, he wasn't nothing but happy.

"Look at you, Ollie," Floyd said, placing his hands on Ollie's hips. He loved seeing Ollie's hair soaking wet, raindrops trickling down his face. "You're so handsome like this."

"You are, too," Ollie responded, smiling up at him with so much contentment, Floyd couldn't hold back from lifting him up in the air.

Ollie wrapped his legs around him, and everything was as it ought to be.

"I'm taking you to the bedroom," Floyd said, a playful hitch in his voice.

Ollie caught his mouth in a kiss.

Once they had both stripped down to their last layers of clothing, which posed a challenge since they were both soaking wet, Floyd hopped onto the bed and pulled Ollie on top of him, wetting the sheets, too. As soon as he raked a hand through Ollie's still-wet hair, his cock started to stiffen, and it wasn't long before they were lost in their pleasure, with Ollie thrusting his hips on top of him. Floyd liked seeing Ollie take what he wanted, pleasure-wise. Not that Ollie was selfish in that way, but it sparked a unique kind of passion inside of him to see Ollie be so confident and comfortable. Floyd had the thought that Ollie was probably hungry—hungry for love and acceptance and all the rest of the things it seemed he had never received—and if Ollie needed to focus on himself and his pleasure, Floyd was plenty fine with it. Ollie could take whatever he needed from him.

Typically, this meant that Ollie came first, and then Floyd either pleasured himself or, more often, Ollie touched him and helped him come, too. Floyd could sense that Ollie still wanted more. But Floyd couldn't make himself ready for more just yet.

When they were both spent, Floyd wrapped Ollie up in his arms and let Ollie rest his head on his chest.

"Thank you for helping me earlier," Ollie said, his voice soft. "It was nice of you to kill the worm so I wouldn't have to."

"Yeah, I'm a real nice worm killer, huh?"

Ollie poked his side. "Shhh . . ."

Floyd poked him back, which made Ollie squirm. He seemed not to appreciate that too much, which made Floyd start to poke him some more to be funny.

"Stop, stop, sweetheart," Ollie choked out as Floyd continued poking. "Please."

Floyd stopped, though he had to resist the urge for one more poke.

"Really, I wanted to make sure you knew that I appreciate all the ways you care for me," Ollie said.

Floyd smoothed back Ollie's hair and kissed his forehead.

"I been thinking 'bout something," Floyd said, and Ollie looked up at him. "I remember you said that you left New York for silly reasons, but you never told me more than that. What were them silly reasons? I bet you I wouldn't even think they were silly."

"Just that my family wasn't very nice to me. Not that they were especially rough with me or anything, but they weren't very loving. I think they thought I was a nuisance. I'm sure I was in some ways. I'm fairly certain that they only put up with me because they couldn't have other children and, well, they wanted someone to take over for my father eventually, so . . ." Ollie shrugged. "So, they kept me alive and educated me and made sure I knew how to look presentable. But they never really cared for me, sweetheart. Ugh, it sounds so childish to me now."

"No, I think I understand."

"I feel silly because . . . because I left home and cut these people out of my life for not loving me the way I wanted to be loved, which . . ." Ollie climbed up to settle on Floyd's chest. "Which sounds so pathetic. You and Effie have *real* stories with *real* hardships. Both of you had real reasons for leaving your old lives behind. Big, important, impactful, meaningful reasons. Mine seem so . . . small."

Floyd hugged Ollie closer as sadness clutched at his heart. It hurt to hear Ollie talking about his pain that way, making it smaller. Because it seemed like Ollie wasn't hurt in one big way, but in a lot of little ways. Even though paper cuts were small, cuts like those could still hurt plenty, especially if a person had a whole bunch of them. He hoped he could make Ollie see it that way.

Floyd kissed Ollie's head and said, "Remember when you were a breaker boy for a little while?"

"How could I forget?"

"Well, remember how you had a whole ton of cuts from the slate and the rocks and such?"

"Yeah?"

"I reckon your life has kind of been like that. Even if you weren't never hurt in one big way, like someone crushing your foot with a whole heap of coal, it sounds like you were hurt in a lot of little ways, like when the pieces of sharp slate leave a bunch of little nicks in your skin. I can imagine how having enough of those kinds of cuts could hurt you so bad that it'd make you feel like you need to leave that life behind." Floyd caressed Ollie's back with his fingertips. "Ain't nothing wrong with wanting to stop the hurt, Ollie."

Ollie was silent for a moment, and Floyd started to feel worried that he might not have liked that comparison so much, but then Ollie looked up at him with tears in his eyes. For a few seconds, Floyd lay there waiting for those little pieces of sadness to tumble down his cheeks, but they stayed right where they were. Floyd felt a little tug on his heart, thinking that maybe Ollie still wanted to keep some of that pain inside.

But then Ollie said, "Thank you, sweetheart," and the tears started to fall.

With a feather-light touch, Floyd wiped them away with his thumb, happy that he could take care of Ollie like this.

"You're a real wonderful person, Ollie. I wish your parents had seen that."

In response, Ollie pushed himself up on his elbow and captured Floyd's mouth in another kiss, one that somehow had a lot of softness behind it, while still overflowing with urgency. Hooking a hand behind Ollie's head, Floyd tried his best to match that liveliness, and the two of them kissed for a long, long time.

Later, when Ollie had fallen asleep, Floyd was still holding him close, thinking 'bout how perfect it was that the two of them were spending the whole night together. Burying his nose in Ollie's hair, Floyd breathed in his scent and thought back to the way they had been physically close for hours and hours. Never before had Floyd ever kissed someone so long and so passionately. Not even Matt.

As soon as that troubling thought entered in Floyd's head, the copperhead came back, writhing and twisting in his stomach, and Floyd had to squeeze his eyes closed to try to shut out the pain.

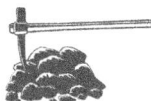

It was a hot, balmy Saturday toward the end of August, and Floyd was helping Effie clean up from their late lunch. Soon, Ollie would be coming over, not to play checkers or to listen to some of Floyd's banjo playing, but to come with Floyd and his family to James Donohue's house, where there was to be a special summer event. Floyd was real excited for it. James said they'd have ice cream and a magician and a puppet show and all sorts of family-friendly things. Floyd suspected there'd be dancing, too. While Floyd had never taken to it, Effie loved moving her feet to some fast music, especially with her friends from church. Floyd hoped he could see Ollie dance, too, even if it was with Effie and not with him. Ollie seemed like the type, what with that constant energy of his.

While Floyd was putting the ceramic bowls back in the cupboard, he started chuckling to himself as he thought about Ollie's seemingly endless energy. It wasn't only that Ollie liked to talk nonstop, but *phew*, he had a lot of energy in the bedroom, too. Seemed like Ollie kept Floyd up late near every chance he had. And then, many times, Ollie'd wake up early wanting even more.

It wasn't that Floyd minded. Not at all. He liked their closeness. Over the last weeks, Floyd and Ollie had been spending the night at Ollie's place more often than not. Effie, the angel that she was, never seemed to mind, though Josephine seemed a bit jealous sometimes. She seemed to be wondering what Ollie's house had that was so special. Floyd supposed they'd have to tell her something real about it all, eventually. But not yet.

As Floyd put the silverware back in its place, he couldn't help but feel a twinge of upset. It was hard to think about the intimacy he and Ollie shared sometimes. It seemed that the closer Floyd felt to Ollie, the farther he felt from Matt. Floyd knew he ought not to have felt that way. Matt wasn't there no more. It wasn't like Floyd was betraying him or nothing. So why was he feeling so bad about Ollie touching him in that way? It wasn't that he always felt bad about it, either. Only sometimes. Only when he realized that he hadn't thought about Matt in a while. Or when he let himself think about the fact that what he and Ollie were doing together, he and Matt hadn't never done together. It made him feel like he was leaving Matt behind. Like Matt hadn't been special. But Matt had been special. He still *was* special.

Floyd sighed. And Ollie was special, too.

Knocking interrupted Floyd's thoughts. He turned to see Ollie poking his head inside.

"Hello, hello," Ollie said, smiling.

Josephine ran over to him. "Mister Oliver, Daddy said there's gonna be ice cream!"

Ollie sucked in a breath, feigning surprise. "Ice cream?!"

"Have you ever had ice cream?"

"Only all the time in New York. We were lucky enough to have a bunch of ice cream parlors nearby."

"What's an ice cream parlor?"

"It's . . . well . . . a shop that sells ice cream."

Floyd cut in, "Imagine if the company store sold ice cream, Jo."

"Oh!"

"We only have it in town once in a while," Floyd explained to Ollie. "Fred and James bring the ice and the cream in from a city somewhere. It's probably expensive."

"Who makes it here?" Ollie asked.

"Couple of people volunteered to head to Donohue's early. I participated once a few years ago. It was pretty fun. We made a batch with strawberries."

Josephine squealed. "It was the *best*."

Ollie raised an eyebrow. "I suppose you haven't had it since?"

"No, not since I was five," Josephine answered. "Mama said it'll be even better this year. They're making it with maple syrup!"

"Sounds tasty," Ollie confirmed.

For some reason, this made Floyd start thinking 'bout the time Ollie had called *him* tasty, and then suddenly it was way, way too warm inside the house.

"Well, let's head over," he said, hoping to rid himself of the filthy thoughts.

"Just a minute," Effie said, drying her hands. "I need to fetch my hat from the back room."

Ollie walked over to Floyd and touched the top of his head, ruffling his hair a bit.

"What about you?"

"I suppose I can't be the only one without a hat, huh?" Floyd said, smiling at the way Ollie was still touching his hair. It made him want to touch Ollie's, too, which had become one of his favorite things.

"You'll look handsome either way," Ollie said, finally taking his hand away and turning back toward Josephine, who was smiling up at them. "Isn't he handsome, Josephine?"

"Yes," Josephine confirmed. "Daddy is very handsome. And Daddy says you're handsome, too, Mister Oliver. I heard him saying that to Mama a few times."

Floyd snorted. Gee, maybe they'd have to learn Jo not to talk about him and Ollie so much. He wondered what sorts of strangeness William must be telling his parents by now. Neither Margaret nor Leonard had said nothing to him about it yet. They probably thought Jo was spinning tall tales, is all. Hopefully, anyway.

Effie came out from the back room wearing her wide-brimmed straw hat.

"What do you think, fellas? Does it look nice enough with this here dress Floyd bought for me over in Charleston?"

"You look real pretty, Effie," Floyd said, staring at her with a kind of wonderment. Sometimes, he was still a little taken aback by her beauty. It wasn't the same kind of admiring he felt toward men, but Effie was prettier than even the nicest painting. He supposed he should tell her that more often. "Even prettier than a sunset."

"Thank you," Effie said, now absolutely beaming.

Ollie must have noticed the change, too. "Well, yeah, with a smile like that, especially."

Effie's cheeks started looking a bit rosy. It was nice to see her like this, though it made Floyd feel sad for her, too. He sometimes wished there was some way he could feel toward her what he felt toward Ollie. Because Effie ought to have been blessed with a husband who was the way he was supposed to be. For the most part, Floyd hadn't had a problem with his liking men. He had made peace with it in his youth. But in moments like this, Floyd found himself feeling a touch bad about it. He hoped Effie was still happy in the life they had together.

Ollie touched his back and said, "Do you want your hat?"

"Yeah," Floyd said, shaking his head, as though to shoo away the unexpected bout of sadness. "I'll wear it."

When Effie handed it to him, she caught his eye and looked at him in a way as though to ask if everything was fine. After a moment, Floyd nodded. Effie's mouth pinched at the corner like she wasn't believing him.

"Oliver, would you mind walking ahead with Josephine?" Effie asked. "I want to talk to Floyd about something real quick."

"Of course not," Ollie said. He held out his hand for Josephine. "Come on, Jo."

It was nice that Jo had taken to holding Ollie's hand sometimes. After Ollie and Jo left, Effie looked at Floyd expectantly.

"Are you happy, Effie?"

"Why're you asking me that? Of course I'm happy."

"With me sleeping over at Ollie's so much, you know . . ."

Floyd looked at his shoes. It pained him to keep looking at her.

"I know you ain't leaving me, Floyd. Is that what this is about?"

"Yeah, maybe. Or . . ."

"Or what?"

"Ain't you want a normal husband?"

"No," Effie said, very matter-of-factly. "I like my strange husband. He treats me well and provides for me and—"

"Anyone can do them things."

"*And* he's my best friend in the whole world. And now I'm so lucky that I got a new friend, too. His name is Oliver. He's sweet and funny and makes my husband real happy."

Floyd could feel the heat blooming on his cheeks. He had to fight to contain a smile.

"Stop that," he said, looking away again.

"Now my strange husband keeps coming home with expensive-looking silk undergarments, too. Makes me feel like we're living in some mansion over in Bramwell or something."

Floyd's eyes snapped up to meet Effie's teasing little smile. In retaliation, he snatched her hat and flung it across the room.

"Hey!"

Effie turned to fetch it, but Floyd caught her arm.

"You swear you ain't upset about me and Ollie?"

"Yes, I swear," she said, like she was real tired of Floyd's bullpoop. "I'm happy for you. And I'm happy for me, too. Because I like Oliver. Josephine likes him, too. I told you a long time ago that I was happy with our marriage. I still am. I like my life the way it is, you hear?"

"Mmm . . . yeah, I suppose," Floyd said, releasing her. "Better find your hat before the wind blows it away again."

"Oh, is *that* what happened?" Effie said, picking it up off the floor. "Time to find Josephine and Mister Oliver."

Floyd smiled warmly. "Yeah, let's head out."

Hands joined together, they walked across town.

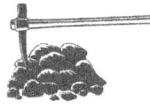

Hours later, the entire town was still having fun in James Donohue's big backyard, enjoying music and food and even a secret bit
of moonshine that had found its way to the party, though Floyd
hadn't found it himself yet. So far, Floyd, Effie, and Ollie had
only been following Josephine around as she had fun watching the
puppet show and seeing the magician (who, she said, was only a bit
more magical than Mister Oliver), and of course, they had all eaten
plenty of ice cream. It had been a real nice night.

Now, though, Josephine was with William and his siblings,
trying to catch lightning bugs over toward the edge of Donohue's
property. With the band playing, Floyd supposed it would probably make Effie happy if he asked her to dance.

Holding out his hand, he said, "Come on, Effie."

Effie looked down at his hand like it was covered with coal dust.
"Are you trying to ask me to dance with you?"

"Uh, yeah. Unless you ain't want to?"

"What kind of invitation is that?"

"What do you mean?"

"It ain't romantic at all!"

"Romantic? Effie, what in the . . ." Floyd huffed. "We're married!"

Ollie pushed Floyd's hand away. "Excuse me, miss, but I
couldn't help but notice you from across the ballroom."

Floyd blew out a puff of air. "Ballroom? Ollie, we're standing
on a patch of dirt."

Ollie ignored him. "And I have to say, you are as beautiful as
the moon." He looked over at Floyd. "Which, everyone knows, is

exceedingly more beautiful than something as completely unre-
markable as the sun." And then back at Effie, who was now barely
containing her laughter. "Would you make me the luckiest man in
the entirety of West Virginia by sharing this dance?"

"Oh my," Effie said, very clearly exaggerating how supposedly
touched she was by this pile of horsefeathers. "Now *that* is an
invitation. Yes, Oliver, of course I will."

Floyd cocked an eyebrow at Ollie, who shrugged and shook his
head as if to say, *"You bungled that, sweetheart,"* only with a bunch
more expletives.

"It's like you've never been to a cotillion before," Ollie said,
leading Effie away.

"Ollie, I'm not even sure what that is," Floyd said through a
laugh.

For the next couple of songs, Floyd stood by and watched Ollie
lead Effie around the so-called ballroom. It made his chest swell
and his heart ache, but in a happy kind of way. He loved seeing the
two of them have fun together.

But somehow, it was making him a little sad, too. Even though
Ollie looked nothing like Matt—Ollie was taller and leaner and
had that beautiful yellow hair—seeing Effie and Ollie being so
close made Floyd think of the years the three of them had all spent
together before—

Floyd closed his eyes. It still hurt to even think about it.

When Floyd opened his eyes again, Ollie was smiling one of
those sweet smiles of his, the ones that made him look so innocent,
even with all that schooling he'd had and places he had been to, and
Floyd replied to that big, beautiful smile with a wink.

Which made Ollie bite down on his bottom lip in this sweet
way. Floyd loved how sweet Ollie could be sometimes. Or maybe
all the time. He was lucky to have found someone who had all this
unique adorableness about him. Yet, he still missed Matt plenty.

He missed the way that every smile of Matt's had felt like a present meant only for him because of how stoic he had typically been otherwise. He missed Matt's low laugh and the way Matt had been fascinated by the most random things—pocket watches and stamps and coins and such. If only he could see Matt again. Just one more time.

As the next song started to play—a slow one, one that was heavy on the viola—Floyd let his eyes wander over to where Jo was playing, and he tried to focus on the little flashes of light from the lightning bugs, rather than the heaviness in his heart. Toward the edge of the woods, he could still see the beautiful blue-purple color of the tube-flowers that bloomed every summertime, and over the next couple of minutes, he watched the colors fade while the sun started to set.

Slowly, Floyd's thoughts traveled back to his childhood, back to when he and Matt had liked to catch lightning bugs, too. Back then, Matt had been in the habit of smushing them. He had liked to see the way they continued to shine on skin or rocks or whatever he had smashed them either with or on. But Floyd hadn't liked that. He felt pathetic remembering it now, but he really hadn't liked Matt hurting those poor bugs. Floyd remembered how he had eventually worked up the courage to tell Matt how sad it was making him.

At first, Matt hadn't seemed to care much, which had been a bit disappointing at the time. Floyd had hoped for some kind of acknowledgment or apology. But then, later that afternoon, Floyd had found Matt by the edge of the shrubbery where they had been watching them lightning bugs before, lining up a whole bunch of pebbles in a row. *"What're those?"* Floyd had asked. *"Headstones,"* Matt had replied, as though Floyd ought to have known that. Matt had always been like that—expecting everyone else to know what he was thinking, like maybe he thought that everyone else was living inside his head, too. *"For what?"* Floyd had asked. *"Lightning bugs. I squished a lot of them."* And then Matt had looked up at Floyd and said, *"I'm sorry I killed them, Floyd. I never meant to make you sad."* After that, Floyd had helped Matt with the little lightning bug memorial or whatever it was.

Floyd was still holding on tight to this memory when he turned his attention back to Ollie and Effie, who were swaying together only a few feet away.

When the song was over, Ollie and Effie parted.

"Well, that was fun," Effie said, coming back over to Floyd. "I'm pretty sure everyone thinks Oliver's fixing to steal me away from you, though."

"Impossible," Ollie said. "I couldn't steal you even if I tried. Floyd's the real catch. Anyone with eyeballs can see that."

Floyd shook his head. "You're lucky the music's still playing loud enough to keep people from hearing that."

"Eh, I'm always making strange comments. I think everyone knows that by now."

Which was probably true. Ollie was becoming a real miner. Everyone in Rock Creek knew Ollie. Everyone seemed to like him, too.

Effie took Floyd's hand.

"We better try one dance. I ain't lying about the way it'll look if people see that I spent all night with Oliver and not with you."

"Yeah, I suppose you're right," Floyd said before remembering that he was probably supposed to ask her in a nice way. "Effie, will you make me the luckiest man in the whole world by sharing a dance with me? Heck, you're as pretty as the sun and the moon and the stars all combined."

Ollie scoffed in a playful manner.

"Of course," Effie said, smiling up at him.

And so, Floyd and Effie shared a dance. Floyd wasn't as coordinated as Ollie, but he tried his best, and Effie seemed to have fun even with Floyd knocking knees with her a couple of times.

When the song was over, Effie told them that she had to fetch Josephine to put her to bed. Floyd offered to find her instead, but Effie protested, telling him to spend some time with Ollie.

After Effie and Jo left, another slow song started playing. Floyd wished that he and Ollie could sway together. But of course, that wasn't in the cards for them. It'd never be.

Ollie kicked a rock and said, "So, should we head back to my house or . . . ?"

"Yeah, let's."

On the way, they talked about the types of ice cream Ollie had tried back up in New York. It made Floyd wish he could visit with Ollie someday. He'd have liked to have a window into that part of Ollie's life.

When they reached Ollie's house, Floyd started up the steps, but Ollie stopped in front of the porch and knelt down.

"Lightning bugs are my favorite," Ollie said, coaxing one of them to land on his hand.

"Mine, too," Floyd said, coming to kneel beside him.

Slowly, Ollie sat back on his butt, keeping his arm steady as he did so that the little bug would stay on his hand. Once Ollie was settled, he held out his other hand and the lightning bug flew over and landed on it like them two were friends already.

Ollie smiled. "What should we name him?"

"Name him?"

"Do you think he looks like a George?"

"He looks like a bug," Floyd said with a laugh.

"Yeah, maybe not George," Ollie said, lifting his hand like he really was trying to find the perfect name for a little insect that would probably fly away in thirty seconds. "How about Carl?

I think Carl suits him." Ollie brought his hand closer to Floyd. "Hold out your palm for him."

"He'll fly away."

"Nah, I don't think so. Carl likes us now. He knows we won't hurt him."

Ollie's words made Floyd's stomach seize. Still, he held out his hand. Sure enough, Carl walked right into it, stopping in the middle of his palm.

"See?" Ollie said. "One time, I walked a whole six or seven city blocks with one on my forearm. I named that one James."

Floyd's stomach was still rolling in an unpleasant way. He hardened his jaw, trying not to let it show.

"What do you think of Floyd, Carl?" Ollie asked. He held out his index finger and pressed it to Floyd's palm. Carl climbed onto it. "He's a sweetheart, isn't he?"

Floyd's throat was starting to tighten. Ollie's tenderness toward the little lightning bug was so beautiful, so funny, so kind. It was everything Floyd loved about Ollie. And yet, in that moment, Floyd hated it, too. Ollie was the opposite of Matt in so many ways.

Floyd inhaled a shaky breath. He needed some space from Ollie right now.

"I need to spend more time with my family, Ollie," Floyd said suddenly. "I been staying here too much."

"Oh." Ollie's tone cut Floyd like a knife. "Yeah, that's, uh, that's fair."

"We'll see each other tomorrow. After church."

"I can come to church," Ollie offered. "Or . . ."

"Don't," Floyd said curtly before catching himself and softening his tone. "I know it ain't something you enjoy."

"Alright," Ollie said, looking away. "After, then."

"Yeah, you can come over. Effie and Jo will like that."

"Effie and Jo."

"I will, too," Floyd added, which was still true. "Goodnight, Ollie."

He hopped to his feet.

"Goodnight, Floyd."

All the way home, Floyd fought back tears. Every minute with Ollie seemed to be pushing him farther from Matt. He wondered what in the heck he was supposed to do.

Chapter Twelve

Oliver

By the time Oliver woke, it was nearly noon. He hadn't been able to fall asleep until three or four in the morning. For hours, he had tossed and turned, unable to move past the strangeness of the previous evening. Oliver couldn't understand what might have happened to make Floyd want to leave in such a hurry.

Normally, whenever the two of them needed to part for a while, Floyd liked to take his time before leaving. In the mornings, before Floyd left to see Josephine off to school, he liked to hold Oliver's face in his hands and plant tiny kisses over his cheeks and nose and forehead, as though he needed to provide Oliver with enough of them to last until they could be alone again. God, how he missed those kisses now. He hadn't even realized how much he had been treasuring them before they had been taken away. He hoped Floyd would still kiss him like that the next time they saw each other.

After washing up, Oliver cooked himself some eggs for breakfast. While they sizzled in the skillet, he prepared an extra strong batch of coffee. He couldn't wait to see Floyd again. Hopefully, spending time together would help Oliver see that he had been overthinking everything. Ever since waking, Oliver had been telling himself that Floyd was allowed to spend evenings with his family. Besides, it had been an especially long night. Dancing had been tiring. Chatting with the townsfolk had been tiring. Oliver could hardly blame him for wanting to have a proper night of rest before church in the morning. Everything was probably fine.

When the eggs were finished, Oliver scooped them onto a plate and practically inhaled them, his body pleading for the energy. As soon as the coffee was cool enough, Oliver chugged it down (mildly scorching his tongue in the process). He left the dishes on the counter to clean some other time. Now buzzing with nervous energy, Oliver shoved his arms into his blue suit jacket before throwing on his new blue fedora, and then he hurried over to Floyd's house.

Nearing Floyd's, Oliver could see Effie sitting outside on the porch on a rocking chair. Josephine was kneeling in front of the steps, sketching with a long stick. Oliver caught Effie's eye and waved. Effie waved back.

"Hi, Oliver," she called.

Josephine looked up and smiled. "Hi, Mister Oliver!" She hopped to her feet and rushed over. "Why didn't you sit with us in the pew today?"

"I slept late," Oliver said sheepishly. "I missed church altogether, I'm afraid."

Josephine's brow furrowed as though this was very upsetting news.

"I'm never allowed to miss church."

"Yes, well, I think it's probably best if you follow your parents, not someone like me."

Effie started down the steps. "Josephine, let's not pester Mister Oliver about church."

"Fine," Josephine sighed with a slight roll of her eyes.

"Where's Floyd?" Oliver asked as Effie approached.

"Napping. He couldn't sleep much last night for some reason."

"Oh. I'm sorry to hear that," Oliver said, trying not to sound too bothered by the news.

"He fell asleep sitting in the pew this morning. Snored and everything 'til I woke him up."

Oliver wished he had witnessed the scene.

"I *may* have had something to do with it," Oliver admitted. "I'm sorry."

"Did something happen last night? I was surprised that he came back so early."

"I'm not really sure. I think I must have upset him somehow."

"Well, I'm sure you'll fix things soon enough."

"I hope so." Oliver cleared his throat. "I should probably head back home, then, if Floyd is asleep."

"You can stay if you want."

"Yeah?"

"Why not? I was thinking of making a skillet cake."

"Oh, but, uhm, I'm not sure I'd be much help with that. I haven't ever tried to make one before."

"All the better. I can teach you."

Her kindness was already helping him feel a bit better about the situation with Floyd. Surely Effie wouldn't want him to stay if Floyd had hinted that something was wrong with their relationship.

"I'd love that," Oliver said, a wonderful warmth spreading through his chest. He was so touched that she wanted to spend time with him.

Effie bent down to talk to Josephine. "I think enough time has passed since you tried to find the circus. If you'd like, you can play with William today."

Josephine's face lit up. "Really?!"

"Really."

Josephine made a funny squealing sound and started running off.

"Bye, Mama! Bye, Mister Oliver!"

"Bye, Josephine!" Oliver hollered back, now smiling again. He looked back at Effie. "Well, let's cook, then."

Together, Oliver and Effie walked back to the house. Then Effie took out everything they'd need—a skillet, a mixing bowl, a whisk, and a bunch of ingredients from the cupboards.

"Have you ever had applesauce cake before?" Effie asked, setting the applesauce on the counter.

"Can't say that I have."

"It's one of Floyd's favorites. Mine, too."

Oliver thought he'd better pay extra close attention, then.

Over the next half hour, Effie helped Oliver measure out the various ingredients, and then Oliver mixed them in the bowl. All the while, Oliver's whole body buzzed with happiness. It felt like Effie was really becoming his friend. How incredible it was! Oliver could hardly believe that in the span of a few months, he had not only found a boyfriend, but a few friends, too—Roy, with whom Oliver still liked to play pool sometimes; Effie, who seemed to enjoy playing chess with him; and Aunt Betty, with whom he had been corresponding through letters. Life in Rock Creek was so much better than life in Cleveland or New York had ever been.

While Oliver and Effie waited for the cake to finish cooking, the two of them started chatting about their childhoods, keeping their voices low so as not to wake Floyd.

Effie told a few stories about her life back in McDowell County, reminiscing about how she and Floyd had become friends. Apparently, their families had owned farms next to each other's, and so, it had been natural for them to play together. In their second year of school, Floyd had become friends with Matt. And then, of course, Effie had become friends with Matt, too.

"When the three of us became friends, there was a time when we all wanted to marry each other," Effie said, shaking her head and chuckling. "Ain't that something?"

Oliver smiled a little. "It is."

"But then, when we were eight or nine, Floyd came up to me one day and said, *'Effie, I think I only want to marry Matt now. I hope you ain't mad.'* I was a little hurt by it, but of course I never told Floyd that. Days later, I was still a little upset when Matt came up to me to ask the same thing, but about Floyd. I think that was the moment that I realized they were in love or something and so, I wasn't really bothered by them not wanting to marry me no more."

"In love? At nine?" Oliver asked, having trouble imagining such a strange occurrence.

"Yup, very," Effie said, as though this wasn't the most extraordinary thing in the world. "It was a child-like kind of love for a while, with them secretly pecking each other on the cheek on occasion and squabbling about marbles and fishing and other petty things, but that love never faded. It matured with them. Years later, when they were both working in the mines together, they were as in love as ever. Or probably more in love than ever."

"Wow, that's incredible," Oliver said. "Very romantic."

Why hadn't Floyd talked about Matt this much? Sure, Oliver had been a smidge upset over the fact that Matt had been more of Floyd's equal in the mines, but had Oliver's reaction really been enough to make Floyd feel like he couldn't ever talk about someone who had obviously been so important to him? Who still *was* important to him?

Effie's hand came to settle on Oliver's shoulder.

"Something wrong?"

"Uhm, not really, but . . ." Oliver sucked on his bottom lip for a few seconds, trying to work out how to phrase what he wanted to say. "Does Floyd ever talk about Matt with you?"

"Not much," Effie said, sadness in her voice. When Oliver looked over to meet her eyes, his chest tightened. It seemed like every ounce of her earlier happiness had vanished. He wanted to say that he was sorry for prying, but then Effie continued on. "Oh, Oliver, Matt's passing hurt Floyd so much. I never even know how to bring it up with him. When I try, he becomes so tight-lipped. I'm not sure if he's ever even let himself cry over it. I reckon that's my fault, in a way, because only a week or so after Matt's passing, I came to tell him that I was pregnant. We left for Rock Creek so fast and . . ." She let out a long sigh. "Life has been a whirlwind ever since. I mean, I know we've had time to ourselves once Jo is in bed, but I haven't ever pushed him to try to talk about Matt in earnest. We've certainly talked *around* Matt plenty, but . . ."

Oliver took Effie's free hand and squeezed it.

"Don't blame yourself, Effie. I can't even imagine how scary everything must have been for you back then. You had to focus on yourself. And on Jo."

Effie squeezed back before letting go.

"Thank you."

Both of them became lost in their thoughts as the cake finished cooking. Oliver's heart hurt for Floyd, but truthfully, he wasn't entirely sure how to help Floyd through his loss. He thought maybe he ought to try to bring Matt up himself, to encourage Floyd to talk about him again. Maybe that was what Floyd needed.

Oliver turned to Effie and asked, "Would you mind if I went to see Floyd? I know it's your bedroom and everything, so I completely understand if you're uncomfortable with it."

"Go ahead."

Oliver crept into the bedroom, the floorboards creaking beneath his feet as he shuffled across toward the bed and carefully sat on the edge of the mattress. Floyd only stirred. For a few moments, Oliver sat completely still, trying not to wake him. He wanted to admire Floyd for a little while—the way the side of his face was smushed into the pillow, the way some of his brown locks had fallen to cover his forehead, the stubble upon his chin—and then finally reached up to sweep the hair off his face. Floyd's eyes fluttered open.

"Ollie?" Floyd asked, his voice thick with sleep.

"I was making a cake with Effie, but I wanted to visit you."

Floyd hummed and said, "Applesauce cake?"

"Yeah," Oliver said softly.

"I like that one," he said through a yawn.

Oliver's smile broadened as Floyd turned and rubbed his face into the pillow before rolling back over to face him. Even with bags under his eyes and his hair a mess, Floyd was so handsome.

Oliver's stomach fluttered from nervousness as he readied himself to try to bring up Matt.

"While Effie and I were cooking, we, uhm, we talked about Matt a bit."

"Yeah?"

"Yeah." Oliver reached for Floyd's hand, which was sticking out from beneath the thin brown blanket. "If you ever need someone to talk to about—"

"Nah, I'm . . . I'm fine, Ollie." Floyd let go of Oliver's hand and then started to stretch. "Actually, I want to be by myself for a bit. Just feeling so tired right now."

"Oh." Oliver's throat tightened. "Of course."

After placing a soft kiss on Floyd's forehead, Oliver left. Out of politeness, he stayed with Effie for a little while so that they could share some of the cake in the kitchen, but his mind was elsewhere.

Why was it that Floyd suddenly seemed so . . . so far away? Even though he was only one room over, Oliver felt as though there was a whole chasm between them. It had to be because of Matt. Or well, because of Floyd's feelings for Matt. Oliver had offered his ear. But Floyd hadn't seemed to want it.

If Floyd wouldn't talk about Matt, then what was Oliver supposed to do? Maybe Floyd had been keeping Oliver away on purpose ever since they had confessed their feelings for each other. Floyd still hadn't let him work with the explosives. Floyd still hadn't initiated more with Oliver in bed. And now . . .

No, Floyd wasn't pulling away, was he?

While Oliver munched on the cake, he tried to consider the possibility. If Floyd's love for Matt had been—or, hell, still was—one with the sort of passion and timelessness that could usually only be found in the most fantastical of storybooks, Oliver couldn't understand how he was ever supposed to compete. Whereas Floyd and Matt's love had been, from the sound of Effie's stories, as deep and everlasting as the earth's oceans, Floyd and Oliver's brief entanglement seemed, in comparison, as transient and shallow as a rain puddle. It made Oliver wonder when Floyd would tire of him. Because eventually, Floyd would realize that Oliver wasn't Matt and that he would never be Matt and, well, that would be that, wouldn't it?

Oliver set his fork back on the table.

"Effie, I think I'll head home. I'm feeling a bit tired myself."

"Alright, well, feel free to come back for some more cake later, if you want."

Oliver faked a smile. "Thank you."

Oliver walked home, kicking a rock as he traveled, each swipe of his foot sending it tumbling ahead on the path, creating little clouds of brown dust. His pant legs became messier with each step, the plumes of brown clinging to the fabric. Along the way,

Oliver tried to tell himself that the slight transformation he sensed in Floyd was merely a trick of the mind—the result of his insecurities making him extra sensitive to even small changes in Floyd's behavior. He and Floyd were fine. Floyd was tired. Everyone felt tired sometimes.

By the time Oliver reached home, his muscles were completely spent from being so constantly tense. Weary and nervous and sad, Oliver collapsed onto the bed without even first removing his shoes.

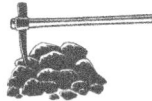

One week later, Oliver was standing in front of Aunt Betty's house praying to whoever might listen that his relative would have some advice for him. Because Oliver had truly become lost. Over the week, Floyd had rejected every single invitation Oliver had extended for the two of them to spend time together without Effie and Jo present. Sure, the two of them still worked together, but Floyd went straight home once they were finished with their shifts. One time, Oliver had eaten supper with Floyd's family and even then, Floyd had been more reserved than ever, barely showing Oliver even the tiniest bit of care. It wasn't that Floyd had been unkind to him. No, Floyd was never unkind. He was still sweet, but that sweetness had been tempered for sure.

Somehow, Oliver must have messed everything up back at the summer party. He wasn't sure how, but it was clear to him now that Floyd's interest in romance had vanished—poof!—like magic. Oliver nearly smiled at the irony of that. Presenting Mister Oliver, Master Magician: he can make people's love for him disappear.

God, he hoped Aunt Betty would have some wisdom to offer him. It wasn't as though Oliver could talk to anyone else. Roy? Effie? Not a chance.

Nervousness continued to percolate inside him, bubbling in Oliver's veins, causing him to fiddle with the buttons on his sleeves. Figuring that he'd better head inside before he inevitably ruined his suit, Oliver started up the walkway.

This time, when Aunt Betty answered, she seemed more pleasantly surprised than merely confused.

"Hello, Oliver," she said, the faintest hint of a smile on her face. "I thought I requested that you provide some notice when you wanted to visit next."

"Yes, I know, but it was a last-minute decision to come here. I need some . . . help." Oliver smiled meekly while Aunt Betty looked at him with skepticism. "May I come in?"

"You may, but I need a couple of minutes first."

"I can wait."

Aunt Betty closed the door. Five minutes later, she opened it again.

"Come in."

Oliver followed her to a small sitting room, and they both sat in chairs in front of an unlit fireplace. She had two small tumblers filled with what looked to be illegal brandy waiting for them. It was curious that she seemed not to have a servant. Oliver's own family had always had hired help—a nanny, a maid, and a woman who cooked and cleaned and helped out in various ways. Clearly, Aunt Betty had the money for servants. It seemed strange for her not to have one. But then, Aunt Betty had always been strange.

Oliver reached for his drink and took a couple of sips in rapid succession. He and Aunt Betty sat in a comfortable-enough-yet-still-a-bit-awkward silence for a few minutes.

Finally, Oliver said, "Do you remember that the last time I came here, I hinted that I might have been messing up my life?" Oliver asked. "Well, I'm pretty sure I've somehow managed to make everything even worse now."

"I'm sorry to hear that," she said.

Even though her words were sweet, her tone seemed off. Cold, even. Even though Oliver tried to himself that he was imagining it, he couldn't help but wish for some kind of throw blanket to pull over his shoulders.

He continued, "Yes, well, now I'm confused as to what I'm supposed to do. I'm in a relationship with someone, but I'm worried I've messed up somehow because, over the last week, they've become so . . ." Oliver looked over to see that Aunt Betty was tapping her foot. Once again, he tried to ignore the potential hint that she was completely uninterested in hearing what he had to say. "Distant. I think my friend might not care for me the same way that I care for them."

"Mmm . . ." Pursing her lips, Aunt Betty looked at her tumbler. Oliver fidgeted in his seat while he waited for her to respond. "Well, I hope it works out."

God, her voice was practically *dripping* with disinterest. He hated this. She was talking to him as though it was a chore. It was how everyone had always talked to him. Everyone except for Floyd. And Effie. And Jo. Roy and John weren't bad either. Actually, most everyone in Rock Creek was fairly lovely. Why on earth was he trying to cultivate a relationship with this woman? Because she was family? Oliver supposed he should have seen this coming.

"Christ, why'd I have to mess everything up?" Oliver set his tumbler back on the table and stood. "And I shouldn't have come here. It's obvious how little you care." He started back toward the entryway, muttering, "No one in our family has ever cared for me. I have no idea why I thought you'd be any different."

He took another two steps before Aunt Betty spoke again. "Oliver," she called out. "I'm sorry."

He stopped and waited.

She continued, "Long ago, I told myself I wouldn't ever put myself in a position to be pushed around by one of our family members ever again. So, yes, I was set on keeping our relationship fairly superficial, but Oliver, I seem to have forgotten that you left, too. I think that merits a second chance."

"I'm not either of your brothers. I promise."

"You're right." She gestured to the empty chair beside her. "Sit."

So Oliver sat. Aunt Betty studied his face for a few seconds before setting her tumbler on the side table.

"Alright, Oliver, I'd be happy to try to offer you some wisdom if I can," she said, folding her hands in her lap. "Tell me a bit more about this woman you're seeing and what happened that may have caused her to start pushing you away."

"I think they might have realized that I'm not . . . enough."

"Not enough?" Aunt Betty asked with a slight tilt of her head.

"Not when compared to his—" Oliver sucked in a breath, his eyes widening in horror before he clapped a hand over his mouth. "Fuck," he cursed, the swear word muffed by his palm.

Surprisingly, Aunt Betty's expression remained relatively stoic—her mouth a straight line, eyes boring into him. Oliver was too scared to even move. Damn, she would probably throw him out of her house as soon as she found her voice.

Instead, Aunt Betty raised both her eyebrows and said, "His?"

Oliver swallowed thickly as he tried to recover.

"Come on, be . . . be scandalized," he managed to say. "I know you're probably struggling to hide your shock and awe. Not, you know, the happy kind, either."

With a shrug, Aunt Betty said, "I'm not scandalized."

Oliver crooked a suspicious eyebrow. "Why not?"

Aunt Betty pursed her lips ever-so-slightly, and then her eyes flitted over to the stairwell outside the room.

"Do you know why I left New York?" she asked, looking over at Oliver again.

Oliver shook his head. "No. Not that I haven't wondered."

"Tell me, why'd you choose Rock Creek?"

"Well, uhm, I knew that you lived in Charleston, and I knew that our family friend Frederick Donohue owned the town so—"

"I'm not sure if you remember this, but I was supposed to marry Frederick."

Oliver's mouth fell open.

"Oh my God," he said. "No, I hadn't remembered, but now . . . wow, I can't believe I had forgotten."

"Well, you were young. I can hardly blame you for not being interested in learning who one of your relatives was supposed to marry," she said with a wave of her hand. "Obviously, that never came to be. I fell in love with Mary, Frederick's sister. Our families tried to keep us apart. You may remember that I came to New York for a little while. Meanwhile, Frederick was upset with his parents for how they reacted, and he left for West Virginia, taking Mary with him. Mary and I kept writing to each other. I wrote to Frederick, too. It wasn't long before he felt secure enough in his business to help Mary and I start our life here."

Oliver took off his hat, raked a hand through his hair, and put his hat back on again. He was so stunned he nearly repeated the nervous tick a second time.

"I can't believe it," he said after a moment.

"So, you see, you having a relationship with a man isn't so scandalous to me."

"Wow, I . . ." It felt as though Oliver's tongue had become knotted in his mouth, preventing him from forming normal sentences. Aunt Betty had fallen for a woman! No wonder she had run from the family. "I'm so sorry you had to run."

"Yes, well, I have my own little family here. Mary and Frederick and James."

"And me?"

She smiled warmly. "And you."

"I wish I could explain how much that means to me."

"I know how much it means to you," Aunt Betty said. "Remember, I'm an Astor, too."

"Yes, that's true," Oliver said before heaving a sigh. "I thought I had created a little family, too, but . . . God, I'm so worried I'll lose Floyd."

"Floyd is the name of the man you're seeing?"

"Right."

"Did you try to talk to him about how you feel?"

"Not . . . yet."

"I think that might be a sensible first step, then," she said with a playful look in her eye, one that suggested that she was teasing him a little. Oliver huffed a laugh. Aunt Betty had teased him! What a strange visit this was.

"Yes, well, I can try, but I haven't been able to convince him to spend time alone with me for the last week or so. Not that I let him know how important I think it is or anything, but . . ." Aunt Betty raised an eyebrow in response to what he had said, making Oliver feel a tiny bit foolish. He supposed that maybe he had been too busy catastrophizing to make a real effort to talk to Floyd about the changes he had sensed in their relationship. Maybe Floyd really *had* only been missing his family. Oliver threw his head back and sighed very loudly. What a nincompoop he was! "Alright, maybe things *aren't* that bad. Or maybe they are?"

"But you aren't sure."

"No, I'm not. It's . . . well, we were spending so much time together and then, suddenly, it stopped. We still see each other in the mines—he's my butty, which is like a mining partner—and we still talk and laugh and everything, but you know, we're basically always in public. I can't kiss him in public. I can't try to have some kind of lengthy, intimate conversation while we're shoveling coal. Fuck, I need to try to talk to him. Maybe tomorrow. Once we're through with work, I'll . . . I'll tell him that it's important. Maybe everything is fine between us."

"I hope it's nothing," Aunt Betty agreed.

"Do you mind if we chat for a little while longer? Take my mind off everything temporarily?"

"Not in the least," Aunt Betty said. "But . . . would you like to meet Mary?"

"Really?" Oliver asked, lifting a hand to his chest. "I'd love to."

Aunt Betty excused herself and left for the stairs. Oliver picked his nails nervously while he waited for her to return. Glancing around the room, Oliver caught sight of himself in the mirror and his eyes found his beautiful blue fedora—the one Floyd had purchased for him. Even though Oliver was terrified of Floyd's potential rejection—petrified that the man with whom he had fallen in love would tell him that he simply couldn't love him back—Oliver knew he had to confront him about the recent changes in their relationship. But, God, how he hoped Floyd loved him, too.

Floyd had awoken something in him, something that he had never felt before, something he hadn't even thought he was capable of feeling. For years, Oliver had read Shakespeare and Austen and Tolstoy and so many other writers, finishing (or, well, nearly finishing) each love story only to be left wondering what the hell was wrong with him. Love? Romance? What in God's name were those? He may as well have been reading a foreign language. But Floyd—Floyd was his Goddamned Rosetta Stone. And now Oliver understood love and passion and romance and, fuck, how could he ever live life without them again? He could move one thousand miles away and part of him—maybe even the most important part of him—would still be back in West Virginia with Floyd.

He had to try to make Floyd see that they belonged together. Oliver wasn't Matt, but . . .

But maybe he was enough.

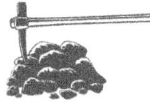

While Oliver took the coal elevator into the mine the following morning, his stomach started rolling like he might throw up. In only a few hours, Oliver would press Floyd to talk. And then he would know the truth. God, it was terrifying to be vulnerable like this, to know Floyd was holding Oliver's heart in his hands.

Floyd was waiting for Oliver by the brass board.

"Hey, you," Oliver said with as much tenderness as he could muster, hoping he could somehow silently communicate the word "sweetheart" in public.

"Hey, Ollie," Floyd said with a sigh, one that maybe suggested that he was tired of Oliver's presence already.

Jesus.

"Uhm . . ." Oliver swallowed, pushing past the feeling of unease. Maybe, before they talked, Oliver could try to remind Floyd of his commitment to their relationship. And his commitment to Rock Creek, too. He could show Floyd how far he had come. "Do you think you could show me how to work with the black powder today?"

"Ollie—"

"Please," Oliver begged. "I want to try. Let me try."

Floyd rubbed his chin in that way he always did when he was thinking something over.

"Yeah, you can try."

Oliver let out a breath, relief washing over him. Even though this offer would have probably seemed inconsequential to others, Oliver knew how important this was. Until now, Floyd had been so resistant to Oliver working with the black powder. Oliver could hardly believe that Floyd had finally relented. He had to be careful not to let Floyd down.

After they reached their workstation, Floyd let Oliver make the holes in the coal seam, and once Oliver was finished, Floyd showed him how to roll the black powder into the paper cartridge before helping him insert the copper needle. Oliver's hands shook the entire time. Even though Floyd must have noticed, he never let on, neglecting to offer even one word of comfort or encouragement, which was so completely unlike him that Oliver had to bury the urge to cry.

Later, once the needle had been removed and the fuse had been set, Floyd let Oliver be the one to call out "fire in the hole!" three times and then light it. He and Floyd took cover. Ears covered, Oliver braced himself for the blast, every single second seeming to stretch on into eternity. He couldn't wait for it to be over, like maybe the blast would not only obliterate the coal wall, but whatever barrier Floyd had erected between them, too.

BANG!

After the smoke cleared, Oliver looked to Floyd for approval.

All Floyd said was, "Well, then, time to shovel."

He walked away, leaving Oliver by himself in the darkness, save for the light of his own headlamp. For a few painful seconds, Oliver considered leaving. He wondered why he was bothering to fight for what they had—or what they had *once* had—when Floyd clearly wasn't willing to do the same. He wondered how and why he would ever fight alone.

But then, when Oliver looked over at Floyd, Floyd paused his shoveling and looked back at him, and thanks to the focused light of Oliver's headlamp, Floyd was the only thing Oliver could see in the darkness. And, Christ, he was beautiful. He was standing there, illuminated, his small smile shining like a beacon of hope. Oliver's breath caught. He knew, then, that he couldn't stop fighting for their relationship. Not yet, and maybe not ever.

"What are you waiting for?" Floyd asked, sounding a little like his old self again. "Come help me with this."

"Sorry," Oliver said, walking over. He came next to Floyd and leaned in close, heart hammering, unsure how Floyd would react to what he was about to say because who the hell knew what had been running through the man's mind for the past week. "Guess I lost myself in you."

"Yeah," Floyd said, his sweet smile broadening the tiniest bit. "I know how that is."

Just like that, everything seemed perfect again.

Their lovesick stares were broken by the sound of approaching footsteps.

"Hey, Floyd. Hey, Oliver," Roy said, John following close behind.

"Hey," Oliver said, scooping up his first shovel's worth of coal.

Roy asked, "Did you hear what happened over by the county line?"

"No, what?" Floyd asked back.

"Some of the union miners from outside of Charleston were marching over here."

Oliver's stomach seized. Jesus, not now, not when it seemed like he and Floyd were finally mending their bond. Wasn't there a better time for Roy and John to spread this news? Or, well, maybe not considering the subject matter. Underground, they were out of earshot from the folks who might have been Chafin's spies. Still, the timing was terrible. Couldn't they talk about this tomorrow?

"Over to Logan?" Floyd asked.

"Yup."

"Why?"

Roy rocked back on his heels. "Well, I heard they were trying to free them strikers who're behind bars in Mingo County, but first, they thought they'd hang Chafin, probably because they'd have had to cut through our county to reach the poor miners over there, anyway."

"*Hang him?!*" Floyd spluttered.

"Yup," Roy said with a shrug. "I'd have probably helped if I had known sooner."

Floyd shook his head in bewilderment. "What happened?"

Meanwhile, Oliver's stomach was in knots. Hopefully, Donohue Coal and Steel wouldn't be impacted by this. Floyd had made it crystal fucking clear that he'd more or less implode if faced with some kind of change for his family.

"Chafin stopped 'em. Of course."

John chimed in. "Roy's making it sound easy, but our fellow miners put up a struggle."

"Oh yeah, there was a huge battle."

Oliver couldn't hold back a scoff. "Battle?!"

Roy nodded. "Yup. People shooting at each other and everything."

"I heard Chafin's recruits had even set up machine guns," John said.

"Where'd this happen?" Oliver asked.

Roy clicked his tongue before answering, "Over at Blair Mountain. Not sure if you've been there yet. It's a mountain ridge between Boone and Logan Counties."

"People are saying that Chafin even had bi-planes. Dropped bombs on people."

"God, that's horrible," Oliver said.

"Yep. Federal troops came, though, and put a stop to everything," Roy said. "I wonder if them miners'll try again. Heck, I reckon I'd fight, too. Everybody in Rock Creek ought to."

Oliver opened his mouth to say something—something about how every single miner everywhere deserved better—but then he caught sight of Floyd.

Poor Floyd was standing there completely frozen, staring off into the nearest tunnel. While Roy and John kept up their back-and-forth, Oliver continued to watch Floyd, and only seconds later, he realized that Floyd's hands had started to tremble.

Oliver knew he'd better shoo Roy and John away before they noticed, too. Damn. Floyd was probably worried that his family might have to leave—leave the coal company, leave the coal industry, or hell, even leave West Virginia.

Oliver spoke up. "Uhm, say fellas, we have a lot more coal to shovel. We've barely even started filling our car. Do you think we could chat about this a little later?"

"Yeah, sure," Roy said. "We ought to find our butties anyway, but we thought you'd want to hear the news."

"Definitely," Oliver said through a strained smile. "Thank you for always taking the time to relay information from your relatives, Roy. Lord knows Donohue wouldn't want us miners knowing about the struggle."

Luckily, Oliver's comment must have seemed sincere enough because Roy and John left after they had exchanged a few parting words. Floyd waved to them half-heartedly as they left for one of the other tunnels. Once Roy and John were out of sight, Floyd flung his shovel to the side and placed his hands flat against the rocky black wall, finally surrendering to whatever it was that he was feeling. Oliver rushed over, throwing his shovel off to the side, too, and placed a hand on Floyd's back.

"I'd put money on the UMWA not taking hold in West Virginia now," Oliver said, trying to be encouraging. "I wouldn't worry too much, Floyd. I can't imagine that there will be future unrest here in Logan. I mean, hell, federal troops were involved!" Oliver started moving his hand in small circles, hoping it would provide some comfort, though he wished he could be more openly affectionate. "I'm sure your family is safe. I'm sure your *life* is safe. I wouldn't think anything would change because of—"

"Ollie . . ." Floyd choked out, flexing his fingers and pressing into the black rocks. Oliver winced. "I can't listen to none of this right now. I can't stand here listening to you trying to make me feel better with these kind-sounding words." He turned to face Oliver, hurt in his eyes. "Not when I know how you really feel."

"What are you talking about?"

"Don't pretend you wouldn't want the UMWA coming here, changing things. I still catch them little comments of yours, the ones about the coal company cheating us."

"What, me pointing out that the price of corn at the company store is three cents higher than it is in the city?" Oliver asked, fighting to keep the frustration from his voice.

Why in God's name was Floyd trying to pick a fight right now? Oliver had been trying to help him feel better!

"What's the point of saying something like that?" Floyd asked.

"What do you mean, 'what's the point?' It's a fact!" Oliver spat, unable to contain his fast-rising temper. "Floyd, why are you picking a fight? Why are you pushing me away?"

Floyd bent over to pick up his shovel, but before he could scoop up even one shovel's worth of coal, Oliver snatched it from him and threw it aside.

"Talk to me!" Oliver shouted.

"Not now, Ollie," Floyd said curtly, pushing past him to retrieve his shovel again.

Oliver hurried ahead to block him.

"What the hell happened over the last week, Floyd?"

"Nothing."

"You were barely yourself with me!" Oliver yelled, fury and sadness swirling inside him, making his voice shake. "And now you're pushing me away!"

"What are you talking about? No, I ain't."

"Yes, you are! Can you really not see it?!" Oliver yelled, and Floyd's only response was to curl his lip. "It's about Matt, isn't it? You're mad because I'm not Matt."

"Ollie, that's enough," Floyd snarled.

"Matt is *dead*, Floyd! Jesus Christ, why am I being forced to compete with someone who will never be anything less than perfect in your eyes? Matt can't ever mess up because Matt isn't here! But I *am*! And, God, I am fucking trying to *be with you*. I'm trying to be . . . to be *perfect* for you!" Oliver felt a tear roll down his cheek and quickly wiped it away. "I am *in love* with you, sweetheart! I am here and I am alive and I am in love with you." Another couple of tears escaped. "And I think you love me, too."

Covering his mouth with his hand, Floyd turned away. Oliver could tell that he was fighting to hold something back—whether crying or yelling, Oliver wasn't sure.

More tears tumbled down Oliver's cheeks. He let them. He let them because they kept coming, one after another, and there wasn't any point in trying to hide them anymore.

Lowering his voice to a whisper, Oliver stepped forward and said, "Floyd, sweetheart, please stop pushing me away."

After a moment, Floyd turned to face him, tears in his bright blue eyes.

"I need you to leave."

"What?"

"I can't . . . I can't . . ."

"Sweetheart, please—"

"Go home, Ollie."

Oliver wondered what exactly Floyd meant by that.

Floyd turned to pick up his shovel. Oliver stood frozen for a few seconds, still trying to accept what Floyd had said.

And what Floyd hadn't said.

After retrieving his pickaxe and shovel, Oliver started down the corridor. Fuck. Floyd was hurting. Oliver *knew* he was hurting. Why wouldn't he let Oliver comfort him? Why was he putting up these Goddamn walls?

When Oliver reached the elevator, he froze, Floyd's words echoing in his mind. *Go home, Ollie.* Christ, that would be the easier route, wouldn't it? Head home. Hell, head back to New York. Embrace the future that was supposed to have been his and forget Rock Creek had ever happened. But . . .

But Oliver loved Floyd.

Leaning against the wall, Oliver let out a sigh. Maybe Floyd would come around. Maybe once he had some time to himself, he would want them to make up, like he had wanted them to make up after they'd had the fight in the music store.

Oliver called over to the boy manning the elevator.

"Do you know Floyd Bennett?"

He tilted his head a bit. "Maybe?"

"Huge man. Taller than I am, even. But broader, too. Strong as a, well, as a mule. Stubborn as one, too. With brown hair and blue eyes." Oliver scrunched up his nose when he realized that the boy wouldn't be able to see Floyd's hair color or eye color very well here in the mine. He shoved a hand in his pocket and pulled out every bit of scrip he had in there. "Here," he said, handing the boy the money. "I need to know when he's leaving. Try your best to spot him. Ask men their names when they leave, maybe. If you find him, I want you to tell him to wait for me up near the entrance and then I want you to come and find me. I think I'll be sorting coal. Not my favorite thing, but . . ." Oliver shrugged. "What do you think? Can you help me?"

Eyes wide with what looked to be a mild form of shock, probably because Oliver had shoved the equivalent of seven or eight bucks in his hands, the boy nodded furiously.

"Yes, sir!"

"Good."

Oliver turned to find the breaker room. Once he was there, the kid-boss turned to him, eyes narrowed with suspicion.

"Why're you back?" he asked.

"Just am," Oliver answered with a shrug. "Mind if I sit for a while?"

"Not as long as you're working."

"Yeah, I'll work."

So, Oliver sat. Hours ticked by, and Oliver continued to help sort the coal. Every time he cut his hands on the slate, his eyes teared up embarrassingly and he thought about heading home. But he wasn't so sure where that was anymore.

Shortly before four, the kid-boss approached him.

"Are you fast?" he asked.

"I have long legs," Oliver answered.

"Good enough. We need someone to help Billy."

"Floyd's old butty?"

"He's one of our spraggers. He usually works with Chester, but Chester had to leave. Must be sick or something. He was throwing up everywhere."

"Oh," Oliver said, making a sour face. "So, you want someone to be a spragger?"

"If you can. Everyone else in here's too young. They'd probably be slow. Get their fingers shorn off."

"Yikes." Oliver stood up. "Just tell me what to do. I'm sure I can manage it."

"Good."

The kid-boss led Oliver over to Billy, who explained to him how spragging worked. Apparently, he and Oliver would need to shove some long pieces of wood—called sprags, incidentally—through the wheels of the approaching coal cars, which would in turn slow the cars. It seemed simple enough. He had already had a vague sense of the task but had never seen the spraggers in action before. Typically, he and Floyd hooked their car up to some other cars when they were finished, and then they rode the elevator up the mine shaft, where they'd find their car again so it could be weighed. It would be interesting to see the entire process. Hopefully, Floyd would be impressed by Oliver's willingness to learn more about the mines. He tried to see this as one more way to prove to Floyd that he was really committed to their life here.

Oliver's first two attempts at spragging went rather well. Even though the cars were fast, Oliver's height worked to his advantage, at least in this particular area of the mine, where the ceilings weren't too low. He'd never be able to help in some of the more challenging areas. But that wasn't what was needed, for now.

But then, on Oliver's third attempt, he missed one of the wheels, nearly injuring himself when he tried to insert the sprag. Determined to fix it, Oliver snatched another wooden piece from the pile and bolted ahead toward the car, which had started rolling faster.

"Forget it!" Billy called.

Oliver ignored him. He could do this. He *knew* he could.

Coming up alongside the car, Oliver tried once more. Not only did Oliver miss inserting the sprag, but he tripped over his own two feet and slammed into the car, hurting his shoulder and nearly falling onto the Goddamn track. When Oliver looked up, the car was practically flying. It was traveling much, much too fast. Oliver could sense that it was at risk of toppling over. He bounded forward, unsure what he would even try to do, because how could you slow a car that weighed over one hundred tons?

Just as Oliver came close to the car, it hopped over the track.

"Shit!" Oliver yelled, stumbling backward, only barely dodging the car as it careened into the wall.

Sure enough, it toppled, and coal dumped out onto the floor.

Seconds later, Billy came up beside him.

"Jeez, Mister, you nearly got yourself crushed to death."

"I realize that," Oliver said. "So, what happens now?"

"Well, we can try to shovel it into a new car, but I think whoever's car that was will probably be real mad on account of having to wait for the weighing."

"God, the two of us shoveling? We'll be here for hours."

"Probably."

"What if . . ." Oliver fished around in his pocket for his wallet and pulled out a fifty-dollar bill. He handed it to Billy. "Here. Can you ensure that makes its way to whoever's car that was? And . . ." He took out a five. "You can have that. I'm sorry I wasn't a very helpful spragger."

"It ain't scrip," the boy said. "How do I spend it?"

"Just take it to the company store and tell Charlie he can yell at me later."

Oliver moved to slide his wallet back into his pocket and winced. Fuck, he had *really* messed up his shoulder. Now that the excitement of the whole ordeal had passed, tremors of pain were rippling up and down the length of his arm. He wondered how he'd even manage to work tomorrow.

"Did you hurt yourself?" Billy asked.

"Yeah," Oliver said, sucking in a breath. "But I'll be alright."

"Should we still shovel the coal?"

"Just leave it. I'll talk to Frederick or whoever I need to."

"Who's Frederick?"

"You know, Frederick," Oliver repeated before coming to his senses. "Donohue."

"You know him?"

"Old family friend."

Billy wrinkled his nose. Oliver understood the sentiment.

"Well, I think I'll head home," Oliver said. "It has been a really challenging day."

"Alright," Billy said. "See you tomorrow, Mister."

"Call me Oliver," he said. "And yes, I'll see you tomorrow, Billy."

Oliver walked back to the elevator. He found the boy he had been talking to earlier.

"Did you see Floyd?" Oliver asked, his voice weary.

"Not yet."

"Alright, well, you can forget it, then. God, Floyd had wanted me to leave in the first place. I should have left right then and there. I should have listened!"

"Can I keep the scrip?" he asked.

"What?" Oliver blurted out, his mind foggy from pain. "Oh. Yes. Keep it. Sorry for the trouble."

Once Oliver returned to the surface, he started for home, the soreness in his shoulder torturing him with every step.

Chapter Thirteen

Floyd

FLOYD'S THROAT WAS TIGHT as he rode the elevator to the surface, his muscles tense from trying to hold in his upset for hours on end. He hadn't even managed to find a replacement butty for the remainder of his shift. It hadn't mattered to him that it was against the rules to work alone. It had been too hard to think of working with anyone else, both because he missed Ollie and because he was still on the verge of tears. He couldn't let others see him this way. Them horrible words—*Matt is dead*—they had struck him with the force of a bullet. Now all Floyd wanted was to be alone so that he could bleed.

Once Floyd found his car, he stood beside it to wait for his turn at the weigh station. It looked like there was some kind of hold-up. One of the senior men who worked in the mines—a man with silver hair named Ed Allen—looked real upset, mumbling curses and tapping one of his feet. Probably Ed had been waiting for his car for a while. It happened sometimes. Maybe it was stuck somewhere underground. Floyd hoped it would all be sorted out soon. He was teetering on the edge of crying or screaming or maybe even both. He couldn't let these fine folks be witness to his inevitable, eventual outburst.

Folding his arms in front of his chest, Floyd tried to hold in his upset for a little while longer. Not two minutes later, little Billy Davis came running toward the weight station.

"Sorry, Mister Allen," Billy huffed, catching his breath. "Accident."

Floyd crooked an eyebrow.

"Where's my God-dang car?" Ed asked.

"I was working with that yellow-haired man—uh, Mister Oliver—and the car tipped over."

Floyd's stomach sank, plummeting so far and fast it felt like it had fallen to the bottom of the mine shaft. He pushed forward to the front of the line.

"What happened?"

"Mister Oliver was helping me chase them coal cars with the sprags."

Floyd's heart was hammering in his chest while he sucked in a series of sharp inhales. "And a car tipped?!"

"Well, yeah, but—"

"Was Ollie hurt?!"

"Yeah, but—"

"Where is he?!"

"Home, I think."

Immediately, Floyd took off running, leaving his coal car behind and, therefore, leaving his earnings behind, too. As Floyd neared the main road, his hat flew off, but he refused to stop for it. None of these things mattered no more. Bounding through town, Floyd's mind was racing even faster than his legs, horrible scenes flickering through his mind with every step, like one of them flip books, only the pictures were mismatched, showing Ollie with a crushed hand or a broken leg or missing fingers. Sometimes, Floyd even pictured poor Ollie suffocating beneath a pile of coal, though that wouldn't make no sense since Ollie had somehow made it home. Still, Floyd couldn't stop imagining these horrible things.

Floyd had some vague sense that he was still supposed to be sore at Ollie for hollering in the mine—for calling him sweetheart in public and talking about Matt the way he had—but he couldn't even care about those things now. All Floyd cared about was making sure that Ollie wasn't hurt too bad. He couldn't hardly believe that he had wasted so much time afeared of letting himself be with Ollie. Floyd had been letting his worriment over forgetting Matt take over his mind. Ollie had been right. Floyd *had* been pushing him away. He had been so afeared of losing Matt that he hadn't even been thinking 'bout how he could have lost Ollie. Forever.

As soon as Floyd reached Ollie's house, he began pounding his fist on the door, bouncing on the balls of his feet while he waited. When Ollie hadn't opened up in less than twenty seconds, Floyd started hitting the wood even harder.

"Ollie!" Floyd yelled, so terrified he felt like he might burst out of his skin. "Ollie, open up! Are you in there? Are you hurt?"

Finally, Ollie opened the door.

"Hi," Ollie said, sounding sheepish.

Floyd's eyes started roaming over Ollie's body, searching for injuries. He seemed fine, somehow, though still filthy from work.

Pressing a hand flat to Ollie's chest, Floyd shoved him backward into the house and followed, kicking the door shut with the heel of his boot.

Ollie started saying, "Sweetheart, I'm sorry for—"

But Floyd placed one hand on either side of his face and cut him off with a hard, impassioned kiss, pressing their lips together with a force that nearly knocked Ollie back again. Heck, he was kissing Ollie so hard that it was barely even a kiss anymore. It was more like he was fixing to meld their faces together.

Once Floyd was satisfied that he had nearly kissed Ollie to death, he pulled away, and then both of them were panting from the intensity of it.

"You're safe," Floyd said, tipping their foreheads together. "Dog-gone-it, Ollie, I nearly lost myself to worriment on the way over here."

"Yes, I'm safe. I'm fine," Ollie said. "Mostly."

"Mostly?"

Floyd's hands fell to Ollie's shoulders, and Ollie let out a sound in between a scream and a cry, causing Floyd to recoil.

"Sorry," Ollie eked out. "Shoulder."

"How'd you manage that?"

"I'm not sure if you know this, but it's very hard to stop a one-hundred-ton coal car once it starts careening out of control. If you've ever considered trying to somehow catch it with your body, I really cannot stress enough how horrible of an idea that is."

Floyd's hands flew to cover his mouth, stifling a cry, and his entire body started to shake, images of the mine collapse in McDowell flitting through his mind.

Over the next few seconds, Floyd's body continued to tremble, his muscles eventually vibrating with so much intensity it seemed like a right miracle that he was still standing.

"I'm safe," Ollie said, reaching up to touch Floyd's forearms. "I'm hurt, but I'm safe." But Floyd could tell that Ollie was fighting back a wince. "Floyd, sit," Ollie said, his voice soft. "I'm safe."

While Ollie kept repeating those two wonderful words, Floyd moved past him into the kitchen area, now barely even hanging on to the present. More and more images of his past flashed in his mind, making him feel lightheaded. But Floyd forced himself to push through it. Because Ollie needed him now.

"You ought to be resting," Floyd said, whirling back around to face him. Only then did he notice the cuts on Ollie's hands. "Gosh, Ollie, what happened to your hands? Were you sorting coal?"

Ollie hooked his hands behind his back like he wanted to hide them. "Yeah, I was. Before I became the world's sorriest excuse for a spragger, that is."

All of a sudden, Floyd's teeth started to chatter, too, shaking right along with the rest of him.

"W-we need some g-goose grease," he said.

Ollie started toward him. "I have some, actually, but, uhm, I couldn't open it. You know, my shoulder . . ."

"I c-can open it for you."

"Sweetheart—"

Ollie reached out to stop him, but Floyd side-stepped his outstretched hand. Somehow, he managed to make it to the counter to fetch the jar, though his legs still felt so wobbly.

"Let me try one more—" Ollie's words were interrupted by the pop of the lid. "Don't worry about taking care of me. You're the one who should be resting. Look at you. You're shaking."

Once Floyd had the ointment ready, he pointed to the couch, wordlessly instructing Ollie to take a seat.

"Nah, I'm f-fine. I'm not the one hurt. N-not like you," Floyd said, coming to meet Ollie on the couch. "Gosh, your p-poor hands."

But the moment Floyd plopped himself onto the cushion, his trembling became worse. Ollie wrapped him up in a hug, hissing once, probably from the pain in his shoulder.

"S-sorry," Floyd said. "I was so worried on the way over. I think my b-body must be reacting funny to the fright I was feeling before. I k-kept picturing such horrible things. I k-keep picturing them now, too."

Ollie stroked Floyd's back and hushed him.

"I know, I know," he said.

"I'm so sorry, Ollie. I n-never ought to have treated you like that—screaming at you and telling you to leave."

"I shouldn't have yelled at you either, sweetheart," Ollie murmured next to Floyd's ear before pulling back and looking him in the eye. "I had it in my head that you were pushing me away. And, well, maybe you were, but I'm sure it wasn't intentional. I probably overreacted. I'm really sorry."

"I *was* pushing you away. Sort of on p-purpose, too."

"Oh," Ollie said, his voice sad and far away.

Floyd took a breath to calm himself and then he stuck his trembling fingers in the solidified fat. Taking Ollie's hands in his own, Floyd began working the salve onto his skin.

Minutes passed. Finally, Floyd's shaking started to slow, stopping only once those horrible memories stopped flashing in his brain. Thankfully, once Floyd's shaking stopped, his teeth stopped chattering too.

"Wasn't because of something you did," Floyd said, still massaging one of Ollie's hands. "Or because I ain't want to be with you no more. *Of course* I still want to be with you, Ollie, but . . ." He heaved a sigh. "But sometimes, when I'm with you, it feels like I'm losing Matt. And I know that he ain't here no more. I know he's . . ."

Floyd trailed off, one last image of the blocked tunnel flashing in his mind and cutting off his words.

"Don't force yourself to say it, Floyd."

"No, I need to." Floyd sucked in a long inhale through his nose and blew it out slowly, telling himself that he needed to face this. He'd been running from his sadness for much too long. "I know Matt is . . . I know Matt is dead." His voice cracked when he said it, right along with his heart. Tears sprang to his eyes, the pain in his chest now so intense he could barely breathe. Inhaling a shaky breath, he said, "Sorry. I never said it aloud before." As soon as the last word tumbled out of Floyd's mouth, he started to cry, and in only seconds, he was bawling, crying a whole eight years' worth of tears at once, and then his body started shaking from sadness instead of fear. "I ain't never said it," he repeated through a sob.

Ollie pulled his hands away, and then Floyd felt Ollie's arms wrap around him. Floyd fell into them, burying his face into the crook of Ollie's neck before a tiny squeak reminded him about Ollie's injury. And so, Floyd moved lower, first resting his head on Ollie's chest, and then letting it fall onto Ollie's lap, curling his legs up onto the couch in the process. He cried and cried and cried.

"I'm here, sweetheart," Ollie said, softly stroking Floyd's hair.

Those words had Floyd thinking of everything Ollie had said back in the mine, reminding him of the fact that he could have lost Ollie, too, which then had him crying even more. How could he have been such a fool?

Ollie, unaware that Floyd was now crying about nearly losing him, too, not only about having lost Matt, said, "I'm so sorry you lost him."

And Floyd wondered how Ollie could be so wonderful?

Over the next few minutes, Floyd continued to let himself cry. Tears poured from his eyes in a steady stream.

In between his sobs, he said, "I'm so sorry, Ollie."

"Don't be," Ollie said sweetly.

"Why'd he have to die? Why'd Matt have to die?" Floyd choked out. "He was my best friend."

"I know," Ollie said, caressing Floyd's wet cheek.

"I love him," Floyd said even though he felt so horrible for it. Ollie was right here loving him and caring for him and still, Floyd was crying about his lost friend. "I'm sorry for that. I'm sorry that I miss him."

"No, sweetheart. Don't ever be sorry for that."

"But you were right. You're here and Matt's not. And I been treating you so bad."

"You haven't been. Really." Ollie cupped Floyd's cheek to tilt Floyd's head so that he could look up at him. "And I *never* meant that you shouldn't miss him."

"What am I supposed to do with it, Ollie? I know it probably makes you feel bad that I still think about him, that I want to think about him, but I'm afeared that if I ain't careful, I'll forget him. And I never want to forget him."

"I won't let you forget him."

"Don't it make you sad that I love him?"

"No, not anymore," Ollie said. "For a little while, maybe, but that was wrong of me. I was feeling insecure. It wasn't ever really about the fact that you love Matt, but that I felt like you weren't letting me be your partner—your real partner—in the mine."

"I was only trying to keep you safe," Floyd said, sitting up. "I never told you this, but Matt . . ." He buried his head in his hands. "We were working together when I left to buy some black powder. Matt wanted to stay behind to collect some more coal, and there was . . ." Floyd felt a pinching in his chest, the memory cutting through him like a knife. "Oh God, Ollie, there was a cave in."

"Oh, fuck, I . . ." Ollie took Floyd's hand and squeezed. "I wish I knew what to say. I'm so sorry, sweetheart."

"I only ever wanted to keep you safe, Ollie," Floyd said through a sniffle.

"Gosh, Floyd, I know. I know that now. I won't let my insecurity hurt you like this again."

"Just tell me when you're feeling like that."

"I will. And I won't ever be sad about your love for Matt again. I promise." Ollie released Floyd's hand and started stroking his cheek instead, the back of his fingers caressing his skin. "Please never feel like you can't talk about him."

Floyd took Ollie's hand away from his face, worried that his stubble might irritate the redness, even though the majority of Ollie's injuries were on his palms.

"I won't," Floyd said before kissing Ollie's knuckles.

"For the last few weeks, I've been feeling like you were keeping something from me. Like you were keeping *yourself* from me. Because you hadn't been talking about Matt as much."

"Because I thought it'd hurt you. You seemed so sad when you found out Matt was my butty."

"I know," Ollie said. "I'm so mad at myself for that. Anytime you want to talk about Matt, I'll listen. Anytime you want to be sad about Matt, I'll be sad with you. Or not. Sometimes it's nice to be sad alone. I can understand that. So, it's, well, whatever you want, really. Just, please, let me in. Don't push me away like that."

"I won't push you away," Floyd said, leaning forward to kiss their foreheads together. He took a moment to breathe in Ollie's scent—sweet and musky and perfect—and then straightened up again. While it was true that he had picked a fight with Ollie intentionally, the subject matter—the scuffle between the miners and the coal operators and Chafin—really *had* been upsetting him. He figured it was time to tell Ollie the truth about everything, no matter how horrible it might make him seem. "I reckon I ought to tell you something else. Something that might make you not want to be with me no more."

"Nothing could make me not want to be with you," Ollie said. "You're my sweetheart."

"Maybe not once you hear this," Floyd said, shame creeping up the back of his neck, burning his skin and reddening his cheeks. "I . . . well, I heard that the UMWA wants to make things safer for us miners. Which is the right thing to do, I *know* it's the right thing to do, but . . . but it ain't fair to Matt." Floyd choked a sob but held the rest in, briefly covering his mouth with his free hand to try to keep himself from crying. Some seconds passed before he could remove it and continue. "I can't know whether some of them safety measures the UMWA is fighting for would have helped Matt, but it still makes me mad to think there could be changes. Because it's too late for him. I *hate* that it's too late for him."

"I'm so sorry." Ollie squeezed his hand. "For what it's worth, I think it's probably normal to feel the way you do. Or if it's not, well, who cares? Not me, certainly. I still love you. You're still my sweetheart, Floyd. You'll always be my sweetheart."

"Thanks, Ollie. I feel so bad for feeling this way. It's one of the reasons why I'm so upset whenever people bring up the UMWA maybe taking hold here in West Virginia. Everyone out here deserves better. I *know* that. I want better things for everyone, but—"

"But Matt deserved better, too."

Meeting Ollie's kind eyes, Floyd nodded. He wondered how he could be so lucky to find someone who seemed to understand. Minutes passed while Floyd let the wave of sadness recede, Ollie rubbing the back of Floyd's hand with his thumb in the meantime.

"Thanks, Ollie," Floyd finally said. "I'm feeling better now."

"Floyd, love," Ollie said, reaching up to cup Floyd's cheek. "I hope you won't dwell on the way things have been between us for the last week. I completely understand why you were pushing me away. And why you've been so mad whenever people have brought up the UMWA. I'm not mad at you. Not even a little." He tapped Floyd's nose with his index finger in a playful sort of way. "I *will* be mad at you if you stay mad at yourself, though. I can't have you beating yourself up for it. I've only experienced one slap from you and holy hell, was it painful."

Floyd huffed a short laugh, wiping the tears from his eyes. Ollie knew how to be funny at the exact perfect times.

"I won't," Floyd said. "I won't beat myself up, but more importantly, I won't never push you away like that again."

Ollie's mouth twisted up into a wry smile. "So you *will* push me away like that again."

Floyd had to restrain himself from shoving Ollie backward a little.

"I really missed you," Floyd said, and Ollie leaned forward to share a kiss. Feeling Ollie's soft lips on his own, Floyd let out a sigh, though eventually he forced himself to break their kiss so that he could look into Ollie's beautiful brown-green eyes. He kissed Ollie's nose and chin and cheek. "Gosh, I want to kiss you all over. I need to show you how much I missed you."

"Good," Ollie said, his smile so big his eyes were crinkling in the corners. "Because I want to kiss you all over, too."

Seeing Ollie's eye wrinkles—the little crevices in his coal-stained face—made Floyd remember how filthy both of them were. As he studied Ollie's skin, he hummed to himself and thought about how nice it might be to wash up together.

"Maybe we ought to clean ourselves first," Floyd said.

"Probably."

"I reckon a warm rag would feel nice on your shoulder, too."

"I like that idea."

"I'll fix everything up for us. You stay here and rest."

"You want me to try to rest on this lumpy couch? Fuck, sweetheart, I can't believe you'd want to punish me like that."

"Shut up, Ollie."

Ollie's hand flew to his chest. "It's like a knife to my heart."

Laughing, Floyd otherwise ignored that and set to work preparing the water, fetching some from the water pump and warming it on the stove. He filled the tin bath near to the brim.

When Floyd was finally finished, he called Ollie over. Ollie started to undress himself, but Floyd could tell that moving so much was bothering his shoulder, and so, Floyd worked to unfasten the rest of Ollie's shirt buttons himself. After Ollie's button-down shirt was off, Floyd worked to undress himself, too. Soon, they were both in their work pants, which Floyd then started to remove, his heart pitter-pattering from excitement the entire time.

Once they were both only wearing their undergarments and Floyd could see the outline of Ollie's half-hard cock beneath the silk fabric, he realized that he was finally ready for something more.

"Can I take these off?" Floyd asked, tugging on the front button.

"Yeah?"

"Only if you want me to."

"Of course I want you to."

Working the first button, Floyd could see that Ollie's cock had already begun to stiffen some more. His own cotton undergarments were becoming tighter, too. As soon as Floyd unfastened the final button, Ollie's cock sprang free. Floyd stared at it for a while, forgetting to breathe.

"I, uh, I hope it's . . . satisfactory?" Ollie said, probably because Floyd was being so quiet.

For some reason, Floyd couldn't think of what to say. He just kept staring in wonderment at the beautiful sight before him. After a few more seconds of wordless staring, he had the sense to force himself to find a compliment, though Floyd thought that whatever he said would never really be enough.

"You have a real handsome cock, Ollie."

Ollie laughed. "Really?"

"Yeah. I'd touch you, but I ain't clean yet."

"Well, then, we better wash up."

Floyd reached for the cloth, but Ollie stopped him.

"What about you?" Ollie asked, moving his hand to the buttons on Floyd's one-piece undergarment. "Not that you have to, of course. It's perfectly fine if you aren't ready for that yet."

"I am. Just forgot, is all."

As Floyd unfastened the buttons, his stomach started to roll all over the place. Even though Ollie had touched him a couple of times, Ollie still hadn't *seen* him. All of a sudden, Floyd felt worried for some reason. Ollie's cock was pretty, like the rest of him was pretty. His own cock had never seemed very pretty to him. He hoped Ollie would like it.

As soon as Floyd's cock was visible, he looked up to see Ollie's reaction, only to be met with what he thought were the hungriest, most lustful looking eyes he had ever seen.

"Jesus, sweetheart," Ollie said, the corner of his mouth curling up into the most adorable half-smile. "Is that really for me?"

"All for you," Floyd said, his stomach flip-flopping when he said it.

Floyd was still wriggling out of his undergarments when one of Ollie's hands came up to snake around his neck. Ollie's mouth claimed his with a kiss. Lips still locked with Ollie's, Floyd fumbled for the washing cloth. Once he found it, he plunged his hand into the water and then broke their kiss so that he could wring it out properly.

He touched the cloth to Ollie's shoulder, coaxing forth a thankful-sounding moan.

"Thank you for suggesting this," Ollie said. "God, that feels so nice."

Floyd sighed. "I'm sorry you were hurt today. I ought to have protected you."

"From my own clumsiness?"

"It was wrong for me to send you away like that," Floyd said, removing the cloth to reveal a smattering of black and blue and purple. Leaning forward, he lightly touched his lips to the newly formed bruise. "I hope I ain't hurting you now."

"Not at all."

Floyd kissed Ollie's shoulder once more and then submerged the cloth in the water.

Over the next few minutes, Floyd slowly ran the cloth over Ollie's body, feeling like he was not only cleaning away the sweat and the coal dust, but everything that was bad about the last week. After Floyd finished cleaning Ollie's body, Ollie took the rag from him and cleaned Floyd's. He moved real slow, probably because of his shoulder, but Floyd wondered if maybe Ollie was trying to savor this time together, too.

"You're so beautiful, sweetheart," Ollie said in the kindest, most tender voice.

It felt nice to be admired in the way that Ollie was admiring him. Even though Floyd liked himself plenty, it was still a nice feeling to know that Ollie liked him plenty, too.

"Bedroom?" Ollie asked when he was finished.

"Yeah," Floyd said, taking the wet cloth and dropping it into the water. "Let me carry you."

Ollie wrapped his arms around Floyd's neck, and Floyd hoisted Ollie into the air, reminding himself not to move too fast. Ollie's legs wrapped around him, and Ollie nuzzled the side of Floyd's face.

"Thank you," Ollie whispered.

Soon, they were in bed together, and Floyd climbed on top of Ollie, which was kind of new for them. Ollie probably couldn't hold himself up much because of his shoulder, though, so Floyd wasn't minding the newness, really, even though he normally loved when Ollie took control. Floyd started peppering kisses all over Ollie's face and neck and chest, pausing for a moment before moving lower.

"I want to take care of you," Floyd said. "Can I?"

"I'd like to take care of you, too," Ollie said, some sadness in his voice.

Floyd came up to kiss that sadness away, first lightly pressing his lips to Ollie's hurt shoulder and then kissing him once on his plump, pink lips.

"We'll figure something out even with your shoulder like that," Floyd said. "But let me care for you first. I been pushing you away when you needed me to love you. I feel so bad about that. I want to show you how important you are to me, Ollie. I want you to know how much you mean to me."

Ollie pulled Floyd in for another kiss. Floyd continued to kiss him for a while, rolling his hips to massage his erection against Ollie's thigh. He was so happy, so excited for the two of them to be close again that he could feel himself inching toward the edge already.

Remembering that he wanted to focus on Ollie, Floyd broke their kiss and moved lower on the mattress, coming to hover above Ollie's cock.

"Tell me what you need."

CHAPTER FOURTEEN

OLIVER

TELL ME WHAT YOU need.

For those first few seconds, Oliver had trouble finding his words. What did he need? Anything. Everything. For the majority of his life, people had been telling him what he needed—the salad fork, not the fish fork; piano lessons, not cello; a homburg, not a fedora; and on and on—and now Floyd was sweetly hovering above his cock, asking what it was that he needed. God, Floyd looked so magnificent like that—his eyes hungry, his hair a mess, his lips slightly pursed.

"Kiss me," Oliver finally managed.

Before Oliver could even clarify that he meant on his cock, Floyd's lips brushed the tip and the sensation made Oliver shudder, excitement rolling through his body like thunder. Floyd wrapped a hand around Oliver's length, slowly pulling back the foreskin, and then he planted another kiss on Oliver's naked head.

"Oh, sweetheart, your lips are so soft," Oliver said, enthralled by the sight before him.

Floyd kissed him once more.

"Can I lick you, Ollie?" Floyd asked, his low voice husky and raw.

Oliver kind of wanted to kick him for that. Why the hell was he even asking? But then, Oliver looked into Floyd's big blue eyes, so wide and caring, and realized how much he loved that Floyd was considerate enough to ask. He was probably the most selfless person Oliver had ever met. Oliver could ask him to do whatever he wanted, and fucking hell, he would do it, too.

"Yes, sweetheart, I'd love that."

Oliver watched Floyd's tongue slowly encircle the head of his cock. Feeling the wet warmth slide over his skin sent hot tremors of pleasure rippling through him, each exquisite enough that Oliver thought he might finish on the spot.

"I want you to take me into your mouth," Oliver said before realizing that he'd better be more specific since he was already so close. "Slowly. Please."

As soon as Floyd's mouth was around him, Oliver sucked in a breath. Bucking his hips, Oliver clutched the sheets tightly, as though they could tether him to the earth, even though with every passing second, Floyd's beautiful mouth was bringing him closer to heaven. Floyd bobbed his head. Once. Twice. Three times. With each repetition, Oliver's cock moved farther toward the back of his throat. On the fourth, Floyd made a little choking sound, and, *fuck*, it was so perfect, Oliver thought that he might collapse.

"Shit," Oliver rasped.

"Hm?"

Floyd was looking up at Oliver with slightly teary eyes, his lips still stretched over the head of Oliver's cock, and Oliver was hit with a fierce rush of fondness.

"Just trying to say that it feels nice," Oliver said, reaching to sweep a hand through Floyd's hair. "You're doing so well, sweetheart. I love it. Keep going."

Floyd turned his attention back to Oliver's cock, continuing to take him into his mouth, his nose bumping Oliver's pelvic area with every few bobs of his head.

"Use your hand, too," Oliver said. "Please."

As soon as Floyd's strong hand wrapped around his shaft, Oliver lifted his hips off the mattress, nearly climaxing. God, Floyd was so strong. It was evident even in what was a fairly light grip.

"Christ, Floyd, you're incredible," Oliver moaned, his hips lifting once more.

Floyd removed his mouth, and a thin thread of spittle lingered, stretching between the head of Oliver's cock and Floyd's lips for the briefest second before falling away. It was probably the single most exciting thing Oliver had ever seen in his life.

"Oh, shit," Oliver whispered, his eyebrows knitting together, warm heat pooling low.

"Do you want me faster?" Floyd asked, his voice rough.

"Yes, yes, oh my God, yes," Oliver responded in a pleading tone. "I'm so close."

Floyd obliged.

In seconds, Oliver's hips were squirming against the mattress, the feeling of pressure making his cock ache for release. Exhaling a ragged breath, Oliver threaded his fingers through Floyd's locks, unable to hold the least bit still anymore. When his hips rose up again, one of Floyd's forearms came to rest across Oliver's pelvis, pinning him down.

"Oh, God," Oliver said, barely able to stop himself from begging Floyd to remove it. He tried to let Floyd hold him in place but couldn't. "It's too much. I can't take it. I . . ."

All of a sudden, Oliver's thigh started to shake, something that had never happened in intimacy, and then his cock started to pulse. He cried out Floyd's name, followed by a whispered string of expletives, and emptied himself into Floyd's mouth.

When Floyd pushed himself to his knees, Oliver saw that magnificent cock of his sticking straight out, the moist head practically crying for attention.

"Come up here, sweetheart," Oliver said.

He struggled to sit up as Floyd walked up toward Oliver on his knees. Soon, Floyd's cock was right in front of him. He moved to touch it but stopped himself.

"Can I take care of you now?" Oliver asked.

Floyd nodded. "Yeah."

As soon as Oliver's hand was on Floyd's cock, he let out the most exquisite moan. Oliver was only able to rub him a few times before Floyd scooted forward more, urging his cock toward Oliver's lips. After a pause, Oliver kissed the head, but then moved his mouth away.

"Oh, God, Ollie, *please*," Floyd said.

"Language," Oliver chastised playfully. "Naughty."

Floyd's thumb brushed Oliver's lips. "Please."

"Of course."

So, Oliver took Floyd into his mouth, and over the next few minutes, Floyd slowly but surely lost himself to pleasure, moaning words like "shit" and "Jesus," even once saying the wonderful phrase "I love seeing my cock in your mouth, Ollie," which wasn't too naughty, Oliver supposed, though it was still Goddamn wonderful to hear.

When Floyd came, Oliver happily swallowed every drop.

Floyd climbed off him and collapsed onto the bed. Dazed and happy, Oliver rolled onto his side—onto his uninjured shoulder—to face Floyd, who immediately reached up to touch his hair.

"Ollie," Floyd said, threading his fingers through it. "I love you."

Oliver smiled. "I love you, too, sweetheart." Oliver closed his eyes to bask in the perfection of this moment. "God, I love you so, so much."

As Oliver let himself enjoy the soft care of Floyd's touches, he found his mind circling back to Floyd's love confession—the one for Matt. It hurt Oliver's heart to know that Floyd had been hurting for so long, both before Oliver had met him, and then, all throughout the time when the two of them had been falling in love. It was so heartbreaking to know that Floyd had been keeping so much love and loss inside of him. Oliver never wanted Floyd to feel like he had to lose Matt in order to keep him. Or that by being close with him, he was losing someone who had been so very important in his life.

"I meant what I told you earlier," Oliver said. "About never letting you forget Matt."

Oliver could tell by the look on Floyd's face how much that meant to him. After one more brush through Oliver's hair, Floyd hooked his hand around the back of Oliver's neck and pulled him in for a soft kiss on the lips—an unspoken "thank you."

Maybe a few weeks ago, Oliver would have left it at that. His insecurities would have prevented him from wanting to really follow through with that promise, especially if it involved talking about the person he had come to think of as a bit of an adversary. But Oliver had overcome much of that. After all, Floyd had spent the last half hour trying very hard to impress upon Oliver just how *much* he cared for him. Now it was Oliver's turn to show Floyd the same.

"Sweetheart," Oliver began, his heart beating faster in his chest, feeling both excited and scared to have Floyd talk about the love that he had lost, "can you tell me about him?"

Floyd sat up on his elbow. "Really?"

"Yes," Oliver said. "Please."

"What do you want to know?"

"Anything. Everything. All I know so far is that he liked to collect pocket watches and stamps and coins. Oh, and that he was a miner."

Oliver watched Floyd's hand come up to stroke his chin, which was such a fucking lovable habit of his. Oliver knew it meant that Floyd was being thoughtful about his response.

Floyd eventually said, "He was shy. Quiet."

"Quieter than you, even?"

"Yeah," Floyd said with a snort. "Hard to believe, huh?"

"Nah, you're not so quiet. Only compared to me, maybe."

"Matt was blunt, too."

"Wow, if *you're* calling him blunt—"

"I know." Floyd was chuckling now, which made Oliver feel so happy. God, he loved hearing Floyd be so open about Matt like this. "Hm, what else can I tell you?" Floyd ran a hand over his face and hummed. "He had this real coarse hair. Copper color." Suddenly, Floyd had a strange look about him, like he had only just realized something important. "Copper color. Jeez." He started to laugh.

It was making Oliver smile even more. "What?"

"Ah, I can't tell you."

"Come on, yes, you can."

"*Don't* laugh."

"Well, that I can't promise, especially now that you've told me *not* to!" Oliver started chuckling. "See?"

"Well, when I met you, I kept . . ." Floyd snorted. "I kept having this stomachache whenever I was with you. I think it was because I was feeling bad about liking you. Whenever it happened, I would . . ." Floyd pointed a finger at him. "*Don't* laugh."

"Alright, alright, tell me."

"I'd imagine that there was a snake in my stomach, like a copperhead."

"Gross," Oliver said, laughing a little.

"It's real hard not to shove you right now," Floyd warned, though from the way his whole face was lit up with happiness, it was clear that he was having fun. "Anyway, I think I pictured a copperhead because of Matt. You know, his copper-colored hair. Like Matt was mad about me liking you."

Oliver wrinkled his nose. "Well, that's a little sad. I feel bad if Matt is up there in heaven hating me for being with you."

"Oh, he ain't mad now," Floyd said, taking Oliver's hand and kissing it. "No more copperhead."

"Phew." Oliver squeezed Floyd's hand. "Well, so, tell me more about him, then."

"Hm, well, he liked everyone. Or . . . I need to think of how to say it. Sexually, Matt *could* have liked anyone."

Oliver thought for a moment. "Do you mean that Matt thought men and women were both attractive?"

"See, you're better at putting things into words than me."

"I thought you two were together since you were kids. How do you know Matt found both sexes attractive?"

"He'd tell me," Floyd said, bursting out laughing. "Golly, I hated that."

Now Oliver was laughing. "He'd *tell* you?"

"Yep. Matt'd come right up to me and ask, *'What do you think of Ruth Walker?'* and I'd say *'What do you mean, what do I think of her? She seems nice enough, I suppose.'* And Ollie, I swear to you he'd respond with something like, *'I think she's handsome. I like her butt, too.'*"

Oliver couldn't stop cackling. "Oh my God, Floyd, you must have been so mad."

"It took some time for that sort of thing not to bother me, especially once we were saying I love you to each other," Floyd said with a shake of his head. "He wasn't trying to be hurtful or nothing. Just honest. Looking back, I think Matt had some trouble understanding how other people might have felt about things he said or did. But if you told him something upset you, he'd come around and say sorry. Well, most of the time." Floyd rolled his eyes. "Never could seem to stop telling me who he thought was handsome."

"Jeez, I'm sorry."

"Ain't your fault. I stopped minding over time. When we were older, I kind of made a game out of it. I'd try to work out who Matt might have thought was handsome at one time or another. I'd see someone, and instead of wondering whether or not I found them attractive, I'd try to figure out if Matt might like them. I'd even ask him if I was right or not."

"Wise beyond your years. Or foolish. I'm not sure which."

Floyd made a face that Oliver knew was probably supposed to be a threatening one—furrowing his brows and narrowing his eyes—only he was still smiling too much for it to be convincing. Holy hell, he was adorable.

"I really would shove you if you weren't injured," Floyd said.

"I'll remind you to punish me somehow when it's better."

Floyd reached up to stroke Oliver's cheek. "You and Matt ain't barely alike."

"Is that one of the reasons you pushed me away?"

"Mm-hmm. It felt like I was betraying him in some way."

"Do you think Matt would have hated me?"

Floyd chewed on his bottom lip, thinking.

"I think Matt would have told me that he thought you had a nice butt," Floyd joked.

"Nice butt *but* talks too much, right?" Oliver teased right back, and then Floyd ruffled up his hair.

"Nah, you talk exactly the right amount. I love it." Floyd started kissing Oliver's arm. "Matt wouldn't have hated you. You're a kind person, Ollie. He'd have seen that."

"Thank you," Oliver said, a little amazed that he was able to accept the compliment without immediately wanting to push back. "Floyd, I love you."

Finally, Floyd stopped kissing Oliver's arm. "And I love you, Ollie."

Somehow, Oliver was able to accept that, too.

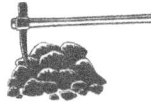

Hours later, Oliver was pacing back and forth from the bedroom to the living room, basically ready to explode with excitement for Floyd to come back.

Moments later, there was a knock. After hurrying over, Oliver threw open the door and lunged forward, flinging his arms around Floyd and knocking him back a step, a spark of pain shooting out from his shoulder in the process.

Oliver made a little "eep" sound from the sudden surge of pain before saying, "What took you so long, lunkhead?"

Floyd chuckled next to his ear, and the low reverberations of Floyd's laughter sent tingles up Oliver's spine.

"Missed me that much, huh?" Floyd patted Oliver on the back. "Come on, Ollie, inside."

Reluctantly, Oliver let Floyd go before they went inside.

"Someone could have seen us, silly," Floyd said, and Oliver was relieved that he sounded more playful than mad. "I had to put Jo to bed, and then I wanted to talk to Effie."

"Was Effie upset that you missed supper?"

Instead of responding, Floyd held up one of his fingers, signaling Oliver to wait. After fishing around in his pocket, he pulled out two nails.

"She told me you can be the one to use 'em," Floyd said. "Last thing she needs is to clean up a bunch of blood off the floor."

Oliver snorted. "Ah, so you told her about our whole Dostoevsky thing."

"Yup."

With a shake of his head, Oliver thumbed over his shoulder toward the kitchen.

"Would you set those down somewhere, please? I'm clumsy enough to follow through with stabbing one of us if you keep holding onto them."

Floyd headed over to the kitchen. After setting the nails on the countertop, he picked a piece of paper and the envelope that Oliver had left there earlier.

"What's this?"

"Just a letter from my Aunt Betty. I've been writing to her."

"Ah, I remember you said you went to visit her."

"Yeah, she's . . . Floyd, she's wonderful. I mean, maybe she's a bit terse sometimes, but she's kind," Oliver said. "I'm really happy to have her in my life again. I can't believe I found someone in my family who isn't terrible. I'm so thankful for it."

Looking at the envelope, Floyd nodded, smiling warmly.

"Yeah, me, too, Ollie. I'm real happy for you."

Oliver came up behind him and wrapped his arms around him.

"Sweetheart, I missed you," Oliver said softly, close to Floyd's ear. "Can I show you how much I missed you?"

Without even a word, Floyd whirled around and captured Oliver's mouth in a kiss.

CHAPTER FIFTEEN

FLOYD

ONE MORNING IN SEPTEMBER, Floyd left Ollie's house early to find some breakfast for the two of them—something easy for Ollie to cook before they went to work together. Moving through the company store, Floyd started humming a tune to himself, happy that everything had been so much better over the past weeks. Ollie and he were so much more open with each other now. Honesty had made their relationship stronger than ever.

While placing eggs into his basket, Floyd felt a hand come to rest atop his shoulder.

"Morning, Floyd," Roy said.

Even though Roy's tone was friendly, there was an edge to it. He was narrowing his eyes like he was waiting to scrutinize Floyd's response, too.

"Morning, Roy," Floyd said, trying not to let on that Roy was making him uncomfortable. "How're the wife and kids?"

"Fine. How's your wife?"

"Uh, not bad," Floyd said. Obviously, there was more to Roy's comment than was being said. Floyd hoped he could change the subject. "Do you always shop so early?"

"Sometimes." Roy crossed his arms over his chest before looking around the store, maybe confirming that it was empty except for the two of them and Charlie, who was behind the register. In a whispered voice, he said, "I seen you sleeping over at Oliver's house a few times these past weeks."

Floyd's blood ran cold, fear starting to prickle his skin.

"Naw, we like to play cards late sometimes, is all."

Pursing his lips, Roy hummed like he was thinking that over, and then he clicked his tongue and said, "You know, our homes, them walls ain't as thick as you might think." Floyd swallowed thickly, shame and fear closing around his throat. "Ain't a problem for me, Floyd, so long as you keep it private. Other people, they might not take too kindly to that sort of relationship. I like you, and I like Oliver, too, so I'm taking the time to warn you. You two best be more careful. You never know who might be watching. Or listening."

Roy turned and left, not even waiting for a response. Little colorful spots began obscuring Floyd's vision, his heart beating so ferociously that he could hear the blood whooshing past his eardrums. He finished shopping as fast as he could.

When he arrived back at Ollie's house, Ollie was sipping a mug of coffee at the breakfast table.

"I hope you're ready for my mediocre eggs. Assuming you found some," Ollie said cheerfully as Floyd kicked off his boots. When Floyd looked up, the two of them locked eyes, and Ollie's face fell. "Something's wrong."

"Yeah," Floyd admitted, setting the poke on the floor before pulling out a chair. "Roy knows about us."

"I'm sorry—what?"

"I seen him at the company store this morning. He, uh, must have heard something." Floyd cleared his throat. "Something interesting."

Oliver's hands flew to cover his mouth.

"Oh my God," he said, the words muffled by his palms.

Floyd reached over to pull them away.

"Roy won't say nothing. But we need to be more careful."

"God, I wish we could be ourselves here. Or, hell, anywhere."

"Me, too," Floyd said, a heaviness in his heart.

Ollie slid a mug of coffee across the table to Floyd. As Floyd moved to sip it, Ollie took the eggs from the poke and brought them over to the stove. One by one, he took them out of the pickling lime and rinsed them in some water.

While Ollie cooked, Floyd read over the newspaper. Still not a peep about the whole battle that had taken place over at Blair Mountain. Seemed like the coal companies in the region were trying to keep the news from reaching the miners, which was kind of silly since the miners had lost the battle, but, well, the coal companies probably were concerned about their image.

Funny how certain images were so important to keep.

"Hey, Ollie?"

"Just a second," Ollie said before cursing under his breath. "Well, so much for over easy. Scrambled it is."

Smiling, Floyd shook his head. Jeez, he couldn't have loved Ollie more in that moment if he had tried.

"Take your time."

A couple of minutes later, Ollie came back to the table with two plates of eggs.

"I'm sorry about my faux pas with the yolks. They're kind of half-scrambled, half-overcooked now."

"Ah, they look tasty enough," Floyd said, which wasn't really true, but eggs were eggs. He started prodding them with his fork, though his stomach was still too sour from his encounter with Roy to eat. "Gosh, I wish people were more accepting."

"Sweetheart, can I ask you something?"

"Anything."

Rather than bursting out whatever it was he wanted to ask, Ollie started chewing on his bottom lip, which was pretty unlike him. Floyd could tell how nervous he was. Hoping to provide some kind of reassurance, Floyd reached for Ollie's hand, lacing their fingers together.

Seconds ticked by on the clock, and then Ollie said, "Well, it looks like there's no chance of UMWA taking hold here in Logan County or maybe even in West Virginia now that the whole horrible fight happened, and sweetheart, I want something better for us. I like mining together. Really. I love working with you. I love the challenge of mining. I love the way your butt looks when you're shoveling coal." Floyd couldn't help but let out a little snort at that. "But I want a better life for us, especially now that I know that we need to be more careful not to let on about what we are to each other. I mean, will you even be able to stay over anymore?"

"I . . ." Floyd's words caught in his throat. Truthfully, he had no idea whether they'd be able to spend as much time together now, especially not overnights. "I can't say."

"Our community here, everyone has been very nice to me, but it's so small, and people here, they probably won't ever accept us. And now, it feels like everyone is watching us." Ollie's voice shook a little when he was saying this, which hurt Floyd's heart. "I'll stay here forever if that's what you want, but . . . would you ever want to start a new life somewhere else? With me? And Effie and Jo, too, of course. I know you said you never wanted to leave the coal industry, though, so I completely understand if—"

Floyd found himself answering without the slightest bit of hesitation, wanting nothing more than to be with Ollie and to relieve him of the sadness he was feeling. "Yeah, Ollie, I'd like that."

"Really?" Ollie's eyes started tearing. "Well, where? I think I have enough money to take us wherever you want within reason. Oh my God, I still can't believe it. Really?"

"Yeah, really. I can't stand the thought of not spending nights with you no more. I want a better life for us, too." He pushed his chair out and tugged on Ollie's hand, coaxing him to come closer, and as soon as Ollie stood, Floyd pulled him onto his lap. "But I won't take your money."

"Ugh, sweetheart, please stop being stubborn about money."

"Well, I suppose I could let you help a little, but I been responsible for Effie and Jo for forever. I been the one to take care of them all these years."

"Which is why you should allow me to help. I want to take care of you. And that wonderful family of yours. Effie is such a treasure to let us be together. I owe her everything—more wealth than I could ever even *dream* of cobbling together."

"I'll think on it."

"Stubborn as a mule," Ollie said with a sigh. "Alright, yes, please think about it."

Floyd looked up at Ollie, who bent down to nuzzle their noses together, and then Floyd rested his head against Ollie's chest, letting his thoughts wander as Ollie stroked his hair.

"Are you scared of starting over?" Ollie asked.

"Yeah, a little," Floyd said. He took a slow breath in and out through his nose, trying to calm his hammering heart. "It's hard not knowing our future. Like whether we'll find a place where we can be together. Or whether we can make a new home for the four of us."

"It's like our path forward is completely unknowable. Like we're inside of a rickety coal elevator, heading for the bottom of the mine." Ollie cupped Floyd's chin and lifted it, forcing Floyd to meet his eyes. "But maybe that's fine for us, sweetheart. We're coal miners. We make our own light." Ollie smiled sweetly. "We'll make it through."

"I hope so," Floyd said, smiling back at him and feeling some of his fear fade. "I feel like I can make it if I have you with me, Ollie."

"You'll have me forever."

Floyd pulled Ollie in for a kiss. Ollie'd have him forever, too.

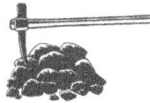

One hour later, Floyd left for home. He and Ollie thought that they ought to skip work so that Floyd could talk to Effie about everything. Floyd had come up with an idea for where they all could move to, but Effie would need to agree to it. If Effie wanted to stay in Rock Creek, then they would stay, even if it meant that he and Ollie would have to live without seeing each other as much.

By the time Floyd reached the house, Jo had already left for school. Effie was up on a step stool reorganizing one of the cupboards. When she heard him come in, she looked over her shoulder, one of her eyebrows raised inquisitively.

"Why're you back here so early? Did you forget some of your work supplies?"

"Nah, me and Ollie ain't working today. I need to talk to you about something."

"Oh." Effie climbed off the stool. "What is it?"

"Let's sit for this," Floyd said, heading to the couch. "Ain't nothing bad. Don't worry."

"Alright."

After sitting beside him, Effie smoothed out her dress. Floyd took one of her hands.

"I want you to know that our family comes first. Always."

"Floyd, you're scaring me a little."

"But I need to tell you that I feel a forever kind of way about Ollie. It's why I been spending so much time with him, staying over and such, but I need to be more present for you and Jo, too. So, now I'm trying to work out how I can both be with Ollie and make sure you never feel like you're raising Jo all by yourself."

"I never feel that way."

"I know, but *I* feel that way. I hate that I sometimes can't make it back before she heads off to school. I hate that I'm not here for her when she wakes up in the night."

"You're here for supper and evenings and weekends."

"I want more. In a whole bunch of ways, I want more. I want to find me a safer job. I want to be able to spend nights with Ollie without prying eyes."

"Prying eyes? What're you talking about?"

"Roy seems to know 'bout us," Floyd admitted, which elicited a small gasp from Effie. "He said he wouldn't tell no one, but he warned me that I ought to be more careful."

"Oh, Lord."

"So, I been thinking, what if we move somewhere else?"

"Won't we have the prying eyes problem wherever we live?"

"Yeah, we will, but maybe not as bad if we have some real land." Effie narrowed her eyes, probably trying to work out what he was suggesting. "What would you say to me taking up farming? I know enough from when I helped out my folks. Even when I worked as a breaker boy and such, I still spent plenty of weekends helping my pop."

"I . . . I mean, I . . ."

"I know it'd be a change, but I thought maybe we'd like having the space. If we move somewhere new, no one needs to know that

Ollie and me are what we are. Maybe we can tell people we're related. Or maybe we won't say nothing, and no one will even ask."

"So, you want Oliver to live with us?"

"We can buy a big house. Bigger than this one."

"How are we supposed to afford all this?"

"Ollie can. Not that I'm happy 'bout taking his money, but it's probably the only way. He has enough for a few acres of land. Heck, he has enough that even leaner years shouldn't be a problem for us." Floyd's eyes flitted over to the bookcase. "I can find me some money, too. Enough for a few pieces of farm equipment, maybe, or a couple of horses or mules. Think of it, Effie, we can farm oats like both our families used to, maybe raise some chickens, plant a few fruit trees. We could be so happy living like that. I know we could."

"So, you and Ollie'd run a whole farm?"

"We could try. You know, they even have them self-propelled harvesters now. I remember my folks wanting one before we left so they wouldn't need so many horses or farmhands," Floyd said. "I know our farm couldn't be too big if it was only me and Ollie, but we would run it fine."

"When'd you start thinking about this?"

"Only this morning. But years ago, me and Matt had talked about running our own farm. I'd be . . . well . . . I'd be living out our future this way. Used to be that I thought Matt would be mad at me if I ever left the coal industry without him, but now, I reckon maybe he's happy to see me happy. I like to think that he's up there in heaven feeling proud of me for finding someone as nice as Ollie. And for continuing to take care of you and Jo, too."

Floyd squeezed Effie's hand as he waited for her response.

"What would we tell Josephine? Would we tell her about you and Ollie?"

"I reckon we'd have to." Floyd ran his free hand over his face. "Golly, that's a scary thought. Do you think she'll hate me?"

"She'd never hate you. Ever."

"We'd have to tell her not to tell no one. Do you think she could keep a secret like this?"

"I'm not sure. Hopefully she can. For everyone's sakes." Effie blew out a forceful sigh, shaking her head. "Floyd, this plan of yours, you're making it sound simple, but it ain't without risk."

"I know. But I want to try." Floyd stared into Effie's uncertain baby blues. "Just like them miners over in the other counties have been fighting for a better life, I'm ready to fight for my better life, too. I have to hope we'll have more luck than they had. I know we could lose a lot. But, Effie, I really, *really* want to try."

Effie thought for a minute before blowing out a breath. "Alright, Floyd Bennett, I reckon we can live on a farm."

Floyd's face broke into the biggest smile. Gosh, he was so happy. Smiling back, Effie pulled him in for a hug.

"Well, that means I only have one more thing I need to do today." Floyd pulled back and walked over to the bookcase. He took out Matt's coin-collecting book. "I suspect it'll mean that you'll need to find a couple more nails, though."

"Oh yeah? Why's that?"

Effie was still smiling so big, her entire face lit up with what looked to be excitement. It made him happy to see it.

"Because I might not be back for supper. I'm heading to Charleston."

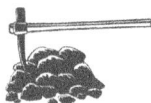

Standing on the front porch of Betty Astor's home, Floyd took a moment to compose his thoughts. Golly, was he lucky to have been blessed with such a sharp memory. Without even meaning to, he had remembered the name of Betty Astor's street, coupled with her house number. All it had taken was seeing these things written out on that envelope he'd found on Ollie's kitchen counter. At the time, he hadn't known how much he'd soon need them.

Now, even though Floyd had no way of knowing whether Ollie's relative might be willing to purchase Matt's coin collection, he still had to hope that he could convince her to buy it from him. Floyd felt certain that Betty could eventually sell the coins herself and make a profit. Floyd, though, couldn't very well afford the time it would take to find individual buyers his own self. He simply couldn't be frittering money away on newspaper advertisements. He had no time to seek out the various coin collectors in West Virginia who might be interested in purchasing one or two of Matt's coins. He was ready for his future to start *now*.

After one more long exhale, Floyd knocked. Moments later, someone who he assumed was Ollie's Aunt Betty answered.

"Hi. Are you Ms. Astor?" he asked.

"Yes?"

"I'm a friend of Ollie's."

One of her eyebrows ticked up ever-so-slightly. "Are you Floyd?"

"Oh, uh, yeah. I mean, yes, ma'am. I wasn't aware that Ollie already told you 'bout me."

"How can I help you?"

"I have a proposition of sorts."

"Oh?" she remarked, sounding intrigued.

Floyd nodded. "Mm-hmm."

"Hm. Come in."

As Floyd followed her through her house, he had to fight to keep his hands from shaking. Something about her made him real nervous. Aside from Ollie and the Donohues, Floyd hadn't really spent much time with people who had a lot of money. Seeing the way Ollie's Aunt Betty carried herself and the large home she lived in was making him feel small. He wondered how silly he'd seem to her offering Matt's coin-collecting book. It looked like she could afford plum near anything she wanted. What need would she have for the bit of extra money could make from these little old coins?

Aunt Betty led him to a room filled with books. Floyd had never seen so many in one place before. He reckoned there was probably more knowledge on only one of the shelves than he had stored up in his entire brain.

They took a seat next to one another on a soft green couch.

Floyd cleared his throat and said, "I came here to see if you would be interested in purchasing this here coin-collecting book. I know you probably ain't a coin collector, but I need the money faster than I could make selling each of these my own self. I thought that maybe you could take your time finding some buyers here in Charleston or even elsewhere in West Virginia. You ought to be able to make some sort of profit that way."

"And for what purpose do you need the money?"

"I'm trying to buy a farm for my family, ma'am."

Wordlessly, Aunt Betty held out her hand—a silent request to look through Matt's book. Floyd hesitated for a few seconds before handing it over. When the book left his possession, it felt a little like he had lost a piece of himself. It took some effort not to let it show. Holding his breath, Floyd watched her flip through the pages.

After looking at a couple, she asked, "Are you and Oliver happy together?"

"Uh, excuse me?" Floyd felt heat blooming on his cheeks. "What?"

"If you're worried about me being scandalized by two men having a romantic relationship, you can rest assured that I am not." Floyd hesitated before eventually managing a nod in response, and then Aunt Betty continued on. "So, I will ask you one more time: Are you and Oliver happy together?"

"Yes. Very."

"Then why on earth would you want to leave Rock Creek? Won't Oliver miss you?"

"He's coming with me. I want us to buy a farm together."

She hummed. "Mostly with his money, I assume."

Floyd's face was still burning, though now it was from shame. "Yeah. Mostly."

"And you said you have a family?"

"Yes, ma'am. I'm married to my best friend Effie. We have a little girl named Josephine." Floyd reached up to scratch his head. "I know how strange this must sound, but Effie and me are only friends. She knows about Ollie. In fact, she likes him. I talked to her about everything before coming here. She ain't got a problem with me and Ollie running a farm together."

"Why not continue to live in Rock Creek, though?"

"Well, I want something better for us. All of us. Me and Ollie can't really be together in such a small community. Everyone's homes are close together, and everybody knows everybody's business. It's not like me and Ollie can pretend that we're related neither. Everyone knows we only met earlier this year. Somebody in town came to me recently and, well, it seems like me and Ollie were probably being a bit too obvious about, uh, about what we are to each other." Floyd bounced his leg as he tried to think of how to phrase what he wanted to say. "I want the two of us to be together. I can't keep spending every workday pretending that he's not . . . that he's not what he is to me. I can't keep pretending I'm not in love with him. I want to live life more honestly than that.

And I reckon having some land to ourselves—some small acreage and our own farmhouse—could help."

Something he said must have struck a chord with her. All of a sudden, she was smiling warmly, the harsh lines of her face seeming to soften, and before Floyd could even utter another word, she reached over to pat his knee.

"I, too, value honesty, but people like us often cannot live our lives honestly, can we?"

Floyd shook his head, not entirely understanding what she meant. Aunt Betty patted his knee twice more and stood. When she left the room without explanation, taking the coin-collecting book with her, Floyd started twiddling his thumbs, wondering if he had somehow ruined everything.

Minutes later, Aunt Betty returned with a handsome woman by her side. Aunt Betty's companion was shorter than she was, with mousy brown hair, cut to her chin, and big brown eyes.

"Floyd, this is my friend, Mary," Aunt Betty said.

Floyd's eyes flew wide. "Oh!" He scrambled to his feet and held out his hand. Mary shook it, and Floyd looked over at Oliver's Aunt Betty before sputtering the first words that popped into his head. "You're like me."

Aunt Betty laughed. "Yes, that's one way to put it."

"Sorry, I've never met a woman who was . . ." He shook his head, still shocked and bewildered by this. "Does Ollie know?"

"Yes, he knows," she confirmed with a nod. "Mary here is Frederick Donohue's sister. I'm sure you've heard this by now, but Frederick was a friend of our family's." Floyd's mouth hung open as she continued on. "Frederick was the one who helped Mary and I start our life together here."

"Fred Donohue?!"

Floyd had a hard time believing that Frederick effing Donohue, as Ollie would have called him, had been so charitable.

"Yes," Aunt Betty said with a shrug, chuckling. "Surprising, I know. Frederick certainly has his flaws." She looked over at Mary again, her eyes suddenly filled with a whole lot of tenderness. It made Floyd happy to see that such a stern-looking woman had a lot of care inside her, only it was reserved for special people, like the woman she loved. After a moment, she looked back at Floyd. "When Oliver first showed up here, I was worried that he may have turned out like his father. For the entirety of his short visit, I was nervous that Mary would come home from the shops and I'd have to think of how to explain who this woman was. Mary and I are very careful about who we tell. When Oliver visited a second time, I had Mary hide away upstairs, and then, once Oliver let it slip that he was in love with a man, I introduced them."

"Ollie never told me."

"I'm sure he felt like it wasn't his place. Floyd, I liked what you said about living life honestly. Or, as honestly as people like us can in this world. I'm very glad that Oliver found someone like you—someone who seems to have integrity, someone who seems to be loyal to his family, someone who is honest. Henry, Oliver's father, is very much your opposite. I was pleased to learn that, even though Oliver is Henry's son, he seems to have matured into a kind, if not somewhat eccentric, person. In his case, the apple seems to have fallen fairly far from its tree."

"Rolled all the way to West Virginia," Floyd said with a nod, the corner of his mouth pulling up into a small smirk.

Aunt Betty hummed. "Indeed." She held up the coin book. "Shall we talk numbers?"

"Yes, ma'am. I'd like that."

As soon as they reached the couch, Floyd asked if he could see the book one last time. Heart heavy, he flipped through the pages, stopping when he reached the page with the illegible tin-colored coin. When his eyes flitted over to Matt's favorite one—the Flying

Eagle penny—he said a silent farewell. *I need to move forward now. Don't worry, though, Ollie'll never let me forget you. Not that I would have on my own. But his promise helps. I still love you, Matty. I always will.* Eyes brimming with tears, Floyd inhaled a quivering breath and removed the Ollie coin from its pouch.

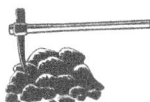

Hours later, when it was completely dark outside, Floyd hopped off the train and started through town. From up the road, Floyd could see Ollie's house, the little oil lamp on his porch shining like a beacon of hope. Seeing the way it twinkled—the lone light in the darkness—Floyd thought about what Ollie had told him about them making their own light. It really was true, wasn't it?

When Floyd reached the edge of Ollie's property, Ollie flung open the door.

"I have half a mind to pummel you for being so late. I was worried," Ollie said, sounding more relieved than mad. "Effie said you went to Charleston for some reason?"

"Yup," Floyd said, coming up the stairs. "I got a surprise for you."

"It's not a hat, is it?" Ollie asked as Floyd walked around him. "I kind of hope it is."

"Nope. Ain't a hat. It's better, I think." Floyd opened his wallet and took out the check. He handed it to Ollie, whose mouth immediately fell open. "I reckon we can buy ourselves a farm now. Not that this is enough for everything or, well, even most of everything, but I couldn't let you be the sole provider."

"I . . . what . . ."

Watching Ollie stumble over his words had Floyd beaming with pride. He couldn't help but puff out his chest a little.

"I sold Matt's coin-collecting book to your Aunt Betty."

Ollie shook his head. "What?"

"Don't worry, I kept the most important one."

Floyd reached into his pocket and took out the Ollie coin. With a flick of his thumb, he sent it sailing over to Ollie, who only barely managed to catch it. Slowly, Ollie turned it over in his hands, which then immediately started to tremble.

"Sweetheart . . ." Ollie's eyes were tearing up, which was making Floyd want to cry, too.

"I couldn't sell the Ollie coin," Floyd said, not even caring that a couple of tears were starting to escape. He hadn't never cried so much in his whole life as he had over the last weeks.

"Because it's trash," Ollie choked out, his cheeks becoming wet from tears.

Floyd came over and wrapped his arms around Ollie, pulling him close.

"Nah, it's the most valuable one, silly." He kissed the side of Ollie's head. "And our future is more important to me than all the rest of them old coins."

Ollie started sobbing, squeezing Floyd in return. Floyd let him cry for a while before pulling back to find Ollie's face with his hand.

"Are you ready to be a farmer with me, city boy?"

Ollie sniffled. "If you'll have me. I know nothing about farming, Floyd. Not one Goddamn thing. But I'll learn. I'll try to be a proper farmer. For you."

"No need to be a proper one, Ollie. Regular is fine."

With a soft chuckle, Ollie hooked a hand behind Floyd's head and pulled him in for a kiss. As their lips moved together, Ollie scrambled to place the check and the coin onto the table behind him, and then Floyd hoisted him up into the air.

As soon as they reached the bed, Floyd sat on the mattress, setting Ollie on top of him. They resumed their kissing, and soon, both of them fell backward. Floyd scooted up toward the headboard. With Ollie rolling his hips, they continued kissing each other, staying in it for so long that Floyd's lips started to feel sore. Unable to keep waiting, Floyd reached for the top button of Ollie's shirt, but then Ollie broke their kiss, his eyes suddenly uncertain.

"Sweetheart, what if we try something new?"

"Sure," Floyd said, already knowing exactly what Ollie was fixing to ask.

"Can I . . . uhm . . ."

Floyd interrupted. "Do you want to fuck me, Ollie?" he asked with a wolfish smile.

"Oh my God!" Ollie exclaimed, eyes wide with shock, a hint of a smile underneath his very fake astonishment. "I've ruined you."

"Not yet, you haven't. I thought that's what you were proposing, though—to ruin me."

Ollie threw his head back and laughed for a few seconds before stopping to look back at Floyd with a very hungry smile.

"You're fucking right that's what I'm proposing."

Before Floyd could respond to that, Ollie was kissing him again, more intensely than before, and then Ollie moved to strip off his own clothes. Floyd could have sworn he heard Ollie snap a few buttons off his shirt in the process. Meanwhile, Floyd worked to remove his own clothing. Once they were naked, Ollie ran off to the kitchen and soon returned with a bottle of oil.

"I'm no expert, but I've been experimenting on my own here and there, and I think we'll need this."

Floyd snorted. "I know. I've experimented plenty myself."

"Jesus, sweetheart, I think that's the most arousing thing I've ever heard you say." Ollie pointed to the bed. "Lie back."

As soon as Floyd was comfortable, Ollie climbed on top of him. He started kissing Floyd's neck, slowly making his way lower. When he reached Floyd's outer thigh, instead of moving up to kiss his rock-hard cock, Ollie took a pause.

"I want to try something," he said.

"Sure, whatever you want."

"Can I lick you . . . lower?"

"Lower?"

"Right."

"Where—" Floyd started to say, but he cut himself off the moment he felt one of Ollie's fingers tap his hole. "Oh!" Suddenly, his head started to swim from nervousness. "Are you sure?"

"Yeah, uhm, is that too strange?"

"No, but . . ."

"I promise I'll stop if you hate it."

"I ain't worried that *I'll* hate it, I'm worried that *you'll* hate it. I mean, it's . . ."

"I know I won't hate it," Ollie said. "I've been thinking about it when I pleasure myself. I mean, Floyd, your butt is very sweet."

"*That* part is sweet?"

"Well, alright, maybe sweet isn't the perfect word. Adorable? Nah, not that either, maybe. But . . ." Ollie started lifting Floyd's legs. "Can we try it?"

"Uh, yeah," Floyd said, his heart thundering from unease. "Sure."

As Floyd pulled his legs up toward his chest, his body started burning from embarrassment, his previously hard cock becoming soft.

"Ollie . . ." Floyd swallowed hard, preparing to tell Ollie they'd better try some other time, but then Ollie looked up at him with the biggest, most hopeful eyes.

"Alright, so, this part *is* kind of adorable," he said.

Floyd tried to shove Ollie backward with his heel. "Stop."

"I'm being serious, sweetheart! I think you must have the most adorable butt hole in the entire world."

Floyd laughed a little. "Ollie! What in the heck kind of comment is that?"

"Can I *please* kiss you now?"

Floyd supposed he ought to let Ollie try, especially if he was strange enough to think his pucker was sweet or adorable or something.

"Yeah. Go on."

As soon as Ollie's tongue brushed his opening, Floyd let out a sigh, one that was sort of mixed with a moan. Because, wow, the firm-yet-wet feeling of Ollie's tongue felt so unexpectedly nice. Ollie's hands came to rest on the underside of Floyd's thighs as he buried his face closer, prodding Floyd's hole with his tongue more intensely, nearly pushing it inside. Floyd's cock began to stiffen.

"Oh . . ." Lost in his pleasure, Floyd couldn't think of one stinkin' thing to say.

Ollie paused. "Do you like it?"

"Yeah," Floyd breathed, still barely able to speak.

As soon as Ollie went back to licking him, Floyd shifted his hips, his throbbing cock now begging for release. He moved to touch himself, but Ollie's hand shot out to stop him.

"Just try to enjoy this, sweetheart," Ollie said. "Don't make yourself come yet."

"Uh-huh," Floyd managed, still in awe of how much he really *was* enjoying himself.

Gosh, how could Ollie's tongue feel so nice?

Suddenly, Ollie's fingers were on his opening, urging him open a little, and then he flicked his tongue over the hole once more, the sensation sending a little wave of pleasure rippling through Floyd's body and making him shudder.

"Oh, God, Ollie," Floyd moaned. "How?"

How could this possibly feel so incredible?

Ollie chuckled to himself and continued to move his tongue. When he eventually stopped, Floyd let out a pathetic little whine.

Ollie said, "I'm sorry, but I think I might not be able to resist the urge to fuck the mattress much longer if I keep licking you." He picked up the bottle of oil from the mattress. "Can I try one of my fingers instead?"

Still in a bit of a daze, Floyd nodded.

Ollie poured some oil on his hand. Floyd stopped breathing the moment Ollie started pressing his finger inside. Ollie's finger hadn't even made it past the middle knuckle before Floyd cried out, the breath he'd been holding rushing out of him in one big *whoosh*.

"I'm not hurting you, am I?" Ollie asked.

Floyd shook his head. Soon, Ollie's whole finger was inside. And Floyd was ready to tell him how incredible it felt when Ollie crooked his finger a little, finding that perfect spot that could make Floyd see stars. Floyd let out a hungry moan instead.

Ollie continued to move his finger. Each tiny motion was enough to make Floyd's muscles tense and shiver.

"God, Ollie, I . . ." Floyd clenched his fists. "I'll come."

"Should I stop?"

"Y-yeah," Floyd stammered, though part of him wanted Ollie to keep going. "I want you inside me now."

"Hold on," Ollie said. "One more finger, maybe. I'm nervous I'll hurt you otherwise."

Once Ollie's second finger was inside, Floyd squeezed his eyes shut. Because he knew that if Ollie moved too fast, he'd never last more than a second or two.

"Slow," Floyd begged. "Gentle."

Gingerly, Ollie moved his fingers a couple of times—in and out—and then, when Floyd was teetering on the edge, he retracted them. Floyd let out a long breath. Ollie took a while to slick himself with oil, which was maybe intentional so that Floyd could take the time to calm himself a little, and then walked forward on his knees. Floyd lifted his legs to rest them on Ollie's shoulders.

Ollie pressed his cock against Floyd's hole.

"Ready, sweetheart?" Ollie asked.

"Very ready."

When Ollie started to push himself inside, Floyd's heart began fluttering, fear suddenly twisting in his stomach. He wasn't even sure why he was feeling nervous about this type of intimacy. He knew Ollie would never hurt him. Not intentionally. But within seconds, the fear had become so intense that Floyd had started to feel a little lightheaded.

"Sweetheart, I think you're forgetting to breathe."

"Oh." Floyd took a few breaths. Sure enough, they helped. "Yeah, I'll . . . I'll remember that."

"Keep breathing," Ollie instructed, pushing forward more.

Once the head of Ollie's cock slipped inside, Floyd's hand shot out to clutch Ollie's forearm, causing Ollie to pause.

"Does it hurt?"

"Not much, but some. Uhm, maybe you can wait a bit." Floyd couldn't help but feel a bit bad for making Ollie stop. He'd been so sweet to pleasure Floyd with his tongue and fingers before this. "I'm sorry if this ain't what you thought it would be."

"What do you mean? It's perfect."

"Yeah? Even though I can't even let you move yet?"

"We're learning together, sweetheart. I'm so happy that we're even trying this."

"Me, too." Floyd reached up to stroke Ollie's cheek.

Ollie snatched Floyd's hand and kissed it. Floyd tried to concentrate on relaxing, and the kindness in Ollie's eyes helped him not feel so bad about how much time was passing. Eventually, once Floyd felt more comfortable, Ollie shifted his hips forward, pushing the rest of his member inside. Thankfully, there was no pain, only fullness.

Floyd nodded encouragingly. "It ain't hurting no more. Go ahead."

When Ollie started to rock his hips, Floyd finally relaxed. Because holy heck, it felt incredible. Even with Ollie's soft movements, Floyd started losing himself in their love, every one of Ollie's light thrusts bringing a new wave of pleasure, each rippling throughout his body and making his head swim.

"Does it feel nice?" Ollie asked sweetly, his forehead etched with concern.

"Better than nice," Floyd said. "I love it."

"Yeah?"

"You can try harder if you want."

With Ollie's next thrust, Floyd sucked in a breath, his hands twisting the sheets. Ollie must have been encouraged by that because he kept up with the harder and faster pace. Floyd closed his eyes and let the world fall away until the only thing that existed was the beautiful feeling of fullness.

Minutes later, while Floyd was still lost in his bliss, Ollie clutched tight to Floyd's shoulder and pushed forward more forcefully, and his thrust caused a sudden surge of pleasure to streak through Floyd's body like lightning. Enlivened by the sensation, a ragged moan tumbled forth from his lips. Ollie's hand came to rest on his cheek.

"Shhh, you're being too loud," Ollie scolded, though there was a levity in his voice.

"I know, I know," Floyd breathed, still barely keeping it together. "But, Ollie, I'm so close."

"Really?" Ollie asked, pausing for a moment. "But you're not even touching yourself."

Immediately reeling from the lack of movement, Floyd placed his hands on Ollie's hips. Without even thinking, he tried to urge Ollie to move again.

"Please," he said, a pleading edge to his voice. "More."

"God, I've never seen you like this," Ollie said, that teasing hitch in his tone that Floyd knew all too well. "Is it really that—"

"Ollie, *please*," Floyd begged, still pathetically trying to move Ollie's hips.

"Alright, sheesh," Ollie chuckled, punctuating that "sheesh" with a rough thrust that coaxed forth another one of Floyd's moans. He knew Ollie was fixing to scold him, even before the next "Sweetheart, shhh!"

But somehow, Floyd couldn't bring himself to care. Ollie continued to fuck him, and Floyd continued to moan, pressure and pleasure mixing and building, causing his cock to throb. For a moment, Floyd considered touching himself, but he couldn't even fathom focusing on something other than these current sensations, every one more intense than every other he had experienced in his life.

Ollie's next forceful thrust sent Floyd over the edge.

"Oh, God, Ollie," Floyd cried out, his cock starting to pulse. "Oh, fuck."

His cock was still pulsing when Ollie let out a moan. Floyd opened his eyes to see Ollie's face contorted with pleasure, his eyes squeezed shut, blond hair a mess.

"I'm coming, too," Ollie rasped, holding tight to Floyd's thighs.

Feeling Ollie empty himself inside him, Floyd let out a long breath and murmured, "Dang, Ollie, that feels so nice, you coming inside me like that."

Ollie seemed a bit lost for a few seconds, recovering from his pleasure with a faraway look in his eye, before he said, "Yeah? Good. Because I . . . wow, yeah, we need to keep doing that."

Chuckling, Floyd scrambled to find Ollie's hand.

"I love you," Floyd said, squeezing it, thinking 'bout how wonderful everything was. Especially Ollie. "You're perfect."

"I'm really not."

"You really are. You're perfect, silly—the perfect man for me."

"I love you." Ollie's smile broadened. "Even though that new nickname you came up with is completely terrible. I love you so much, sweetheart."

He was looking at Floyd with such wonderment, it sent Floyd's heart a-flutter. Afterward, Ollie snuggled up on top of him, resting his head atop Floyd's chest. Floyd stroked his soft yellow hair and spent the whole next hour wide awake, excited for their future.

CHAPTER SIXTEEN

OLIVER

WEEKS LATER, OLIVER WAS fiddling with the key while he tried to unlock their new farmhouse, his excitement morphing into frustration when minutes had passed and yet he *still* hadn't heard a click. He tried to yank the key back out so that he could try one more time, but now he couldn't do that either.

"Just my luck," Oliver muttered. He looked over his shoulder to see Effie, Floyd, and Jo staring at him expectantly. "I think we might need to break into our own house."

"Let me try," Floyd said, coming forward.

Oliver scoffed, feigning upset. "As though it's my fault that this lock is shi—" He caught himself. "—immy proof," he said instead.

Floyd snorted. "Shimmy proof?"

"Yup. Shimmy proof."

With a laugh, Floyd wiggled the key, and then Oliver heard a click. Damn.

Oliver threw up his hands. "Ugh. Of course."

"Well, come on, you two," Floyd said to Effie and Jo as he and Oliver stepped inside. "Ollie and me been itching to show you the house."

Right away, Josephine ran in past them.

"Mama! It's stupendous!"

Which made Oliver feel like his heart might burst clean out of his chest.

Effie smirked at him. "Is that one of the many words you been teaching her?"

"I *may* have peppered in the word stupendous in the middle of our checkers matches from time to time," Oliver said with a smirk of his own. "It's so fun to hear her pick these up."

Floyd said, "Like when she called supper *absolutely delectable*."

"Yeah, I liked that," Effie said. "Now enough playing with words, I want a tour."

As soon as the three of them were inside, Josephine ran over to Floyd, who scooped her up into the air, making her laugh.

"Ain't she a little heavy for you now, Floyd? She's eight," Effie said.

Floyd looked over at Oliver. "Nah, I lift heavier things."

Oliver whispered to Effie, "He means people."

Effie chuckled.

"Hush up, Ollie!" Floyd chastised.

But Josephine was tickled by this. "Daddy, you can lift Mister Oliver?! I want to see!"

"No," Floyd said. "Mister Oliver was being silly, is all."

"Oh, yes, you know me," Oliver said through a laugh.

"Can I see our bedroom now?" Josephine asked Floyd.

He set her down. "*Your* bedroom, Jo. I told you, this place is big enough for you to have your own room."

Josephine squealed and ran to the stairs. Floyd followed, leaving Oliver and Effie by themselves. Hooking his hands behind his back, Oliver watched Effie survey the room. From the way her eyes were sparkling, Oliver could tell that she liked it, maybe especially the pink and yellow flower wallpaper.

"Would you like to see the kitchen?" he asked after a while.

"Sure."

Oliver held out his arm and Effie linked hers with it.

"It's so nice having such a refined man around," Effie said, a little playfulness in her voice.

But Oliver's stomach fluttered unpleasantly. Sometimes, he still worried that he was ruining everything, especially when it came to Effie.

"Are you sure?" Oliver asked as they walked to the kitchen. "We still have some time to back out of the purchase. I mean, everything has been moving so quickly the last couple of weeks. I can only imagine how hard it is for you to have your entire world turned on its head like this. If you'd like, I could try to purchase a small home in the city so that I won't be in the way. I'll still help on the farm, of course, but, Effie, your family—"

"Our family," Effie corrected. "You're part of the family now, Oliver."

"Oh, but I'm not, really. I'm Floyd's . . ." Oliver could feel the heat rushing to his cheeks. "God, I'm like . . . I'm like a piece of slate mixed in with the coal."

"You're not."

"I'm so worried that me being here is hurting you."

Effie shook her head. "We couldn't have bought this farm without you."

"You wouldn't have had to. You'd have been happy—"

"Floyd was never happy. Not like he is now."

"And what about you? And Jo?"

"Jo loves you," Effie said. "When we told her that you and Floyd were together, she was smiling from ear to ear. Now, I never told Floyd this, but I been putting it in Josephine's head ever since she was little that love can look all sorts of ways. I thought that . . . well . . . that if she ever found out about Matt, she shouldn't be surprised. I never wanted her to be confused or mad or to think it was wrong. I never wanted her to look at Floyd with nothing but love."

"Oh, Effie, that's so kind of you. Floyd's so lucky to have you. *I'm* so lucky to have you." Biting his bottom lip, Oliver studied her face for a moment. "Are you sure you're happy, too?"

"I'm very happy. And if you think Floyd hasn't asked me that one thousand times himself, you're crazy. Me and him have talked about this 'til we were both blue in the face."

"Just tell me if you're ever unhappy and I promise I will try to fix it. Even if that means I have to leave. I swear I will move mountains to make sure you're happy again."

"I can't see that happening. I love our family."

Oliver's throat tightened, every positive emotion in existence seemingly bubbling to the surface at once. *Our family.* He could scarcely believe it. He had a family. One that was so much better than the Astors had ever been.

"Me, too," he said softly.

Once Oliver composed himself, he showed Effie the kitchen, which was much larger than the one she'd had back in the company town. While Effie was busy exploring the cabinets, Floyd and Josephine returned from upstairs.

Oliver knelt down. "So, what did you think of your new room, Jo?"

"It's big!"

"Yeah? What else?"

"It's real nice."

"Nice? Is that the best word you can come up with?"

Josephine pursed her lips for a moment, thinking.

"Phenomenal?"

"I like that better. Sounds much more exciting that way."

Josephine grinned—a big, toothy smile; one that was made even better by the fact that she was missing one of her front two teeth—and then proceeded to run over to Effie so that she could beg her mama to come see it, too. When Oliver stood back up, Floyd put his hands on Oliver's waist, pulling him close.

"Are you preparing Jo for college or something?"

Oliver shrugged. "Not intentionally, though I'd certainly pay for her tuition."

"Ain't that a little strange considering the fact that you never even finished college yourself?"

"Oh, Josephine's more focused than I ever was."

Floyd clicked his tongue. "Yeah, she's something special."

"Agreed."

Whistling, Floyd looked around the kitchen. "Can you believe we own this? It's even bigger than the farmhouse my parents had."

"And we'll fill it with books and music and—"

"Music? What, my banjo?"

"Sweetheart, I'm buying us a phonograph. And I'm buying myself a piano because I refuse to let you be the only musician in this house. Don't try to argue with me about it."

"I won't. I want to hear you play," Floyd said. "Heck, I'm excited for it."

"Soon the two of us will be playing music together," Oliver said before leaning forward for a soft kiss. As soon as they parted, Oliver reached into his pocket. He had thought he'd hold the surprise until later that evening, but he now realized he couldn't hold off that long. Hell, he couldn't even stand to wait one more minute. "I have something for you. Close your eyes." Floyd only *sort of* closed them. "Sweetheart, I can see you peeking through those pretty lashes of yours. Close them properly, please."

Floyd snickered. "Dang."

One moment later, Oliver held out his hand.

"Ready."

As soon as Floyd opened his eyes and saw the coin in Oliver's hand, his face fell, which was pretty much the exact opposite of the reaction Oliver was trying for. Oliver started to pull his hand away, but Floyd reached out and caught his wrist.

"Is that . . ."

"It is." Oliver nodded, still unsure whether or not Floyd was happy about the present.

As Floyd took the coin out of Oliver's palm, his expression stayed unreadable—his eyes wide with surprise, but his lips a hard line.

"Ollie . . ." he whispered, studying the coin. When Floyd looked up to meet Oliver's eyes, his baby blues were shimmering with tears, but Oliver couldn't yet tell whether they were happy tears or sad ones. "Why?"

"I couldn't let you have the Ollie coin without the Matt coin. You need both."

When Floyd looked back at the coin, still not yet smiling or otherwise looking pleased, Oliver's stomach twisted and tightened, making him wonder whether Matt might be upset with him. Perhaps it hadn't been his place to retrieve the coin. Swallowing his shame, Oliver opened his mouth to apologize, but then, before he could, Floyd hooked a hand behind his head and pulled him in for a kiss, one so passionate and fierce that Oliver could barely breathe.

When Floyd broke away, he said, "Sorry I keep nearly kissing you to death."

"Does this mean you like the present?"

Floyd tipped their foreheads together. "I love it."

"Really?"

"Of course," Floyd said, now smiling madly.

"Are you sure? You barely looked happy before."

"I was too touched, is all. I can't believe you found this."

"It was nothing. Just had to ask Aunt Betty who had pur-chased it."

"I hope it wasn't too expensive to retrieve it."

"Don't worry, the collector was reasonable."

"Gosh, I love it so much," Floyd said, sniffling while he studied the coin some more, rotating it in his hand.

Oliver leaned in to nuzzle Floyd's nose. "Oh, sweetheart, I'm so happy you like it. I was worried. You know, I think I understand what you mean about the copperhead now."

"What?"

"Well, when I was waiting for your reaction, it felt like my insides were twisting together, and I had the thought that maybe Matt was upset with me."

"Oh, Matt's probably mad because he never bought me nothing this thoughtful," Floyd said, and Oliver was so happy to see how Floyd could talk about Matt so easily now. "Or maybe he was mad that I wasn't reacting the right way." Floyd kissed him once more. "Don't worry about Matt, you hear?"

"Yeah."

"Don't worry that I won't like whatever else you ever buy for me neither."

"Even if it's the latest and best phonograph? One that costs a whole bundle of money?"

"Even then."

"Even if it's—"

"Sweet, silly Ollie," Floyd said, interrupting. "Yes. Even then."

"But you have no idea what I was *fixing to* say."

"I know, but I promised myself I wouldn't argue with you about money no more. I think buying this house—this *home*—helped me with that. I reckon we love each other too much to keep squabbling over money." Floyd reached up to caress Oliver's cheek with the back of his fingers, still clutching the Flying Eagle in his palm. "You and me are forever. We're family."

Oliver snatched Floyd's hand and kissed it.

Family.

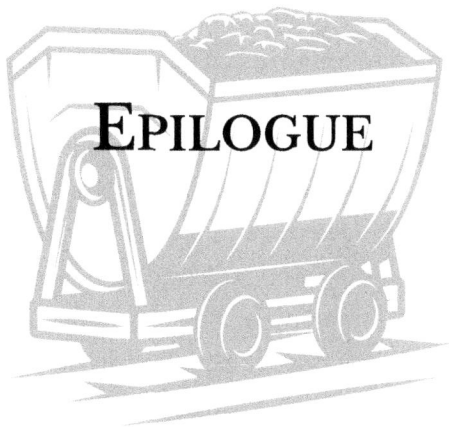

EPILOGUE

Floyd

Eight months later . . .

WHILE OLLIE AND JO cleaned up in the kitchen, Floyd and Effie were sitting on the floor across from each other in the living room with a chessboard between them. Even though it had only been a couple of weeks since Effie had taught Floyd how to play, Floyd was already becoming a bit of an expert, which seemed to bother both Effie and Ollie to no end, but in a playful sort of way. Floyd could kind of tell that they were having fun playing with him, even if he had nearly beaten both of them by now. Ollie said that he and Effie ought to try to soak up the victories while they still could because they wouldn't last much longer.

Furrowing her brow with what looked like intense concentration, Effie moved a piece.

"Remember, you ain't allowed to take that back," Floyd taunted.

"Stop it, Floyd," Effie chastised, one corner of her mouth turning up a bit, which told Floyd that she was fighting a smile. "I know you're just trying to scare me."

"Naw, never." Floyd moved his rook and captured Effie's bishop. "See."

"Am I supposed to feel better that it was a real warning?"

"Of course."

As Effie sighed, Ollie and Jo came back from the kitchen.

"Thank goodness," Effie said, pushing herself to stand. "I need a break from playing. Do you want to take over for me, Oliver?"

"I'm not really in the mood for a beating."

Floyd pouted. "Why won't no one play with me?"

"Let's play something we're equally talented at instead. Or, well, not *equally* talented, exactly, but something trickier for us to compare ourselves to each other." Ollie held out his hand to help Floyd up. "Music?"

Floyd took Ollie's hand. "I'd like that."

While Floyd tuned his banjo, Ollie set himself up at the piano. Josephine walked back and forth between them.

Effie asked her, "Which one do you want to learn first?"

"I can't choose."

Floyd had a feeling that Jo wanted to learn piano. Sometimes, he'd catch her sitting at the bench when she thought no one was looking, pressing on the keys real lightly, probably hoping that no one would hear her. He couldn't hardly blame her for wanting to learn piano. It was a real impressive-looking instrument, and Ollie played it so well. It was likely that Jo was afeared of hurting someone's feelings if she chose, especially if she chose Ollie. Jo had been choosing Ollie more and more often.

Many nights, she'd request for Mister Oliver to read her a bedtime story. Sometimes she'd pick him to play checkers with, too. Not only was Jo choosing Ollie a lot, but Effie had been spending a bunch of time with Ollie, too. Ollie had been learning her a little piano here and there, and the two of them still really liked to play chess.

But Floyd wasn't bothered by none of this. It made him happy to see them take to Ollie so much. After the lonely life Ollie'd had, he needed to be chosen first sometimes. Or maybe a lot of times.

"Jo, you can sit with Ollie tonight," Floyd said, nodding over to him. "It's easier to share a piano than a banjo."

Jo smiled. "I can?!"

"Yup."

She ran over to the bench, but paused, and then whirled to hurry back over to Floyd. She threw her arms around his neck and hugged him. He squeezed her back.

"Go on," he said, releasing her.

For the whole next hour, Floyd and Ollie played songs together. Or sometimes Floyd and Ollie and Jo, with Jo being responsible for hitting a couple of notes here and there, while Effie put her feet up and relaxed on the couch. Sometimes, Ollie looked over his shoulder and threw Floyd a wink, which was real sweet, and one time, Jo noticed and copied, which was even sweeter, though it seemed like Jo was trying to tease them.

Eventually, it was time for Jo to be tucked in, and this time, she asked Effie to read to her. Floyd and Ollie had to stop playing so they wouldn't keep her awake, but luckily, they had set up the new phonograph in the back room, on the opposite end of the house from Jo's bedroom, and if they closed the door, they could play some music without bothering no one.

After Ollie wound up the phonograph, which was a newer portable type that looked more like a wooden suitcase than a listening device, he came over to Floyd and took his hand.

"Come on," Ollie said. "Dance with me."

"Can't we cuddle up on the loveseat instead?"

"Nope," Ollie said, placing a hand on Floyd's shoulder.

At first, the two of them tried a Foxtrot, but Floyd still had some trouble not crushing Ollie's feet, and so, they eventually started swaying instead, resting their heads together and moving more slowly than the song called for.

"Feels more like we're trying to rock ourselves to sleep," Floyd teased.

"I like it," Ollie said, with a wistful kind of tenderness in his voice that made Floyd's heart melt a little.

Floyd hummed and said, "Yeah, it ain't bad, I suppose."

After a moment, Ollie said, "I'm so happy, sweetheart."

"Me, too."

Soon enough, Ollie was yawning.

"I think you were right about us rocking ourselves to sleep."

"Early morning tomorrow. We ought to head up soon."

Ollie shuffled his feet closer, positioning himself so that their bodies were nearly pressed up against each other, and said, "Just a little while longer."

"Worse comes to worst, I can carry you up the stairs."

"Don't try to excite me," Ollie mock-scolded. "We have an early morning tomorrow."

"Ollie, you keep me up late nearly every night with that energy of yours. I took your excitement into consideration already."

Ollie laughed next to his ear. "Are you poking fun of me?"

"Maybe."

"Lunkhead," Ollie said with an exaggerated scoff.

"Shut up, Ollie," Floyd said through a low chuckle.

After Ollie stopped swaying, he brought his face closer to Floyd's, pausing when their mouths were only a couple of inches from each other, and then, in the sweetest, most playful voice, said, "Make me."

And, of course, Floyd couldn't very well refuse. He captured Ollie's mouth in a passionate kiss. When the music finally faded, they broke the kiss at the same time, and then they were both smiling big, silly smiles at each other. Floyd could feel the happy energy in the room, like it was leaking out from their bodies.

"Ready for bed?" Ollie finally asked, still a little breathless.

"Yeah, *bed*," Floyd teased.

Ollie squeezed his butt. "I can meet you upstairs, sweetheart. I need some water first."

"Go ahead," Floyd said. "I'll wait here."

After Ollie left for the kitchen, Floyd walked over to the phonograph to close it. Standing in front of the box, his eyes found the frame hanging nearby—the one with the Ollie coin and the Matt coin side-by-side—and took some time to enjoy the sight.

Nowadays, Floyd was able to talk about Matt more easily. Even though his heart still hurt from losing him, Floyd had found that keeping Matt's memory alive with stories was helping a whole lot with the pain. What helped even more was that Ollie and Effie and even Jo had started to mention Matt more often, too. Sometimes Ollie would pester Floyd for stories. Sometimes Effie and he would reminisce. These talks reminded Floyd that even though he had moved on from coal mining, even though he had made a new family for himself, he could breathe easy. Because Matt hadn't been forgotten. He never would be forgotten. He was still loved.

"Goodnight, Matty," Floyd said softly to the coin on the wall.

Seconds later, Ollie poked his head inside and strummed his palms on the doorframe.

"Coming up, sweetheart?"

"Yeah. Just talking to Matt."

"Oh." Ollie smiled sweetly. "Well, take your time, then."

"Nah, I'm finished." Floyd came over and caught Ollie by the wrist, pulling him close. "Want me to carry you?"

"God, yes."

So Floyd lifted Ollie up, and Ollie hooked his legs around Floyd's torso. Floyd couldn't resist balancing Ollie's weight in his left arm so that he could reach up and move his fingers through Ollie's soft yellow locks.

Ollie let out a peaceful-sounding sigh. "Let's head upstairs, sweetheart."

And then Ollie touched their lips together, and the only thing Floyd could think about was how lucky he was to have met Ollie—this beautiful person who had helped him face his long-buried pain; this sweet, silly man with whom he had fallen in love.

Oliver

Two months later . . .

Rocking back on his heels, Oliver knocked twice on Aunt Betty's front door. Moments later, she opened it, her typically stoic expression replaced with the faintest hint of a smile.

"Oliver," she said, and then she was smiling so wide her eyes were crinkling in the corners. "How was the circus?"

"Fantastic."

Josephine chimed in from behind him. "Aunt Betty, we saw a man flying through the air and another who made himself into a pretzel! And then we *bought* a pretzel, too."

"Oh my, that sounds wonderful," she replied, moving to the side.

Josephine bounded into the house, and Oliver could hear her fading calls of "Aunt Mary! Aunt Mary! We saw the pretzel man like Mister Oliver said we would!" Meanwhile, Aunt Betty welcomed Effie and Floyd with a short, warm embrace. When she turned to Oliver, she wrapped her arms around him, too, only it wasn't a short embrace, but a long one, one that was so heartfelt, so sincere, Oliver could barely hold himself together for it. After only a few seconds, his legs started feeling wobbly, as though they had been transformed into two noodles.

"I'm so happy you stopped by," she said as they parted. "It's always nice to see all of you together."

Oliver took a breath to compose himself. It still felt so foreign to receive that kind of physical affection from anyone other than Floyd (and maybe from Josephine, who had taken to sitting close with him while he read to her some evenings).

"Well, we love visiting," he said.

Effie remarked, "Josephine is real fond of Mary."

"Mary loves children. Especially your Josephine."

Aunt Betty led them into the library room where Josephine and Mary were starting to play cards. Floyd left for the kitchen to fetch everyone some club soda, which Aunt Betty and Mary often liked to serve, and Effie started browsing the bookshelves. Soon, Floyd returned with a large bottle of club soda and several small glasses on a tray.

Watching the scene, Oliver took a long breath, his chest expanding like every second of his new reality was filling him up with more love than he thought he'd ever have in a lifetime. He wasn't alone. Not anymore. None of these wonderful people ever made him feel bad for talking too much or making silly jokes or filling up half of a bedroom with his selection of clothing and hats. They loved him. And he loved them, too.

Josephine's voice broke through his overly sentimental thoughts.

"Mister Oliver?"

"Hm?"

"Did you really try to run away and join the circus when you were little? Aunt Mary said I made it up. But I remember you telling me that."

Oliver chuckled. "You're *almost* right. I can't blame you for forgetting the specifics. I think you were half asleep when I told you the story." He rocked back on his heels again. "No, I never ran away. I wasn't as brave as you, Josephine. Gosh, I *still* can't believe you snuck off to Charleston by yourself. On a train, too," he said with a playful wag of his finger. "Me, on the other hand, well, I was too scared to venture off of our property when I was your age, mostly because my parents forbade it, and so I started my own circus."

Mary raised both of her eyebrows. "Your own circus?"

"It's the reason I've mastered so many magic tricks. Magic was my special skill. I'm not sure if I had yet realized that magicians were a whole separate entity with their own shows and everything, rather than being circus performers, but well, I knew I couldn't be a lion tamer or a trapeze artist, and so I thought that coin and card tricks would be the next best thing."

"Who else was in your circus?" Mary asked, though from her tone Oliver could tell that she was only humoring him.

Oliver had noticed Mary often looked at him like he was some silly kid, which, he supposed, she wasn't entirely incorrect about in some ways.

"Oh, tons of people. I had the largest circus in Cleveland."

Jo's face was scrunched up in confusion. "Really?"

"Yes, but I'm sad to say that no one came to see us. Probably because everyone except for me was invisible." At that, Mary burst out laughing. Oliver could hear Effie chuckling nearby. He thought he ought to explain the silliness to Jo. "Get it? No one came to *see* us?"

Jo wrinkled her nose and said, "Mister Oliver!" though then she laughed a little, too.

Floyd came up beside him, his arms crossed over his chest, and cocked an eyebrow.

"Invisible circus performers?"

Oliver smiled and shrugged. "Oh, it's not that strange. Is it?"

"Only a little," Floyd said before whispering, "It's sweet, too."

Oliver's cheeks started to burn. It was incredible that Floyd's sweet comments could still overwhelm him sometimes.

Over the next few hours, everyone spent time together in the library—telling stories, playing cards, watching a few of Oliver's silly magic tricks—and then Oliver, Effie, Floyd, and Jo left to return to their farm outside Charleston, traveling by car. Oliver had purchased one not long after they had moved so that they could visit Aunt Betty and Aunt Mary more easily.

After they arrived, Effie and Oliver cooked some stew together (Oliver was becoming more proficient with cooking nowadays, which was perfect because he loved that some nights, Effie could take time to herself while he cooked instead), and then Oliver went out back to the barn so that he could feed his new cat, Colonel Whiskers II. He stayed out back to pet him for a little while and then went back inside so that he could have supper with his family.

Later that evening, once Oliver had finished reading to Josephine, he retrieved a book from the living room before heading back up to his shared bedroom with Floyd. He came in to find Floyd sitting up in bed playing with a nickel.

"Have you mastered that coin trick yet?" Oliver asked in a teasing tone, remembering that it had taken him days to master it himself.

"Yeah, I think so."

"What?" Oliver asked, inadvertently letting the door slam a little too loudly behind him. "No, you haven't. That's impossible."

"Why's it impossible? You were reading to Jo for nearly an hour."

"Yes, one hour. *Only* one hour." Oliver hopped on the bed. "Show me."

And then Floyd held up the coin, flicked his wrist, and made it disappear. Oliver's mouth fell open. He stared at Floyd with complete astonishment for about twenty fucking seconds before smacking Floyd's hand, causing the coin to fall.

"I can't believe you!" Oliver exclaimed. "How?!"

Floyd shrugged. "Wasn't hard, is all."

"Ugh."

Floyd flashed a smile, one that looked a tiny bit smug, before nodding toward Oliver's book.

"What are you reading?"

"*The Brothers Karamazov* by Dostoevsky." Oliver held it up for Floyd to see. "It's the one I never finished."

"Are you trying to finish it so you can have your revelation?"

"I'm surprised you remember that. Or, well, maybe I shouldn't be surprised since you can learn coin tricks in record time and memorize musical numbers after only hearing them once, which I am *still* unbelievably envious of you for, by the way." Oliver sighed. "But, no, I'm not reading it for the revelation."

"Because you still believe people can't be nothing but terrible?"

"Can't be nothing but terrible," Oliver repeated. "God, sweetheart, you're too perfect for words sometimes."

Floyd nudged him with his foot. "Ollie. Answer."

"Alright, fine. I'm not reading it for the revelation because I already *had* that revelation. Way back when I had supper with you for the first time. It was like you were serving my own words right back to me. I remember it so clearly. I was sitting with everyone at the table trying to hide the fact that it felt like my heart was being crushed in a vice."

"Or maybe squeezed by a snake," Floyd suggested with a little playful raise of his eyebrows. "How'd we serve your words back to you?"

"You were all so nice." Oliver rested his head against Floyd's chest. "Oh, Floyd, I can't believe I wasted so much of my life being lonely, thinking that everyone else in the world was probably horrible." He heaved a forceful sigh. "But it was only my family and their friends, I suppose, who were horrible. And, when I was small, the kids at school, too." Oliver craned his head to look up at Floyd. "Sweetheart, my silly story about the circus was true. I had a bunch of invisible friends. And now I have a real friend in Effie and a real Josephine—whatever she's supposed to be to me—and a real you."

"And you always *will* have us."

Oliver sat up to plant a soft kiss on Floyd's lips. "Thank you, sweetheart."

"I'm so happy you ain't lonely no more, Ollie."

"Me, too," Oliver said, turning to rest his back against Floyd's chest. He readied the book in his lap. "Do you want to read with me over my shoulder?"

"Nah, I'll probably be too slow since I'm so out of practice. How about you read the story out loud to me? That way, I can listen to that nice voice of yours."

"Do you want a long, rambling summary first?"

"Extra long and extra rambling," Floyd said before kissing the side of Oliver's head.

"Perfect."

So, Oliver spent the next chunk of forever talking Floyd's ear off. Every so often Floyd would nuzzle him or kiss him or thread his fingers through his hair, and Oliver never once worried that Floyd thought he was babbling too much. Finally, he had found someone who not only accepted his eccentricities but celebrated them.

Snuggled with Floyd in their farmhouse bed, Oliver finally knew what it was to be loved.

ABOUT THE AUTHOR

Logan Sage writes historical MM romance with plenty of sweetness, a little heartache, occasional humor, and hard-earned happily ever afters. Her work explores themes like healing from loss, finding the courage to fall in love, learning to love oneself, and overcoming trauma.

Readers who enjoy stories with historical settings will be sure to like Logan Sage's romances.

Logan Sage harnesses her love of learning in order to paint rich, immersive worlds for her readers to fall into. She especially enjoys writing love stories between everyday people, and typically sets her stories in the 20th century, mostly in the United States.

When she's not writing or reading, Logan Sage enjoys working, cooking, and spending time with her supportive family.

Follow her on Instagram: @logan.sage.adams

Join her Facebook Group: Logan Sage Adams – MM Romance Readers

Subscribe to her newsletter: www.logansageadams.com

Printed in Great Britain
by Amazon

60876306R00184